Evidence-based Equine Nutrition: A Practical Approach for Professionals

AF903939

Evidence-based Equine Nutrition: A Practical Approach for Professionals

Editors:

Teresa Hollands BSc (Hons), MSc (Animal Nutrition) PhD, RNutr, FHEA

Senior Lecturer (Veterinary Nutrition)
Department of Veterinary Clinical Science, School of Veterinary Medicine,
University of Surrey, Guildford, UK

Lizzie Drury BSc (Hons), MSc (Equine Science), RNutr

Senior Nutritionist and Assistant Director
Saracen Horse Feeds, Aylesford, Kent, UK

CABI

CABI is a trading name of CAB International

CABI
Nosworthy Way
Wallingford
Oxfordshire OX10 8DE
UK

Tel: +44 (0)1491 832111
E-mail: info@cabi.org
Website: www.cabi.org

CABI
200 Portland Street
Boston
MA 02114
USA

Tel: +1 (617)682-9015
E-mail: cabi-nao@cabi.org

A catalogue record for this book is available from the British Library, London, UK.

ISBN-13: 9781789245110 (paperback)
9781789245127 (ePDF)
9781789245134 (ePub)

DOI: 10.1079/9781789245134.0000

Commissioning Editor: Alexandra Lainsbury
Editorial Assistant: Lauren Davies
Production Editor: James Bishop

Typeset by Straive, Pondicherry, India
Printed and bound in the UK by Severn, Gloucester

Contents

Contributors List

Nikki Bell
The Donkey Sanctuary, Devon

Dr Faith Burden BSc (Hons), PhD
Executive Director of Equine Operations, The Donkey Sanctuary, Devon
https://www.thedonkeysanctuary.org.uk/research/contributor/2130
https://uk.linkedin.com/in/faith-burden-972b3362

Lizzy Drury BSc (Hons), MSc, RNutr
Senior Nutritionist and Director, Saracen Horse Feeds, Aylesford, Kent
https://uk.linkedin.com/in/lizzie-drury-bb264129

Rod Fisher BVSc, MRCVS
Abbey Equine Clinic, Abergavenny

Dr Teresa Hollands BSc (Hons), MSc (Animal Nutrition), PhD, RNutr, FHEA
Senior Lecturer (Veterinary Nutrition), School of Veterinary Medicine, University of Surrey, Guildford
t.hollands@surrey.ac.uk
https://www.surrey.ac.uk/people/teresa-hollands
https://uk.linkedin.com/in/dr-teresa-hollands-r-nutr-65747227

Louise Jones BSc (Hons), MSc, RNutr
Scout Farm,
louise@scoutfarm.co.uk
https://uk.linkedin.com/in/louise-jones-7ba34060

Bryony Witherow BSc (Hons), MSc, FHEA, RNutr
Lecturer, Writtle University College; and Owner Director, Practical Equine Nutrition
briony@practicalequinenutrition.co.uk
https://writtle.ac.uk/profiles/profile.cfm?stID=2625&nofooter=1

Authors' details

Mrs Nikki Bell, BSc (Hons), MSc
Senior Researcher (Europe) – Nutrition & Care, The Donkey Sanctuary, Devon
https://www.thedonkeysanctuary.org.uk/research/contributor/2105
https://www.linkedin.com/in/nikki-bell-43a753a0/

Nikki has over twenty-five years of practical experience working with equines and holds a first-class honours degree in Equine Science from the University of the West of England (UWE) and a Masters with distinction in Applied Equine Science from the Royal Agricultural University (RAU). Nikki joined The Donkey Sanctuary in 2011 and has held the position of Senior Researcher for the last eight years, focusing on projects to improve donkey and mule health and welfare. Nikki specialises in nutrition and parasitology and is a registered animal medicines advisor (RAMA). She also leads The Donkey Sanctuary's nutrition advice service offering impartial and practical advice to donkey owners globally. Nikki has co-authored ten peer-reviewed articles, produced many educational resources and guidelines and has produced an online course on donkey nutrition for The Donkey Sanctuary's virtual learning environment (VLE). Nikki has contributed to the chapter on donkey nutrition for this book.

Dr Faith Burden, BSc (Hons), PhD
Executive Director of Equine Operations, The Donkey Sanctuary, Devon
https://www.thedonkeysanctuary.org.uk/research/contributor/2130
https://uk.linkedin.com/in/faith-burden-972b3362

Faith is a senior leader in the animal welfare sector with a PhD in infectious diseases.
She specialises in equine welfare operations and has worked for The Donkey Sanctuary since 2004, expanding and developing their research programmes and technical support services. She has co-authored over 75 peer-reviewed articles and book chapters and is globally recognised as an expert on the health and welfare of donkeys and mules. Her expertise encompasses sanctuary care, welfare outreach, veterinary services, education and technical support services.

Faith is passionate about ensuring that good welfare practices are driven by sound scientific evidence and that this is at the heart of operational decision making.

Faith has a particular passion for nutrition and is a firm believer that species appropriate nutrition is fundamental to good welfare. She has worked with commercial feed companies and care providers to design and produce donkey-friendly products, and to implement positive changes for many thousands of donkeys globally based on cutting edge science.

Lizzie Drury, BSc (Hons), MSc, RNutr
Senior Nutritionist and Associate Director, Saracen Horse Feeds
Lizzie.drury@saracenhorsefeeds.co.uk
https://uk.linkedin.com/in/lizzie-drury-bb264129

Lizzie leads the technical and nutrition team at Saracen where she has worked for over 20 years and is responsible for providing nutrition support, including to many Olympic riders as well as members of Team GB. She manages feed formulations, product innovation and development, working in collaboration with the world leaders in equine nutrition research – Kentucky Equine Research (KER).

She works closely with academia and clinicians, providing lectures to many colleges, universities and veterinary practices. Lizzie travels extensively, consulting and lecturing in Poland, the UAE and many other European countries. Her particular area of interest is the performance horse but, being very much a practical nutritionist, Lizzie enjoys working with all levels and abilities of horse owners and riders to help provide the support to people to get the best out of their horses and enjoy them.

On a personal level, Lizzie started riding when she was 9 years old, having a particular interest in dressage. She has two horses that she trains and competes at British Dressage; her pride and joy is her Hanoverian chestnut gelding, Ferdi, and together they have progressed through the levels from Novice level to Advanced. Her second horse is a young 6-year-old homebred who is third generation from her parents' Irish Draught Hunter. Lizzie lives with International Show Jumper Philip Spivey and their daughter, Alexa. Philip is known for producing and competing up to Nations Cup level on the talented horse Romonov II. Philip concentrates on producing young horses at their new showjumping base in Suffolk, helping them to reach their full potential, aided by an on-site nutritionist!

Their daughter enjoys riding her cheeky Welsh mountain pony, Taffy, and aspires to follow in her dad's footsteps.

Rod Fisher, BVSc, MRCVS
Abbey Equine Clinic, Abergavenny

Rod Fisher qualified from the University of Bristol and started mixed veterinary practice in Abergavenny. After a period of general practice in Australia, he returned to Abergavenny to develop the equine department.

Rod recently retired as a director of Abbey Equine Vets in Abergavenny but remains a consultant. He was Team Vet for the British Endurance Team from 1989 to 2001 and Team Vet to the Team GB Para-Equestrian Dressage Team from 2001 to 2020.

He is on the FEI's recognised list of Veterinary Surgeons in the disciplines of Endurance and Eventing and enjoys an active role in officiating in both spheres.

He has a particular interest in sports medicine and has a number of publications covering a range of subjects. His philosophy is to look at the whole horse and to prevent rather than just cure, monitoring horse health, nutrition and fitness.

Dr Teresa Hollands, BSc (Hons), MSc (Animal Nutrition), PhD, RNutr, FHEA
Senior Lecturer (Veterinary Nutrition), School of Veterinary Medicine, University of Surrey, Guildford
t.hollands@surrey.ac.uk
https://www.surrey.ac.uk/people/teresa-hollands
https://uk.linkedin.com/in/dr-teresa-hollands-r-nutr-65747227

All little girls love ponies, who doesn't dream of owning one? My dream came true on my eighth birthday – an early Christmas present.

I called my first pony Kelpie, because he was a little Welsh 13.2 (I was in the Kelpie (Welsh for pixie) pack at Brownies). I shared him with my friend who lived on a farm and so did Kelpie but every other week he was all mine.

I went on a week's course with him to learn to ride and look after him. I can still remember the first canter I ever had; I just couldn't stop giggling and went home with a massive grin on my face. I was hooked!

Two years later, my friend discovered boys and Kelpie became all mine. Summers of Pony Club camps and winter working rallies filled my days, in between homework and school. He kept me sane through my O-levels and broke my heart when I had to sell him. He introduced me to friends who shared the passion and who several decades later, despite children, geography and jobs, remain my friends bound by a common interest.

My 'bestest' pony left my life because Topic joined it. A 7/8th Thoroughbred chestnut gelding with loppy ears, Topic (posh name Mr Top Coat) introduced me to 'grown up' eventing and BSJA.

He took me to Hickstead when we qualified for the Schools' Showjumping Championships; he represented Bucks (I went too) on a Young Rider's BSJA Training Scholarship; we qualified for Foxhunter Regional Finals in style by coming first at Bucks County. Even my father started to understand 'why horses'.

Competing became less early mornings, more civilised as we moved up to Grade C, then he got navicular syndrome and my world came tumbling down. X-rays and warfarin treatment meant he still competed with that huge heart of his for another year and it was my vet who inspired me to consider veterinary science as a career. But I had to say goodbye to Topic and although I didn't make it as a vet, my curiosity to learn about the biology and science of the horse has never diminished.

Maybe (a 16 hh TB 4-year-old mare) was the first horse I bought with all my own money, working through university to pay for her; my intention was to bring her on during my placement year and then sell her. But she ended up coming to the Isle of Man with me, to my first and my second job, and 23 years later I was still her 'mum'.

My horse experience gave me lifelong friends, opened the door for my career, kept it open and has given me the hands-on knowledge that allows me to translate the biology and science I have since learnt during my BSc, MSc and PhD for my career at Belvoir Horse Feeds, Dengie Horse Feeds, Dodson and Horrell, School of Veterinary Medicine and Science, Nottingham and The School of Vet Med, University of Surrey.

Louise Jones, BSc (Hons), MSc , RNutr
louise@scoutfarm.co.uk
https://uk.linkedin.com/in/louise-jones-7ba34060

In 1999, Louise qualified with a BSc (Hons) in Equine Science, specialising in breeding science, graduating with an MSc in Equine Science in 2000. In 2007, Louise gained registered nutritionist (RNutr) with the Association for Nutrition (AfN); she is currently one of only a handful of registered nutritionists specialising in equines.

Over the years Louise has worked as a nutritionist with some of the most widely recognised feed and supplement manufactures; she spent over a decade with Dodson & Horrell before joining Top Spec as Senior Nutritionist and then became UK Head of Equine for Connolly's RED MILLS and Foran Equine.

Louise's extensive knowledge and experience is well recognised, and she is regularly invited to speak at conferences and contribute to the equine press. She has authored and co-authored several conference proceedings and abstracts. Louise has been a member of the British Equestrian Trade Association (BETA) Feed Committee since 2016.

Louise has an extensive understanding of stud, clinical and performance horse nutrition, and has worked with trainers, breeders and riders in the UK, Continental Europe and the Middle East. Her main area of interest is how optimal nutrition can influence the equine athlete throughout their life.

Briony Witherow MSc BSc (Hons), PGCERT, FHEA, RNutr (Animal)
HE Lecturer, Writtle University College; and Owner Director, Practical Equine Nutrition
briony@practicalequinenutrition.co.uk
https://writtle.ac.uk/profiles/profile.cfm?stID=2625&nofooter=1

A graduate of Aberystwyth University and the Royal Agricultural College, the early part of Briony's career was spent in the commercial sector, as senior nutritionist at one of the UK's major feed companies. Briony went on to achieve registered nutritionist status with the Association for Nutrition (AfN) and started her own equine nutrition consultancy, Practical Equine Nutrition. Based in Cambridge, Briony currently works as an equine nutritionist through her private consultancy and lectures at degree and postgraduate level in Equine and Animal Science at Writtle University College.

During Briony's career as a nutritionist she has worked in various disciplines and yards, with a range of horse owners, from leisure riders to high-level international and Olympic performance riders and leading British breeders.

Briony consults nationwide for leading forage and supplement producers, including quality assurance matters (including FEMAS and NOPS) as well as technical support and product development. In addition to this, she supports private clients including stud and performance yards and private owners.

Briony has written peer-reviewed articles for leading equine veterinary journals in addition to content for many of the UK's leading equestrian publications such as *Horse & Hound*; *Horse & Rider*; *Pony Magazine*; *Horse*; *Equine Health Magazine* and *British Breeder Magazine*. Her specialist interests centre on promoting a 'forage first' mentality to feeding, and a holistic approach to nutrition, working closely with other paraprofessionals to optimise performance in every horse, whether the aspirations be performance or otherwise.

In her spare time, Briony has a PRE gelding which she rides and competes, and a Welsh section A which she drives.

Forewords

Foreword by Carl Hester

The nutrition and feeding of horses have changed significantly over the years, not just with respect to the amount of knowledge and research that is now available to riders, owners and grooms but also the huge array of different products and supplements that are available and on the market.

We all strive to get the best from our horses and to ensure their health and their wellbeing in the hope that in doing this we will achieve our best results and have horses that are able to perform and recover to the best of their ability and have long and successful careers. I am proud to be able to look out of my window at home and see the heads of horses who have been with me since the very beginning and are still here today – horses that have travelled the world and won countless medals and who have contributed so much to equestrian sport. They have thrilled and encouraged people and given many riders and owners hope. Being able to have these horses living out their veteran years out of the competition limelight but seeing them still healthy and active is a testament to good nutrition playing its part and adapting to the different life and training stages of horses to meet their changing needs. Nutrition is a contributing factor of the huge jigsaw of expertise that works together for the health of horses but most importantly the love of horses.

This book brings a fantastic insight into how to feed your horse that is not based on hearsay or myth; it has worked well to bring the science and the research together to justify and explain how to feed horses.

Lizzie and Teresa have worked in the field for many years, listening, observing, and accruing experience and knowledge to be able to advocate the correct and sensible feeding of horses. They have succeeded in bringing all of this practical experience together supported by the evidence into one book that will help all equine professionals understand why they are doing what they are doing and to feed horses with confidence.

This book is the product of determination of two equine nutritionists and enthusiasts and is a must for any clinician, equine student or professional that will allow riders and trainers like myself to be able to concentrate on the riding and leave the professionals to fuel my horses correctly.

Carl Hester, MBE

Carl Hester's Medal tally from 2009:

2009 European Championships Team Silver; 2010 World Equestrian Games Team Silver; 2011 European Championships Team Gold; 2011 European Championships Individual Silver (Special); 2011 European Championships Individual Silver (Freestyle); 2012 Olympic Games Team Gold; 2013 European Championships Team Bronze; 2014 World Equestrian Games Team Silver; 2015 European Championships Team Silver; 2016 Olympic Games Team Silver; 2017 World Cup Finals Individual Bronze; 2018 World Equestrian Games Team Bronze; 2020 (2021) Olympic Games Team Bronze; 2021 European Championships Team Silver

Carl is also an Honorary Fellow of the British Horse Society and was awarded an MBE for his services to Equestrianism.

*

Foreword by Tim Mair

This is an important book. Throughout my career as an equine vet, I have appreciated the importance of equine nutrition in both health and disease, but I have found it difficult to put the theories of nutrition into practice. At university, I was taught about the basics of equine nutrition, but understanding how to translate knowledge of the energy and nutrient requirements of healthy and sick horses into the practical, day-to-day feeding recommendations has been extremely challenging. This book will fill an important gap in the published literature on feeding both well and ill horses. By the fact that you are reading this book, I suspect that you are also looking for some practical, down-to-earth advice about the nutritional management of horses in both health and disease. If this is the case, then you won't be disappointed.

I have known both Lizzie Drury and Teresa Hollands for many years and have always been impressed by their extensive knowledge and practical approach to equine nutrition. The authors have successfully managed to combine their experience and common-sense approach to equine nutrition with research and published data to produce a practical, evidence-based book that will be a valuable source of information to equine veterinarians, veterinary and bioscience students, professional horse owners and many others. There is no doubt that this book will rapidly become a treasured and well-thumbed addition to my own library and I am sure that it will be consulted on many occasions when looking for advice about the nutritional management of the horse.

Tim Mair BVSc PhD DEIM DESTS DipECEIM AssocECVDI FRCVS

Acknowledgements

Without Lizzie, this book would not have happened. She was offered the commission after CABI heard her present at The London Vet Show on the 'Practical management of obesity and client engagement'.

If that approach had been made 10 years ago, the book in its current form would not have happened, because Lizzie and Teresa were working for competitive horse feed manufacturers, making collaboration too awkward. That is not to say that their paths did not overlap, with both writing for *Your Horse* magazines, doing the same show circuits and often looking after different horses on the same yard, particularly in the build-up to London 2012.

The collaboration became stronger when Teresa, starting at The University of Surrey School of Vet Med, contacted the main horse feed manufacturers for support for the students (thank you to Saracen, Dodson & Horrell, Baileys, Horsehage, Honeychop, Spillers and Dengie) and the rest is history.

Neither of us could have completed this book without our co-authors, nor CABI's patience and support as deadline after deadline slipped. We never really stopped to appreciate how large a project writing a book is – the time it entails and trying to fit around what were more than full-time jobs during a pandemic.

We are particularly grateful to Lottie Payne for her patience and time in the uploading of photographs and guidance and advice to Lizzie, who now feels much more confident and up to date with some of the latest computer technologies. To Steph and Lucy for reading through almost all of the completed chapters and helping with some figure illustrations and spreadsheet excellence. We would also like to thank Priscilla Robinson in Dubai, for her incredible photography of some of our case studies and also for her support and encouragement throughout this whole process. Priscilla was one of Lizzie's first sports horse clients in the Middle East and has been a huge driving force behind the improved education in equine feeding and feed management in the Middle East.

And of course neither of us would have been in the position to write the book without the thousands of horses, clients, vets and industry professionals with whom we have worked, learnt, swapped ideas and been challenged by – thank you one and all.

Lizzie Drury and Teresa Hollands

This book is an accumulation of over 35 years working as an equine nutritionist; it would not have happened without the support and friendship of so many within the veterinary profession, the animal feed business and the wider equine community.

Mr Tim Henson from Belvoir Horse Feeds who had the confidence to respond positively to a begging letter to support me on my MSc in Animal Nutrition. That led me to write another letter to Dr Derek Cuddeford to ask to do my thesis with him at The Royal Dick School of Veterinary Science (he accepted – I was free labour, after all) which was the start of my learning journey on critical evaluation, being encouraged to challenge every research paper and study design; Derek was my mentor in my early career.

It was at Edinburgh that I made friends and colleagues for life who encouraged me to work with vets to support them in providing diet advice: Professor Bruce McGorum and more recently Dr John Keen as well as many of the equine hospital staff, too many to mention. Inviting me to teach on 5th-year electives meant I could visit Angie McDougall every year with free lodging at Heather's. Angie let me lodge with her while I was in Edinburgh back in the mid-1980s, remaining one of my 'bestest' friends as well as my 'go to' for checking if my advice was relevant and understandable for clients.

To the whole team at Dengie for taking a punt on a greenhorn, supporting me in my new role as an Animal and then Equine Nutritionist, and to John Sharpe for head hunting me (I said no a few times first) to join Dodson and Horrell as Senior Technical Marketing Manager.

To everyone at Dodson and Horrell for letting us fly, enabling us to become the largest manufacturer of horse feed in the UK, for encouraging positive interaction and provision of CPD for Vets, the development of The Internal Conferences on Feeding Horses (funding our international speakers who agreed to speak twice a day for 5 days around the country, on the road every night; Drs Joe Pagan and Andrew Clarke; Professors Stephanie Valberg, Phil Johnston, Katherine Houpt, Sarah Ralston, and Chris Politt – you are amazing) as well as providing an R&D budget, the first pennies spent on a weighbridge so that Julie Ellis and myself could spend two summers at shows and pony club camps to develop our scientifically validated weight tape, with the larger proportion spent at Hannover/Leipzig Vet schools with Professors Manfred Coenan and Ingrid Vervuert further developing my scientific rigour, and finally for supporting me on my PhD (Dr Jeremy Burn – I would not have succeeded without your critical support), which I combined with continuing to work three days a week – it was a blast working with Deborah Lucas, Louise Jones (nutritionists in crime), Elli Farrington, Amanda Renoir our technical sales team and Helpline, always hungry for knowledge and ensuring we kept up to date – working with Team GB for London 2012, specifically the Para dressage was a huge privilege. What an era!

To Professors Josh Slater and Mark Bowen, both of whom came along to clinical clubs as students for the free pizza and then organised for me to teach equine nutrition in curriculum when they became staff at Cambridge, RVC and Nottingham Vet schools; Professor Sandy Love for doing the same at Glasgow. And Professors Cathy McGowan and Derek Knottenbelt for letting me teach 5th-year electives at Liverpool Vet School and for lecturing at our roadshows that were the International Conferences on Feeding Horses and Laminitis Awareness 2010 and 2011. To Derek K also for all CPD he organised (including Ukraine, Czech Republic and Estonia), letting me teach nutrition, and to Professor Sarah Freeman and others at Nottingham for enabling me to support 3rd-year projects, which we published.

Of course, equine nutrition is wasted if it stays in academia, it needs to be applicable and understandable by horse owners. My journey in doing that was started by Karen Bush, editor of *Equestrian World* who I met when I was horse sitting for a mutual friend whilst doing my MSc, and then continued by Lesley Bayley, editor of *Your Horse* magazine, Marian O'Sullivan, editor of *Horse and Rider*, and Arnold Garvey, editor of *Horse and Hound*, Clare Thomas and Liz Benwell of ETN and Carolyn Henderson, all of whom commissioned so many articles that I have lost count.

The other great educators I have had the privilege to work with include BHS (thank you Emmeline Hannelly, amongst others), World Horse Welfare (Tony Hall, Sam Chubbuck, Basil Hayes – hours of The Right Weight, filming and supporting 3rd-year vet student projects as well as a few drinking hours at BEVA). The Equine Team at Boehringer for partnering on 'Talk about laminitis', 'Care about Cushings' and the fat scoring – so important to disseminate to horse owners.

Every single vet who has supported me: I am a little nervous naming anyone because you have all been so supportive and such fun to work with. Many have moved on from the practices where we spent many a client evening – I learnt so much from you and your clients – but Helen Whitbread, Lesley Barwise Monro, Rod Fisher, Jane Nixon, Wendy Furness of equine XLVets, Madeline Campbell, David Catlow, Andy Durham and Dr Alex Dugdale (for many a debate), Dr Tim Mair and Dr Nicky Holdstock, and Kiern O'Brian come to mind for the longevity of contact (and I have your mobile numbers).

And finally, the team at The University of Surrey School of Veterinary Medicine, specifically Professor Rob La Ragione for whom I taught horse nutrition as an external, and Professor Sue Lanham New for responding so positively to my vision of integrating nutrition as an essential part of preventive medicine within the curriculum. I don't dare name any individuals at Surrey because I am still there, but everybody at The Vet School and School of Biological Science (and I don't distinguish between academics and support staff) working on the coalface have helped me develop into an academic teacher (sort of), have responded so positively to my insistence that you cannot practise vet med without nutrition, to all the students who have borne with me in the journey and every single one of you who talk about fat scoring and nutrition every time you see a horse.

Actually not quite finally, the last word has to go to family, friends and horses – my mother for hours and months or years of mucking out horses, taking me to shows and encouraging me in my riding; my bruv and sis for tolerating being dragged to shows, my husband who met me when I was doing my PhD and became my rock, Dr Sarah Leno whom I have known since I was 10 whose mutual passion for horses has meant we are still mates. My horse experience gave me lifelong friends, opened the door for my career, kept it open and has given me that hands-on knowledge that allows me to translate the biology and science I have since learnt. New foals still bring a smile to my face, fat little ponies still make me sad, the sound of horse trotting along the road still whets my appetite and there is nothing as exhilarating as cantering through the waves. Horses moulded my life.

Teresa Hollands

This book has been one of my most challenging achievements to date and without all of the people who have been there and supported me on my journey as an equine nutritionist it would never have happened. My career really started after an evening in West Sussex, when I met the then Sales and Marketing Director at Saracen Horse Feeds, Jim Scott, who saw something in me and offered me my first equine nutritional role and the rest is history. He drove my ambition to always be better and never let obstacles get in my way. He was also the person who first mentioned the name Dr Teresa Hollands, a nutritionist whom he held in high regard. Teresa at that time (unbeknown to her) became the nutritionist that I wanted to be and whenever I was featured in a *Your Horse* Q&A or a minor editorial piece where Teresa was the main author, was a huge privilege to me. I had during this time never met Teresa personally, and this did not happen until she moved to Surrey University and in this time we quickly became firm friends and I learnt that we actually had a lot in common with regards to our approach and ethos to equine nutrition – she had taught me well!

When I was offered the opportunity to write this book, I very rapidly realised that this was no task that I could manage on my own and so when Teresa accepted the offer to write with me, I was to say the least overwhelmed and honoured. To write with the nutritionist who I have looked up to throughout my career has been amazing. Teresa has been an absolute rock throughout this process and known when to push me, when to tell me off and when things are really good and I literally cannot thank her enough. When are we going to do the next one?

Throughout my career I have been so fortunate to work with so many amazing riders, owners and of course horses from literally all levels of experience and all over the world, and I still never take any of this for granted. Riders such as Carl Hester, Spencer Wilton, Gareth Hughes, Charlotte Dujardin, Catherine Dufour, Harrie Smolders, and the list goes on, have enabled me to experience the highest level of training and competition and the stresses and unexpected that can happen at this level.

The horses involved have taught me that things do not always follow the rule book and that you must think quickly and outside of the box. The first horse to really do that was Carl Hester's ride, Escapardo. This horse was the start of my elite performance horse career and to him I will be forever grateful. I also have learnt so much from my grassroots clients, horses and ponies, who are our everyday clients. They bring something new every day and maybe one day I will put together a book of all my past and present horse and pony clients, their incredible stories, journeys and successes.

I have been exceptionally privileged to work with some of our world's greatest vets and nutritional expertise, including Tim Mair and the team at Bell Equine, Richard Hepburn, whom I have dragged across the Middle East with me, scoping numerous numbers of endurance horses, and Nivaldo Meneghetti, with whom I have worked throughout my whole Middle East experience and career. And of course the team at Kentucky Equine Research US and Australia. These people have helped to shape my career and I hope will continue to do so, as every day is a new day to watch, listen and learn.

My career has been nurtured and supported by Saracen Horse Feeds, who have allowed me to drive my own career path, learn by my mistakes, support my continued education and over the past long 2 years of writing this book have been bearing with me through this process. For this I am so thankful, and I hope that I can help repay this by supporting our next generation of nutritionists so that they can go on to experience everything that I have been so fortunate to see.

Lastly, my family! Wow, the tears, the tantrums, the late, late nights and 5 am starts to do 'book work', as it became known, is what they have had to endure, and yet their support and calmness enabled me to just keep going. My gorgeous daughter, Alexa, who kept saying, 'Mummy, you can do this and you are brilliant,' which meant I could not give up. Philip for bearing the brunt of my tears and tantrums and just pouring the wine or serving supper, with no judgment or complaints. Mum and dad for just believing in me. This book is for you, thank you.

To all of my friends who have listened and read and just been there!

Lastly to every single horse and pony, no matter how big or small and whatever you are doing, your smell, your beauty, your strength and pure brilliance is why I am doing what I do and I hope that this book helps others to understand you better so that you can be fed and managed in the best way.

Lizzie Drury

Glossary of Abbreviations

AA (amino acids)
AAFCO (Association of American Food Control Officials)
ADG (average daily gain)
ADH (antidiuretic hormone)
AfN (Association for Nutrition)
AGE (advanced glycation end-product)
AI (artificial insemination)
AIC (Agricultural Indus(tries) Confederation)
APR (acute phase protein)
ATM (adipose tissue macrophages)
BCAA (branched-chain amino acid)
BCS (body condition score)
BETA (British Equestrian Trade Association)
BFS (body fat score)
BFS/BCS (body fat/condition score/scoring)
BFT (back fat)
BHA (British Horseracing Authority)
bpm (beats per minute)
BW (bodyweight)
CCP (critical control point)
CDP (conditioning programme)
cfu (colony-forming unit)
CHO (carbohydrate, i.e. hydrated carbon)
CK (creatine kinase)
CL (corpus luteum)
CLI (chronic low-grade inflammation)
CLS (crown-like structure)
CNS (cresty neck score)
COX (cytochrome c oxidase)
CP (crude protein)
CPD (Continuing Professional Development)
CT (computerised tomography)
D1C (Day One competence)
DAG (diacylglycerols)
DBC (dried brewer's grain)
DCAB (dietary cation–anion balance)
DCP (digestible crude protein)
DE (digestible energy)
DEXA (dual-energy X-ray absorptiometry)
DHA (docosahexaenoic acid)
DIO (diet-induced obesity)
DMI (dry matter intake)
DOD (developmental orthopaedic diseases)

DOMS (delayed-onset muscle soreness)
EBEN (evidence-based equine nutrition)
EBM (evidence-based medicine)
EBN (evidence-based nutrition)
EBVM (evidence-based veterinary medicine)
ECF (extracellular fluid)
ECG (electrocardiogram)
ECM (extra-cellular matrix)
EDT (equine dental technician)
EGGD (equine glandular gastric disease)
EGUS (equine gastric ulcer syndrome)
EMS (equine metabolic syndrome)
ER (exertional rhabdomyolysis)
ESC (ethanol-soluble carbohydrate)
ESGD (equine squamous gastric disease)
ET (embryo transfer)
EU (European Union)
FA (fatty acid)
FEFAC (European Feed Manufacturers Federation)
FEI (Fédération Equestre Internationale, International Federation for Equestrian Sports)
FFA (free fatty acid)
FFDCA (Federal Food, Drug, and Cosmetic Act
FFL (full fibre length)
FOS (fructooligosaccharides)
FPT (failure of passive transfer)
FSA (Food Standards Agency)
GC (growth curve)
GEH (Gesellschaft für Ernahrungphysiologie (**GfE**))
GHCL (glucosamine hydrochloride)
GIT (gastrointestinal tract)
GLUT (glucose transporter)
GRAS (Generally Recognised As Safe)
GS (glucosamine sulphate)
GYS (glycogen synthase)
HACCP (Hazard Analysis and Critical Control Point)
HDL (high-density lipoproteins)
HOYS (Horse of the Year Show)
HR (heart rate)
HRM (heart rate monitor)
HRV (heart rate variability)
HS (high starch)
HYPP (hyperkalaemic periodic paralysis)
iCa (ionised calcium)
ICF (intracellular fluid)
ICMSF (International Commission on Microbiological Substances for Foods)
Ig (immunoglobulin)
IGF (insulin-like growth factor)
IgG (immunoglobulin G)
IL-1 (interleukin-1)
INRA (Institut National de la Recherche Agronomique)
IR (insulin resistance)
IRS (insulin receptor substrate)

ISO (International Organization for Standardization)
KER (Kentucky Equine Research)
LGCI (low-grade chronic inflammation)
LMICs (low- and middle-income countries)
LS (low starch)
LT (lactate threshold)
LW (liveweight)
M (maintenance)
ME (metabolisable energy)
MECC (making every contact count)
MG (muscle gain)
MHO (metabolically healthy obesity)
miRNA (microribonucleic acid)
MJ DE (megajoules of digestible energy)
MOOC (multiple online open-access course)
MS (medium starch)
MSBP (molassed sugar beet pulp)
MSK (musculo-skeletal)
NASC (National Animal Supplement Council)
NDF (neutral detergent fibre)
NEFA (non-esterified fatty acid)
NEWC (National Equine Welfare Council)
NFE (nitrogen-free extract)
NG (nasogastric intubation)
NGO (non-governmental organisation)
NI (neonatal isoerythrolysis)
NIR (near-infrared)
NIS (nutritionally improved straw)
NO (nitric oxide)
NOAEL (no observed adverse effect levels)
NOPS (Naturally occurring prohibited substances)
NRC (National Research Council)
NSAID (non-steroidal anti-inflammatory drug)
NSC (non-structural carbohydrate)
OA (osteoarthritis)
OCD (osteochondrosis)
PARNUT (PARticular NUTritional purposes)
PCV (packed cell volume)
PFPT (partial failure of passive transfer)
PPID (pituitary pars intermedia dysfunction)
PSSM (polysaccharide storage myopathy)
PTH (parathyroid hormone)
PUFA (polyunsaturated fatty acid)
PV (plasma volume)
QC (quality control)
QIQO (quality in equates to quality out)
RAT (retroperitoneal adipose tissue)
RCT (randomised controlled trial)
RCVS (Royal College of Veterinary Surgeons)
RER (recurrent exertional rhabdomyolysis)
RH (relative humidity)
ROM (range of motion)

RTU (real-time ultrasonography)
RUS (real-time ultrasound)
SAA (serum amyloid A)
SAT (subcutaneous adipose tissue, subcutaneous fat)
SB (Standardbred)
SBP (sugar beet pulp)
SC (stud cubes)
SCFA (short-chain fatty acid)
SDF (synchronous diaphragmatic flutter)
SI (small intestine)
SJ (showjumper)
SL (sweat loss)
SMF (skeletal muscle fat)
SOCS (suppressor of cytokine signalling)
SOD (superoxide dismutase)
SOP (standard operating procedure)
SUL (safe upper limit)
TB (Thoroughbred)
TBF (total body fat)
TBX (Thoroughbred cross)
TG (triglyceride)
TLR (toll-like receptor)
TNF (tumour necrosis factor)
TSP (total serum protein)
UFAS (Universal Feed Assurance Scheme)
UFET (urinary fractional excretion test)
VAT (visceral adipose tissue)
VDMI (voluntary dry matter intake)
VFA (volatile fatty acid)
VO_2 (oxygen consumption)
VO_2max (maximal oxygen consumption)
WBC (white blood cell)
WMD (white muscle disease)
WSAVA (World Small Animal Veterinary Association)
WSC (water-soluble carbohydrate)

1 Why This Book?

Teresa Hollands

School of Veterinary Medicine, University of Surrey

Learning Objectives

LO1 List the importance of nutrition in terms of prevention and health promotion.
LO2 Describe how nutrition affects all the body systems.
LO3 Describe how vets work with nutritionists and where to access professionally qualified nutritionists.
LO4 Select reliable sources of nutritional information.
LO5 Describe where nutrition fits into the RCVS Day One competencies.
LO6 Describe the importance of being evidence based.

At the end of this chapter, you will be able to summarise the importance of a team-based approach to evidence-based preventive nutrition.

Why is Nutrition Important?

Owning or working with horses is an important part of many of our lives. In the UK, 3 million people ride and the population of horses is estimated as 847, 000, (BETA, 2019). Horses help keep us fit, provide us with companionship and a sense of purpose and are good for our mental health (Burgon *et al.*, 2018).

Keeping an animal lean by feeding a balanced diet is the only scientifically proven intervention for healthy longevity (Roth *et al.*, 2000; Lawler *et al.*, 2008; Fontana and Hu, 2014; Adams *et al.*, 2016) and yet owners struggle with the fact that feed and vet bills are one of the highest expenditures associated with horse ownership (Stowe, 2018). Horses are living longer (Hotchkiss *et al.*, 2007; Ireland *et al.*, 2011), with many clients retiring their older horses but keeping them for life (Brosnahan and Paradis, 2003). Whatever the age or performance level of the horse, its nutrition should never be compromised, because every system in the horse's body (and that of every animal, including humans) is either directly or indirectly affected by nutrition.

There is no doubt that poor and inappropriate nutrition impacts on the health, performance and welfare of every horse, thus the science of nutrition should provide the basis to any advice on the art of feeding. It is vital that all professionals use evidence-based nutritional information to support the health and performance of all horses as part of their preventative medicine armour.

Communicated correctly, vet and feed bills will be seen as a preventative measure and a vital expenditure in maintaining the performance and health of all the equids in our care. Opinions on nutrition are often very personal, perhaps because feeding animals and ourselves is a daily activity and the consequence of getting it wrong takes several years to develop. In the UK, 31% of horses and ponies suffer from chronic long-term inflammatory disease (Robin *et al.*, 2015) associated with inappropriate nutrition yet only 35% of owners recognise the disease (Ireland *et al.*, 2012). It is essential that everyone who interacts with or cares for the horse – be it the owner, the vet, the farrier, the judge, or the trainer – takes responsibility for staying up to date and practising evidence-based preventative medicine, of which nutrition is key.

DOI: 10.1079/9781789245134.0001

Clients' needs from their vets and advisers are changing and there is a generational difference in the way they want to interact with advisers and obtain their information (Parrott, 2004; Larkin, 2014). Advisers need to react to this demand, get the basics right and make every contact count (Lawrence *et al.*, 2018; Lynden *et al.*, 2018) to support nutritional understanding and improve equine health at relatively low cost.

This chapter sets the scene for the book, which aims to provide not only graduating vets with enough information to meet their day one competencies, but also any professional who wishes to discuss with owners the evidence behind their nutritional advice and to provide case-based examples of 'the art and management of feeding equids'.

The Role of Nutrition in Preventive Medicine

Size of the market

There are 58 million equines in the world, including 7 million in the EU (eurogroupforanimals.org) and 9.2 million in the USA (Table 1.1). If you add in working equids (donkeys and mules), then the worldwide total is 112 million equids (horses, donkeys, mules) (Upjohn and Wells, 2016). In the USA, 60,000 horses (15%) are feral (Schoenecker *et al.*, 2021).

The UK horse industry contributes £8.5 billion/year to the national gross output (British Equestrian, 2021); it has one of the highest levels of horse ownership per capita in Europe (Tables 1.2 and 1.3); it is world renowned for its Thoroughbred (TB) racing industry (Table 1.1) and was ranked by Longines[i] in 2022 as 3rd in the world for training highest-ranked horses.

Despite this success, there has been a 8% decrease in the number of Thoroughbred breeders, mainly because their operation was unprofitable (TBA, 2018), with feed and veterinary costs being cited as one of the major cost centres (Fig. 1.1).

Obviously, every one of these horses needs to be fed and consequently horse owners in the UK spend an average of £610/horse/year; with an estimated total UK expenditure on all types of feed in

Table 1.1 The size of the equine industry across the world

Country	Horse type	Number of horses	Contribution to economy	Number of people riding or supported by horses	Evidence base
UK (2017)	Thoroughbred breeding	9000 broodmares 4778 foals	£427 m	19,000 jobs 3318 breeders	TBA (2018)
USA (2005)	All	9.2 million Racing: 844,531; Showing: 2,718,954; Recreation: 3,906,923; Other: 1,752,439 Horse use: 68.6% pleasure/trail riding; 31.1% idle, retired, or otherwise not working; 27% dressage; 23% lessons and training	$39 billion	2 million own horses 238,000 are involved in breeding, 481,000 in competing	Deloitte Consulting (2005) Stowe (2018)
Canada (2010)		963,500	$19 billion	76,334 jobs	Equine Canada (2010)
Australia	Thoroughbred	21,500 broodmares 700 stallions (20% of horses)	$1.143 billion	4200 breeders 6 state breeders organisations	AgriFutures Australia, (2018)
Australia	All	221,000 (2006) Feral horses 400,000	$6.3 billion		Ninmo (2018)
France	All			2 million riders	Fédération Française d'Équitation (2022)

Table 1.2 Number of horses per 1000 persons by continent (Gilbert *et al.*, 2018)

Continent	Number of horses	Number of people ('000)	Horses per person ('000)
Africa	4,240,612	921,073	4.6
Asia	14,256,852	3,936,535	3.7
Europe	6,489,242	729,420	8.9
Latin America and Caribbean	8,562,285	184,854	46.4
North America	9,586,060	335,175	28.7
Oceania	374,657	33,559	11.1
South America	15,225,273	371,658	41
TOTAL	58,734,981	6,512,274	9.1

Table 1.3 Horse populations in European countries (European Council, 2009; Liljenstolpe, 2009; Liljenstolpe and Andersson, 2009)

Country	Number of horses	Horses per 1000 people	Horses per hectare
Great Britain	1,000,000	16.6	41
Germany	1,000,000	12.1	28
France	900,000	14.3	16
Spain	559,598	12.8	11
Netherlands	400,000	24.5	96
Poland	320,000	8.4	10
Belgium	300,000	28.5	98
Italy	300,000	5.1	10
Sweden	280,000	30.9	6
Denmark	150,000	27.6	35
Austria	100,000	12.1	12
Ireland	80,000	19	11
Finland	77,000	14.6	2
Czech Republic	64,126	6.3	8
Hungary	60,000	6	6
Norway	45,000	9.6	1
Serbia	350,000	17.5	3
Greece	27,000	2.4	2
Slovenia	22,000	11	11
Latvia	13,600	5.9	2
Slovakia	8,000	1.5	2
Estonia	4,900	3.7	1
Luxembourg	4,490	9.7	17
TOTAL	7,570,714		

2019 of £638.2 million (BETA, 2019). It is important that we are able to advise owners how to spend wisely and to be able to answer their question: 'Is this the right feed for my horse?'

The Importance of Nutrition in Terms of Health Promotion

Despite nutrients being essential for every process in the body – and indeed life itself – and the massive amount of nutritional information available on the internet (a Google search for 'nutrition horses' in December 2022 resulted in about 58.7 million results), we continue to see a worldwide increase in a non-communicable disease caused by poor nutrition, resulting in obesity. The disease is chronic low-grade inflammation. In the UK, the cost of obesity, which is ranked as one of the top three global social burdens generated by human beings, is £47 billion (Dobbs *et al.*, 2014). Our horses are no exception. In horses, chronic inflammation (Wellen and Hotamisligil, 2003; Reynolds *et al.*, 2019) increases the risk of numerous diseases, all of which can be mitigated by appropriate nutrition.

- 57.3% of Canadian horse owners identified hay and concentrates as the areas in which their expenses had increased the most (Stowe, 2018). Although feed and veterinary fees are two of the highest costs for owners, repositioning feed as preventive medicine should mitigate some of these costs. Sections of the industry are moving towards recognising nutrition's role in the health and performance of horses.
- As part of their 5-year strategy, the Australian TB industry has a short-term aim to achieve 'Improvement in prevention of dietary related diseases of horses' and in the longer term to 'Communicate strategies for prevention of dietary related disorders' (AgriFutures Australia, 2018).

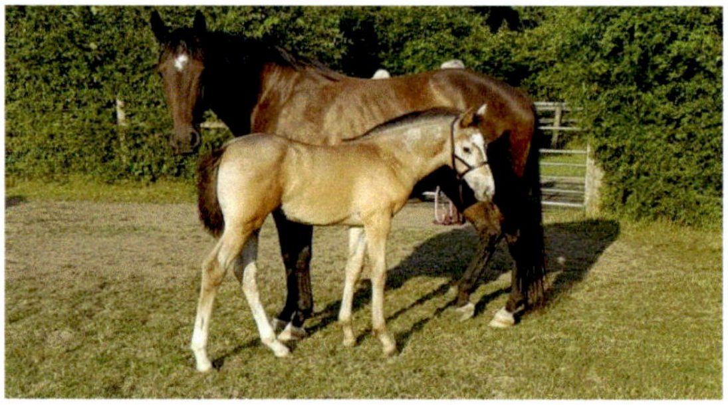

Fig. 1.1 Setting nutritional targets as part of preventive medicine.

Good nutrition supports a healthy musculoskeletal system and healthy longevity, reduces risk of diseases and micronutrient deficiencies and, if the diet is fed properly, will replicate the normal feeding behaviour of the horse and support gut health.

All domesticated equids (working or pleasure) have a need for a suitable diet and a need to exhibit normal behaviour patterns when eating (Animal Welfare Act, 2006; DEFRA, 2018). Ninety-five per cent of vets care for 2% of this equine population (M. Appleby, personal communication, 2017) and it is your responsibility (RCVS, 2020) to be able to advise clients how to feed their horses to ensure healthy longevity and to recognise that nutrition is an essential cornerstone of preventative medicine (Box 1.1).

Preventive Nutrition

The only scientifically validated intervention for supporting healthy longevity and, by inference, performance is maintaining a lean body mass (Roth *et al.*, 2000; Lawler *et al.*, 2008; Fontana and Hu, 2014; Srikanthan and Karlamangla 2014; Adams *et al.*, 2016). We also know that every system in the body is either directly or indirectly affected by nutrients and the delivery of the diet.

From foal – epigenetics

Nutrition has an impact on the foal even before it is born. Many mares are overfed but undernourished during their first two trimesters, relying mostly on grass, which can provide twice their calorie requirements but will be deficient in minerals (Jones *et al.*, 2005a,b). Minerals are an essential component of microribonucleic acid (miRNA) (Beckett *et al.*, 2014), which codes certain genes. These genes are inherited from the mare and stallion and if the micronutrients are deficient, then genes involved in energy metabolism are not switched on, increasing the risk of the foal being born with insulin resistance (Sessions-Bresnahan *et al.*, 2018). Native breeds or mares that are kept on poor grazing to control their weight are likely to give birth to low-birthweight foals. In humans and other animals, low birthweight is correlated with increased susceptibility to diabetes, obesity and cardiovascular disease in later life (Barnes and Ozanne, 2011; Koletzko *et al.*, 2012). A low-calorie, low-protein diet has negative effects on DNA methylation and histone modifications of foetal developmental genes (Haggarty *et al.*, 2013). A deficiency in essential fatty acids (omega-3 fatty acids) is associated with aggression in dogs (Re *et al.*, 2008), subopti-

Box 1.1 The importance of nutrition in terms of prevention and health promotion.

Inappropriate feeding management can increase the risk of:

- stereotypy behaviour (Waters *et al*., 2002);
- obesity (Robin *et al*., 2015);
- colic (Gonçalves *et al*., 2002);
- gastric ulcers (Meyer *et al*., 1985, 1986; Luthersson *et al*., 2009); and
- dental pathologies (Khosravi *et al*., 2013).

Appropriate nutrition can minimise the risk of:

- chronic low-grade inflammation (Wellen and Hotamisligil 2003; Reynolds *et al*., 2019);
- dermatological conditions, musculoskeletal problems (Salonen *et al*., 2009) and osteoarthritis (Marshall *et al*., 2010);
- laminitis (Carter *et al*., 2009);
- insulin resistance (Suagee *et al*., 2012; Cao, 2014);
- endothelial changes within blood vessels (Engin, 2017);
- cognitive decline (Pedditizi *et al*., 2016);
- metabolic syndrome (Morgan *et al*., 2015); and
- shortened lifespan (Nagai *et al*., 2012)

It is your responsibility (RCVS, 2020) to be able to advise clients how to feed their horses to maintain healthy longevity, gut health and normal feeding behaviour. You can do this by encouraging them to recognise that nutrition is an essential cornerstone of preventive medicine (Day One competency).

mal cognitive and visual function in children (Kuratko *et al.*, 2013) and, potentially, with an increase in misbehaviour in fat ponies taken off grass (Buckley *et al.*, 2013). Omega-3s are essential for healthy membranes and the brain phospholipid membrane undergoes biochemical changes associated with deficiency in n-3 fatty acids. The adverse effects associated with omega-3s seen in animals is a result of losses in brain hippocampal function (Murthy *et al.*, 2002). Animals recover from losses in brain function when switched to an n-3 fatty acid-adequate diet (Koletzko *et al.*, 2012).

Making every contact count

No owner knowingly feeds their horses inappropriate diets and no owner knowingly has an under- or overweight horse. It is the responsibility of everyone who has contact with the owner and the horse to provide continuous and coherent nutritional support. Lynden *et al.* (2018) studied the role of the farrier in supporting owners with horses prone to laminitis and found that 'the farrier's role as a "conduit" and referral agent to veterinarians and nutritionists for specialist advice and guidance' helped clients to minimise the risk of laminitis. The authors emphasised 'the unique and valuable role farriers have working in partnership with owners and veterinarians to make every contact count in helping to prevent laminitis'. Lynden (2019) described that making every contact count (MECC) in human health care has been effective in delivery of successful weight loss, where nurses, doctors and healthcare assistants support the patients with diet advice, highlighting that Churchill and Ward (2016) argued that all veterinary practice staff, including receptionists, support staff and practice nurses, should have specific and collaborative roles in supporting weight management during different stages of the consultation process.

Owners also look to friends and trainers as sources of nutritional advice when feeding supplements (Gemmill *et al.*, 2015)

Working with nutritionists

- Most feed companies offer a nutritional helpline. Use them to obtain practical feeding advice, forage and feed analysis.
- Many companies employ qualified nutritionists who offer yard support and individual consultations. The best companies are members of British Equestrian Trade Association (BETA)[ii],

are signed up to industry codes of practice and operate under a Universal Feed Assurance Scheme (UFAS)[iii] (see Chapter 8).

- Some companies employ vets; make sure that they have had additional training in equine nutrition.
- Welfare organisations that are members of the National Equine Welfare Council (NEWC)[iv] provide useful help leaflets and resources as do other organisations (Box 1.2).

Working with a team

- Involve your farrier in noting the implications of dietary changes throughout the season; they visit your clients every 6–8 weeks and can spend up to 45 min with them.
- Run weight clinics with feed companies or independent nutritionists. Make sure that you are working with a qualified nutritionist (see Chapter 8, section 'Suitably qualified nutritionists'). They should have a postgraduate degree and a minimum of 3–5 years of experience.
- Involve the whole practice with training through client evenings and Continuing Professional Development (CPD).
- Note the diet, weight and fat score of the horses on every record (see Chapter 2, Figure 2.1: 'A vital card for clients to include basic ration information').
- Develop simple and straightforward help leaflets that do not contain any technical information (Crowe, 2019; Sheats *et al.*, 2019) (see Chapter 2).

Box 1.2 Useful sources of reliable nutritional information

http://www.associationfornutrition.org
http://www.feedipedia.org
http://www.dsm.com/markets/anh/en_US/Compendium.html
http://www.fediaf.org
http://microsteed.com/ker
http://pchorse.se/index.php/en/
https://www.avma.org/Pages/home.aspx
https://www.nap.edu/catalog/11653/nutrient-requirements-of-horses-sixth-revised-edition
https://nrc88.nas.edu/nrh/

- Always follow an evidence-based medicine approach to nutrition.
- Share your nutritional advice with the trainers, physiotherapists and other paraprofessionals who support your clients' horses.

Meeting Day One competences (D1Cs)

The ability to do a nutritional assessment in the UK is a Royal College of Veterinary Surgery (RCVS) core competence for new veterinary graduates.

Incorporating nutritional advice at every visit means that you are also:

- practising evidence-based veterinary medicine;
- distinguishing between facts and fiction by reviewing and evaluating literature and presentations critically;
- developing the understanding behind preventative nutrition by using your professional capabilities to contribute to the advancement of veterinary knowledge, in order to improve the quality of animal care and public health;
- communicating effectively with clients.

Evidence-based Equine Nutrition (EBEN)

One of the main aims of this book is to provide you with the evidence base behind feeding horses. One of the challenges with developing an evidence base in equine nutrition is that it is impossible to isolate nutrition from all the other interacting factors and even more challenging to investigate the effect of isolated nutrients within the clinical setting. Additionally, the methods from some excellent research papers are not always transferable into a busy yard setting. Clients may have entrenched views on feeding based on their own experiences and these should be considered, whilst providing them with evidence to back up your advice. Remember, $n = 1$ is not an evidence base no matter how much personal practical experience you have had in feeding horses, neither does it stand up in a law court, but yours and your client's expertise is actually a key part of evidence-based nutrition (EBN).

The formal definition of evidence-based medicine (EBM) is the 'conscientious, explicit, judicious and reasonable use of modern, best evidence in making decisions about the care of individual patients,

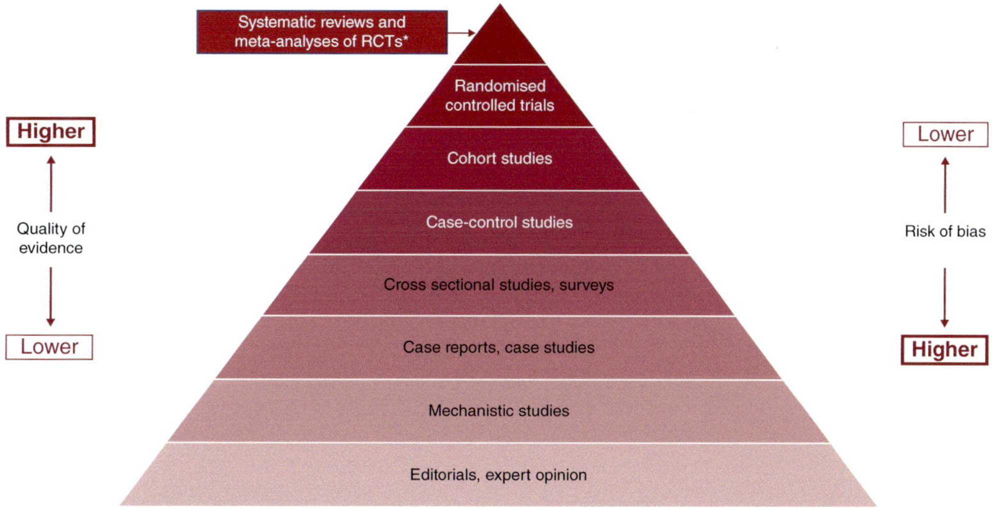

Fig. 1.2 Hierarchy of Evidence pyramid. Source: https://commons.wikimedia.org/wiki/File:Drawn_image_illustrating_the_Hierarchy_of_Evidence.png

integrating clinical experience and patient values with the best available research information' (Masic *et al.*, 2008). It is important that the evidence that you use is obtained in a systematic way and that the evidence is graded based on the quality of the evidence available. In the hierarchy of evidence, randomised clinical trials are seen as being at the top of the pyramid (Fig. 1.2) for drug testing but it is not always the most appropriate way to investigate nutritional questions (Blumberg *et al.*, 2010).

If you want to explore evidence-based veterinary medicine (EBVM) further, a useful website is https://knowledge.rcvs.org.uk/evidence-based-veterinary-medicine/knowledge-summaries/

Bear in mind that medical doctors who graduate from 'traditional medical curriculums progressively decline in their knowledge of appropriate clinical practice, whereas graduates of a medical school that teaches lifelong, self-directed, evidence-based medicine are still up to date as long as 15 years after graduation' (Rosenberg and Donald, 1995).

- Be prepared to accept a variety of evidence.
- The way that you explain the science needs to be memorable for the client to take action (Ratner and Riis, 2014). Simplicity is often key (Sheats *et al.*, 2019). Fig 1.3 illustrates the use of a detailed and simplified diagrams to summarise similar information – sometimes less is more. Your choice might be determined by your client's demographic and learning style.
- Use Knowledge Summaries (Veterinary Evidence) and Critically appraised topics (Equine Veterinary Education).

Summary

You, as the primary care clinician, are key to improving evidence-based equine nutrition (EBEN). Often the nutritionist is consulted after a disease has been diagnosed; retrospective dietary data, body fat score and dietary management are missing, making it impossible to be precise in causality. The World Small Animal Veterinary Association (WSAVA) stated that nutritional history should be the 5th vital sign (Freeman *et al.*, 2011) in small animal consults. The equine practitioner should do likewise by ensuring that nutritional status is an integral part of the clinical examination and both preventative and treatment plans. Chapter 2 provides an overview of the 5th vital sign in equine practice, with subsequent chapters discussing each aspect in more detail.

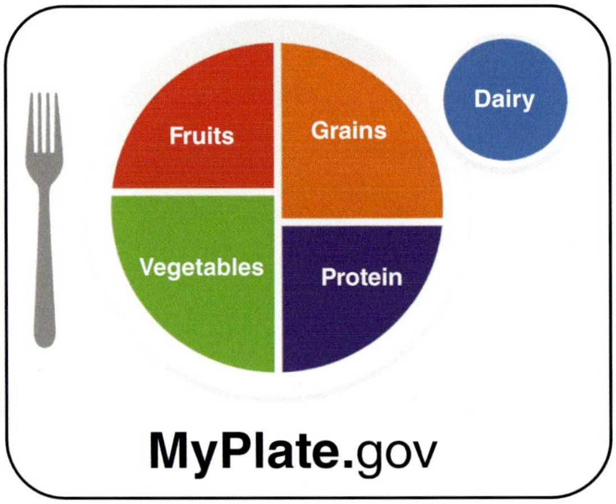

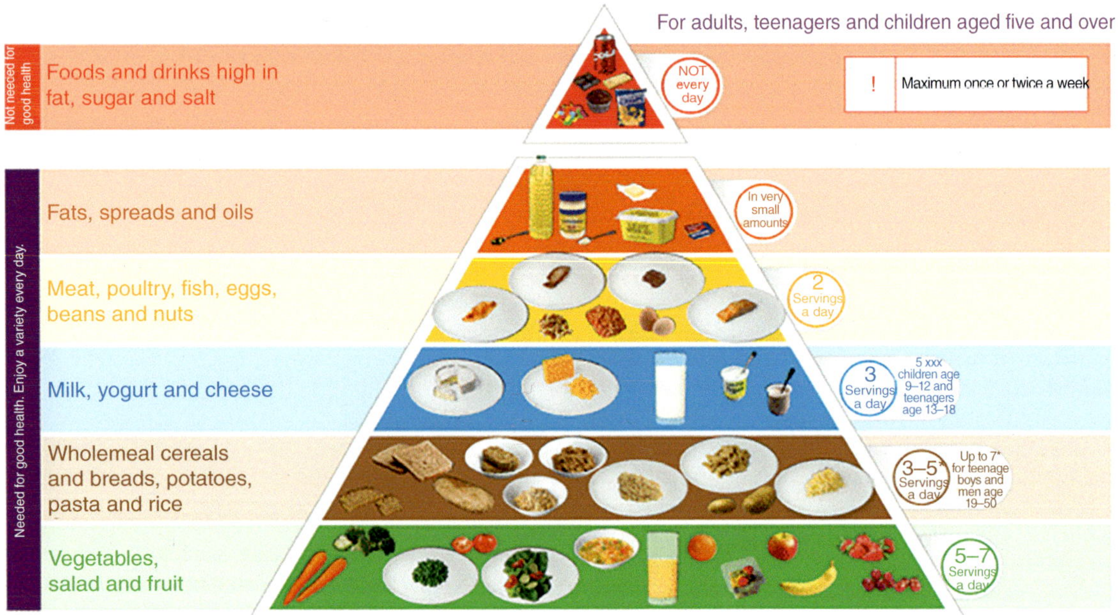

Fig. 1.3 The use of food pyramids (lower image) and plates (top image) to illustrate the usefulness of using memorable science and advice. Lower image (Crown copyright, 2018) available at https://www.safefood.eu/Healthy-Eating/The-Food-Pyramid-and-The-Eatwell-Guide/The-Food-Pyramid.aspx. Top image (copyright US Department of Agriculture) available at https://www.choosemyplate.gov; see also https://www.cdc.gov.

Notes

[i] https://www.ifhaonline.org/Default.asp?section=Resources&area=1

[ii] http://www.beta-uk.org/pages/feed-safety.php

[iii] https://www.aictradeassurance.org.uk/ufas/about-ufas/

[iv] http://www.newc.co.uk/members/

Bibliography

Adams, V.J., Watson, P., Carmichael, S., Gerry, S., Penell, J. and Morgan, D.M. (2016) Exceptional longevity and potential determinants of successful ageing in a cohort of 39 Labrador retrievers: results of a prospective longitudinal study. *Acta Veterinaria Scandinavica* 58, 29.

AgriFutures Australia (2018) Interim Thoroughbred Five Year RD&E Plan Publication No. 17/052, ISBN 978-1-74254-975-0. Available at: www.agrifutures.com.au (accessed 9 May 2022)

Animal Welfare Act (2006) UK Public General Acts, ch. 45. Available at: https://www.legislation.gov.uk/ukpga/2006/45/contents (accessed 9 May 2022).

Appleby, M. (2017) From the horse's mouth; the need for evidence of human and animal benefit. Talk given at World Horse Welfare Conference 2017: Invisible Horses of the Future.

Barnes, S.K. and Ozanne, S.E. (2011) Pathways linking the early environment to long-term health and lifespan. *Progress in Biophysics and Molecular Biology* 106, 323–336.

Beale, L., Maxwell, N.S., Gibson, O.R., Twomey, R., Taylor, B. and Church, A. (2015) Oxygen cost of recreational horse-riding in females. *Journal of Physical Activity and Health* 12(6), 808–813.

Beckett, E., Yates, Z., Veysey, M., Duesing, K. and Lucock, M. (2014) The role of vitamins and minerals in modulating the expression of microRNA. *Nutrition Research Reviews* 27(1), 94–106.

BETA (British Equine Trade Association) (2019) The National Equestrian Survey; Produced for BETA by JDA Research, p. 77.

Blumberg, J., Heaney, R.P., Huncharek, M., Scholl, T., Stampfer, M. *et al.* (2010) Evidence-based criteria in the nutritional context. *Nutrition Reviews* 68(8), 478–484.

Boucher, O., Burden, M.J., Muckle, G. *et al.* (2011) Neurophysiologic and neurobehavioral evidence of beneficial effects of prenatal omega-3 fatty acid intake on memory function at school age. *The American Journal of Clinical Nutrition* 93(5), 1025–1037.

British Equestrian (2021) *Britsh Equestrian Annual Report* 2020–2021, p. 33. Available at: https://www.britishequestrian.org.uk/assets/About%20the%20BEF/Annual%20Report/Annual%20Report/Annual%20Review%2020_21_FINAL_sm.pdf (accessed 19 July 2023).

Brosnahan, M.M. and Paradis, M.R. (2003) Assessment of clinical characteristics, management practices, and activities of geriatric horses. *Journal of the American Veterinary Medical Association* 223(1), 99–103. doi: 10.2460/javma.2003.223.99

Buckley, P., Morton, J.M., Buckley, D.J. and Coleman, G.T. (2013) Misbehaviour in Pony Club horses: incidence and risk factors. *Equine Veterinary Journal* 45, 9–14.

Burgon, H., Gammage, D. and Hebden, J. (2018) Hoofbeats and heartbeats: equine-assisted therapy and learning with young people with psychosocial issues – theory and practice. *Journal of Social Work Practice* 32(1), 3–16. doi: 10.1080/02650533.2017.1300878

Cao, H. (2014) Adipocytokines in obesity and metabolic disease. *The Journal of Endocrinology* 220(2), T47–T59. doi: 10.1530/JOE-13-0339

Carter, R.A., Treiber, K.H., Geor, R.J., Douglass, L. and Harris, P.A. (2009). Prediction of incipient pasture-associated laminitis from hyperinsulinaemia, hyperleptinaemia and generalised and localised obesity in a cohort of ponies. *Equine Veterinary Journal* 41(2), 171–178.

Churchill, J. and Ward, E. (2016) Communicating with pet owners about obesity: roles of the veterinary health care team. *The Veterinary Clinics of North America. Small Animal Practice* 46(5), 899–911. doi: 10.1016/j.cvsm.2016.04.010

Crowe, C. (2019) Are your client notes working for you – how to write for lay people. *Equine Veterinary Journal* 51, 433–434.

DEFRA (2018) Code of practice for the welfare of horses, ponies, donkeys and their hybrids. ISBN 978-1-5286-0172-6 PDF, 1.14MB, 38 pages. Available at: https://www.gov.uk/government/publications/code-of-practice-for-the-welfare-of-horses-ponies-donkeys-and-their-hybrids (accessed 9 May 2022).

Deloitte Consulting LLP (for the American Horse Council Foundation) (2005) *National Economic Impact of the U.S. Horse Industry*.

Devienne, M.F. and Guezennec, C.Y. (2000) Energy expenditure of horse riding. *European Journal of Applied Physiology* 82, 499. doi: 10.1007/s004210000207.

Dobbs, R., Sawers, C., Thompson, F. *et al.* (2014) *Overcoming obesity: an initial economic analysis*. A discussion paper by the McKinsey Global Institute, London.

Engin, A. (2017) Endothelial dysfunction in obesity. *Advances in Experimental Medicine and Biology* 960, 345–379. DOI: 10.1007/978-3-319-48382-5_15.

Equine Canada (2010) *Canadian Horse Industry Profile Study*. Available at: www.equestrian.ca/cfs/files/resources (accessed 1 February 2023).

European Council (2009) Modifications to the Common Agricultural Policy. Official Journal of the European Union. Council Regulation (EC) No 72/2009.

Fédération Française d'Équitation (2022) Horse Riding in France. Available at: www.ffe.com (accessed 9 May 2022).

Fontana, L. and Hu, F.B. (2014) Optimal body weight for health and longevity: bridging basic, clinical, and population research. *Aging Cell* 13(3), 391–400. doi: 10.1111/acel.12207

Freeman, L., Becvarova, I., Cave, N., MacKay, C., Nguyen, P. *et al.* (2011) WSAVA nutritional assessment guidelines. *Journal of Small Animal Practice* 52, 385–396.

Gemmill, R., Agar, C., Freeman, S.L. and Hollands, T. (2015) Factors affecting owners' choice of nutritional supplements for use in dressage and eventing

horses. *Veterinary Record Open* 3, e000155. doi: 10.1136/vetreco-2015-000155
Gilbert, M., Nicolas, G., Cinardi, G. *et al.* (2018) Global distribution data for cattle, buffaloes, horses, sheep, goats, pigs, chickens and ducks in 2010. *Sci Data* 5, 180227. doi: 10.1038/sdata.2018.227.
Gonçalves, S., Julliand, V. and Leblond, A. (2002) Risk factors associated with colic in horses. *Veterinary Research* 33(6), 641–652. doi: 10.1051/vetres:2002044
Haggarty, P., Hoad, G., Horgan, G.W. and Campbell, D.M. (2013) DNA methyltransferase candidate polymorphisms, imprinting methylation, and birth outcome. *PLoS ONE* 8, e68896.
Horsetalk (2007) World horse population estimated at 58 million. Available at: https://www.horsetalk.co.nz/2007/09/12/world-horse-population-58m/ (accessed 9 May 2022).
Hotchkiss, J.W., Reid, S.W.J. and Christley, R.M. (2007) A survey of horse owners in Great Britain regarding horses in their care. Part 1: Horse demographic characteristics and management. *Equine Veterinary Journal* 39, 294–300.
Ireland, J.L., Clegg, P.D., McGowan, C.M., McKane, S.A. and Pinchbeck, G.L. (2011) A cross-sectional study of geriatric horses in the United Kingdom. Part 1: demographics and management practices. *Equine Veterinary Journal* 43(1), 30–36.
Ireland, J.L., Clegg, P.D., McGowan, C.M., McKane, S.A., Chandler, K.J. *et al.* (2012) Comparison of owner-reported health problems with veterinary assessment of geriatric horses in the United Kingdom. *Equine Veterinary Journal* 44, 94–100.
Jones, L., Lax, J. and Hollands, T. (2005a) Analysis of the mineral content of spring summer grazing used for thoroughbred breeding stock in the UK. In: Proceedings of 44th BEVA Congress, Harrogate, p. 368.
Jones, L., Lax, J. and Hollands, T. (2005b) *The Mineral Content of Spring and Summer Pasture Grazed by Young Growing Thoroughbreds in the UK*. Short communication ENUCO, Hanover, Germany.
Khosravi, R., Ka, K., Huang, T., Khalili, S., Nguyen, B.H., Nicolau, B. and Tran, S.D. (2013) Tumor necrosis factor-α and Interleukin-6: potential interorgan inflammatory mediators contributing to destructive periodontal disease in obesity or metabolic syndrome. *Mediators of Inflammation.* 2013, Article ID 728987, 6.
Koletzko, B., Brands, B., Poston, L., Godfrey, K. and Demmelmair, H. (2012) Early nutrition programming of long-term health. *Proceedings of the Nutrition Society* 71, 371–378.
Kuratko, C.N., Barrett, E.C., Nelson, E.B. and Salem, N. Jr. (2013) The relationship of docosahexaenoic acid (DHA) with learning and behavior in healthy children: a review. *Nutrients* 5(7), 2777–2810.
Larkin, M. (2014) The Generation Factor. How the rise of the millennial generation could mean changes in the way veterinarians do business. *Journal of American Veterinary Medical Association News*. Available at: https://www.avma.org/javma-news/2014-11-01/generation-factor (accessed 9 May 2022).
Lawler, D., Larson, B., Ballam, J., Smith, G., Biery, D. *et al.* (2008) Diet restriction and ageing in the dog: major observations over two decades. *British Journal of Nutrition* 99(4), 793–805. doi: 10.1017/S0007114507871686.
Lawrence, W., Black, C., Tinati, T., Cradock, S., Begum, R. *et al.* (2018) 'Making every contact count': evaluation of the impact of an intervention to train health and social care practitioners in skills to support health behaviour change. *Journal of Health Psychology* 21(2), 138–151. doi: 10.1177/1359105314523304.
Liljenstolpe, C. (2009) Horses in Europe. In: *Proceedings of the EU Equus*, Uppsala, Sweden, 29–30 October 2009, p. 23.
Liljenstolpe, C. and Andersson, H. (2009) *Horses in Europe*. PhD thesis, Dept of Economics, Swedish University of Agricultural Sciences.
Luthersson, N., Nielsen, K.H., Harris, P. and Parkin, T.D.H. (2009) Risk factors associated with equine gastric ulceration syndrome (EGUS) in 201 horses in Denmark. *Equine Veterinary Journal* 41, 625–630. doi: 10.2746/042516409X441929.
Lynden, J. (2019) Working above the coronet band: a multi-methods study exploring how farriers support horse owners to prevent and manage laminitis, Ch. 3. PhD thesis, University of Surrey.
Lynden, J., Ogden, J. and Hollands, T. (2018) Contracting for care – the construction of the farrier role in supporting horse owners to prevent laminitis. *Equine Veterinary Journal* 50, 658–666. doi: 10.1111/evj.12950.
Marshall, W.G., Hazewinkel, H.A., Mullen, D., De Meyer, G., Baert, K. *et al.* (2010) The effect of weight loss on lameness in obese dogs with osteoarthritis. *Veterinary Research Communications* 34(3), 241–253. doi: 10.1007/s11259-010-9348-7.
Masic, I., Miokovic, M. and Muhamedagic, B. (2008) Evidence based medicine – new approaches and challenges. *Acta Informatica Medica* 16(4), 219–225.
Meyer, H., Coenen, M. and Gurer, C. (1985) Investigations of saliva production and chewing in horses fed various feeds. *Proceedings Equine Nutrition and Physiology Society*, East Lansing, Michigan, pp. 38–41.
Meyer, H., Coenen, M. and Prost, D. (1986) Feed insalivation and passage in the equine upper intestinal tract. *Journal of Animal Physiology and Animal Nutrition* 56, 171–183.
Morgan, R., Keen, J. and McGowan, C. (2015) Equine metabolic syndrome. *Veterinary Record* 177, 173–179. doi: 10.1136/vr.103226.
Murthy, M., Hamilton, J., Greiner, R.S., Moriguchi, T., Salem, N. Jr and Kim, H.Y. (2002) Differential effects of n-3 fatty acid deficiency on phospholipid molecular species composition in the rat hippocampus. *Journal of Lipid Research* 43, 611–617.

Nagai, M., Kuriyama, S., Kakizaki, M. *et al*. (2012) Impact of obesity, overweight and underweight on life expectancy and lifetime medical expenditures: the Ohsaki Cohort Study. *BMJ Open* 2, e000940. doi: 10.1136/bmjopen-2012-000940.

Ninmo, D. (2018) Feral horses in Australia. Hot Topics in Ecology, Ecological Society of Australia. Available at: https://www.ecolsoc.org.au/?hottopic-entry=feral-horses-in-australia ().

Parrott, R. (2004) Emphasizing 'communication' in health communication. *Journal of Communication* 54(4), 751–787.

Pedditzi, E., Peters, R. and Beckett, N. (2016) The risk of overweight/obesity in mid-life and late life for the development of dementia: a systematic review and meta-analysis of longitudinal studies. *Age and Ageing* 45(1), 14–21. doi: 10.1093/ageing/afv151.

Ratner, R. and Riis, J. (2014) Memorable and actionable guideline. *Proceedings of the National Academy of Sciences* 111(Suppl. 4), 13634–13641.

RCVS (2020) Day One competences. Available at: https://www.rcvs.org.uk/document-library/day-one-competences/; also available at: https://www.rcvs.org.uk/news-and-views/publications/

Re, S., Zanoletti, M. and Emanuele, E. (2008) Aggressive dogs are characterized by low omega-3 polyunsaturated fatty acid status. *Veterinary Research Communications* 32, 225–230.

Reynolds, A., Keen, J.A., Fordham, T. and Morgan, R.A. (2019) Adipose tissue dysfunction in obese horses with equine metabolic syndrome. *Equine Veterinary Journal* 51, 760–766. doi: 10.1111/evj.13097.

Robin, C.A., Ireland, J.L., Wylie, C.E., Collins, S.N., Verheyen, K.L. *et al*. (2015) Prevalence of and risk factors for equine obesity in Great Britain based on owner-reported body condition scores. *Equine Veterinary Journal* 47(2), 196–201. doi: 10.1111/evj.12275.

Rosenberg, W. and Donald, A. (1995) Evidence based medicine: an approach to clinical problem-solving. *BMJ* 310, 1122–1126.

Roth, G.S., Ingram, D.K., Black, A. and Lane, M.A. (2000) Effects of reduced energy intake on the biology of aging: the primate model. *European Journal of Clinical Nutrition* 54(Suppl. 3), S15–S20.

Salonen, L.K., Hollands, T., Piercy, R.J. and Verheyen, K.L.P. (2009) Epidemiology of equine obesity in south-east England: Preliminary findings. *In: Proceedings British Equine Veterinary Association Congress*, vol. 48, p. 247.

Schoenecker, K.A., King, S.R.B., Ekernas, L.S. and Oyler-McCance, S.J. (2021) Using fecal DNA and closed-capture models to estimate feral horse population size. *Journal of Wildlife Management* 85, 1150–1161. doi: 10.1002/jwmg.22056.

Sessions-Bresnahan, D.R., Heuberger, A.L and Carnevale, E.M. (2018) Obesity in mares promotes uterine inflammation and alters embryo lipid fingerprints and homeostasis. *Biology of Reproduction* 99(4), 761–772. doi: 10.1093/biolre/ioy107.

Sheats, M.K., Royal, K. and Kedrowicz, A. (2019) Using readability software to enhance the health literacy of equine veterinary clients: an analysis of 17 American Association of Equine Practitioners' newsletter and website articles. *Equine Veterinary Journal* 51, 552–555.

Smith, D., Mayes, R., Hollands, T., Cuddeford, D., Yule, H. *et al*. (2007) Validating the alkane pair technique to estimate dry matter intake in equids. *The Journal of Agricultural Science* 145(3), 273–281. doi: 10.1017/S0021859607006788.

Srikanthan, P. and Karlamangla, A. (2014) Muscle mass index as a predictor of longevity in older adults. *The American Journal of Medicine* 127(6), 547–553.

Stowe, J. (2018) Results from the 2018 AHP Equine Industry Survey. *2018 American Horse Publications (AHP) Equine Industry Survey sponsored by Zoetis*. pp. 5–8.

Suagee, J.K., Corl, B.A. and Geor, R.J. (2012) A potential role for pro-inflammatory cytokines in the development of insulin resistance in horses. *Animals: An Open Access Journal from MDPI* 2(2), 243–260. doi: 10.3390/ani2020243.

TBA (2018) *The contribution of thoroughbred breeding to the UK economy and factors impacting the industry's supply chain*. Thoroughbred Breeders' Association, Newmarket, UK. Available at: https://www.thetba.co.uk/asset/7333E09E-8D59-4D8D-85280892C37D9113/ (accessed 19 December 2022)

Upjohn, M. and Wells, K. (2016) Challenges associated with informed consent in low- and low-middle-income countries. *Frontiers in Veterinary Science* 3, 92. doi: 10.3389/fvets.2016.00092.

Waters, A.J., Nicol, C.J. and French, N.P. (2002) Factors influencing the development of stereotypic and redirected behaviours in young horses: findings of a four year prospective epidemiological study. *Equine Veterinary Journal* 34(6), 572–579. doi: 10.2746/042516402776180241.

Wellen, K.E. and Hotamisligil, G.S. (2003) Obesity-induced inflammatory changes in adipose tissue. *The Journal of Clinical Investigation* 112(12), 1785–1788. doi: 10.1172/JCI20514.

2 Taking a Nutritional History: An Overview of the 5th Vital Sign

TERESA HOLLANDS AND LIZZIE DRURY

School of Veterinary Medicine, University of Surrey; Saracen Horse Feeds, Aylesford

Learning Objectives

LO1 Evaluate the importance of taking a dietary history.
LO2 List the differences between diet and ration, food and nutrients.
LO3 Describe the implications of digestibility.
LO4 Explain the need for an iterative process.
LO5 Describe some methods of recording the data.

At the end of this chapter, you will be able to provide an overview of the horse and diet details you need to collect to check the horse's nutritional intake.

Integrating Nutrition into Your Practice

The importance of taking a dietary history

Globally governments are starting to recognise that nutrition should be one of the cornerstones of preventative medicine, particularly as the cost and effectiveness of new drugs becomes more constrained due to legislation and resistance. Feeding, exercise and management changes have been recognised as important aspects of preventative medicine in primary health care for the past two decades (US Preventive Services Task Force, 1996); it should be no different in the equestrian population. The association between nutrition and health in horses has been clearly documented (see Chapter 1: 'The importance of nutrition in terms of health promotion'). Vets and other equine professionals are often expected to address nutrition and dietary behavioural issues with their clients in the context of a brief clinical encounter.

Engaging your clients

To engage your clients, you will need to understand the culture that motivates your client and maybe enter a process of negotiation to move them from their current feeding practice to one that is evidence based. Remember that education tends to work well when 'learning is, first, participatory, provocative, communal, and collaborative; and second, when learning is a process of constructing meaning rather than receiving' (Bruner, 1996), especially when dealing with 'millennium' clients. **It is also important to focus on the positive rather than negative, so how to keep horses 'fighting fit' rather than 'fighting the fat'.** Ensuring that nutrition is specifically relevant to your visit and that you address diet at every visit (spiralling and integrating the information) will increase understanding in the same way that understanding increased when nutrition was integrated into a medical curriculum compared with being taught separately (Walsh *et al.*, 2011). And of course, do not forget to record the information (Fig. 2.1).

DOI: 10.1079/9781789245134.0002

Vital Card		
Vital signs	**Average adult horse (at rest)**	**Normal vitals for (name)**
Temperature	37.5–38.5C	
Pulse rate **Heart rate**	36–48bpm 32–36bpm	
Respiration	8–15 breaths/minute	
Capillary refill time	2 secs or less	
Appetite	2.5% BW Forage: concentrates (kg)	
Body fat score /5 Neck/middle/bottom	3, 3, 3	
Bodyweight (kg) Weighbridge/weightape		
Vet Surgery phone number		

Fig. 2.1 Example of a vital card for clients to include basic ration information.

Maybe your practice does not actively encourage nutrition consults and the reasons for this are likely to be similar to those in human medicine: 'lower priority in medical practice for prevention issues in general, time pressures during clinical encounters, and lack of financial incentives for delivery of nutritional counselling' (Devries and Freeman, 2017).

But this is changing, driven in part by the demand from your clients; over 24,000 individuals started a multiple online open-access course (MOOC) in equine nutrition provided by Edinburgh Vet School: 1900 actively participated, 5600 completed and 4000 wanted to do more (J. Murray, personal communication). In an online survey about feeding supplements to performance horses, nearly half of respondents obtained information on nutritional supplements from vets (49.8%) as opposed to internet articles/reviews (39.4%), other horse owners (38.7%), coaches/trainers (36.5%) and nutritionists (33.4%). Respondents ranked the most reliable sources of information in descending order as vets, nutritionists and research studies, with the most influential sources of information as vets, followed by coaches/trainers and nutritionists (Gemmill *et al.*, 2015). Free text responses from the same study indicated that horse owners did not always think that their vets knew enough about equine nutrition.

Using an Evidence-based Approach

One of the consequences of not following an evidence-based approach to feeding horses has been a total misunderstanding as to the causes of laminitis in leisure horses and ponies. Owners fell into the trap of blaming commercial feeds (usually 0.5 scoop/day for a 14.2 hh cob, which provides 5 MJ digestible energy) getting into the hind gut of their horses and causing laminitis. However, obese horses are at 6× greater risk of getting laminitis compared with horses that have a fat score of less than 3.5 (Salonen *et al.*, 2009), because adipose tissue is metabolically active – in the UK, 41% of our ponies and 26% of our horses are either overweight or obese (Robin *et al.*, 2015). This misunderstanding is not helped by owners thinking that their good doers gain weight on fresh air, when in reality their 14.2 hh cob can eat the equivalent of 125 scoops of grass per day (Fig. 2.2) in a 24 h period (Smith *et al.*, 2007), which supplies 113 MJ digestible energy, which is nearly twice their daily energy requirement.

It is essential to appreciate how nutrition can both support performance and aid recovery from loss of function.

Practical application of the skills and keeping up to date with nutritional research will help, as follows.

- Differentiate between behaviour changes in performance horses due to the feeding of large meals resulting in hind gut acidosis and those that might be early warning signs of gastrointestinal disease.
- Determine if general lethargy is a result of long-term micronutrient deficiency or under/oversupply of calories.

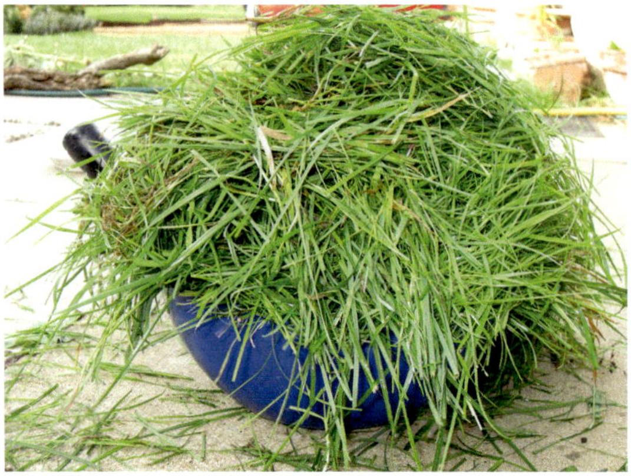

Fig. 2.2 A scoop of fresh grass weighing 0.5 kg.

- Determine if the wrong diet is partly responsible for resentment on tacking up and dullness – a consequence of gastric ulceration.
- Evaluate if the loss of muscle, weight or condition along the neck, back and quarters is due to poor-quality protein or a lack of fibre in the horse's diet (which means that the horse spends more time exhibiting stereotypy than eating).
- Increase the healthy longevity of the horse and reduce the risk of disease.

Clearly, there is an extensive body of literature linking nutrition to health outcomes in the horse and it is an area that vets wished they knew more about (Roberts and Murray, 2014; Parker *et al.*, 2018). It is incumbent upon you to have the knowledge and skills to begin the nutritional conversation with your clients and you should be fully engaged with taking nutritional information as the 5th vital sign (Fig. 2.1). The solution to more complex or specialised nutritional interventions is to work with consultant nutritionists (either company based or independent)

Assessment of the Diet

The diet and ration evaluation are used to identify potential nutritional imbalances that may relate to the health and performance of an individual horse or a group of horses.

Nutrition terminology in common use includes the following.

- **Nutrition** – the interaction between food/nutrients and the body.
- **Nutrients** – chemical components in food involved in a specific structural or functional activity in the body needed for life:
  - Protein, carbohydrates, fats, vitamins and minerals; water
- **Food/diet** – anything edible; everything that the animal eats, normally on a daily basis:
  - Feed/food
  - Feed ingredients
  - Straights, cereals, forages
  - Compounds – complementary/supplementary
- **Ration/meal** – sequence and quantity of food/diet eaten on a daily basis.
- **Feeding behaviour** – eating patterns of individual animals or herds.
- **Dietary history**
  - Collection of evidence to investigate the diet/ration and its interaction/balance (physiology) in relation to health (prevention) and disease (treatment)
  - All foods are a mixture of nutrients but not all foods provide adequate nutrients
- Properly balanced diet needs a mixture of feedstuffs.

The dietary history requires collection of data on the feedstuffs and observation and discussion as to how and when they are fed. There are three key pieces of information needed to check a horse's diet regardless of its workload:

- Forage;
- Concentrates; and
- Supplements.

For each of these, five checks need to be taken:

  - Physical appearance and characteristics;
  - What the feed value is;
  - How it is being fed (feeding management);
  - Quantities; and
  - Checking intake against requirements.

Physical evaluation

Feeds should be stored in closed containers that are clean and dry and that prevent the risk of contamination from rodents, birds, moisture and pests such as mite or grain beetles (see Chapter 8: 'Feed storage'). Supplements such as vegetable oils or natural sources of vitamins should be kept protected from light and high temperatures.

Safe feed storage is dependent upon moisture content of the feed and humidity. During the summer months or in a tropical environment, feed will have a shorter shelf life. Feed should only be stored at a moisture level of below 10–12%. Fungi growth rates increase when humidity levels go above 65% and moisture content of the feed is above 15% (sometimes 9%), depending upon the specific ingredients in the feed (Kabak *et al.*, 2006)

Remind clients that the feed that is coming into the storeroom should be properly rotated and a first-in and first-out system managed. Records of batch numbers and 'best before' dates should also be recorded.

Forage sources, including forages such as straw for bedding purposes, should be kept protected from rain and moisture.

Physical examination of the feed will require investigation of the food source for colour, smell, dust levels (see Chapter 8: 'Appropriate sampling and testing for risk'), presence of weeds or other contaminants and comparison of the feed components. Observation of processing methods is also important and you should help clients recognise steam flaking, extruding and micronisation techniques (see Chapter 5: 'Processing').

What is the feed value?

The nutrient content of feeds can be obtained from the feed labels, nutrient databases and chemical nutrient analyses. During the visit it is helpful to collect or photograph all labels and declarations in case you want to evaluate in more detail later. Commercially bagged feeds are subject to strict regulations for correct feed labelling and nutrient declarations (see Chapter 7: 'How to read a label').

How is it being fed?

Feeding management and environmental factors are key parts of the dietary history process (Table 2.1). High-starch diets are perfectly safe, if they are fed as small starch meals (see Chapter 5: 'Meal size'); dusty forages should be soaked; small-holed haynets slow intake; and feeding balls encourage foraging behaviour. Capturing and understanding the implications of the feeding environment on the horse's eating behaviour and gut health is vital.

Horses evolved to be trickle feeders. If feed is made available to them, horses will eat hourly during the day and every 2–3 h during the night (Houpt, 1982).

Feed intake

It is important to understand that feeds should be fed by weight rather than volume, because of the highly variable densities among feeds. Scales should be an essential accessory of any feed room, both for forages and for compound feeds (Fig 2.3).

Concentrate feeds, e.g. coarse mixes and cubes, vary in weight per unit of volume; and forage sources such as hay slices or flakes will also vary, even within the same harvest. The amounts of all supplements should also be weighed and recorded.

The amount of feed and forage that is consumed is measured by weighing everything that is fed and

Table 2.1 Environmental audit

Who is the primary carer of the horse?
Feeding management (location, frequency)
Forage
Grazing
Concentrates
Is the horse turned out or stabled with multiple horses?
Hours grazing
Hours stabled
Does anyone else feed or care for the horse?
Extent of environmental enrichment (toys, feed balls, tracking systems, all-weather turnouts)
Activity of the horse daily:
• Type of exercise (hacking, schooling, training)
• Amount (frequency, duration)
• Energy level (fizzy, lethargic, lacking stamina)
Environmental stressors (e.g. moving yard, conflict over food resource, uncontrollable outdoor stimuli)

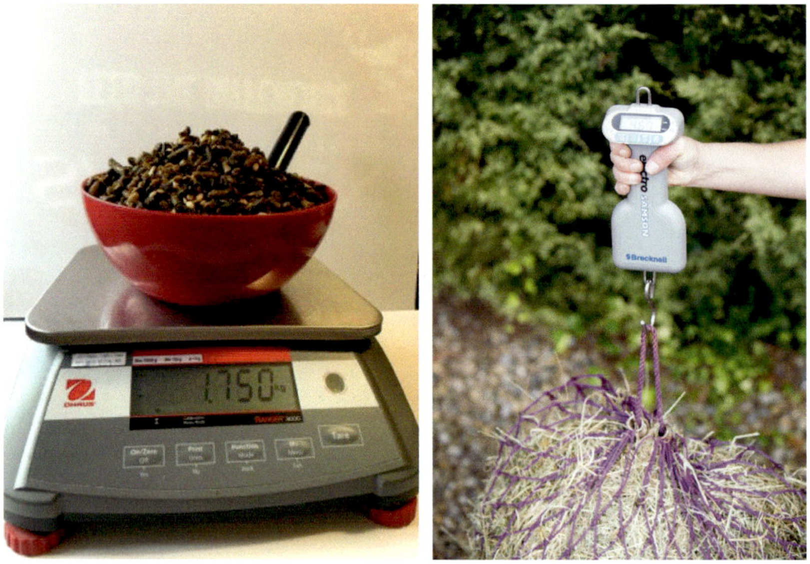

Fig. 2.3 Scales are an essential tool in the feed room.

weighing anything that is leftover. It is more difficult to calculate accurate feed intakes from horses that are fed from the ground or in groups. Where possible, it is advised to try to encourage feeding individually and off the ground for a few days for 'estimations' of feed consumption.

Voluntary pasture intake is more difficult to establish. Pasture intakes are calculated or predicted based on total dry matter intake (DMI) and the quality, quantity and availability of pasture. The DMI of horses and ponies can vary between 1.6% and 3.6% of their bodyweight (BW) (NRC, 2007). When there is excess dry matter available, then horses are capable of eating a mean of 3.74% BW as dry matter, but up to 5% BW (Smith *et al.*, 2007) (Table 2.2).

Ponies appear to have the capability to consume a high proportion of their predicted VDMI in a relatively short period of time when grazing is restricted (Dugdale *et al.*, 2011) and are capable of ingesting nearly 50% of their total daily DMI during only 3 hours of grazing (Ince *et al.*, 2011). It is important to note that the DMIs of the ponies were the same over the 20 hours measured (from the grass and haylage) regardless of how long the ponies were out grazing (Chapter 9, Table 9.4).

When using ration evaluation software programs (see Chapter 10, Table 10.1: 'Various ration packages available across the species'), the contribution of grass to total daily DMI can be predicted either manually or by software. This is often achieved by subtracting the predicted DMI of the other feeds from the predicted total DMI. Consider adjusting those numbers based on the pasture availability, stocking density and time out grazing.

Table 2.2 Example of mean dry matter intake (DMI) of grass as a percentage of bodyweight (% BW) by horses grazing 24/7

Grass intakes	Mean	Maximum	Minimum
DMI (kg)	18.7	26.8	15.9
% BW	3.74	5.2	3.2
98–300 g DM/m2; 8–12% protein; 64–77% digestibility			

Assessment of the Horse

Digestibility and individualism

As well as evaluating the feed, it is necessary to evaluate the response of equines to feed. All digestibility studies provide information for the 'average' horse or mean population and each horse you assess is not 'the average'; thus, on an individual basis, nutritive value is not directly correlated with animal growth or performance level. Digestibility studies provide information on how much of each of the fractions in feed – i.e. starch or energy, protein (amino acids), fats, minerals or vitamins – can be used by the horse for repair, growth and performance; undigested food and by-products of digestion are voided in faeces and urine. In reality the only 'nutrient' that can be measured clinically is energy intake and this is assessed by body fat scoring (see Chapter 3: 'Fat scoring a horse').

Iterative process

Many horses do not need a detailed nutritional assessment. If the horse is working well and if you have recorded a fat score of neck 3/5, middle 3/5, rump 3/5 (5.5/9) and if the horse is being fed adequate forage/fibre and manufacturer's recommended feed, then you may only need to repeat the process every quarter (with the seasons) or with the annual flu/tetanus visit. If you have found that the horse has a body fat score of less than 2/5 or more than 4/5 (< 3 or > 7/9), is lacking muscle, has a nutrition-related disease, is competing at a high level and is breeding, young or aged, then a more detailed assessment is required.

Ration evaluation

Having established what the horse is eating, the next step is to evaluate the ration. There are multiple methods that can be used for ration evaluation, from comparing a limited number of nutrients with the published standards to using computer-based programs that allow the evaluation of multiple nutrients at once.

What is being fed?

Ideally a feed plan is available that details the weight of both the feeds and forages being fed, together with a note of grazing times. It is always a good idea to check:

- that the board/plan is up to date;
- if using scoops, what a 'scoop' looks like (is it heaped or flat?);
- what supplements are in the feed room;
- which brand and product are in the bins;
- in the stables: if hay/haylage is available to the horse and how it is provided; and
- in the paddocks: quantity and type of grass.

It is not enough just to check if the horse is being provided adequate nutrients; you also need to check feeding management to ensure that the diet is providing the enrichment required. Other factors, such as digestive and metabolic efficiency and the 'character' of the horse in respect of whether they box walk, worry etc. and therefore burn more calories, need to be measured as well as bodyweight, fat score and workload (Dekker *et al.*, 2007).

Extrinsic factors, which include weather, environment, rider weight and ability and whether the horse is stabled or not, will also impact on calorie requirements of the individual horse. Extrinsic factors need to be factored into the scientific basis of calorie requirements, together with some flexibility needed for individual horses. The same diet checks should be undertaken regardless of the horse's workload; and, because environmental factors as well as workload will change, diet assessment needs to be an iterative process.

The most basic ration check is to take the horse's bodyweight, calculate how much it should eat, and check recommended intake of the hard feed from the bag; the difference should be hay. This assumes that the feed is being fed at recommended intakes to meet nutrient requirements. The horse's bodyweight (BW) and level of exercise need to be checked, to ensure that they are on the correct feed (Fig. 2.4).

If you wish to check across the nutrient spectrum, including lysine etc., there are several specifically designed computer software programs (see Chapter 10, Table 10.1: 'Various ration packages available across the species') available to calculate the nutrient intake from the total daily ration and compare with nutritional requirements (NRC or KER) for the age and physiological state of the horse (Pagan *et al.*, 1996).

When evaluating and designing feeding programmes for a group of horses, it is helpful to categorise the horses based on their bodyweight, fat score (BFS), reproductive and performance status and age. A representative number of horses can then be evaluated and a ration evaluated for each category, using averages of obtained variables.

Dietary assessment triage

If it is the first time you have included nutrition as the 5th vital sign, then discuss with the client the information that will need to be evaluated to determine if the horse is being fed the appropriate diet (Fig. 2.5).

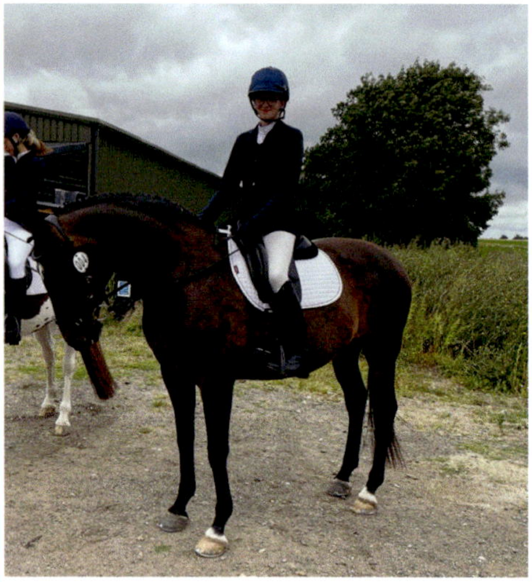

Swift Opposition 15.2hh, 16-year-old mare
Ridden by an amateur rider in Riding Club activities (light work)
525 kg on the weight tape
Body fat/condition score of 6/9
She is on the cusp of being fat but not unexpected in the summer, important she loses the fat in the winter.
She has good energy levels, and the owner would like these to stay the same.
She lives out during the day and is stabled at night.

Quick ration sense check
2.0 kg of Cooling Mix and Herbs
She should be eating 2.5% BW as dry matter, so 13kg
She is out during day so will eat 6.5kg DM grass (would eat 13kg in 16–18hrs if out 24/7)
She should therefore have 13kg minus (6.5kg + 2.0kg) = 4.5kg hay at night
As this is a quick check hay and hard feed have been calculated on a fresh weight basis.

Fig. 2.4 A quick check of energy and dry matter intake in a horse's diet.

Diet history

Feed-specific information should include:

- advantages and disadvantages of different feed-stuffs;
- checking feeding management and comparing with the horse's physiological and anatomical adaptations; and
- the ration.

Feed samples might be needed for lab analysis; forage analysis should be undertaken.

Animal history

Horse information should include:

- weight;
- workload;
- fat score;
- age;
- any perceived dietary intolerances; and
- appropriate and relevant blood tests.

Preparing a report

A diet plan describes which feeds are to be fed; the plan needs to be tailored to the individual horse and you do this by working out a ration (the actual quantities to be fed at each meal). This ration will be adjusted regularly depending upon the body fat score and performance of the horse, although the diet plan may stay the same.

A report should include:

- a summary of the client's concerns and questions;
- details on the way that the diet or the ration needs to be adapted/maintained to minimise the risk of a number of nutritionally related diseases;
- comparison of the intake versus requirements using PCHorse[i] or Microsteed[ii] or against the back of the feed bag, taking into account the horse's bodyweight etc; and
- results from laboratories, an explanation of their meaning and contextualisation of their relevance.

In any of the above processes, you can involve a nutritionist; make sure the process you use is

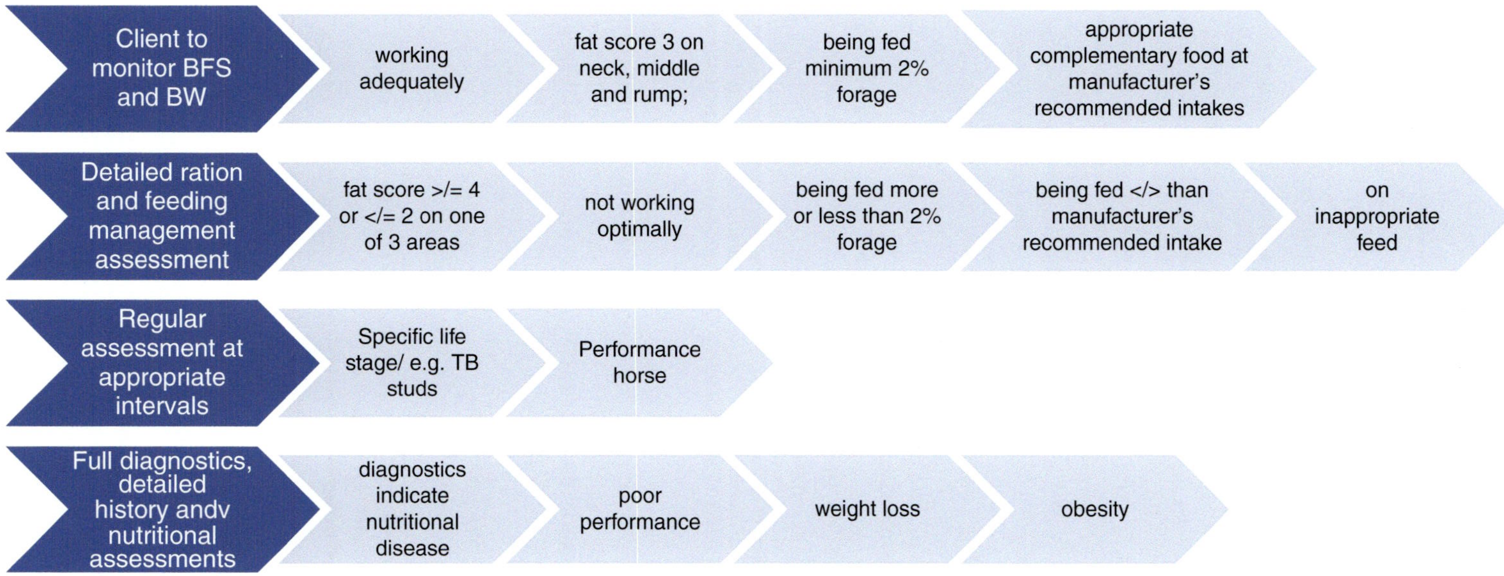

Fig. 2.5 'Triage' of nutritional assessments. In all instances, clients should be trained to fat score and weigh their horses to monitor energy (calorie) intakes and keep records for your next visit. Adjustments to the ration should be made accordingly.

consistent, then you can compare outcome data to demonstrate efficacy. Every contact needs to use the same systematic method and to think critically to provide safe and effective nutritional advice. This advice can then be shared with other paraprofessionals involved in the care of the horse.

Make sure that the diet and ration that you are recommending are evidence based; that they meet the physiological and anatomical adaptations of the horse's gut and that the owner understands the recommendation why you are making it. Do remind them that the impact of diet is rarely immediate; that it affects every system in the horse's body either directly and indirectly; and that diet can minimise disease, make the difference in healthy longevity, and ultimately improve performance, health and welfare.

Recording Data

Once the feeding plan is established, the next important step is to establish a monitoring plan that will follow adjustments to be made as needed. Horses that are in good body condition (fat score 3, 3, 3 out of 5; or 5.5/9 appropriately muscled) and performing well may only need reassessing on a seasonal basis. Encourage owners to monitor their horses at home and to keep quantitative records of any changes. Creating a specific schedule with the client for follow-up via telephone or visit to elicit questions is useful to ensure compliance and adherence to the recommended feeding programme.

Information should be systematically collected and recorded, either electronically or paper based, using a logical approach and an appropriate form. You will be familiar with systematic history taking and nutrition should be part of this history. A database or app that allows you to add nutritional information to the practice's software records will ensure that your recommendations are evidence based and become one of the 5 vital signs.

Adjusting the diet

Some horses and ponies can maintain optimum body condition when provided with free-choice forage, while others will require additional concentrate meal feeding of appropriate amounts to maintain health and performance. Remember that a successful outcome requires adherence to the advice provided, not just on the ration but also on feeding management and any necessary environmental changes.

How to support adherence to a diet ration

Think about using all or any of the following:

- Agree and confirm the use of an appropriate food-measuring device for both the forage and the concentrate feed.
- Find a container that holds exactly the quantity needed for one meal for each component.
- If advising small quantities, then provision of feeding toys slows eating time, mimicking trickle feeding.
- Feed hay in the four corners of the stable or in multiple piles in the field.
- Weigh forage; it often provides 90% of the calories for leisure horses. Haynets can hold between 3 kg to 17kg of hay, yet the client will describe this as a 'haynet'.

Summary

Incorporating a nutritional assessment into your regular visits is critical for maintaining the horse's health, as well as its response to disease and injury. Incorporating a screening nutritional evaluation as the 5th vital sign in the standard physical examination requires a small additional cost and time. This is easily offset by the development of a deeper partnership between yourself, the vet practice and your client, resulting in healthier horses.

Top tip

Nutritional assessment is an important aspect of optimal equine care. Providing guidance, effective assessment, evaluation, monitoring and education can provide an approach that can be efficiently incorporated into clinical practice without additional time or expense.

Notes

[i] https://www.pchorse.se/index.php/en/
[ii] https://ker.com/tools/microsteed/

Bibliography

BETA (2019) *The National Equestrian Survey 2019*. Produced for British Equine Trade Association (Wetherby, West Yorkshire) by JDA Research.

British Equestrian (2021) *Britsh Equestrian Annual Report* 2020–2021, p. 33. Available at: https://www.britishequestrian.org.uk/assets/About%20the%20BEF/Annual%20Report/Annual%20Report/Annual%20Review%2020_21_FINAL_sm.pdf (accessed 19 July 2023).

Bruner, J. (1996) *The Culture of Education*. Harvard University Press, Cambridge, Massachusetts.

Dekker, H., Marlin D., Alexander L., Bishop R. and Harris P. (2007) A pilot study investigating the relationship between perceived and actual workload and estimated energy intake in riding centre horses. *Equine and Comparative Exercise Physiology* 4, 7–14.

Devries, S. and Freeman, A.M. (2017) Nutrition education for cardiologists: the time has come. *Current Cardiology Reports* 19, 77.

Dugdale, A.H.A., Curtis, G.C., Cripps, P.J., Harris, P.A. and Argo, C. McG. (2011) Effects of season and body condition on appetite, body mass and body composition in ad-libitum fed pony mares. *Veterinary Journal* 190(3), 329–337.

Freeman, L., Becvarova, I., Cave, N., MacKay, C., Nguyen, P. *et al*. (2011) WSAVA nutritional assessment guidelines. *Journal of Small Animal Practice* 52, 385–396.

Gemmill, R., Agar, C., Freeman, S.L. and Hollands, T. (2015) Factors affecting owners' choice of nutritional supplements for use in dressage and eventing horses. *Veterinary Record Open* 3, e000155. doi: 10.1136/vetreco-2015-000155.

Geor, R.J., Coenen, M. and Harris, P. (2013) *Equine Applied and Clinical Nutrition Health, Welfare and Performance*. Elsevier Health Sciences, Oxford, UK.

HGCA (2011) *Grain Storage Guide for Cereals and Oilseeds*, 3rd edn. HGCA Guide 52, Agriculture and Horticulture Development Board. HGCA Publications, Kenilworth, UK.

Houpt, K.A. (1982) Feeding problems. *Veterinary Clinics of North America: Equine Practice* 4(7), 17–20.

Ince, J., Longland, A., Moore-Colyer, M. *et al*. (2011) Changes in proportion of dry matter intake by ponies with access to pasture and haylage for 3 and 20 hours per day respectively for 3 weeks. *Journal of Equine Veterinary Science* 31, 230–356.

Kabak, B., Dobson, A.D. and Var, I.I.L. (2006) Strategies to prevent mycotoxin contamination of food and animal feed: a review. *Critical Reviews in Food Science and Nutrition* 46(8), 593–619.

NRC (National Research Council) (2007) *Nutrient Requirements of Horses: 6th Revised Edition*. The National Academies Press, Washington, DC. doi: 10.17226/11653.

Pagan, J.D., Jackson, S. and Duren, S. (1996) Computing horse nutrition: how to properly conduct an equine nutrition evaluation using microsteed™ equine ration evaluation software. *World Equine Veterinary Review Archives* 1(2), 10B1–10B7.

Parker, A., Mastellar, S., Bott-Knutson, R., Daly, R. and Carroll, H. (2018) Upper Midwest veterinarian perceptions and confidence levels regarding equine nutrition topics. *Journal of Equine Veterinary Science* 69, 108–114.

Roberts, J. and Murray, J. (2014) Equine nutrition in the United States: a review of perceptions and practices of horse owners and veterinarians. *Journal of Equine Veterinary Science* 34(7), 854–859.

Robin, C.A., Ireland, J.L., Wylie, C.E., Collins, S.N., Verheven, K.L.P. and Newton, J.R. (2015) Prevalence of and risk factors for equine obesity in Great Britain. *Equine Veterinary Journal* 47, 196–201.

Salonen, L.K., Hollands, T., Piercy, R.J. and Verheyen, K.L.P. (2009) Epidemiology of equine obesity in southeast England: preliminary findings. In: *Proceedings of 48th BEVA Congress*, Birmingham, UK, p. 247.

Smith, D.G., Mayes, R.W., Hollands, T., Cuddeford, D., Yule, H.H. *et al*. (2007) Validating the alkane pair technique to estimate dry matter intake in equids. *Journal of Agricultural Science* 145(3), 273–281.

Walsh, C., Ziniel, S.I., Delichatsios, H.K. and Ludwig, D.S. (2011) Nutrition attitudes and knowledge in medical students after completion of an integrated nutrition curriculum compared to a dedicated nutrition curriculum: a quasi-experimental study. *BMC Medical Education* 11, 58–65.

US Preventive Services Task Force (1996) *Guide to Clinical Preventive Services: Report of US Preventive Services Task Force*, 2nd edn. Williams and Wilkins, Baltimore, Maryland.

3 Horse Information Required to Check Dietary Adequacy as Part of a Dietary History

TERESA HOLLANDS

School of Veterinary Medicine, University of Surrey

Learning Objectives

LO1 Describe the relationship between bodyweight, dry matter (feed) intake and energy requirements.
LO2 Discuss how nutrient requirements change according to workload.
LO3 Explain what techniques can be used to calculate workload, weigh, and fat score horses.
LO4 Explain how to weigh a horse, measure workload and fat score.

At the end of this chapter, you will be able to explain to your client why and how you (i) weigh, (ii) calculate workload and (iii) fat score a horse as part of checking the diet adequacy.

Introduction

Chapter 2 has discussed why taking a dietary history should be a routine part of the clinical examination, not least because it is a key component of preventative medicine. Clearly clients need to know their horse's bodyweight to check feeding guidelines on the back of the bag, but often this is a guesstimate. They overestimate the workload (Hale *et al.*, 2016), underestimate the fat score of their horses (Stephenson *et al.*, 2011) and at the same time do not appreciate that fat scoring is used to check calorie/energy adequacy. A better understanding of the significance of these measurements and their relationship to their horse's digestive system and nutrient requirements should help client compliance.

Bodyweight

Clients are familiar with the use of bodyweight (BW) to calculate their own calorie requirements but generally do not appreciate why bodyweight has a relationship to their horse's appetite or dry matter intake (DMI). It falls to you and the nutritionist to be as evidence-based as possible when collecting this information, which ideally is entered as part of the clinical records.

Bodyweight and appetite

It is well recognised that the gut capacity of herbivores is a constant and direct proportion of bodyweight (Demment and Van Soest, 1985) with bigger animals eating more per $kg^{0.75}$. When fed the same forage, the daily DMI and digestibility of cattle are higher than those of sheep, (g/kg $BW^{0.75}$) because of the longer retention time in their larger rumen (Soto-Navarro *et al.*, 2014) resulting in a more complete fermentation (Reid *et al.*, 1988). Thoroughbreds (TBs) eat more than Shetland ponies, when compared on a kg $BW^{0.75}$ basis, but more intuitively, when compared as a direct pro-

DOI: 10.1079/9781789245134.0003

portion per kg liveweight (kg LW), the Shetlands ate the most, followed by donkeys, TBs and Highlands (Cuddeford *et al.*, 1995). Similar to ruminants, the larger TBs were better able to digest the forages compared with the ponies (Cuddeford *et al.*, 1995), possibly because the rate of passage was slower due to a reduced intake enabling longer retention time in the larger hind gut.

Interestingly, when horses are compared with similar sized cows, the horse eats 63% more (144 g DM/kg $BW^{0.75}$/day) compared with cattle (88 g DM/kg $BW^{0.75}$/day) and the horse extracts more nutrients (78 g DM/kg $BW^{0.75}$/day) from low-quality forages compared with the ruminants (51 g DM/kg $BW^{0.75}$/day) despite being hind gut fermenters (Menard *et al.*, 2002; Duncan *et al.*, 1990).

When comparing species eating ad lib hay, cattle had the highest g DM/$kg^{0.75}$ (hay 95) > sheep (hay 72) > ponies (89) > donkeys (82). All species ate less ad lib straw (g DM/$kg^{0.75}$) compared with hay: pony/donkey (52) > cattle (50) > sheep (36). Horses digested hay better than donkeys, but the donkeys were more able to digest straw compared with ponies (Pearson *et al.*, 2006).

Unless they know the bodyweight of their horse, clients cannot work out the acceptable minimum/maximum DMI or spot decreases in appetite that might be an early warning sign of disease or an indication that feeding management needs changing. Whilst many clients feed on an ad lib basis, they should know the baseline DMI for their horse, which should not be compromised when seeking to reduce calorie intake.

Bodyweight and energy requirements

The maintenance calorie requirement (M) of any animal is also related to their bodyweight (BW) and decreases per kg BW as the animal gets heavier. The commonly used equation to describe metabolic rate over a huge number of animal species (Rucker, 2007) is M = kg $BW^{0.75}$ (Glazier, 2005; Isaac and Carbone, 2010), even though some argue that, if ruminants are removed from the database, the relationship is M = kg $BW^{0.66}$ (White and Seymour, 2005).

Clearly all equations are based on the average horse and there has been some adjustment to the above equation to consider the 'good doer' as well as the 'excitable horse' (Table 3.1). If your client's horse weighs between 125 kg and 856 kg, the NRC (2007) advises using the linear relationship between energy and body mass established by Pagan and Hintz, (1986).

Top tip

If you want a quick check when on the yard, then a mean daily digestible energy intake of 13% BW is a useful compromise and one you can teach your client.

Do not forget that the energy requirements for horses are calculated as apparent digestible energy (DE), unlike those for dogs and cattle that are calculated as metabolisable energy (ME). This means that energy requirement for horses is less accurate, as only the energy lost in faeces is calculated and not the additional loss in urine and metabolic heat.

There has been a move towards improved accuracy by adopting ME for horses (Table 3.2) (Kienzle and Zeyner, 2010; Coenen *et al.*, 2011). ME has not been adopted in the UK and may not be, unless a simple linear relationship can be developed for ambulatory use.

The group working on ME requirements noted that a fit horse might need 15% more maintenance calories compared with an unfit fat horse simply as a reflection of their lean body mass (Coenen *et al.*, 2011). These calculations were based on 5% body fat for a fit horse and 20% body fat for an unfit horse

Table 3.1 Horse's daily maintenance energy requirements (megajoules of digestible energy MJ/DE) depending upon their metabolic type (adapted from NRC, 2007)

Horse bodyweight	Fat horses 12.5 MJ DE/100 kg BW	Normal horses 13.9 MJ/100 kg BW	Nervous/ prone to weight loss 15 MJ/100 kg BW
200	25	28	30.5
400	50	56	60
500	62.5	70	75
600	75	84	90
700	87.5	97	105

Workload

Changes in energy requirements according to workload

As well as increased maintenance requirements the fit horse has an increased energy requirement for work. The workload of horses has been categorised according to maximum heart rate and duration of the workload (Table 3.3), but most clients overestimate the workload of their horse (Hoffman *et al.*, 2009).

For example, when asked to describe their horse's workload (Table 3.3), nearly three-quarters of owners (n = 1207) surveyed face-to-face over 2 years significantly overestimated their horses' workload (Hale *et al.*, 2016), categorising them as being in either medium (n = 407) or hard (n =314) work. Researchers quantified the workload of the same horses by recording weekly type, duration and frequency of work so the horse could be allocated according to NRC (2007) and placed most into the light work category (n =535) (Hale *et al.*, 2016). If you are dealing with clients with leisure horses or competing at amateur competition level, always obtain an example of the horse's typical weekly workload from the client rather than accepting their definition.

The ability to estimate workload level improves with client experience; the perceived workload estimated by instructors at a riding school was not significantly different from relative workload measured by heart rate (Dekker *et al.*, 2007). If you are working with professional riders, then it would be more appropriate to take a more objective approach to measuring workload by measuring heart rate.

Table 3.2 Horse's daily maintenance requirements as metabolisable energy (Coenen *et al.*, 2011)

Breed	Maintenance (MJ ME/kg$^{0.75}$)
Warmbloods	0.52
Thoroughbreds	0.64
Ponies	0.4
Other	0.4–0.5

Measuring workload using heart rate

Heart rate (HR) will increase isometrically with workload, although an excitable horse (Dias Villas-Boas *et al.*, 2016) or an unfit horse will have higher heart rates than expected, due to their increased effort. Smaller horses have higher HR compared with larger breeds based on bodyweight (but not fat score) (Schwarzwald *et al.*, 2012). Day-to-day heart rate variability (HRV) is minimal

Table 3.3 Workloads of horses (adapted from NRC, 2007) in addition to daily turnout

Types of activities	Mean heart rate of entire exercise bout (beats/min)	Duration (weekly)	Workload
Hacking Start of training Show horses Unaffiliated competitions School horses	80	½–1 h/day 6 days a week 40% walk; 50% trot; 10% canter	Light
Affiliated competitions up to Novice Polo, 8th week of training programmes	90	1–2 h/day 6 days/week – regular competitions. 30% walk, 50% trot, 10% canter, 10% jumping, dressage, eventing	Medium
High-goal polo Medium-level eventing, point-to-point	110	> 2 h/day, 6 days/week 20% walk, 50% trot, 15% canter, 15% gallop/jumping etc	Hard
Endurance > 50 miles, National Hunt, > 2 days/week hunting	110–150	Either minimum 1 h/week speed work plus schooling or > 12 h/week slow long work	Very hard

when horses are tied up or loose in a stall, when measured with Polar® HR monitors (HRMs) V800 and Kubios software (McDuffee *et al.*, 2019). Correlation between the heart's rhythm measured by electrocardiogram (ECG) and Polar HRM is improved if the measuring time is increased to 30 min in stationary, non-restrained horses (Ille *et al.*, 2014.)

'Resting' heart rate varied from 36 bpm in the stable to 52 bpm in the field (measured by ECG and a 24 h Polar Equine S810i R-R Recorder (Polar Electro Oy) (Parker *et al.*, 2009).

But when HR is measured at walk over time, there is a significant difference in HRV between an HRM and an ECG, related to the effect of motion on the HR monitor (McDuffee *et al.*, 2019) and loss of contact with the electrodes (Parker *et al.*, 2009).

The agreement between ECGs and Polar HRM is low when HR is measured in exercising horses, e.g. endurance horses (Lenoir *et al.*, 2017), as indeed it is in exercising cattle (Hopster and Blokhuis, 1994). Researchers highlight that, for humans, there are still major challenges regarding HRV that need addressing before portable HTM can be accepted in human health care (Shaffer *et al.*, 2020).

Despite these limitations, heart rate can still be used to provide an indirect, objective measure of oxygen consumption (VO_2) and, together with GPS monitors (Kingston *et al.*, 2006; Fonseca *et al.*, 2010), can provide the client with an expected time to complete set distances to achieve that heart rate.

There is a strong correlation between HR and oxygen consumption in all species and thus HR can be used as an indirect measure of aerobic effort (VO_2) in horses. VO_{2max} is the maximal oxygen consumption of a horse and is reached when the horse is no longer able to transport any more oxygen through its circulatory system or use oxygen in motor muscles. Maximum heart rate (HR_{max}) and oxygen consumption of horses (VO_{2max}) at 200 bpm is highly correlated and repeatable (Evans and Rose, 1988). Although not as repeatable as HR_{max}, HR can also be used to measure the aerobic fitness of a horse during training (Ainsworth, 2008) because of the linear relationship with speed.

HR and submaximal exercise

HR has been validated as an accurate measurement of energy expenditure (EE) during submaximal exercise (Fortier *et al.*, 2014). VO_{2max} and VO_2 during submaximal exercise (2375 m during 3.41 ± 0.47 min at 70% of maximal velocity) were measured directly and calculated from HR. The VO_2 was then used to calculate energy expenditure by multiplying the total VO_2 (measured, or predicted from HR), with its caloric equivalent (4.86 kcal/litre); the difference in EE (2422 ± 390 kcal direct VO_2 and 2630 ± 706 kcal HR) between the two methods was not significant (Fortier *et al.*, 2014). Of course, maximal HR of horses will vary between horses but not within a horse; maximal HRs have been recorded between 201 and 240 bpm (Vincent *et al.*, 2006).

Using HR to estimate aerobic versus anaerobic energy expenditure

Heart rate is correlated with blood lactate level and can be used as an estimate of whether the horse is working aerobically or anaerobically. This is done by measuring the speeds the horse needs to reach to increase blood lactate to 2 mmol/l (V_2/V_{La2}) and 4 mmol/l (V_{La4}) and the subsequent heart rate measured ($HR_{La\ 2}$ and HR_{La4}). In humans, workload is further defined by blood lactate threshold levels (LT):

- LT1 (1 mmol lactate/litre): initial rise above baseline indicating glycolysis and fast twitch fibre recruitment. Most human athletes can exercise for 3–4 h at this level (low-intensity endurance).
- LT2 (2 mmol) is the point of accelerated increase in blood lactate levels indicating a move to a mix of aerobic and anaerobic metabolism, typical of humans in 1 h endurance races (10 km and half-marathons).
- LT4 is unsustainable except for short aerobic bursts of 3–5 min.

Horses are working anaerobically when their blood lactate is between 75% and 85% of their maximum HR_{L200}, normally with an HR higher than 180 bpm (Vincent *et al.*, 2006). Blood lactate ($L200/HR_{L200}$) at maximum HR (200 bpm) can also be measured.

Using heart rate to estimate the horse's workload and lactate levels (Table 3.4) helps the trainer to control training intensities and enables you to tailor the energy supply of the horse's diet to meet either (or both) anaerobic (starch and sugars) or aerobic (fibre and oil) needs of the muscle fibres (see Chapters 5 and 12).

Table 3.4 Summary of heart rate (HR) and lactate levels of horses at various workloads

<table>
<tr><th>Horses</th><th>Workload</th><th>Heart rate</th><th>Lactate</th></tr>
<tr><td>Warmblood showjumpers
1.10 m versus flat work
(Léguillette et al., 2020)</td><td>5 m/s flat canter
8 m/s flat canter
11 m/s flat canter

Time to complete: 59.45 ± 3.43 s; mean speed 6.42 ± 0.35 m/s
Jumping course mean speed (6.42 ± 0.35 m/s) = slower than speed for same HR on track
Jumping exercise imposes > workload than flat work
Mean jumping phase HR > mean HR during the 8 m/s canter</td><td>139.3 ± 12.9 bpm
161.5 ± 36.6 bpm
196.8 ± 9.6 bpm
After jumping: 175.4 ± 13.4 bpm</td><td></td></tr>
<tr><td>Amateur show-jumping horses competing on different levels
(Szabó et al., 2021)</td><td>Winter indoor show-jumping
Oct–Feb against the clock, no jump-off, course length 450–550 m
Difficulty of course (height of jumps): 100 cm (48.3 min), 120 cm (54.5 min), 130 cm (61.4 min)
Speed: 325–350 m/min
Warming up 40 min</td><td><table>
<tr><th>Level</th><th>HR (bpm)</th></tr>
<tr><td>100 cm</td><td>av. 102.5; max. 170.8</td></tr>
<tr><td>120 cm</td><td>av. 110.8; max. 152.9</td></tr>
<tr><td>130 cm</td><td>av. 107.89; max. 152.2</td></tr>
<tr><td>Warm-up (37.8 min)</td><td>av. 88.6; max. 168.6</td></tr>
<tr><td>Rest (4.2 min)</td><td>av. 95.3; max. 143.7</td></tr>
<tr><td>Course riding (1.3 min)</td><td>av. 172.9; max. 193.2</td></tr>
<tr><td>Cool down (11.4 min)</td><td>av. 73.6; max. 126.0</td></tr>
</table></td><td></td></tr>
<tr><td>Young endurance horses (n = 71)
(Younes et al., 2016)</td><td>15 min warm-up (10 min walking, 5 min trotting)
Exercise test 15 (T), 30 (2T) or 45 min (3T) of constant-speed cantering for 4-, 5- and 6-year-olds, 22 km/h (about 110 strides/min); then 500 m gallop at full speed</td><td><table>
<tr><th></th><th>4yo</th><th>5yo</th><th>6yo</th></tr>
<tr><td>At rest HR (bpm)</td><td>45.3</td><td>44.1</td><td>43.8</td></tr>
<tr><td>Mean speed (km/h)</td><td>22</td><td>21</td><td>22</td></tr>
<tr><td>15 min exercise max. HR (bpm)</td><td>148.9</td><td>142.9</td><td>139.2</td></tr>
</table></td><td></td></tr>
</table>

		15 min exercise mean speed (km/h): 22 / 22 30 min exercise max. HR (bpm): 144 / 139 45 min exercise max. HR (bpm): 144.9 HR > in younger horses	
Racehorses (2- and 3-year-olds) (Ebert and Moore-Colyer, 2020)	On horse walker for 45 min, canter 75 min	54.3bpm 103bpm	
Mixed-age unfit Standardbreds (*n* = 18) (young = 6yo, middle-aged = 15yo; old = 27yo) (Betros *et al*., 2002)	Fixed 6% grade at initial speed of 4 m/s for 60 s Increased to 6 m/s for 60 s, incremental 1 m/s increases/60 s until fatigue	**6yo / 15yo / 27yo** Max. HR (bpm) pre-training: 218 / 215 / 185 Run time (s): 389 / 330 / 247 Speed (m/s): 8.5 / 9 / 7 Max. HR (bpm) post-training: 221 / 218 / 189 Run time (s): 400 / 360 / 278 Speed (m/s): 10.5 / 9.5 / 8	
Thoroughbred racehorses (age 9.1±1.9 years) of mixed levels (*n* = 10) (Williams *et al*., 2019)	(a) Maintenance, interval training session at start of week after day off; one or two interval runs at max speed of 25 mph; 11.2 m/s (b) 2× fast work interval training sessions (c) 1× jump training session and 2 h/day on horse walker, total 42 sessions 126 individual gallop runs, each horse mean completion of 4 training sessions (3 interval training repetitions (gallop runs) per training session)	Between 72% and 82% of HR_{max} lower anaerobic threshold of 75%; Average HR threshold of 173 bpm at mean speed 8.1 – 9.5 m/s	

Continued

Table 3.4 Continued.

<table>
<tr>
<td>Stallions (n = 20) (age 5–10 years): Andalusian (AN), n = 9; Arabian (A), n = 7; and Anglo-Arabian (AA), n = 4
(Muñoz et al., 2002)</td>
<td>(i) 1st 3 weeks:
walked for 40 min without rider
(ii) 3 weeks: 45 min trotting without rider in mornings at frequency of 5 days/week; plus pm 3 days/week walking exercises and three 5 min periods of trotting. Two days/week: 60 min dressage
(iii) 2 weeks morning work = 45 min trotting without rider, 5 days/week; pm as previously, + 1 day/week 60 min trot @ 12 km/h
(iv) 8 weeks am 60 min unridden trot; pm 3 days/week walked and trotted for 90 min; 2 days 60 min dressage;
(v) 8 weeks am 60 min unridden trot; pm 3 days/week 15 min walking, 30 min trotting, 15 min galloping; 2 days 60 min track exercises</td>
<td></td>
<td>Mean plasma lactate concentrations at rest, immediately after exercise and after 10 min after exercise at different stages of an exercise programme
Andalusian
<table>
<tr><th></th><th>Before training</th><th>(iii)</th><th>(v)</th></tr>
<tr><td>Rest</td><td>0.89</td><td>0.73</td><td>0.742</td></tr>
<tr><td>After exercise</td><td>22.79</td><td>22.8</td><td>13.24</td></tr>
<tr><td>10 min post-exercise</td><td>15.65</td><td>14.4</td><td>6.752</td></tr>
</table>
Arab
<table>
<tr><th></th><th>Before training</th><th>(iii)</th><th>(v)</th></tr>
<tr><td>Rest</td><td>0.726</td><td>0.732</td><td>0.715</td></tr>
<tr><td>After exercise</td><td>19.16</td><td>12.21</td><td>13.36</td></tr>
<tr><td>10 min post-exercise</td><td>8.739</td><td>9.372</td><td>7.34</td></tr>
</table>
Anglo-Arab
<table>
<tr><th></th><th>Before training</th><th>(iii)</th><th>(v)</th></tr>
<tr><td>Rest</td><td>0.525</td><td>0.605</td><td>0.515</td></tr>
<tr><td>After exercise</td><td>19.74</td><td>12.88</td><td>12.59</td></tr>
<tr><td>10 min post-exercise</td><td>6.968</td><td>5.67</td><td>5.113</td></tr>
</table>
</td>
</tr>
<tr>
<td>Haflinger stallions (2-year-olds)
(n = 6)
(Lindner et al., 2009)</td>
<td>Latin square of 1 of 3 conditioning programmes (CDP) lasting 6 weeks:
21 exercise sessions/CDP of 45 min at speeds to reach 1.5 mm lactate/l blood (v1.5)</td>
<td></td>
<td>Effect of exercise duration at set speeds at blood lactate concentrations of 1.5, 2.5 and 4 mmol/l on mean heart rate and blood lactate in horses
<table>
<tr><th>Mean speed m/s</th><th>To reach blood</th><th>HR bpm:</th><th>LA (mmol/l) 25 min</th><th>LA (mmol/l) 45 min</th></tr>
</table>
</td>
</tr>
</table>

	or 25 mm lactate/l blood (v2.5) or 25 min at speeds to reach 4 mm lactate/l blood (v4)		(continued) lactate conc mmol/l | mean, (range) | exercise: mean, (range) | exercise: mean, (range) 3.1 | 1.5 | 164 (148–176) | n/a | 3.43 (1.6–6.7) 3.5 | 2.5 | 180 (45 min) (153–185) | n/a | 4.6 (1.35–6.85) 3.8 | 4 | 173 (165–195) | 4.84 (2.15–8.45) | n/a
Andalusian horses (4-year-old males) (*n* – 16) (Agüera *et al*., 1995)	3 exercise tests consisting of 4 levels of increasing intensity of 4, 5.5, 7 and 8.5 m/s, each followed by a 5 min rest After conditioning, horses were able to exercise faster before lactate increased, indicating an increased aerobic capacity	Heart rate measured in 3 track tests in Andalusian horses **Heart rate bpm** Test | HRL_2 | $HRLA_4$ Untrained | 133.7 | 149.75 Trained 2 months | 155.54 | 182.9 Trained 4 months | 157.2 | 181.4	Plasma lactate level and velocity indices measured in 3 track tests in Andalusian horses **Plasma lactate mmol/l** | **Velocity m/s** Test | L_{150} | L_{200} | VL_2 | VL_4 Untrained | 4.04 | 23.69 | 4.27 | 6.86 Trained 2 months | 1.71 | 5.86 | 5.51 | 6.9 Trained 4 months | 1.71 | 6.36 | 5.86 | 7.19
Mixed gender, age and breed (43 jumpers, 58 gallopers, 39 trotters, 13 trekking, 2 treadmill, 2 swimming) (Piccione *et al*., 2010)	Jumpers = 350 m with eight obstacles. Gallopers official races of 1500, 1800 and 2100 m. Trotters = 1200 m race with 3 tests of increasing load intensity lasting 3 min, alternated with 1 min breaks. Trekking horses = trekking walk of 40 km with gradients between 850 and 1900 m.		Mean blood lactate (mmol/l) of horses working in different disciplines at rest, straight after exercise and 30 min after exercise **Horse / exercise type (*n*)** | **At rest** | **After exercise** | **After 30 min** Showjumpers | 2.26 | 5.07 | 2.59 Gallopers 1500 m | 0.66 | 2.45 | 2.05

Continued

Table 3.4 Continued.

	Treadmill = 2 min treadmill running test with velocity of 11 m/s and 5 degrees slope. Swim = 3 min swimming session.		1800 m	0.74	10.38	12.2
			2100 m	0.77	12.21	8.45
			Trotters (39)	0.79	2.01	3.02
			Trekking (13)	1.77	3.11	2.76
			Treadmill (2)	0.65	5.22	0.7
			Swimming (2)	0.7	5.8	2.1
			Significant difference between SJ and galloping from rest to exercise and recovery – anaerobic work			

Calculating energy requirements from maintenance on the yard

If the client is unable or unwilling to use heart rate monitors, then it is possible to estimate how much extra energy the horse needs for work by multiplying by a factor based on maintenance requirements, (Table 3.5). This is a simplified way of working out energy that you can do on a visit.

Do remember that the feed manufacturers have taken all the above into account when they formulate feeds and thus 'all' you need to do is to advise the appropriate feed whilst remembering to establish if the horse is consuming excess calories/energy through body fat scoring.

Body Fat Scoring

Monitoring energy intake by body fat scoring

The amount of body fat a horse has is a direct measure of calorie/energy intake. Clients should body fat/condition score (BFS/BCS) their horse fortnightly and of course you will score the horse every time you visit. It is important that you teach clients how to fat score, because most clients use weight tapes (62%), with fewer than 2% reporting the use of BCS (Murray *et al.*, 2015) to measure 'fatness'.

As you know, 'body condition might be correlated with body weight, BUT body fat is generally independent of weight or frame size, indicating that additional information is gained from the BCS' (Burkholder, 2000).

Top tip

- Bodyweight tells your client nothing about the health of the horse, because it provides no evidence as to body composition: is the weight fat or muscle?
- Excess adipose tissue is not restricted to just the leisure horse: dressage and show hunters have significantly higher body fat and cresty neck scores, compared with polo ponies (Pagan *et al.*, 2009), which were positively correlated to higher plasma insulin and triglyceride.

Why body fat scoring?

Body fat score provides additional information to bodyweight and provides a clear indication as to whether the horse is suffering from chronic low-grade systemic inflammation (see Chapter 15) and is equally important and relevant for the performance horse.

Table 3.5 Workload requirements of horses expressed as a factor of maintenance (M[a]) requirements (NRC, 2007)

Workload	Energy requirements over maintenance
Light	M × 1.2
Medium	M × 1.4
Hard	M × 1.9

[a]M can be calculated during a visit as 13% of BW

- Fatter performance horses reach maximum lactate threshold faster than lean horses (Kearns *et al.*, 2002b).
- Fat-free mass is positively correlated with finishing a race more quickly (Lawrence *et al.*, 1992; Kearns *et al.*, 2002a)
- An increase in body fat score:
  - affects metabolic responses in performance horses (Leleu and Cotrel, 2006); and
  - increases asymmetry when moving (Jansson *et al.*, 2021), contributing to a reduction in performance.

So, all horses need to be fat scored and their riders taught to use the score fortnightly.

Despite what you might have read in the horse literature, manual palpation of skeletal landmarks (body fat scoring (BFS) or body condition scoring (BCS)) was developed and validated to measure body fat in production animals, not muscle. 'Cow-calf producers routinely use body condition scores (BCS) to subjectively monitor the body condition, or external fatness, of their cows' (Apple *et al.*, 1999). There is some argument in the literature that once the horse gets to a certain fatness then the palpation does not reflect the visceral fat (Dugdale *et al.*, 2011) – this is the same as cattle, which also have a curvilinear relationship between body fat score and total body fat % (Gregory *et al.*, 1998). On a herd health basis, manual palpation is key because there is a linear increase in back-fat thickness in cattle with the increase in BCS (Schroder and Staufenbiel, 2006); in other words, there is a significant correlation between subcutaneous fat thickness and BCS.

Real-time ultrasound (RUS) has been correlated to back fat (BFT) which is predictive of dissected total body fat (TBF) (Domecq *et al.*, 1995), which is why RUS measurements at predetermined skeletal landmarks are increasingly used in cattle; a change in back fat of 1 mm is equivalent to 5 kg of total body fat (Staufenbiel, 1997; Greiner *et al.*, 2003). In other species, BFS in dogs has been correlated with dual-energy X-ray absorptiometry (DEXA) (Lauten *et al.*, 2001); each incremental increase from BCS4 to BCS9 on a nine-point scale is equal to an increment of 10–15% in DEXA-measured BF% (Munday *et al.*,1994). In cats, BCS has been correlated with DEXA (Speakman *et al.*, 2001; Buelund *et al.*, 2011; Shoveller *et al.*, 2014) and ultrasound (Okada *et al.*, 2017).

In line with the other species, BFS has also been validated in horses with extracted fat and ultrasound (Westervelt *et al.*, 1976; Kane *et al.*, 1987; Gee *et al.*, 2003; Martin-Rosset *et al.*, 2008; Dugdale *et al.*, 2012 and Silva *et al.*, 2016a).

Various ultrasonographic measurements of fat depth recorded over 18 months, including rump fat in both a control group of Shetlands and a group of Shetlands fed excess calories (Siegers *et al.*, 2018), were strongly correlated (ranging from 0.84 to 0.91) to BCS/BFS subcutaneous adipose tissue (SAT); others have also recorded this correlation (Gentry *et al.*, 2004; Quaresma *et al.*, 2013).

One of the arguments against manual palpation of SAT is that it does not reflect internal fat, although this has in part been disproved. Retroperitoneal adipose tissue (RAT) in Shetlands being fed excess calories was 8× thicker and correlated to SAT (1.6–2.2× thicker) compared with the controls (Siegers *et al.*, 2018) and more recently by dissection (Burrows *et al.*, 2013; Baker *et al.*, 2020).

Production animal experimental methods (industry-accepted procedures under the supervision of the Canadian Food Inspection Agency used over the past 20 years) were used to extract fat from horses. There was a strong correlation between BFS (0–9 point score) with kidney–pelvic–heart fat; neck fat depth, absolute trimmed carcass fat and trimmed carcass fat as a percentage of hot carcass weight. 'These data indicate a strong relationship between subjective live BCS and objectively measured carcass fat depots (BFS) in various equine breed types and sexes' (Baker *et al.*, 2020).

Retroperitoneal, and to a lesser extent omental fat depot, increases with an increase in fat scores (Fig. 3.1). Manual palpation of nuchal fat (cresty neck score) had such a strong correlation with EQUIFAT dissected score that the researchers took nuchal fat out of their mathematical model, (Morrison *et al.*, 2017).

Top tip

- 'If an animal looks obese, precise estimation of body composition is of limited clinical value' (Smoliga, 2014). Once the horse is fat, it does not really matter how fat – you just want the owner to recognise that fat cover.
- 'Recognition of overweight or obesity status leading to general weight management recommendations likely has greater clinical impact than attempts to precisely estimate body composition parameters' (Smoliga, 2014).

Why cresty neck score (CNS)?

Silva *et al.* (2016b) acknowledged that the CNS (Carter *et al.*, 2009a) had never been validated with postmortem measurements, (Giles *et al.*, (2015); and subsequently correlated carcass nape fat measurements with photographic image analysis and CNS in horses. Dorsal and medial photos postmortem were standardised and digitised to measure nape fat thickness and total carcass fat was also measured. Silva *et al.* (2016b) established a straight-line correlation between CNS, nape fat thickness and total carcass fat. Others (Briceño *et al.*, 2015; Briceño *et al.*, 2017) have characterised the histology and presence of infiltrative lipomatosis following a CNS of the horses.

It is reassuring to be able to discuss with the client that simple manual palpation is strongly correlated with both adipose and visceral fat but actually does that really matter in your clinical situation?

Top tip

Your clients can distinguish between 'no fat', which feels like a piece of string (fat score 3), and 'excessive fat infiltration', fat that feels like a large bunch of elastic bands (fat score 4), as well as 'dysfunctional fat', where the ligament seems fused to the underlying muscle and cannot be palpated, just bent over (fat score 5).

[a] Measurements of crest fat (cm)	Cresty neck score and 0–5 fat neck score equivalents
0±2.99	0–3
3±5.99	4
6±8.99-12	5

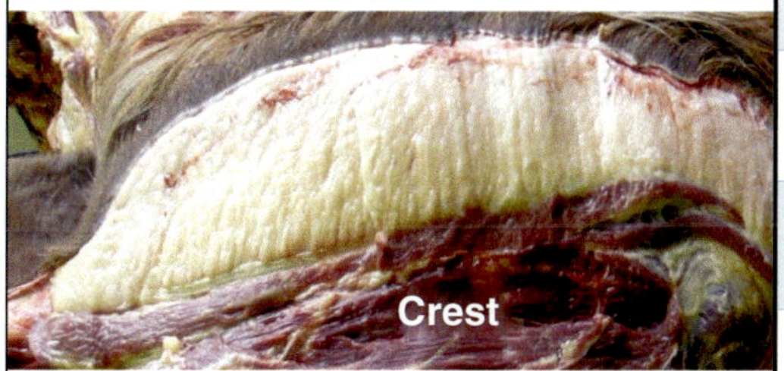

Measurement of omental fat (Equifat score)

OMENTAL FAT
Evaluate ~ 30cm of omentum extending distally from the midpoint of the greater curvature of the stomach

Score	Descriptor	Exemplar
1	No or minimal fat visible	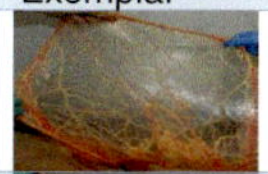
2	Fat in immediate vicinity of the gastroepiploic vessels (GEVs) but vessels still clearly visible.	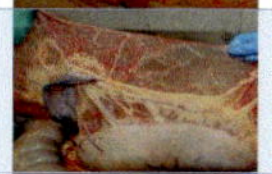
3	Distinct fat deposits around and beginning to fill the spaces between GEVs. GEVs partially obscured by fat.	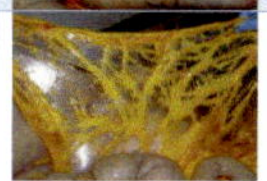
4	Extensive accumulations of fat largely obscuring and filling the spaces between most GEVs.	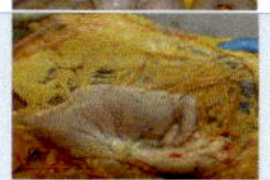
5	Omental peritoneum and GEVs completely obscured by fat.	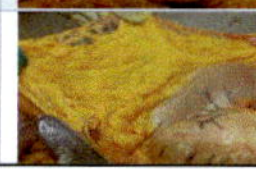

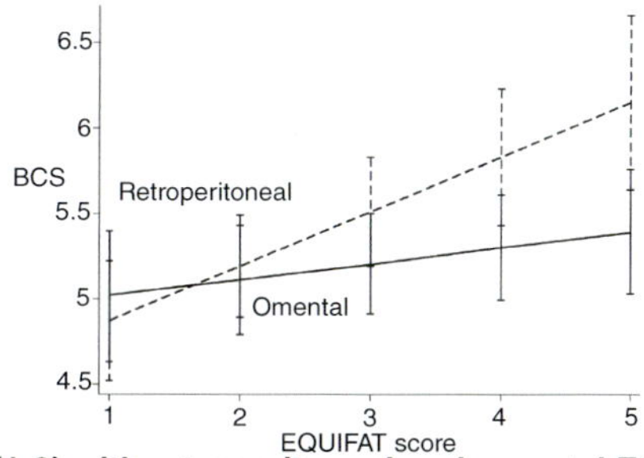

Modelled changes in mean BFS (1-9) with retroperitoneal and omental EQUIFAT scores.

Fig. 3.1 The relationship between subcutaneous, visceral and body fat score in the horse. (Modified from Morrison et al., 2017.) (Crest photo courtesy of Professor Caroline Argo.)

Measuring Horse's Bodyweight

Weighbridges

Ideally a horse will be weighed on a calibrated weighbridge at regular intervals. Most feed companies offer weigh-in days for practices when they bring a portable weighbridge with them. Many 3-star events provide weighbridges (Fig. 3.2) and more practices are investing in their own weighbridges.

Weight tapes

If a weighbridge is not available, then a weight tape offers an alternative. Be aware that not all weight tapes are equally accurate (Ellis and Hollands, 1998) and thus you should encourage clients to use scientifically validated weight tapes, (Ellis and Hollands, 2002) (Table 3.6).

Formulas

You will find that some clients still use a formula to estimate the bodyweight of their horse: [girth^2 (cm) × length (cm)]/11,877 (Carroll and Huntington, 1988), which is accurate for Thoroughbreds (Górniak *et al.*, 2020) but has been superseded by more accurate formulae that have been used to develop weight tapes, (Ellis and Hollands, 2002) and for ponies: [length (cm) ×2.8] + [height (cm) × 4.2] − 606 (Martinson *et al.*, 2014).

Length (L) is from point of shoulder to a line that is perpendicular to the point of the buttock and can be compared with actual BW [G (cm)$^{1.486}$ × L (cm)$^{0.554}$ × H (cm)$^{0.599}$ × N (cm)$^{0.173}$]/3606, where height (H) is taken at 3rd thoracic vertebra, and neck circumference (N) halfway between poll and withers and girth (G) at base of mane hairs. There is also a refined formula for growing miniature horses (< 3 years) (Catalano *et al.*, 2019).

You can appreciate why you might get better compliance from clients using a weight tape.

How to Weigh a Horse

Weighbridge

Setting up

- Ensure that you have a flat even surface and check the bridge using a spirit level.
  - Check that the bridge is calibrated using industry standardised weights annually.
- Allow enough room for the horse to access and exit the bridge in a straight line.
  - Better compliance is often achieved by placing the bridge next to a wall.
- Make sure the weighing scale is fully charged and set to the correct weight ranges.
  - If the scale is not Bluetooth, ensure that the leads are tucked under the bridge and the scale is safe from being trodden on or kicked.

Loading the horse

- If using a scale with an electronic database, ensure that you have entered the horse's details that you need.
- Some horses react to the noise as they walk on the bridge. Just let them keep walking to condition them to the noise and then lead them on again.
- The handler should simply step off the bridge when the horse is standing square (Fig. 3.3)
- The scale normally takes multiple readings to provide a mean which is confirmed when the number stops changing.
  - A light comes on to signify the result.
- Record to the electronic database.
  - As a backup, write the weight down with the horse's details.

Weight tape

Whilst weight tapes are not precise, they are better than a client's estimation of BW, which has been shown to be out by 16 kg for miniature horses, 38 kg for saddle horses, 43 kg for thoroughbreds (Catalano

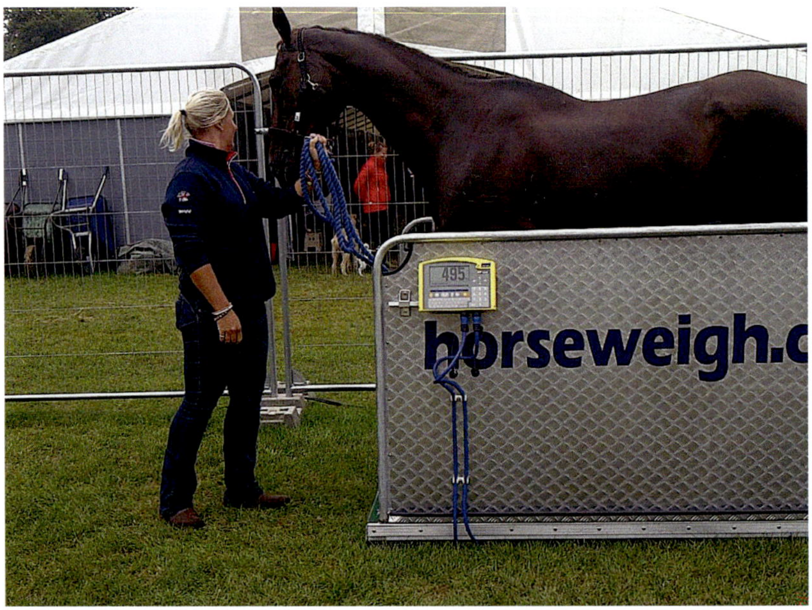

Fig. 3.2 Weighbridges are the most accurate method to obtain a horse's bodyweight.

Table 3.6 A comparison of methods of weighing horses

Method	Accuracy	Number of horses	Breeds	Reference
Morphometric measurements correlated to weighbridge – mean BFS 3, 3, 3	Weight tape used around lower heart girth. Two different formulas used to develop tapes: (i) horses up to 14.2 hh: pony tape estimate of mean (SD) bodyweight (100.5 [6.2] per cent), R^2 0.9; (ii) horses over 14.2 hh: horse tape estimate of bodyweight (98.6 [18.4] per cent), compared with weighbridge, R^2 0.84	2000	Mixed ages, heights and breeds	Ellis and Hollands, (2002)
Morphometric measurements correlated to weighbridge	Most accurate estimates of BW for both Icelandic and Warmblood horses when only heart girth is measured	81	43 Icelandic and 38 Warmblood horses.	Jensen *et al*. (2019)
Morphometric measurements correlated to weighbridge	Wt correlated with girth^2 × length; no weights for 12 hh, 13 hh, 14 hh, nor for horses at BCS 1 or 5; nor 16 hh BFS 5	372	Varying breeds and heights	Carroll and Huntingdon (1988)
Morphometric measurements, weighbridge and various weight formulae		299	Five breeds: ponies, Polish Noble Half Breed, Silesian Breed, Wielkopolski Breed and Thoroughbred	Górniak *et al*. (2020)
Weighbridge, height and body length linear regression modelling	R^2 0.86	629	Adult horses and ponies – four breed types	Martinson *et al*. (2014)
Morphometric measurements, weighbridge	Within 4% of actual BW	619	Adult (> 3 years, nonpregnant) saddle-type (209), adult (249) and juvenile (< 3 years) (61) Miniatures, and adult Thoroughbreds (100)	Catalano *et al*. (2019)

et al., 2019) and 75 kg for warmbloods (Catalano *et al.*, 2016). They provide accurate guides to bodyweight changes due to dehydration that are not significantly different to a weighbridge (Ellis and Hollands, 2017). These changes can be picked up before the client would recognise the changes visually and thus a horse should be weighed fortnightly at the same time of the day (and fat scored) so as not to record diurnal bodyweight changes.

Using the tape

- Stand the horse square on a level surface.
- Check which side of the tape that you are using.
- Gently place the tape at the lowest point of the withers and drop one end of the tape over the back of the horse.
- Gather the tape from under the belly and bring as close to the elbow as possible (Fig. 3.4a).
- Bring the tape up to make a circle around the lower heart girth (the tape should follow a diagonal) (Fig. 3.4b).
- Read the bodyweight where the tape overlaps or as indicated by an arrow (Fig. 3.4c).
- Ensure the tape is tight but not causing an indentation.
- Make sure there are no fingers under the tape.

Ask the client to record date, time and BW and then discuss the patterns when you visit or as part

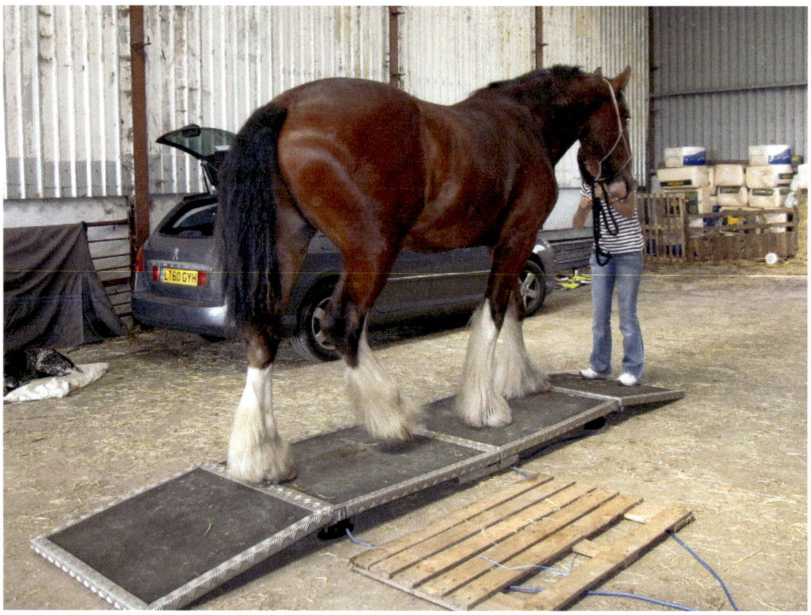

Fig. 3.3 The handler needs to step off the weighbridge before taking a measurement. Note that the leads have been covered by a pallet.

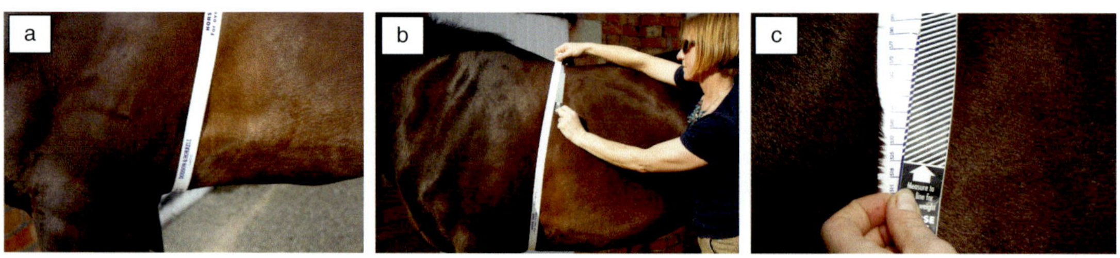

Fig. 3.4 Positioning a scientifically validated weight tape on a horse.

of a phone consult. A body fat score should be recorded at the same time.

Fat Scoring a Horse

Challenges and statements that clients might ask when discussing fat scoring

1. It is not accurate.

- Agree with them.

Visual assessment of body fat is not accurate; you cannot tell how fat a horse is by looking at it. You need to feel (palpate/grope) the fat over the skeleton.

2. You cannot compare across breeds – TB and cob conformations differ.

- Disagree with them.

Fat scoring does not take conformation into account (Fig. 3.5).

3. But my horse is healthy and in good condition.

- Disagree and then agree (to a point).

When horse owners talk about good condition, they are not using the literal translation from the dictionary 'fit for purpose' – neither a thin nor a fat horse is fit for purpose and indeed neither are they healthy.

They are describing the horse's outline, their coat, their feet, their eyes – what they see visually. But they are not distinguishing between fat and muscle that defines that outline of their horse. All you are doing when you teach fat scoring is how to manually palpate fat over the skeleton.

4. It is not precise.

- Disagree with them.

Reassure them that both scoring systems have been tested for repeatability/precision and reproducibility/reliability.

5. It can't be accurate.

- Agree with them.

Fat scoring is not accurate enough to provide an actual body fat percentage.

- And then disagree with them.

It is precise enough to put their horse into a category of fatness which reflects the real-time ultrasound and dissected carcass measurements. There will be some variation, but the research has shown

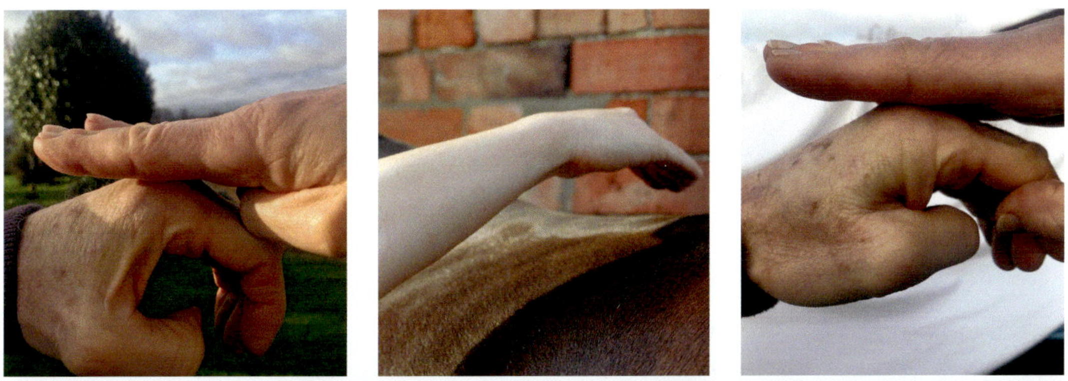

Make a tight fist and place your fingers across the knuckles (backbone) and relax them to curve over the knuckles this is a TB.,

You can also run your fingers over your fingers "to feel the fat over the ribs".

Then loosen your fist, so that your fingers are no longer touching your palm- this widens the 'ribcage' and represents a cob with the larger skeleton

Fig. 3.5 Using your knuckles to show that fat score is independent of confirmation, where your knuckles represent the backbone (middle illustration) and when you relax your hand over your knuckles it will form the same curve shown by the hand over the horse's back.

that variation is acceptable and ensures that manual palpation will put the horse into the right category.

6. But I can see my horse's ribs, so they are not fat.

- You may end up disagreeing or agreeing with them.

It depends upon the score you give the middle and bottom. If you cannot feel the bones in any other area that you are palpating, then the horse is fat.

In this situation, it will help client's understanding if you can teach them the cresty neck score too. Do remind them that it is not just about the ribs; fat around the shoulder, back and bottom are indications that their horses might be producing higher levels of inflammatory substances (Fig. 3.6).

'Ultrasonographic measurements of subcutaneous adipose tissue thickness at the shoulder, lumbar region, and rump are relevant indicators of fatness related with adipokine plasma concentrations and expression of adipokine-related receptors in adipose tissue, and particularly highlight seasonal effects' (Staub *et al.*, 2019).

7. I can't remember all the places to score and the numbers.

- Teach them a simple version of the scores.
- Tell them that you will leave the scoring instructions with them, but if they only have a few minutes to spare it is better they do a simplified score than none.
    - If they can see and feel the bones, the horse does not have enough fat tissue.
    - If they can feel (easily) the bones but not see them (or very slightly), their horse has an ideal fat cover.
    - If they cannot see and cannot feel the bones, their horse has excess fat tissue and is at risk of being chronically inflamed.

You can use your knuckles and palm of your hand (Fig. 3.7) to show them what they should feel as you explain the above.

8. I should average the scores.

- Disagree with them.

Horses, like people, seem to have 'danger' areas where they store more fat. By scoring each area separately, the client can monitor their individual horse. As importantly, it takes the focus away from just the ribs too.

Which fat score?

Whichever score you use, the important thing is to use the score every time you visit.

You will be teaching the client to take the following steps.

- Feel for fat over predefined, scientifically validated areas over their horse's skeleton.
- Allocate a score between 0 and 5 (Carroll and Huntingdon, (1988); Hollands *et al.*, 2009) or 1–9 (Henneke *et al.*, 1983), based on the description of the fat cover over those specific areas of the skeleton. Researchers using both scoring systems record strong correlations between them (Hollands *et al.*, 2009). 'The two BCS systems used in this study were strongly correlated, indicating that both can be used to describe BCS of Icelandic and Warmblood horses' (Jensen *et al.*, 2019).

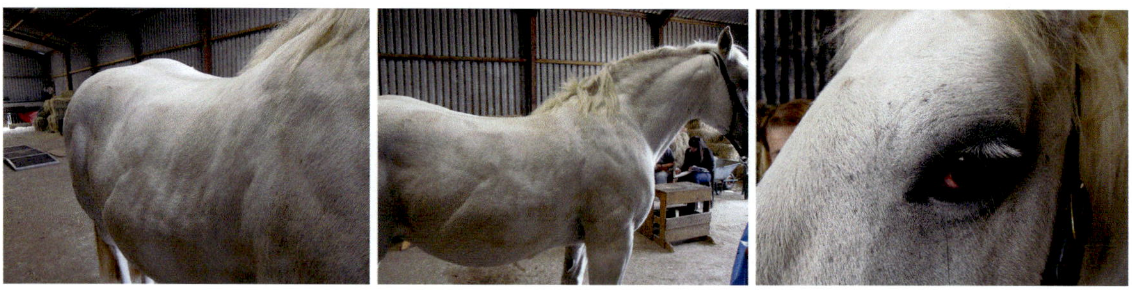

Fig. 3.6 Different distribution of fat showing a fat score of 2 on ribs but 4 on neck and bottom. Ribs can be seen, but large crest, apple-shaped bottom, flat back and fat in the supra orbital fossa.

Risk of morbidity	Unhealthy	Healthy	Unhealthy	Risk of morbidity
Very Thin	Thin	Ideal	Fat	Obese
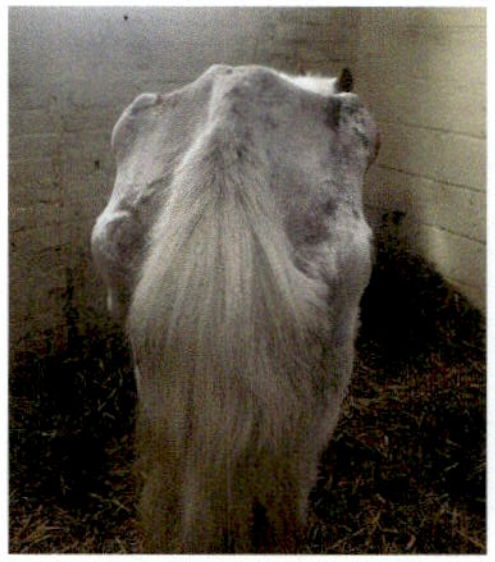	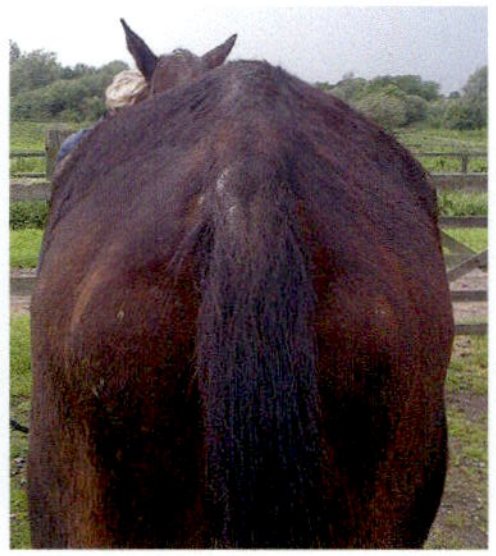	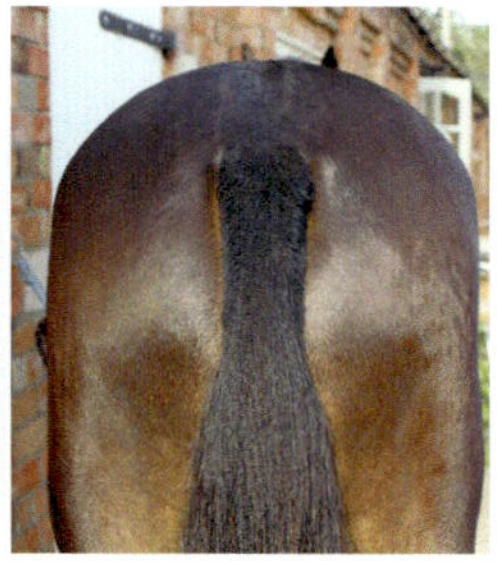	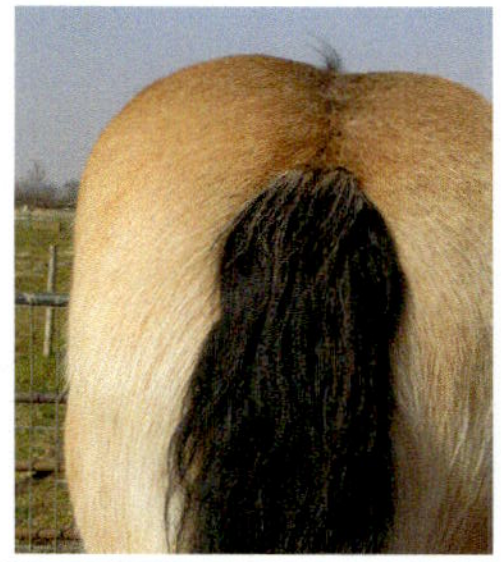	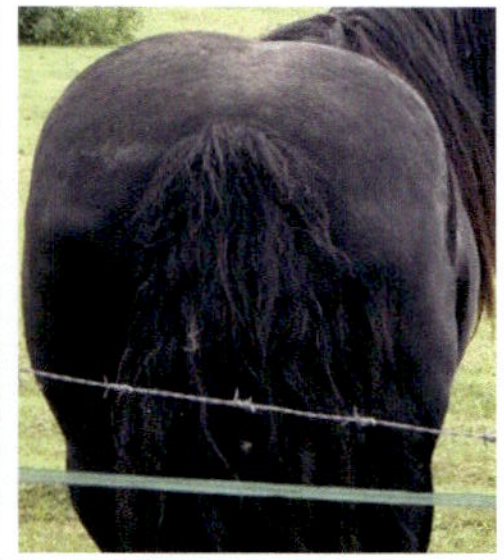
See and feel individual bones on horse (1/5)	See outline of bones, feel all bones (2/5)	Feel but not see bones (3/5)	Can neither see nor feel bones (4/5)	bones-covered with spongy fat cant see or feel (5/5)
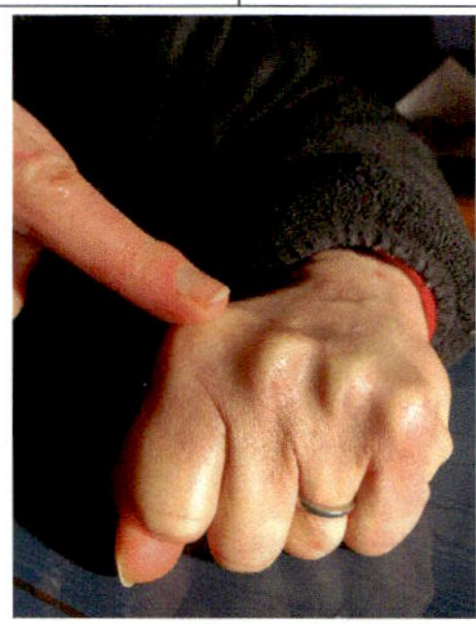		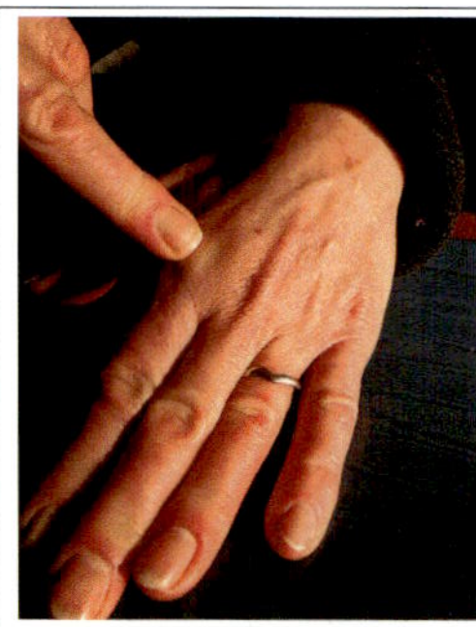	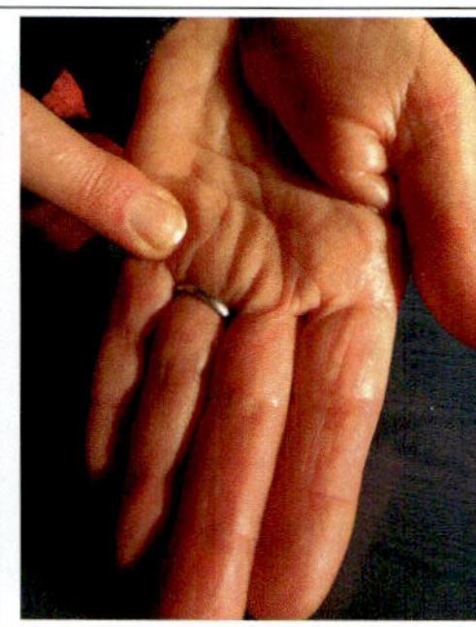	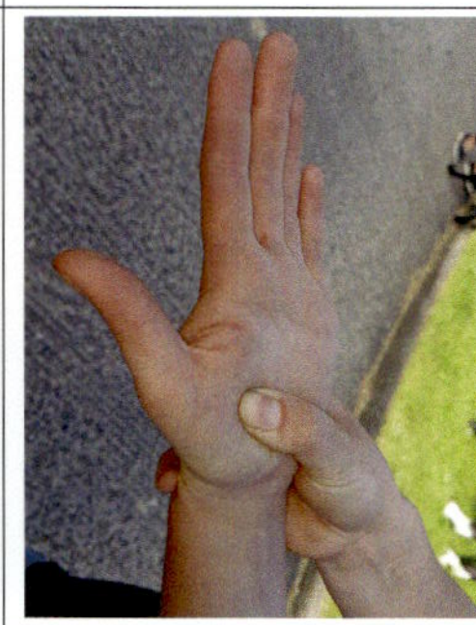
Form a knuckle and run your fingers over the knuckle Can feel and see each knucklebone (1/5)	Relax knuckle slightly; run your fingers over the knuckle Can feel and see outline of knucklebones (2/5)	Flatten your hand and run your fingers over your knuckles, can easily feel but not see bones	Turn your hand over. Run your fingers over the 'back' of your knuckles. Cannot see nor feel bones	Feel the pad of your thumb-spongy and thick layer of fat

Fig. 3.7 Using your knuckles to illustrate thin, okay and fat.

- Use the cresty neck score (Carter *et al.*, 2009b), because fat over the nuchal ligament has been shown to be correlated with several inflammatory cytokines (see Chapter 15: 'Recategorising upper and lower fat in horses').

Regardless of the score you decide to use (1–9, Henneke *et al.*, 1983; 0–5, Carroll and Huntingdon, 1988; modified Henneke (Kohnke, 1992; Hollands *et al.*, 2009), all have been validated and what you palpate on the outside reflects visceral fat (Figs 3.6 and 3.8)

Cresty neck score

Another useful technique for recording fat is the cresty neck score (CNS) (Carter *et al.*, 2009b – if for no other reason than to help clients understand that there is no muscle at the top of their horse's neck: they need to understand that a crest is just fat.

- Try to dissuade them from calling it topline – it is fatline (Fig. 3.9). Anything above the nuchal ligament is fat; there is no muscle there.
- The fat above the nuchal ligament appears to have some relationship with visceral (mesenteric) fat (Morrison *et al.*, 2017) and is strongly correlated with clinical signs of disease and inflammatory markers (Bruynsteen *et al.*, 2013; Burns *et al.*, 2010; Fitzgerald *et al.*, 2019; Blaue *et al.*, 2020).

Top tip

- Find the nuchal ligament.
- Follow it along the neck.
- Establish fat depth above the ligament.

This illustrates to clients just how much fat their horse is carrying in that area.

How to Fat Score

0–5 (modified Carroll and Huntingdon)

1. Divide the horse into three areas (Fig. 3.10):
   - The neck – crest and suprascapular fat deposits
     - Tell the client anything forwards of the withers.
   - The middle – rib area and spinous back fat
     - Tell the client to feel the ribs and backbone.
   - The bottom – sacrum and tailbone fat and subcutaneous fat over the bony prominences of the pelvis
     - Tell the client to feel the hips, pelvis and tail bone.
2. The best way to capture your client's attention is to start with the supra orbital fossa. This measurement been correlated as a sign of increased risk of EMS and thus inflammatory cytokines or IR (Carslake *et al.*, 2021).
   - You will only find fat pads here when the horse has been fat for a long period of time. Fat pads are a clear indicator that the metabolism has changed. If there are fat pads, then increase the neck score by 1.
3. Thirdly, show them how to find their own nuchal ligament.
   - Bend your head forward and pinch the ligament that runs over your spine at your neck.
   - Then show them how to find their horse's nuchal by finding it just behind the poll, pinch it gently and the horse will pull away – then follow it down the neck as far as you can.
4. Share Table 3.7 to enable them to allocate a score to the neck, middle and bottom of their horse.
5. Work with the client – showing, not telling.
   - Either you do the palpation and they match your descriptors to the score;

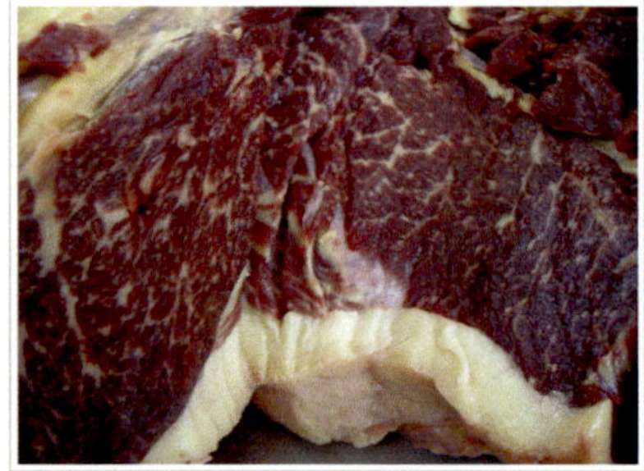

Fig. 3.8 Intra- and intermuscular far in a pony's muscle (courtesy of Professor Derek Knottenbelt). If you can palpate fat under the skin, there will be the same amount in and around all the internal tissues and organs.

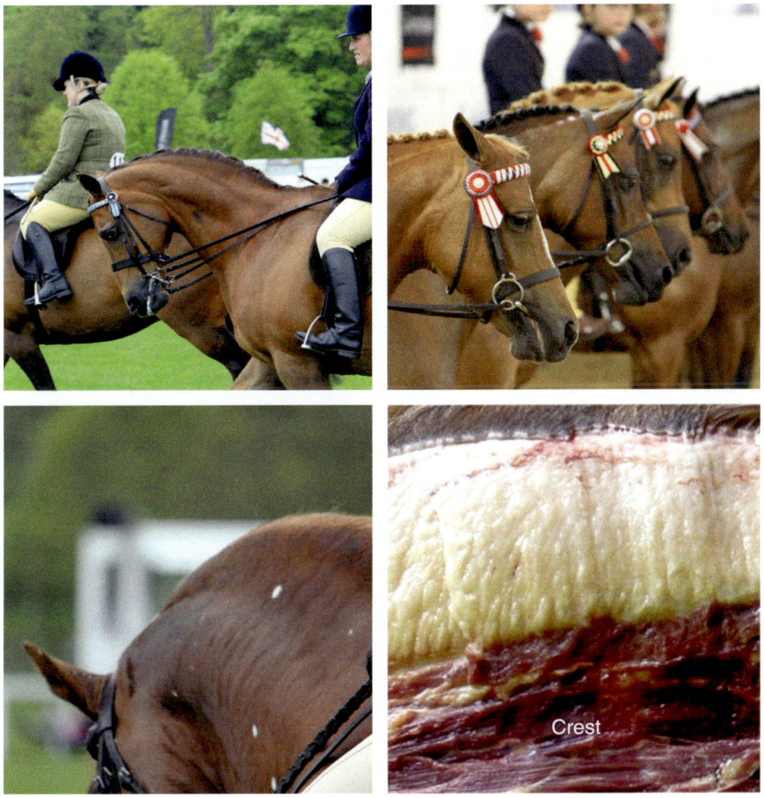

Fig. 3.9 Horses in the show ring with obese necks, commonly termed topline but better described as fatline. (Crest photo used with permission from Professor Derek Knottenbelt.)

- or having chatted them through the technique, let them do the palpation and you read out the score.
- Ask them to set up a record of the neck, middle and bottom scores with the date and then to fat score fortnightly.
  - Score 2 has been included for interest and this is the amount of fat you would expect to palpate in a fit TB.
- It is likely that you will be mostly be using scores 4 and 5, both of which increase the risk of disease and shorten lifespan in the horse.
  - Score 3 – healthy level of fat tissue
  - Score 4 – unhealthy fat tissue
  - Score 5 – extremely unhealthy fat tissue / dysfunctional adipose tissue (see Chapter 15).

Do *not* average the neck, middle and bottom; record a separate score for each

Henneke 1–9 score system

Various papers use either the Henneke technique or the modification of that technique by Kohnke, (1992) that he published in a textbook. Finding a copy of the modified technique has been challenging and Table 3.8 was found in Dugdale (2011).

How to cresty neck score

If you are using the Henneke *et al.* (1983) 1–9 scoring system, which does not differentiate specific areas of fat storage, then it would also be useful to teach your client the cresty neck score (Fig. 3.11). The descriptors are the same as Carter *et al.* (2009a) but the numbers have been modified to reflect those of the 0–5 scoring system.

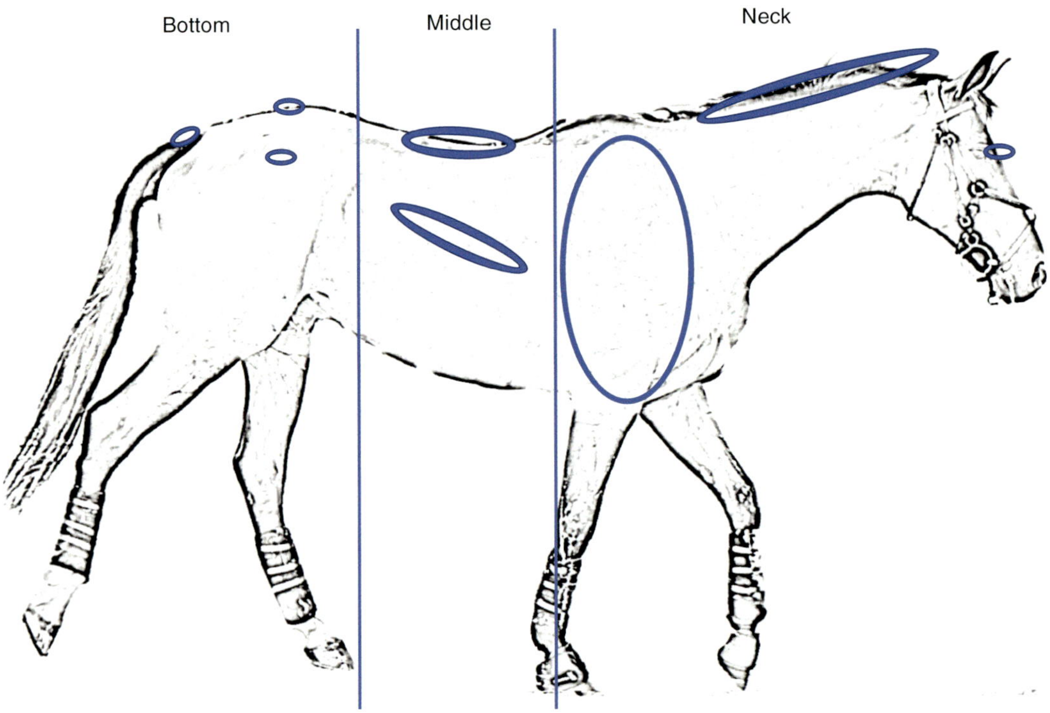

Neck areas to palpate: crest, suprascapular fat and supra-orbital fossa	
Find the nuchal ligament.	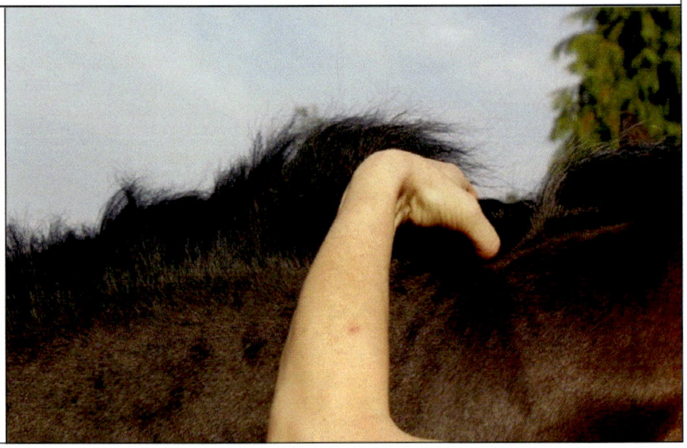

Fig. 3.10 How to identify the areas needed to palpate to fat score (0–5). Examples of positions provided = fat score 3/5 except for pelvis (5/5).

Run your hand down the neck towards the shoulder blade.	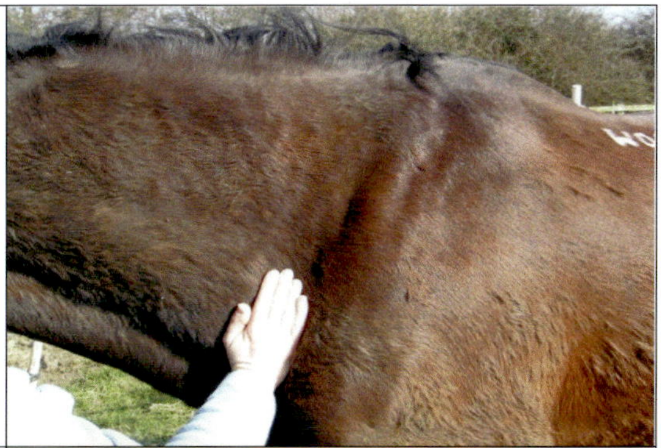
Feel around the shoulder blade and pinch the flesh behind the shoulder blade.	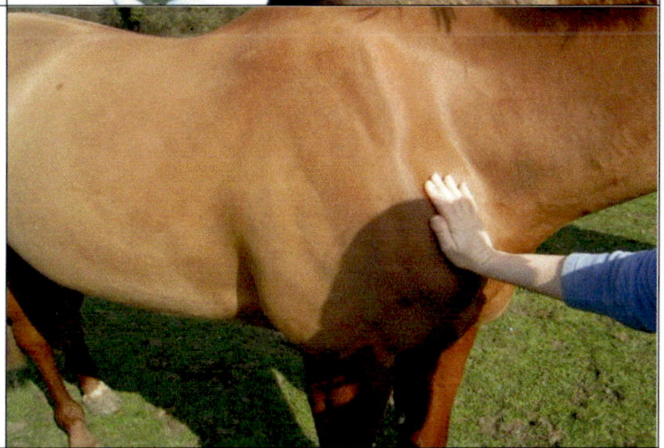
Check the outline of the shoulder blade.	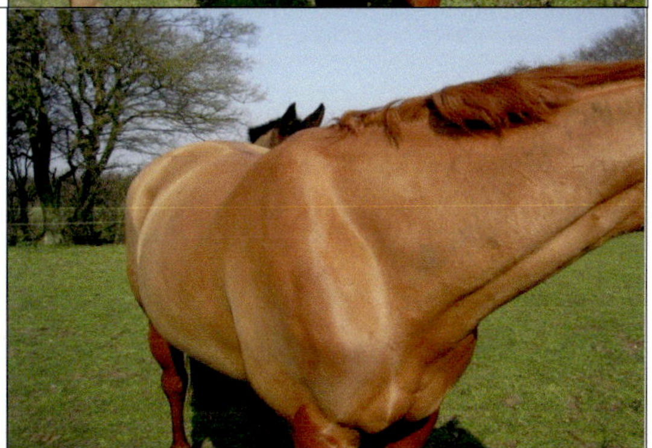 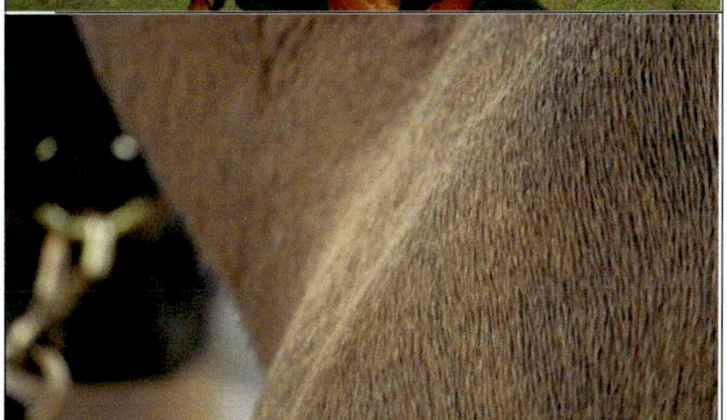
Check above eyes.	
Ask the client to close their eyes and feel around the shoulder blade, could they draw the shape from what they are feeling?	

Fig. 3.10 Continued.

Middle areas to palpate: rib area and spinous back fat	
Run your hand diagonally across the horse's rib cage. Use a firm pressure but not so firm that the horse moves away.	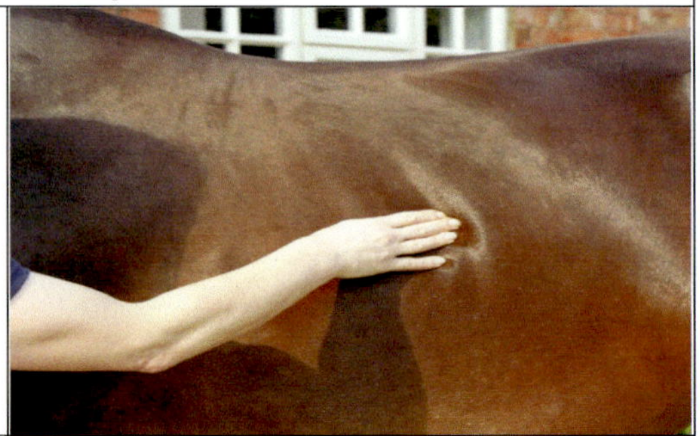
Place your left hand at the lowest point of the horse's withers at 90 degrees to the backbone. Place your right hand directly next to it, with your fingers pointing across the backbone, which should be in the middle of your palm. Remove your left hand.	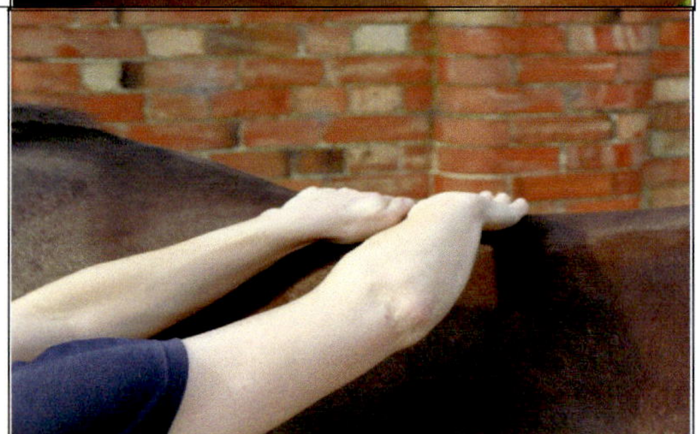
Relax your right hand and note if it stays flat or makes a curve.	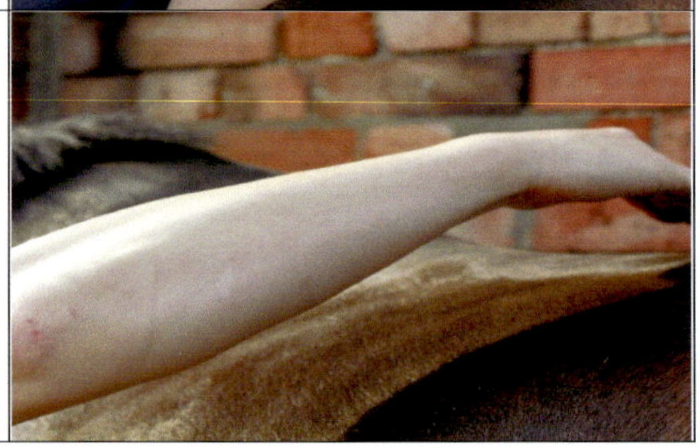

Bottom areas to palpate: sacrum and tailbone, subcutaneous fat over bony prominences of hips and pelvis	
Place your hand flat on the top of the horse's bottom to feel the bones of the pelvis.	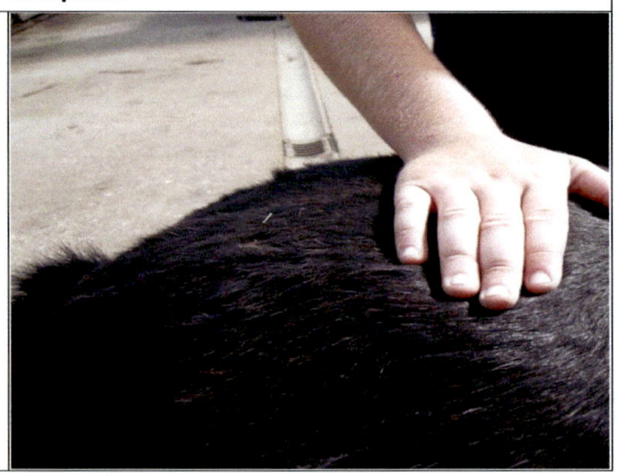

Fig. 3.10 Continued.

Run your hand from the hindquarters onto the tail, feeling for the tailbone.

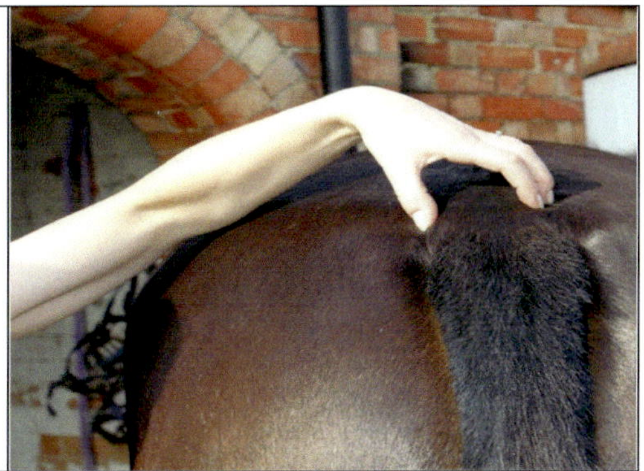

Find the hip bones and curve your hand around the outline of the bone – you are not using your fingertips.

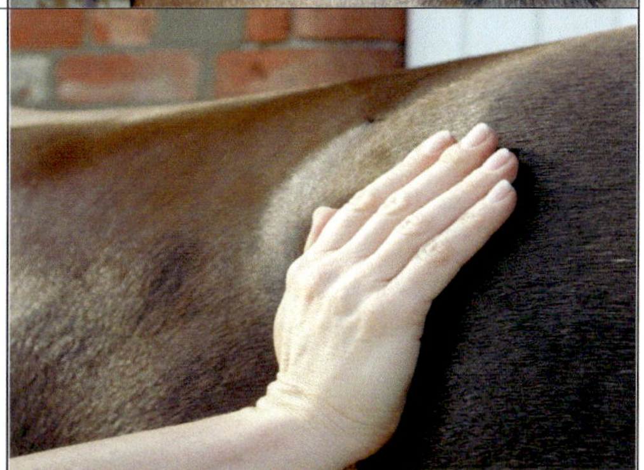

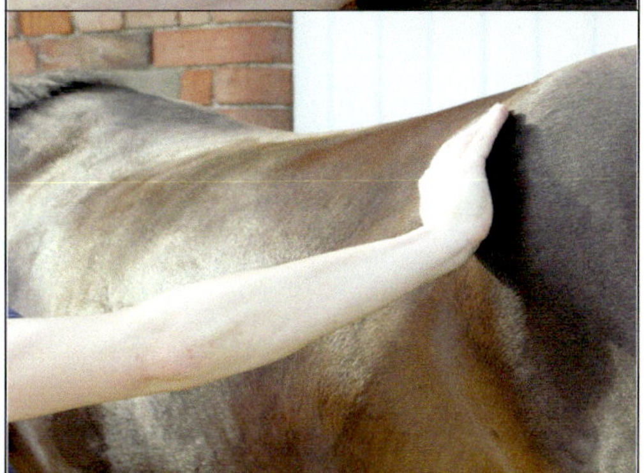

Note the shape of the silhouette of the rump.

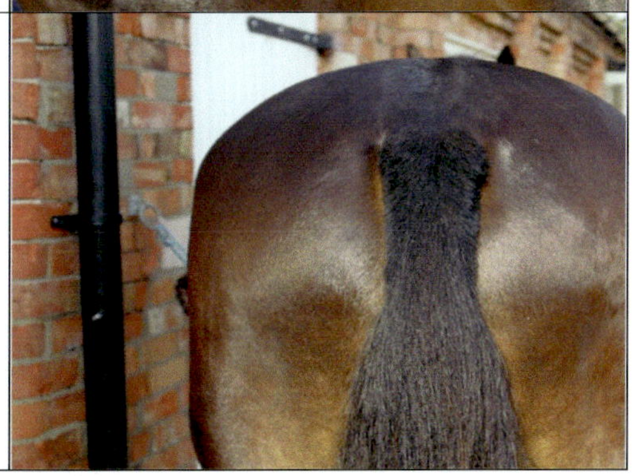

Fig. 3.10 Continued.

Table 3.7 Scoring the fat cover over the horse's skeleton

Neck – mean of the neck and shoulder blade so you might be allocating 0.5 scores
Remember to check if there is a fat pad in the supra-fossa orbital

Score	2	3	4	5
Nuchal ligament With your finger and thumb 'pinch' the nuchal ligament' just behind the poll and continue to follow it down the neck with your thumb and finger *Press your thumb firmly against your finger and squeeze gently*	Feels like a piece of string, or can't be felt	Feels like a plaited string, sits on the top of the neck as there is no fat above. Horse might pull away slightly when palpated	Crest/fat above ligament. The ligament is thick and difficult to follow when a third of the way down the neck. You can pull the crest over the ligament Horse is sensitive to the palpation of the ligament and will often pull away when first 'pinched' at the poll	Very wide and/or firm crest. Might have corrugation (lines) when turning neck towards you Unable to follow the ligament down the neck with the fingers either side as crest is too thick. Horse sensitive to the palpation behind the poll.
Shoulder blade Run hand down neck towards and over scapula *If you are uncertain, close your eyes and imagine you have to draw the outline of the shoulder blade from what you can feel (or not)*	i. When hand is run down neck, stops sharp at the shoulder blade ii. No fat cover but individual bones cannot be seen iii. Outline of scapula easily distinguishable. Scapula cartilage (under withers) rounded. iv. Point of shoulder easily cupped	i. When hand is run down neck, stops at scapula ii. There is a distinct outline to the scapula, although bones cannot be seen. There is less than 2 cm fat behind the shoulder blade iii. Able to cup the point of shoulder	i. When hand is run flat down neck, it does not stop at the shoulder blade as the front of the blade is covered with fat ii. Scapula is covered in fat and so bones cannot be felt iii. It is possible to 'pinch' fat behind the shoulder blade; more than 2 cm iv. Point of shoulder is very rounded as covered with fat	i. When hand is run down neck, the scapula is indistinguishable from the shoulder ii. Shoulder blade cannot be felt and there is local accumulation of fat pads iii. Roll of fat behind shoulder blade. Sometimes fat behind shoulder cannot be 'pinched', due to excess amount iv Point of shoulder indistinguishable

Middle – mean of ribs and backbone so you might be allocating 0.5 scores

Score	2	3	4	5
Ribs Run your hand diagonally across the horse's rib cage. *Use a firm pressure but not so the horse moves away from your hand*	Just visible and easily felt	Ribs easily felt; only visible when inhaling or turning on a circle	Ribs cannot be felt or only with firm pressure (horse will probably move away from pressure). Ribs not visible.	Cannot feel or see ribs and likely to be pockets of fat over rib cage

Continued

Table 3.7 Continued.

Backbone				
Place your left hand at the bottom of the horse's withers at 90° to the backbone. Place your right hand next to it, with your fingers pointing across (not along) the backbone. Remove your left hand, you are using your right hand. Relax the fingers of your right hand. *This ensures you measure the same place every time*	Individual vertebra can be felt but not seen. Cupped hand forms a rounded V over backbone	Vertebra felt easily but not seen. When hand laid flat along backbone and relaxed, the hand forms a slight cup	Backbone starting to be buried, i.e. gutter starting to form. Hand stays flat on backbone when relaxed	Back is flat with gutter, backbone cannot be seen as is in gutter, 'tabletop back' you can lay a pencil across the back or in the gutter and it stays there
Bottom – mean of pelvis, hips and tail bone so you might be allocating 0.5 scores				
Score	**2**	**3**	**4**	**5**
Pelvis				
Place your hand flat on the top of the horse's bottom to feel the top of his pelvis	Just visible and easily felt	Pelvis bones can be felt easily but not seen	Pelvis bones only found with firm pressure	Cannot feel or see pelvis. Pelvis buried, rump bulging
Hips				
Curve your hand around to feel the outline of the bones	Hips defined but not prominent, can feel bones but skin is supple	Hand can cup around the hip bones and feel them and skin is supple	Cannot feel outline of hips, unable to cup hand around them	Cannot feel hip bones, likely to be cellulite type lumps near hips or a dimpled appearance to the skin
Tail bone				
Run your hand from his hind quarters onto his tail, feeling for his tailbone	Slight cavity under tail. Tail bone easily felt and visible. Rump flat either side of backbone forming a slight 'v' shape	Rump is an upside-down 'c'. Tail bone easily felt	Tail bone cannot be felt. Gutter forming from rump to tailhead; apple shaped	Lumps of fat either side of tailhead. Very deep gutter from rump to tailbone

Table 3.8 Body condition scoring chart 1–9 (Henneke *et al*., (1983) modified by Kohnke (1992) (used with permission)

Condition Score	General condition	Neck	Withers	Loin	Tailhead	Ribs	Shoulder
1	Very Poor	Individual bone structure visible	Bones easily visible no fat	Spine bones visible, ends feel pointed	Tailhead and hip bones very visible	Ribs very visible and also furrows between ribs	Bone structure very visible
Animal extremely emaciated so no fatty tissue can be felt							
2	Very Thin	Bones just visible animal emaciated	Withers obvious very minimal fat covering	Slight fat covering over vertical and flat spine projections. Ends feel rounded	Tail bone and hip bones obvious	Ribs prominent slight depression between the ribs	Bone structure can be outlined
3	Thin	Thin, flat muscle covering	Withers accentuated with some fat cover	Fat build-up half way on vertical spines but only discernible. Flat spine bones not felt	Tailhead prominent hip bones appear rounded but visible. Pin bones covered	Slight covering over ribs. Rib outline obvious	Shoulder accentuated, some fat
4	Moderately Thin	Neck some fat not obviously thin	Withers not obviously thin, smooth edges	Slight ridge along back	Fat can be felt	Faint outline	Shoulder not obviously thin
5	Moderate	Neck blends smoothly into body	Withers rounded over top	Back level	Fat around tailhead beginning to feel spongy	Ribs cannot be seen but can easily be felt	Shoulder blends smoothly into body
6	Moderate Fleshy	Fat can be felt	Fat can be felt	May have slight inward crease	Fat around tailhead feels soft	Fat over the ribs feels spongy	Fat layer can be felt
7	Fleshy	Visible fat deposits along the neck	Fat covering withers is firm	May have slight inward crease down back	Fat around tail head is soft and rounded off	Individual ribs can still be felt	Fat buildup behind shoulder
8	Fat	Noticeable thickening of neck	Area along withers filled with fat	Crease down back evident	Tailhead fat very soft and flabby	Difficult to feel ribs	Area behind shoulder filled in flush with the body
9	Extremely Fat	Bulging fat	Bulging fat	Obvious deep crease down the back	Bulging fat around tailhead	Patchy fat over ribs	Bulging fat
Fat along inner buttocks may rub together. Flank filled in flush							

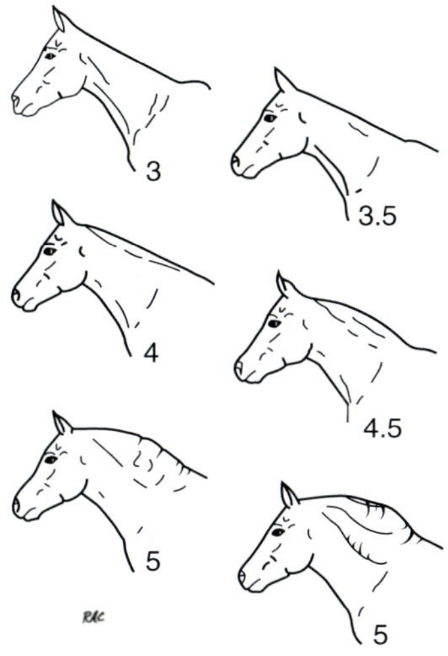

Modified score	Description
3	No visual appearance of a crest (tissue apparent above the ligamentum nuchae). No palpable crest.
3.5	No visual appearance of crest but slight filling felt with palpation.
4	Noticeable appearance of a crest, deposited fairly evenly from poll to withers. Crest easily cupped in one hand and bent from side to side.
4.5	Crest enlarged and thickened. More fat deposited in middle, giving a mounded appearance. Crest fills hand and begins to lose side-to-side flexibility.
5	Crest grossly enlarged and thickened. Can no longer be cupped in one hand or bent to one side. Crest may have wrinkles/creases perpendicular to topline. Crest might be so large it permanently droops to one side.

Fig. 3.11 The cresty neck score (modified from Carter *et al.*, 2009a).

How to Estimate Workload

Table 3.3 provides the best estimation and definitions of the different workloads. It is important that you obtain details on the actual activities the horse does.

- When hacking, is it on the bit, do they trot, how often and for how long?
- Does the horse sweat when working?
- Do they compete, how often and at what level, under rules or local shows?
- Is the horse turned out? For how long, on what sort of grazing and with how many other horses?

A stabled horse uses significantly less calories compared with one out on pasture as it moves less (Graham-Thiers and Bowen, 2013).

> **Top tip**
>
> - Most leisure horses are at maintenance or in light work.
> - Medium work is only applicable if horses are competing under rules or affiliated.
> - Clearly, unless working hunter, all show animals are in light work.

Summary

Measuring, recording and discussing the three key pieces of information with your client every time you visit increases their compliance and understanding. The information provides a scaffold for preventative medicine and is key to the successful feeding and performance of all horses, regardless of their workload.

It changes their perception of you from someone who pays a fleeting visit and sends a bill, to a vet that knows their horse, who is keen to follow progress and who wants to minimise the risk of disease aside from any nutritional issues. **A diet consult should be billable – it is a Nutritional Prescription – it is preventable medicine.**

Bibliography

Agüera, E.I., Rubio, M.D., Vivo, R., Santisteban, R., Muñoz, A. *et al.* (1995) Blood parameter and heart rate response to training in Andalusian horses. *Revista Española de Fisiología* 51(2), 55–64.

Ainsworth, D.M. (2008) Chapter 3.2: Lower airway function: responses to exercise and training. In: Hinchcliff, K.W., Raymond, J., Geor, R.J. and Kaneps, A.J. (eds) *Equine Exercise Physiology*. W.B. Saunders Co. Ltd, Philadelphia, Pennsylvania.

Apple, J.K., Davis, J.C., Stephenson, J.D., Hankins, J.E., Davis, J.R. and Beaty, S.L. (1999) Influence of body condition score on carcass characteristics and subprimal yield from cull beef cows. *Journal of Animal Science* 77(10), 2660–2669.

Baker, L.A., Burrows, A.M., Nonella, K.J., Pipkin, J.L., Holmes, L.D. *et al.* (2020) Relationship between live body condition score and carcass fat measures in equine. *Translational Animal Science* 4(4), txaa179. doi: 10.1093/tas/txaa179.

Betros, C.L., McKeever, K.H., Kearns, C.F. and Malinowski, K. (2002) Effects of ageing and training on maximal heart rate and VO_{2max}. *Equine Veterinary Journal* 34(S34), 100–105.

Blaue, D., Schedlbauer, C., Starzonek, J., Gittel, C., Brehm, W., Blüher, M., Pfeffer, M. and Vervuert, I. (2020) The influence of equine body weight gain on inflammatory cytokine expressions of adipose tissue in response to endotoxin challenge. *Acta veterinaria Scandinavica* 62(1), 17. https://doi.org/10.1186/s13028-020-00515-5

Briceño, A.M., Sanchez, A.M. and Arevalo, J.P. (2015) Infiltrative lipomatosis in neck and colon in a Spanish pure breed horse. *Brazilian Journal of Veterinary Pathology* 8(1), 14–17.

Briceño, A.M., Sánchez, A.M., Angulo, J.M., Sánchez, A.E. and Arévalo, J.P. (2017) Diagnostic tools for the study of the cresty neck in horses. *International Journal of Applied Research in Veterinary Medicine* 15(1), 41–49.

Brown, H., Marlin, D., Alexander, J.A. and Harris, P. (2007) A pilot study investigating the relationship between perceived and actual workload and estimated energy intake in riding centre horses. *Equine and Comparative Exercise Physiology* 4(01), 7–14.

Bruynsteen, L., Erkens, T., Peelman, L.J., Ducatell, R., Janssens, G.P. Harris, P.A. and Hesta, M. (2013) Expression of inflammation-related genes is associated with adipose tissue location in horses. *BMC Veterinary Research* 9, 240. doi: 10.1186/1746-6148-9-240.

Buelund, L.E., Nielsen, D.H., McEvoy, F.J. *et al.* (2011) Measurement of body composition in cats using computed tomography and dual energy x-ray absorptiometry. *Veterinary Radiology & Ultrasound* 52, 179–184.

Burkholder, W.J. (2000) Use of body condition scores in clinical assessment of the provision of optimal nutrition. *Journal of the American Veterinary Medicine Association* 217, 650–654.

Burns, T.A., Geor, R.J., Mudge, M.C. *et al.* (2010) Proinflammatory cytokine and chemokine gene expression profiles in subcutaneous and visceral adipose tissue depots of insulin-resistant and insulin-sensitive light breed horses. *Journal of Veterinary Internal Medicine* 24, 932–939.

Burrows, A.M., Baker, L.A., Holmes, T.J., McEvers, K.J., Nonella, L.D. *et al.* (2013) Relationship between live body condition score and internal kidney, pelvic, and heart fat measurements in equine carcasses, Proceedings of the 2013 Equine Science Society Symposium. *Journal of Equine Veterinary Science* 33(5), 361–362.

Carroll, C.L. and Huntington, P.J. (1988) Body condition scoring and weight estimation of horses. *Equine Veterinary Journal* 20, 41–45.

Carslake, J.B., Pinchbeck, G.L. and McGowan, C.M. (2021) Equine metabolic syndrome in UK native ponies and cobs is highly prevalent with modifiable risk factors. *Equine Veterinary Journal* 53(5), 923–934. doi: 10.1111/evj.13378.

Carter, R.A., Geor, R.J., Staniar, W.B., Cubitt, T.A. and Harris, P.A. (2009a) Apparent adiposity assessed by standardised scoring systems and morphometric measurements in horses and ponies. *Veterinary Journal* 179, 204–210.

Carter, R.A., McCutcheon, I.J., George, L.A., Smith, T.L., Frank, N. and Geor, R.J. (2009b) Effects of diet-induced weight gain on insulin sensitivity and plasma hormone and lipid concentrations in horses. *American Journal of Veterinary Research* 70(1), 1250–1258. doi: 10.2460/ajvr.70.10.1250.

Castejón, F., Rubio, D., Tovar, P., Vinuesa, M. and Riber, C. (1994) A comparative study of aerobic capacity and fitness in three different horse breeds (Andalusian, Arabian and Anglo-Arabian). *Journal of Veterinary Medicine Series A* 41(1–10), 645–652.

Catalano, D.N., Coleman, R.J., Hathaway, M.R., McCue, M.E., Rendahl, A.K. *et al.* (2016) Estimation of actual and ideal bodyweight using morphometric measurements and owner guessed bodyweight of adult draft and warmblood horses. *Journal of Equine Veterinary Science* 39, 38–43.

Catalano D.N., Coleman, R.J., Hathaway, M.R., Neu, A.E., Wagner, E.L. *et al.* (2019) Estimation of actual and ideal bodyweight using morphometric measurements of miniature, saddle-type, and thoroughbred horses. *Journal of Equine Veterinary Science* 78, 117–122. doi: 10.1016/j.jevs.2019.04.008.

Clauss, M., Steuer, P., Müller, D.W., Codron, D. and Hummel, J. (2013) Herbivory and body size: allometries of diet quality and gastrointestinal physiology, and implications for herbivore ecology and dinosaur gigantism. *PLoS ONE* 8(10), e68714.

Coenen, M., Kienzle, E., Vervuert, I. and Zeyner, A. (2011) Recent German developments in the formulation of energy and nutrient requirements in horses and the resulting feeding recommendations. *Journal of Equine Veterinary Science* 31(5–6), 219–229.

Costa, A., Hetherington, M. and Oliveira, A. (2021). Maternal perception, concern and dissatisfaction with child weight and their association with feeding practices in the Generation XXI birth cohort. *British Journal of Nutrition* 127, 1106-1116. doi:10.1017/S0007114521001653

Cuddeford, D., Pearson, R.A., Archibald, R.F. and Muirhead, R.H. (1995) Digestibility and gastro-intestinal transit time of diets containing different proportions of alfalfa and oat straw given to Thoroughbreds, Shetland ponies, Highland ponies and donkeys. *Animal Science* 61(2), 407–417.

Dekker, H., Marlin, D., Alexander, L., Bishop, R. and Harris, P. (2007) A pilot study investigating the relationship between perceived and actual workload and estimated energy intake in riding centre horses. *Equine and Comparative Exercise Physiology* 4(1), 7–14.

Demment, M. and Van Soest, P. (1985) A nutritional explanation for body-size patterns of ruminant and nonruminant herbivores. *The American Naturalist* 125(5), 641–672.

Dias Villas-Boas, J., Martins Dias, D.P., Ignacio Trigo, P., Aparecida dos Santos Almeida, N., Queiroz de Almeida, F. *et al*. (2016) Behavioural, endocrine and cardiac autonomic responses to a model of startle in horses. *Applied Animal Behaviour Science* 174, 76–82. doi: 10.1016/j.applanim.2015.10.005.

Domecq, J.J., Skidmore, A.L., Lloyd, J.W. and Kaneene, J.B. (1995) Validation of body condition scores with ultrasound measurements of subcutaneous fat of dairy cows. *Journal of Dairy Science* 78(10), 2308–2313. doi:10.3168/jds.S0022-0302(95)76857-6.

Dugdale, A.H.A. (2011) Aspects of adiposity in ponies. PhD thesis, The University of Liverpool.

Dugdale, A.H.A., Curtis, G.C., Harris, P.A. and Argo, C.M. (2011) Assessment of body fat in the pony: part I. Relationships between the anatomical distribution of adipose tissue, body composition and body condition. *Equine Veterinary Journal* 43, 552–561.

Dugdale, A.H.A., Grove-White, D., Curtis, G.C., Harris, P.A. and Argo, C.M. (2012) Body condition scoring as a predictor of body fat in horses and ponies. *Veterinary Journal* 194, 173–178. doi: 10.1016/j.tvjl.2012.03.024.

Duncan, P., Foose, T.J., Gordon, I.J., Gakahu, C.G. and Lloyd, M. (1990) Comparative nutrient extraction from forages by grazing bovids and equids: a test of the nutritional model of equid/bovid competition and coexistence. *Oecologia* 84, 411–418.

Ebert, M. and Moore-Colyer, M.J. (2020) The energy requirements of racehorses in training. *Translational Animal Science* 4(4), txaa196.

Ellis, J.M. and Hollands, T. (1998) Accuracy of different methods of estimating the weight of horses. *Veterinary Record* 143, 335–336.

Ellis, J.M. and Hollands, T. (2002) Use of height-specific weigh tapes to estimate the bodyweight of horses. *The Veterinary Record* 150(20), 632–634.

Ellis, J. and Hollands, T. (2017) A preliminary investigation into the use of weightapes for the detection of dehydration in the performance horse. In: *Proceedings 40th BEVA Annual Congress* 221.

Evans, D.L. and Rose, R.J. (1988) Determination and repeatability of maximum oxygen uptake and other cardiorespiratory measurements in the exercising horse. *Equine Veterinary Journal* 20(2), 94–98. doi: 10.1111/j.2042-3306.1988.tb01467.x.

Evans, D.L., Rainger, J.E., Hodgson, D.R., Eaton, M.D. and Rose, R.J. (1995) The effects of intensity and duration of training on blood lactate concentrations during and after exercise. *Equine Veterinary Journal* 27(S18), 422–425.

Fitzgerald, D.M., Anderson, S.T., Sillence, M.N. and de Laat, M.A. (2019) The cresty neck score is an independent predictor of insulin dysregulation in ponies. *PLoS ONE* 14(7), e0220203. doi: 10.1371/journal.pone.0220203.

Fonseca, R.G., Kenny, D.A., Hill, E.W. and Katz, L.M. (2010) The association of various speed indices to training responses in Thoroughbred flat racehorses measured with a global positioning and heart rate monitoring system. *Equine Veterinary Journal* 42, 51–57.

Fortier, J., Goachet, A., Deley, G. and Julliand, V. (2014) Quantification of energy expenditure in field conditions: comparison of direct VO2 versus VO2 estimation from heart rate measurements. *Equine Veterinary Journal* 46, 12–12. doi: 10.1111/evj.12267.

Gee, E.K., Fenessy, P.F., Morel, P.C.H., Grace, N.D., Firth, E.C. and Mogg, T.D. (2003) Chemical body composition of 20 thoroughbred foals at 160 days of age, and preliminary investigation of techniques used to predict body fatness. *New Zealand Veterinary Journal* 51, 125–131. doi: 10.1080/00480169.2003.36351.

Gentry, L.R., Thompson, D.L., Gentry, G.T., del Vecchio, R.P., Davis, K.A. and Del Vecchio, P.M. (2004) The relationship between body condition score and ultrasonographic fat measurements in mares of high versus low body condition. *Journal of Equine Veterinary Science* 24, 198–203.

Giles, S.L., Nicol C.J., Rands, S.A. and Harris, P.A. (2015) Assessing the seasonal prevalence and risk factors for nuchal crest adiposity in domestic horses and ponies using the cresty neck score. *BMC Veterinary Research* 11, 13.

Glazier D.S. (2005) Beyond the '3/4-power law': variation in the intra- and interspecific scaling of metabolic rate in animals. *Biological Reviews of the Cambridge Philosophical Society* 80(4), 611–662. doi: 10.1017/S1464793105006834.

Górniak, W., Wieliczko, M., Soroko, M. and Korczyński, M. (2020) Evaluation of the accuracy of horse body weight estimation methods. *Animals* 10(10), 1750.

Graham-Thiers, P.M. and Bowen, L.K. (2013) Improved ability to maintain fitness in horses during large pasture turnout. *Journal of Equine Veterinary Science* 33(8), 581–585.

Gregory, N.G., Robins, J.K., Thomas, D.G. and Purchas, R.W. (1998) Relationship between body condition score and body composition in dairy cows. *New Zealand Journal of Agricultural Research* 41(4), 527–532. doi: 10.1080/00288233.1998.9513335.

Greiner, S.P., Rouse, G.H., Wilson, D.E., Cundiff, L.V. and Wheeler, T.L. (2003) The relationship between ultrasound measurements and carcass fat thickness and longissimus muscle area in beef cattle. *Journal of Animal Science* 81(3), 676–682. doi: 10.2527/2003.813676x.

Hale, C.E., Hemmings, A.J. and Randle, H. (2016) Accuracy of horse workload perception by owners when compared to published workload parameters. *Journal of Veterinary Behavior* 15, 94.

Henneke, D., Potter, G., Kreider, J. and Yeates, B. (1983) Relationship between condition score, physical measurements and body fat percentage in mares. *Equine Veterinary Journal* 15, 371–372.

Hoffman, C.J., Costa, L.R. and Freeman, L.M. (2009) Survey of feeding practices, supplement use, and knowledge of equine nutrition among a subpopulation of horse owners in New England. *Journal of Equine Veterinary Science* 29(10), 719–724.

Hollands, T., Ellis, J.M., Allen, D.E. and Salonen, L. (2009) An assessment of 2 visual methods of fat scoring in the equine to determine the most suitable for client recognition of obesity in their horses. *Proceedings of 48th BEVA Congress*, p. 247.

Honore, E.K. and Uhlinger, C.A. (1994) Equine feeding practices in Central North Carolina: a preliminary survey. *Journal of Equine Veterinary Science* 14(8), 424–429.

Hopster, H. and Blokhuis, H.J. (1994) Validation of a heart-rate monitor for measuring a stress response in dairy cows. *Canadian Journal of Animal Science* 74(3), 465–474. doi: 10.4141/cjas94-066.

Ille, N., Erber, R., Aurich, C. and Aurich, J. (2014) Comparison of heart rate and heart rate variability obtained by heart rate monitors and simultaneously recorded electrocardiogram signals in nonexercising horses. *Journal of Veterinary Behavior* 9(6), 341–346. doi: 10.1016/j.jveb.2014.07.006.

Isaac, N.J.B. and Carbone, C. (2010) Why are metabolic scaling exponents so controversial? Quantifying variance and testing hypotheses. *Ecology Letters* 13, 728–735. doi: 10.1111/j.1461-0248.2010.01461.x.

Jansson, A., Gunnarsson, V.Þ., Ringmark, S., Ragnarsson, S., Söderroos, D. *et al.* (2021) Increased body fat content in horses alters metabolic and physiological exercise response, decreases performance, and increases locomotion asymmetry. *Physiological Reports* 9(11), e14824.

Jensen, R.B., Rockhold, L.L. and Tauson, A.H. (2019) Weight estimation and hormone concentrations related to body condition in Icelandic and Warmblood horses: a field study. *Acta Veterinaria Scandinavica* 61. doi: 10.1186/s13028-019-0498-5.

Kane, R.A., Fisher, M., Parrett, D. and Lawrence, L.M. (1987) Estimating fatness in horses. In: *Proceedings of the 10th Equine Nutrition and Physiology Symposium*, Urbana, pp. 127–131.

Kearns, C.F., McKeever, K.H., Kumagai, K. and Abe, T. (2002a) Fat-free mass is related to one-mile race performance in elite standardbred horses. *The Veterinary Journal* 163, 260–266.

Kearns, C.F., McKeever, K.H., John-Alder, H., Abe, T. and Brechue, W.F. (2002b) Relationship between body composition, blood volume and maximal oxygen uptake. *Equine Veterinary Journal* 34, 485–490.

Kienzle, E. and Zeyner, A. (2010) The development of a metabolizable energy system for horses. *Journal of Animal Physiology and Animal Nutrition* 94(6), e231–e240. doi: 10.1111/j.1439-0396.2010.01015.x.

Kingston, J.K., Soppet, G.M., Rogers, C.W. and Firth, E.C. (2006) Use of a global positioning and heart rate monitoring system to assess training load in a group of thoroughbred racehorses. *Equine Veterinary Journal* 38(S36), 106–109.

Kohnke, J. (1992) *Feeding and Nutrition: the Making of a Champion*. Birubi Pacific, Australia.

Lauten, S.D., Cox, N.R., Brawner, W.R. and Baker, H.J. (2001) Use of dual energy x-ray absorptiometry for noninvasive body composition measurements in clinically normal dogs. *American Journal of Veterinary Research* 62, 1295–1301.

Lawrence, L.M., Jackson, S., Kline, K., Moser, L. and Biel, M. (1992) Observations on body weight and condition of horses in a 150-mile endurance ride. *Journal of Equine Veterinary Science* 12, 320–324.

Léguillette, R., Bond, S.L., Lawlor, K. *et al.* (2020) Comparison of physiological demands in Warmblood show jumping horses over a standardized 1.10 m jumping course versus a standardized exercise test on a track. *BMC Veterinary Research* 16, 182. doi: 10.1186/s12917-020-02400-9.

Leleu, C. and Cotrel, C. (2006) Body composition in young standardbreds in training: relationships to body condition score, physiological and locomotor variables during exercise. *Equine Veterinary Journal* (Suppl. 36), 98–101.

Lenoir, A., Trachsel, D.S., Younes, M., Barrey, E. and Robert, C. (2017) Agreement between electrocardiogram and heart rate meter is low for the measurement of heart rate variability during exercise in young endurance horses. *Frontiers in Veterinary Science* 4, 170. doi: 10.3389/fvets.2017.00170.

Lindner, A., Mosen, H., Kissenbeck, S., Fuhrmann, H. and Sallmann, H.P. (2009) Effect of blood lactate-guided conditioning of horses with exercises of differing durations and intensities on heart rate and biochemical blood variables. *Journal of Animal Science* 87(10), 3211–3217.

Martin-Rosset, W., Vernet, J., Dubroeucq, H., Arnaud, G., Picard, A. and Vermorel, M. (2008) Variation of fatness and energy content of the body with body condition score in sport horses and its prediction. In: Saastamoinen, M.T. and Martin-Rosset, W. (eds) *Nutrition of the Exercising Horse*. Wageningen Academic Publishers, Netherlands, pp. 167–176.

Martinson, K.L., Coleman, R.C., Rendahl, A.K., Fang, Z. and McCue, M.E. (2014) Estimation of body weight and development of a body weight score for adult equids using morphometric measurements. *Journal of Animal Science* 92(5), 2230–2238.

McDuffee, L., Mills, M., McNiven, M. and Montelpare, W. (2019) Establishing statistical stability for heart rate variability in horses. *Journal of Veterinary Behavior* 32, 30–35. doi: 10.1016/j.jveb.2019.05.003.

Menard, C., Duncan, P., Fleurance, G., Georges, J.Y. and Lila, M. (2002) Comparative foraging and nutrition of horses and cattle in European wetlands. *Journal of Applied Ecology* 39, 120–133.

Morrison, P.K., Harris, P.A., Maltin, C.A., Grove-White, D. and Argo, C.M. (2017) EQUIFAT: a novel scoring system for the semi-quantitative evaluation of regional adipose tissues in Equidae. *PLoS ONE* 12(3), e0173753.

Munday, H.S., Booles, D., Anderson, P. *et al.* (1994) The repeatability of body composition measurements in dogs and cats using dual energy X-ray absorptiometry. *Journal of Nutrition* 124 (Suppl.), S2619–S2621.

Muñoz, A., Riber, C., Santisteban, R., Lucas, R.G. and Castejón, F.M. (2002) Effect of training duration and exercise on blood-borne substrates, plasma lactate and enzyme concentrations in Andalusian, Anglo-Arabian and Arabian breeds. *Equine Veterinary Journal Supplements* (34), 245–251.

Murray, J.-A.M.D., Bloxham, C., Kulifay, J., Stevenson, A. and Roberts. J. (2015) Equine nutrition: a survey of perceptions and practices of horse owners undertaking a massive open online course in equine nutrition. *Journal of Equine Veterinary Science* 35(6), 510–517. doi: 10.1016/j.jevs.2015.02.005.

NRC (National Research Council) (2007) *Nutrient Requirements of Horses: Sixth Revised Edition*. National Academies Press, Washington, DC. doi: 10.17226/11653.

Okada, Y., Kobayashi, M., Sawamura, M., and Arai, T. (2017) Comparison of visceral fat accumulation and metabolome markers among cats of varying BCS and novel classification of feline obesity and metabolic syndrome. *Frontiers in Veterinary Science* 4, 17. https://doi.org/10.3389/fvets.2017.00017

Pagan, J.D. and Hintz, H.F. (1986) Equine energetics. 1. Relationship between body weight and energy requirements in horses. *Journal of Animal Science* 63(3), 815–821. doi: 10.2527/jas1986.633815x.

Pagan, J.D., Martin, O.A. and Crowley, N.L. (2009) Relationship between body condition and metabolic parameters in sport horses, pony hunters and polo ponies. *Journal of Equine Veterinary Science* 29(5), 418–420.

Parker, M., Goodwin, D., Eager, R., Redhead, E. and Marlin, D. (2009) Comparison of Polar® heart rate interval data with simultaneously recorded ECG signals in horses. *Comparative Exercise Physiology* 6(4), 137–142. doi: 10.1017/S1755254010000024.

Pearson, R., Archibald, R. and Muirhead, R. (2001) The effect of forage quality and level of feeding on digestibility and gastrointestinal transit time of oat straw and alfalfa given to ponies and donkeys. *British Journal of Nutrition* 85(5), 599–606. doi: 10.1079/BJN2001321.

Pearson, R., Archibald, R. and Muirhead, R. (2006) A comparison of the effect of forage type and level of feeding on the digestibility and gastrointestinal mean retention time of dry forages given to cattle, sheep, ponies and donkeys. *British Journal of Nutrition* 95(1), 88–98. doi: 10.1079/BJN20051617.

Piccione, G., Messina, V., Casella, S., Giannetto, C. and Caola, G. (2010) Blood lactate levels during exercise in athletic horses. *Comparative Clinical Pathology* 19(6), 535–539.

Quaresma, M., Payan-Carreira, R. and Silva, S.R. (2013) Relationship between ultrasound measurements of body fat reserves and body condition score in female donkeys. *The Veterinary Journal* 197, 329–334.

Reid, R.L., Jung, G.A. and Thayne, W.V. (1988) Relationships between nutritive quality and fiber components of cool season and warm season forages: a retrospective study. *Journal of Animal Science* 66(5), 1275–1291.

Robergs, R. and Burnett, A. (2003) Methods used to process data from indirect calorimetry and their application to VO_{2max}. *Journal of Exercise Physiology* 6(2), 44–57.

Rucker, R.B. (2007) Allometric scaling, metabolic body size and interspecies comparisons of basal nutritional requirements. *Journal of Animal Physiology and Animal Nutrition* 91, 148–156. doi: 10.1111/j.1439-0396.2007.00681.x.

Schroder, U.J. and Staufenbiel, R. (2006) Invited review: Methods to determine body fat reserves in the dairy cow with special regard to ultrasonographic measurement of backfat thickness. *Journal of Dairy Science* 89(1), 1–14. doi: 10.3168/jds.S0022-0302(06)72064-1.

Schwarzwald, C.C., Kedo, M., Birkmann, K. and Hamlin, R.L. (2012) Relationship of heart rate and electrocardiographic time intervals to body mass in horses and ponies. *Journal of Veterinary Cardiology* 14(2), 343–350. doi: 10.1016/j.jvc.2012.03.001.

Shaffer, F., Meehan, Z.M. and Zerr, C.L. (2020) A critical review of ultra-short-term heart rate variability norms research. *Frontiers in Neuroscience* 14, 594880. doi: 10.3389/fnins.2020.594880.

Shoveller, A.K., DiGennaro, J., Lanman, C. *et al.* (2014) Trained vs untrained evaluator assessment of body condition score as a predictor of percent body fat in adult cats. *Journal of Feline Medicine and Surgery* 16, 957–965.

Siegers, E., De Ruijter-Villani, M., Van Doorn, D., Stout, T. and Roelfsema, E. (2018) Ultrasonographic measurements of localized fat accumulation in Shetland pony mares fed a normal v. a high energy diet for 2 years. *Animal* 12(8), 1602–1610. doi: 10.1017/S1751731117003251.

Silva, S.R., Payan-Carreira, R., Quaresma, M., Guedes, C.M. and Santos, A.S. (2016a) Relationships between body condition score and ultrasound skin-associated subcutaneous fat depth in equids. *Acta Veterinaria Scandinavica.* 58(Suppl. 1), 62. doi: 10.1186/s13028-016-0243-2.

Silva, S.R., Payan-Carreira, R., Guedes, C.M. *et al.* (2016b) Correlations between cresty neck scores and post-mortem nape fat measurements in horse, obtained after photographic image analysis. *Acta Veterinaria Scandinavica* 58(Suppl. 1), 60. doi: 10.1186/s13028-016-0241-4.

Smoliga, J.M. (2014) If an animal looks obese, precise estimation of body composition is of limited clinical value. *Journal of the American Veterinary Medical Association* 245(5), 484–485.

Soto-Navarro, S.A., Lopez, R., Sankey, C., Capitan, B.M., Holland, B.P. *et al.* (2014) Comparative digestibility by cattle versus sheep: effect of forage quality. *Journal of Animal Science* 92(4), 1621–1629.

Speakman, J.R., Booles, D. and Butterwick, R. (2001) Validation of dual energy x-ray absorptiometry (DXA) by comparison with chemical analysis of dogs and cats. *International Journal of Obesity Related Metabolic Disorders* 25, 439–447.

Staub, C., Venturi, E., Cirot, M., Léonard, L., Barriére, P. *et al.* (2019) Ultrasonographic measures of body fatness and their relationship with plasma levels and adipose tissue expression of four adipokines in Welsh pony mares. *Domestic Animal Endocrinology* 69, 75–83. doi: 10.1016/j.domaniend.2019.02.002.

Staufenbiel, R. (1997) Konditionsbeurteilung von Milchkühen mit Hilfe der sonographischen Rückenfettdickenmessung. *Prakt. Tierarzt coll. vet* 27, 87–92.

Stephenson, H.M., Green, M.J., Freeman, S.L. (2011) Prevalence of obesity in a population of horses in the UK. *The Veterinary Record* 168(5), 131–131.

Szabó, C., Vizesi, Z. and Vincze, A. (2021) Heart rate and heart rate variability of amateur show jumping horses competing on different levels. *Animals: An Open Access Journal from MDPI* 11(3), 693. doi: 10.3390/ani11030693.

Villas-Boas, J.D., Dias, D.P.M., Trigo, P.I., dos Santos Almeida, N.A., de Almeida, F.Q. *et al.* (2016) Behavioural, endocrine and cardiac autonomic responses to a model of startle in horses. *Applied Animal Behaviour Science* 174, 76–82.

Vincent, L., Newton, J.R., Deaton, C.M., Franklin, S.H., Biddick, T. *et al.* (2006) Retrospective study of predictive variables for maximal heart rate (HRmax) in horses undergoing strenuous treadmill exercise. *Equine Veterinary Journal, Supplement* (36), 146–152. doi: 10.1111/j.2042-3306.2006.tb05531.x.

Westervelt, R., Stouffer, J.R., Hintz, H.F. and Schryver, H.F. (1976) Estimating fatness in horses and ponies. *Journal of Animal Science* 43, 781–785. doi: 10.2527/jas1976.434781x.

White, C.R. and Seymour, R.S. (2005) Allometric scaling of mammalian metabolism. *The Journal of Experimental Biology* 208(Pt 9), 1611–1619. doi: 10.1242/jeb.01501.

Williams, J., Kenworthy, K., Jones, T., Marlin, D. and Tabor, G. (2019) The role of heart rate monitoring to assess workload during maintenance interval training in National Hunt racehorses. *Journal of Veterinary Behavior* 30, 54–60. doi: 10.1016/j.jveb.2018.12.003.

Younes, M., Robert, C., Barrey, E. and Cottin, F. (2016) Effects of age, exercise duration, and test conditions on heart rate variability in young endurance horses. *Frontiers in Physiology* 7, 155–166.

Young, L.E., Marlin, D.J., Deaton, C., Brown-Feltner, H., Roberts, C.A. *et al.* (2002) Heart size estimated by echocardiography correlates with maximal oxygen uptake. *Equine Veterinary Journal Supplement* 34, 467–471.

4 Diet Details: the Evidence Behind the Practice. What Are Forages? Factors Affecting Feed Value and Intake

TERESA HOLLANDS

School of Veterinary Medicine, University of Surrey

Learning Objectives

LO1 Explain forages.
LO2 Define fibre.
LO3 Explain what affects digestibility and intake of forages.
LO4 Classify forages depending upon their conservation.
LO5 Give examples of how forages are preserved.
LO6 Compare and contrast the role of alternative fibre sources.
LO7 Explain how to take a forage sample for analysis.

At the end of this chapter, you should be able to recognise common forages in the provision of the horse's nutrient requirements (energy, protein, vitamins and minerals) and their role in maintaining the health of the horse.

The Importance of Forage in the Horse's Diet

Every client knows that forage is the most important part of their horse's diet and in some instances it might be providing over 90% of the energy (calories) and nutrients that their horse eats. Despite this awareness, few get it analysed, many do not weigh it, and some do not realise that the difference in quantities of fibre in forages will have implications that might affect gut health and therefore the performance of their horse.

What Is Forage?

Forage is defined as 'edible parts of plants, other than separated grain, that can provide feed for grazing animals or that can be harvested for feeding' (Forage and Grazing Terminology Committee (1991), cited by Wilkins, 2000). The fibre in the forage cell walls is the main source of carbohydrates for horses, which the bacteria in the horse's guts (predominantly hind gut) ferment to produce substances called volatile fatty acids (VFAs); in human nutrition these substances are called short-chain fatty acids (SCFAs). The VFAs are absorbed out of the horse's gut into the horse's body cells where they are taken to cells and the liver before being converted to glucose. There is not a specific 'nutrient' requirement for fibre, but the horse's gut is designed to process food for 16–18 h out of 24 h, including being able to chew and produce saliva for this duration. Forage should provide a minimum of 50% of the dry matter intake even in competition horses. Whilst forages provide the structural carbohydrates that are essential for the health of the

DOI: 10.1079/9781789245134.0004

horse's hind gut (Table 4.1) not all fibre is forage; whole-grain cereals can provide up to 45% of a person's fibre intake (Sawicki *et al.*, 2017), which has proven health benefits for our bacteria. This cereal fibre (wheat feed, oat feed) can be included in pellets or coarse mixes and is of equal importance for the health of the horse's hind gut as forage fibre. Processed fibre requires less chewing, so it will not produce as much saliva or completely satisfy the horse's psychological need to chew compared with unprocessed fibre. Additionally, the reduced fibre length increases the rate of passage through the gut (Cymbaluk and Christensen, 1986; van Weyenberg *et al.*, 2006).

What Is Fibre?

Fibre is the common name for plant cell wall carbohydrates such as cellulose, hemicellulose and lignin that cannot be digested by mammalian enzymes (Table 4.2). Fibre is the cell wall of plant cells. Cell contents are highest in young plants and decrease as the forage matures. The cell wall increases as the forage matures, in order to provide structural support for the stem as the forage gets taller.

Historically dietary fibre was defined by human nutritionists as 'the sum of lignin and polysaccharides that are not digested by endogenous secretions of the digestive tract of man' (Trowell *et al.*, 1976).

Table 4.1 A summary of forage and the constituents of plant cell walls (fibre)

Forages are constructed of plant cells.
- The cells have a lumen and cell wall.
- The lumen is the inner part of the cell where sugars and proteins are housed.
- The space between cells is the middle lamella.
- The middle lamella is a structural polysaccharide high in pectin and it binds plant cells together, similar to cement between bricks.

Cell walls (fibre) = hemicellulose, lignin, cellulose, non-cellulosic and pectic polysaccharides, proteins, phenolic compounds and water.
- The major components (> 90%) are polysaccharides/carbohydrates
- Two wall types surround plant cells: primary wall and secondary wall.
- The primary wall in young cells provides flexibility and basic structural support, protecting the cell.
- The thicker durable secondary wall lies between the primary wall and plasma membrane. It is deposited when the cell has stopped growing and dividing and it is an adaptation to enable upright growth.

Cellulose
- Water-insoluble carbohydrate found in both primary and secondary cell walls.
- Fibrous structure enables the maintenance of structural integrity.
- Linear chain of glucose (sugar) units with β 1-4 linkages.
- Linkages broken by bacterial cellulase predominantly in hind gut but some in small intestine.
- The microorganisms break open the cell wall and access polysaccharides from cell contents. They use cell contents as a fuel/energy source which allows them to ferment the cellulose and other cell wall fractions.

Pectins
- Predominantly in the primary cell wall.
- Confers expansion, strength.
- Fermented in small intestine.

Hemicellulose
- More complex structure, with several different types of sugars bound by β 1-4 linkages.
- Closely associated with lignin.
- Highly digestible if it is not lignified.

Lignin
- Major component of the secondary cell wall, limits digestion of plant matter polysaccharides.
- Plant matures, lignin content increases; grasses accumulate lignin in their stems as they mature.
- Digestion is limited when high lignin.
- Plant ages = shift in the type of lignin being deposited.
- The cross-link of lignin to polysaccharides is the determining factor for digestibility.
- When lignin is cross-linked to the polysaccharides of the plant cell wall (mainly hemicellulose), digestion is dramatically decreased.
- Cross-link forms a barrier that limits microbial access to polysaccharides so cannot ferment the fibre.

These carbohydrates are the structural component of plant cell walls, with mature plants containing more structural carbohydrates compared with young plants. Plants generally contain a mixture of both soluble and insoluble structural carbohydrates – cellulose, hemicellulose, lignin, pectins, β-glucans, pentosans and xylans – which vary according to the type and stage of maturity (Houston *et al.*, 2016).

Table 4.2 The difference between cell walls and cell content of forages

	Components found	Where and how digested
Cell contents Highest in young forages	Sugars, starch, pectin, protein, fats, vitamins and minerals, water	Small intestine Digested by horse's enzymes Some carbohydrates, like fructans, are fermented by bacteria in stomach and small intestine of the horse (Coenen *et al.*, 2006; Respondek *et al.*, 2008; Glatter *et al.*, 2019)
Cell wall		Hind gut
Primary	Cellulose	Digested by bacterial fermentation
Secondary cell wall	Hemicellulose	
Highest in mature forages	Lignin	

Fibre content is measured after extraction with a neutral detergent solution according to the method of Van Soest and Wine (1967) and called neutral detergent fibre (NDF). NDF approximates the total cell wall constituents and can be used to predict how much of the forage the horse will eat and digest.

Horses are herbivores with specifically adapted guts and feeding behaviour to digest cellulose and they need a large percentage of plant cell walls in their diet to maintain their physiological (gut health) and psychological (need to chew) health.

What Affects the Nutritional Value of the Forage Being Fed?

Forages will vary considerably in nutritional value (Table 4.3) dependent upon: (i) availability and season; (ii) species; (iii) growth stage; and (iv) method of conservation and area/country in which grown. Because forage can provide up to 95% of a horse's total nutrient requirements, it is important to understand what affects the nutritional value of forages, so you can explain to clients the implications for their horses in terms of intake, gut health and nutrient availability.

Availability and season – climate change

The availability of forages depends upon their growth. Plants need a soil temperature above 6°C, water, sunshine and nutrients to grow. Whilst there is seasonality to growth, local climate variability will affect growth and nutrient value.

Table 4.3 Typical analysis of common forages fed to horses in the UK

Forage	Estimated digestible energy (DE) (MJ/kg DM)	Protein (% DM)	Lignin (% DM)	Mean NDF (% DM) (indication of fibre digestibility)
Spring grass (meadow)	11.5	22	3.2	49.5
Summer grass	10	10	5	60
Meadow hay	8	7	7	65–70
Haylage (high fibre)	11 7–10[a]	7–10[a]	6	50
Haylage (ryegrass)	14 9–11.5[a]	9–12[a]	5	45
Straw (barley or oat)	5	3.8	8	76–80
Alfalfa (high-temperature dried)	12	18	5	33–45
Dehydrated sugar beet (molassed)	12	9	2	40–47

[a]Data from HorseHage (https://www.horsehage.co.uk/wp-content/uploads/2019/09/HorseHage-Analysis.pdf)

Remind clients to monitor the weather forecast, as grass growth responds rapidly and horses may need to be restricted in their grazing. Cool temperatures slow growth rates and maturity; this reduces the lignin and may result in higher quality at a given age.

Be careful not to assume a certain nutrient value dependent upon season, as this tends to be atypical compared with many papers and books; adjust according to the predominant weather and the management of the forage. Differences in ambient temperature are seldom independent of other variables, such as daylength and moisture conditions, and growth may not be 'typical' of that season.

Warm weather with available water for growth will result in continuous new forage growth regardless of the season. If the client manages the grass through topping (not common unless commercially managed studs) the forage will maintain a high ratio of cell content to cell wall because the grass is not being given the chance to grow tall and mature.

Cool temperatures and short daylengths delay maturation and slow the associated decline in forage quality; high temperatures increase the rate of plant maturation and cell wall lignification (Mueller and Orloff, 1994). Even in 1956, people were aware that the micronutrient content of grasses varies with season – temperate grasses lose 87% carotene and 66% phosphorus, whereas calcium generally increases in grass tissue with advancing season (Oelberg, 1956). Realistically too, very few pastures or conserved forages are single species and so the forages will be at different stages of growth, their plant tissues will vary and therefore the feed value will differ even within a field. Clearly this is a challenge when you think that grass or other forages might provide 90–100% of a horse's feed intake.

Forage species

It is difficult to recognise what grass species are growing at the early growth stage of forages and agronomists are the best experts to refer to, should you need advice. You should be able to identify the common forages fed to horses as the plant matures and produces flowers and seed heads, whether in fields as grass or conserved as hay or haylage. Being able to recognise species allows you to generalise about the nutritional value of the forages (fresh or conserved).

Grasses vary in nutritional value (Table 4.4).

Perennial ryegrass (Fig. 4.1a) is a high-quality species that is often grown for cattle as it is high in energy (calories) compared with meadow grasses such as timothy (Fig. 4.1b), fescues (Fig. 4.1c) and cocksfoot (Fig. 4.1d).

Make sure that the forages being fed are suitable for the workload of the horses that you are assessing. Pastures high in clover will be high in starch; clover is a legume, not a grass, and will have a higher energy content compared with grass. The availability of the grass will also depend upon how well it is managed and the number of horses or other animals eating the paddocks – a large amount of lower feed-value grass can still make a horse fat, if they eat enough of it. Generally, ryegrass will be higher in feed value as it has been bred specifically to maintain the dairy cow, whereas timothy and meadow grasses are lower in all nutrients.

Growth stage

If forages are the horse's main source of nutrients, then the length of time that the forage has been growing will have the biggest impact on whether the horse you are assessing is going to get fat, maintain its fat cover or lose weight.

Forage quality declines with advancing maturity because the cell contents decrease and the percentage of cell wall increases; lignin reduces the fermentation of cellulose and hemicellulose (Smith *et al.*, 1972). It is harder for the bacteria to ferment mature cell walls and the horse might only be able to use 50% of the mature forage; this measure of the forage is known as digestibility. Your clients probably

Table 4.4 Monthly and average crude protein of common grasses fed to horses (adapted from Martinson *et al.*, 2010)

Grass	May	June	July	August	September	October	Seasonal average
Perennial ryegrass	22	20	19.5	22	23	24.5	20.6
Meadow fescue	19	21	15	18	22	21	19
Timothy	17	20	17	21.5	21	21	18

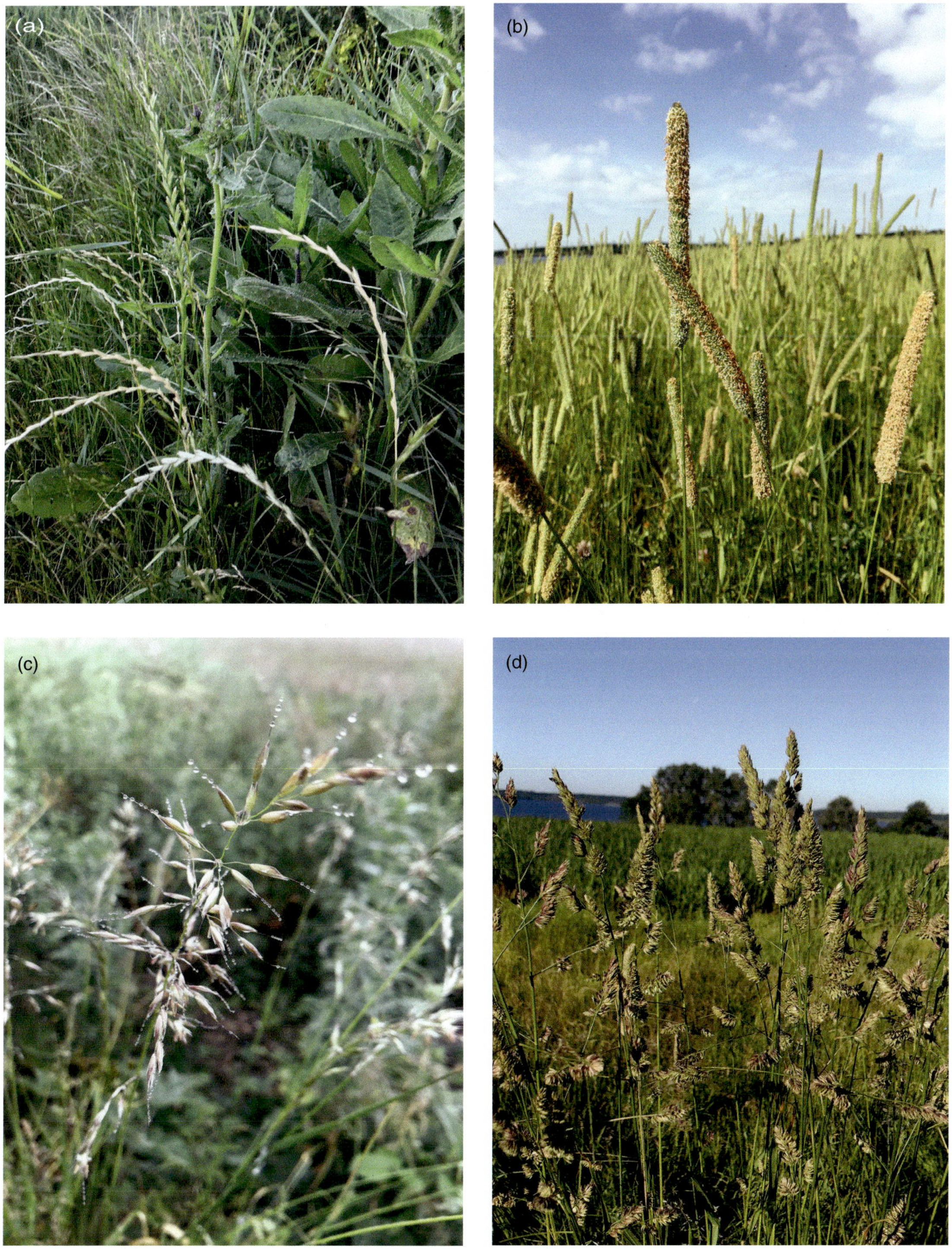

Fig. 4.1 Examples of grass species: (a) perennial ryegrass; (b) timothy; (c) fescue; (d) cocksfoot.

recognise that forage quality is inversely related to the amount of cell wall and lignification, with straw being the lowest in quality and digestibility.

Top tip

- Digestibility (the extent to which forage is absorbed as it passes through an animal's digestive tract) varies greatly.
- Young, leafy grass may be 80–90% digested, while less than 50% of mature, stemmy grass is digested.
- If you read a forage analysis (see Chapter 9: Figs 9.1, 9.2) the number that gives the best indication of digestibility is neutral detergent fibre (NDF).

As forages mature, the proportion of stem cell walls and lignin increase to provide strength to the stem to support the flower and seed head. At the same time, the percentage of leaf decreases (remember that leaves are higher in nutritive value compared with stems).

The fibre in the stem of timothy grass can be as high as 72% NDF (DM) whereas leaf is only 49% NDF; the stem contains 5.8% protein compared with 18% in the leaves (Collins 1988). Most cool-season grasses (growing best between 15°C and 24°C) require a period of cool temperatures (vernalization) for flowering and produce reproductive stems in the spring. Reproductive growth lowers leaf-to-stem ratio. Bear in mind that the forage quality of regrowth of these grasses is greater and changes less over time because they have higher leaf-to-stem ratios than first-growth forage.

How much grass a horse might eat is dependent upon the stage of growth but there are multiple factors that need to be taken into account. You might assume that the more grass there is, the more the horse can eat, but intake is dependent upon whether there is a lot of young grass (high in water/cell contents) or a lot of mature grass (higher in cell walls/fibre). Horses' jaws are well adapted to cropping short grass and can graze even when the grass is as short as 2 cm, unlike cows, which need a sward height of more than 6 cm (Table 4.5).

Clients might assume that horses choose short rather than long grass because of the higher nutrient value of short grass. But the higher digestibility of short grass has to be set against the effort required to obtain the nutrition: short grass requires more bites to consume the dry matter compared with long grass and horses adapt to eating long grass by consuming more per bite (Naujeck and Hill, 2003). In fact, horses when given the choice between grasses of different lengths actually maximise voluntary intake by spending more time eating long grass compared with short grass (Naujeck *et al.*, 2005). Intake will also be influenced by pasture management. Naujeck and Hill (2003) showed that on a well-managed pasture, horses will walk continuously whilst grazing and graze the pasture evenly unless roughs develop due to faecal build up. Ponies, on the other hand, seem to prefer shorter grasses which have a higher digestibility (Gordon, 1989). Intake also depends upon seasonal influences on nutrient quality of the forages. If protein is adequate, horses will select longer grass (tall height/poor quality to maximise dry matter intake (DMI)) but if protein is low, then horses will select shorter grass (lower height/high quality) and so reduce their DMI (Edouard *et al.*, 2010). If horses have access to grasses at different stages of growth (which is possible if clients manage the pasture), then the horses will eat both swards, balancing protein and energy needs with fibre needs (Edouard *et al.*, 2010). Clients need to be aware of these variables and be able to adjust their horses' access to grazing by monitoring their horse's fat scores (see Chapter 3: 'Body fat scoring').

Advising clients to manage the growth stage of their grass

Clients can also manage their pasture to minimise the impact of changing calorie content by cutting the grass.

Perennial ryegrass that is defoliated to the 1 or 2 leaf tiller stage by cutting to 2 cm contains less water-soluble carbohydrates (WSCs) compared with grass cut to 6 cm (Lee *et al.*, 2010); frequently cut grass contains 30–50% less water-soluble carbohydrates in the stubble compared with grass left to grow to 6 leaves, (Lee *et al.*, 2009).

Similarly, taller swards have higher levels of soluble carbohydrates (including starch) than short swards (Siciliano, 2015) and rotational grazing (longer grass) compared with continuous grazing (short grass) was higher in fructans and sugar but lower in protein (Williams *et al.*, 2019).

If clients can keep grass growth to 1 leaf height, then quantities of grass will stay low (15% pasture growth versus 40% at 2 leaf) (Lee *et al.*, 2010). If you are concerned about fructans, which are

Table 4.5 A comparison between the jaw anatomy of herbivores and their ability to graze (adapted from Armstrong, 1993)

	Horse	Cow	Rabbit
Prehension	Lips and incisor teeth, cutting or biting of the vegetation, upper and lower incisors	Long, muscular tongue pulls grass/hay into mouth, shearing it between lower incisors and upper gum (no upper incisors) by upward movement of head and neck	Bite/tear, upper and lower incisors
Jaw anatomy adaptation	Chewing cycle an opening stroke, a closing stroke and a power stroke. Lateroventral movement of the working side during the opening stroke and a marked mediodorsal movement of the working side during the power stroke (Adams *et al*., 2016)	Selection for higher masticatory forces during chewing; and flattening of the molar and premolar profile. Sideways movement of jaw plays an important role in grinding and chewing (Pérez-Barbería and Gordon, 1999)	A crushing movement, jaw maintains a rotation to the working side (occurs in carrot and frequently in pellet mastication), and a shearing movement where the jaw rotates back to the midline, with an occasional slight over-rotation to the balancing side (occurs in hay) (Weijs and Dantuma, 1980)
Sward height	Selective 2 cm. Prefer grass with high digestibility	Slightly selective, > 6 cm rough vegetation	Very highly selective, 1 cm, avoid aromatic and low-digestibility plants
Chewing	Mechanical breakdown Chew 1/s; 3600 chews/h Swallow when < 4 mm (Vervuert *et al*., 2010)	0.2 chews/s; 734 chews/h (Bailey and Balch, 1961) initial consumption, grass not chewed – only after initial fermentation as part of rumination	Rapid intake, 0.96 chews/s; 2.3–8.5 chews/g (Ravosa *et al*., 2015)
Fibre 'digestion'	Physical breakdown of cell walls allows some fermentation in stomach and enzymic digestion of cell contents in small intestine. Fibre fermented in hind gut	Foregut fermentation to break down cell walls – interspersed with regurgitation and 2nd and 3rd chewing cycles until fibre particles (with bacteria attached) small enough to pass to abomasum (true stomach)	Fibre partially fermented in hind gut due to rate of passage and smaller hind gut – consumes faecal caecotrophs – enzymic digestion of bacterial protein, vitamins and minerals and 2nd fibre fermentation

fermented in the small intestine to volatile fatty acids (Coenan *et al.*, 2006) and protective in the hind gut (Respondek *et al.*, 2008), then be aware that they are higher in stubble than in leaves, (Lee *et al.*, 2010) – something we have known since the 1950s (Waite and Boyd 1953) – and if grass stays very short then white clover (which stores starch) finds it easier to compete with the grass (Lee *et al.*, 2009).

Horses grazing short grass (15 cm) ate less grass (0.24–0.66% BW) and had lowered insulin and glucose responses compared to horses grazing long grass (40cm) who consumed 2.36–2.42% BW (Siciliano *et al.*, 2017).

Top tip

Cutting grass maintains it in a regrowth phase (in the spring and autumn), which means the grass uses up its stored WSC and thus keeps the sugar levels lower (and there is less grass for the horse to eat).

You can reassure your clients that the capacity of their horse's small intestine enzymes (disaccharidases sucrase, lactase and maltase) to digest and absorb grass sugars is high when they are grazing (Dyer *et al.*, 2002).

Conservation

There are times through the year when grass growth stops and it is vital that other fibre sources are available to maintain gut health and to replicate the normal eating behaviour of horses. A variety of conserved forages can be fed to horses, including hay, haylage, straw and sugar beet, to provide fibre.

You will find that clients have some interesting ideas about the feed value of conserved forages, when they can be fed and how much should be fed. Do listen but be prepared to explain using an evidence-based approach, probably on more than one occasion. There are two main methods of forage conservation: drying and pickling.

Drying

Grass

Hay is grass that has been grown past flowering and is often cut at seeding stage; it is mature grass, with low levels of sugar and high levels of structural carbohydrates. It is usually cut (depending on the weather) mid to late July but some years late June is not uncommon. It is left to dry in the field for 3–5 days and turned to encourage moisture loss until it is 'dry' (< 15% moisture) (Fig. 4.2).

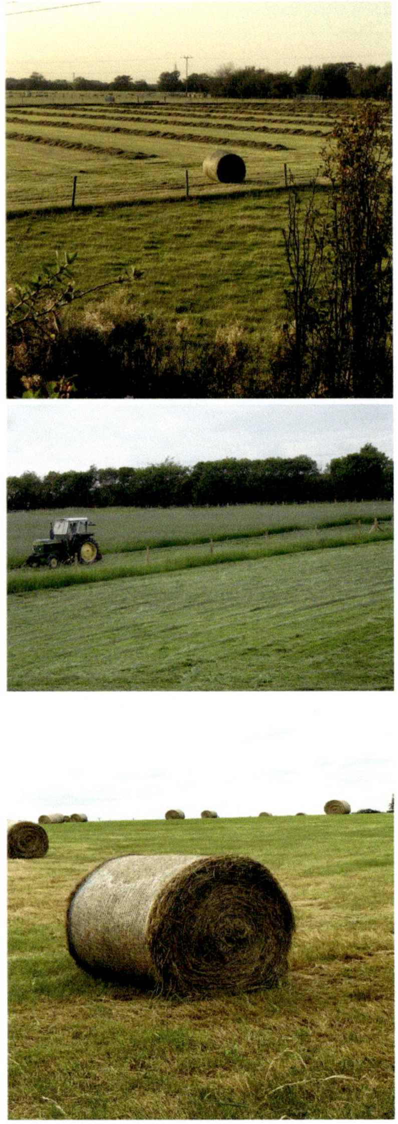

Fig. 4.2 Hay making.

Certain factors can reduce the nutrient content of the grass as it is being dried; these include leaf loss, plant respiration and leaching by rainfall. Clients do not normally have access to the harvesting circumstances unless they have made their own; check the hay for leaf:stem ratios, check the colour and get it analysed (see Chapter 9: 'Interpreting forage analysis'). Grass that lies in the field for more than 2 weeks for curing should not be fed to horses. Physical, biological and chemical changes occur in forage as it dries in the field (Rotz and Muck, 1994), with an increase in mycotoxins rendering it unsuitable for feeding to horses.

Drying stops plant enzyme activity and the grass (now hay) is stable as long as it stays dry. Rewetting of the crop by dew or rain reactivates enzyme activity and the feed value of the hay will be reduced. Soluble carbohydrates are the principal compounds used in respiration with little loss of total nitrogen (N) and fibre. Rain also leaches soluble plant nutrients from the drying grass, having a similar effect to soaking hay (Fig. 4.3)

If hay has not been dried properly, then the grass will continue to respire because the bacteria, yeasts and fungi on the grass are using the moisture to ferment the grass. Fermentation can cause the bales to heat and the dry matter is lost as heat and gases. Damp haybales in the middle of a stack are a fire hazard and of course damp hay should not be fed.

If dry hay is stored under cover (Fig. 4.4), little heating occurs and DM loss over 6 months of storage is about 5% (Rotz and Muck, 1994). Hay stored outside is not normally suitable for feeding to horses and dry matter loss is greater (10–15%) as the hay deteriorates (Fig. 4.5). You can recognise this deterioration as the hay changes to brown in colour and often looks more

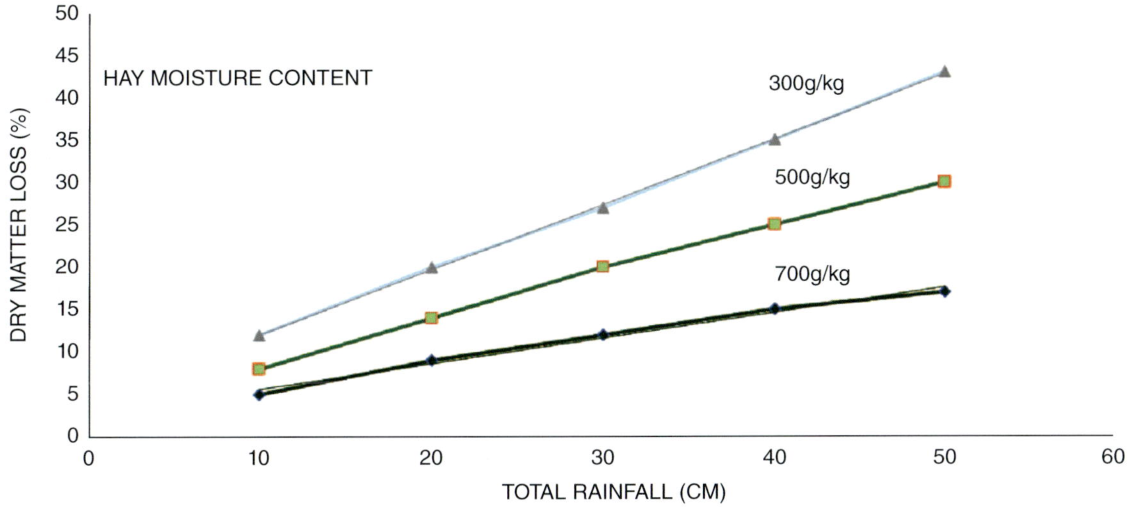

Fig. 4.3 The relationship between hay moisture content, dry matter losses and rainfall. (Used with permission from Rotz and Muck, 1994.)

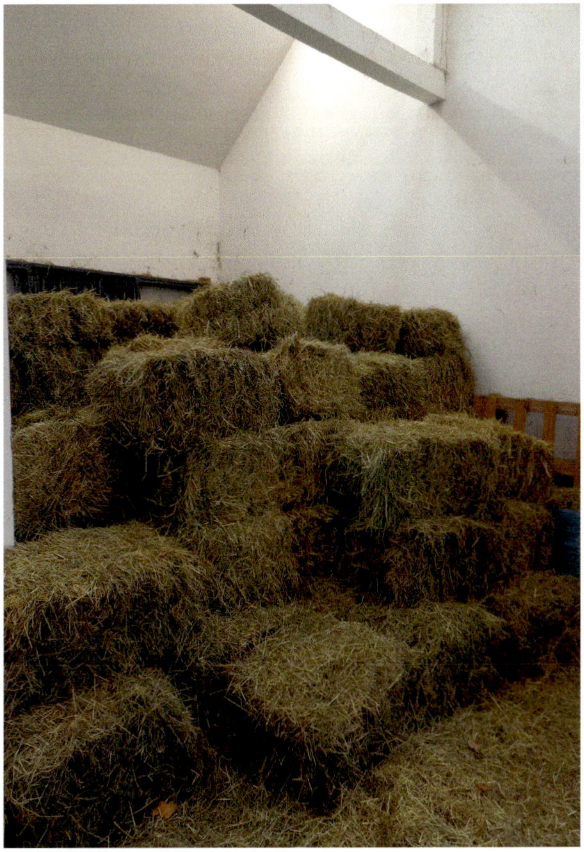

Fig. 4.4 Hay needs storing under cover.

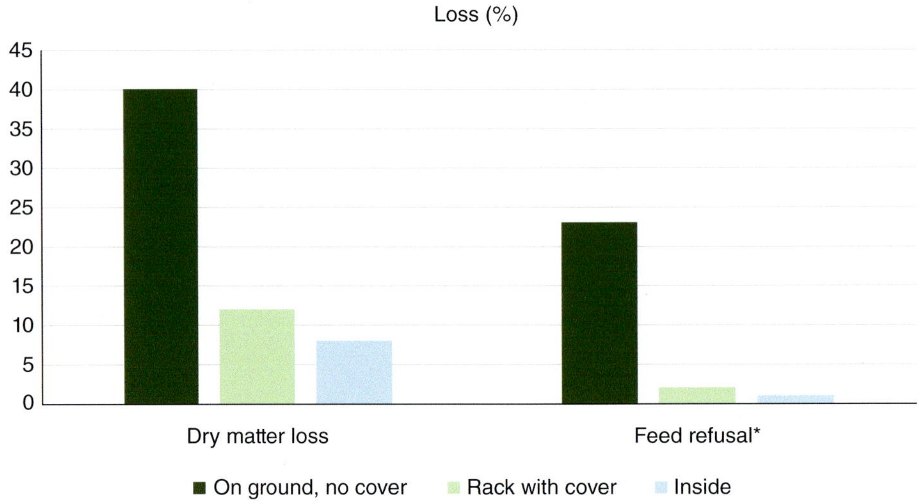

Fig. 4.5 The effect of hay storage on dry matter loss and feed refusal. (Used with permission from Verma and Nelson, 1983.)

like straw. Clearly you should be advising that hay is stored protected from the weather, under cover.

When to advise feeding new hay

Some of your clients might want confirmation as to how soon after harvest they can feed 'new' hay; they think they must wait 6 months before they can feed the hay and can be anxious if they do not have enough hay left from the previous year.

Timing of feeding relative to harvest depends purely on how well the grass was dried and whether the grass is still respiring. Hay that has been dried properly to 85% dry matter (less than 150 g moisture/kg hay) is stable, little respiration occurs and it can be fed as soon as it has been stored in a barn. Hay that is stored wetter than 15% moisture will continue to dry and respire until it reaches an equilibrium at 15%; this hay should not be fed until it is stable.

Do remind owners not to store hay bales directly on the ground, where they will absorb water; stacking and storing on pallets allows air to circulate. In terms of nutrients, over time there is a loss of protein, minerals and vitamins; hay that has lost its green colour is unlikely to contribute much to vitamin requirements as they will have been oxidised. Mineral content will reflect the original grass crop minus any leaching during drying. Once baled, the hay must be protected from the weather and stored under cover to prevent it getting wet.

Even good-quality hay contains a high level of dust (plant fragments, fungal spores, mites and bacteria) that can lead to asthma (previously recurrent airway obstruction).

Straw

Straw is the by-product of cereal production and is the mature stem that is left over once the grain has been thrashed and removed (Fig. 4.6). This forage (stem) is left on the field to dry and then baled and it can be a valuable source of low-nutrient fibre for horses that tend to gain weight and get fat easily. Mixing straw with high-temperature alfalfa or higher-quality hay is very common and is widely marketed as an alternative to other forages for horses. Straw normally costs less per tonne compared with hay, but this may change as it becomes a useful substrate for biofuels.

Similar to other forages, availability will be dependent upon weather. If straw gets repeatedly soaked it will disintegrate and be impossible to bale. Often farmers need to drill new crops and cannot wait for the straw to dry and will plough the straw into the soil. When harvest conditions are challenging, farmers tend to keep the straw for their own livestock rather than sell on the open market and prices will reflect scarcity. The UK produces around 10,000 tonnes of straw (SRUC, 2018). Horses tend to eat less straw compared with hay but straw can

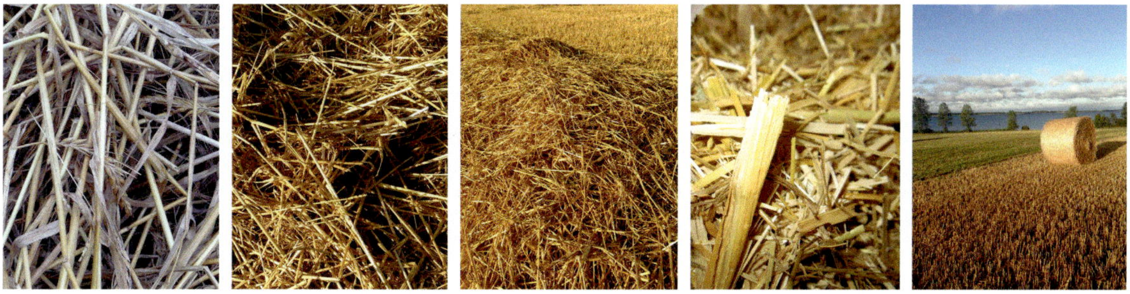

Fig. 4.6 Straw.

Table 4.6 Nutrient values[a] of dried cereal forage crops/straw (% DM)

Forage	Protein	NDF	Lignin	DE MJ/kg DM
Barley straw	3.8 (1.9–6)	80.5 (69–89)	6.5 (4.1–9)	5 (3–6)
Barley hay	8.7 (3.9–13)	53 (31–64)	2.3 (1.4–3)	10 (9–11)
Oat straw	3.6 (2–6)	76 (68–83)	6.5 (5.5–7.5)	8 (7–9)
Oat hay	9 (5–14)	61 (51–73)	4 (2–6.5)	9 (8–10)

[a]Adapted from https://www.feedipedia.org and from commercial lab analysis

still provide excess calories (more than 34–51% of energy requirements) to ponies, whilst only just meeting the energy requirements for donkeys (Pearson *et al.*, 2001). This is because ponies will eat more straw compared with horses and donkeys (Cuddeford *et al.*, 1995), although donkeys can digest and utilise more of the straw compared with horses and ponies due to the slower transit time.

The nutritional quality of straw may vary from year to year due to effects of environmental conditions; weathering will influence composition and quality of the most nutritious parts of cereal residues, and suitability will be determined by the cereal crop. Wheat straw should not be advised for horses, due to the high lignin and silica content, although clients will be happy to tell you about their horses that eat their wheat-straw beds without any adverse effects.

It is important to note that in Canada and America, oat and barley crop chaff is fed. 'Cereal crop chaff consists of smaller particles than straw and contains glumes, hulls, parts of heads, short straw, leaf materials, weed seeds, and whole or cracked kernels separated from harvested grain' (McCartney *et al.*, 2006). Additionally, oat and barley forage/hay might be harvested if the weather indicates that the crop will not grow to completion and the crop is cut whilst the grain is still at a milky stage – this is more digestible and higher in nutrients compared with straw (Table 4.6). Make sure your clients understand your descriptors.

Fermentation

Haylage is grass that has been preserved through fermentation, by excluding oxygen in a similar way to pickling vegetables (onions, gherkins). Haylage is dustless compared with dried grass (hay) and feeding haylage rather than hay (as well as swapping straw for shavings) can halve airborne dust and reduce endotoxin concentrations (Whittaker *et al.*, 2009). Grass for haylage is cut earlier than hay, normally 2 weeks earlier, just as or before the grass comes into flower. The reason that the grass needs to be younger is that the fermentation process needs sugar in the cell contents for the bacteria to 'pickle' the grass. The grass is not wilted/dried for so long, as moisture is also needed for the fermentation process – typically grass is left to wilt to around 50% moisture before being collected and made into small bales (15–20 kg) and around 30% moisture for making into big bales ($^1/_4$–½ tonne).

The grass is wrapped in several layers of plastic to create anaerobic conditions similar to the horse's hind gut. This means that the lactic acid bacteria naturally present on the grass can use the sugars to grow,

> **Top tip**
>
> - Some clients might be wary of the fact that the haylage is lower in pH compared with hay.
>   - Lactic acid is a tasty acid and good conservation relies on its presence.
>   - The acidity of a horse's stomach is considerably lower than the haylage.
> - Generally, a haylage would have a higher pH if the grass was drier, indicating that the fermentation has been restricted because there was not enough water in the original grass crop.
> - The drier the grass when it was cut before it was wrapped, the less complete the fermentation, and so the haylage:
>   - will be less acidic;
>   - have less lactic acid and potentially higher levels of sugar; and
>   - it may be less stable.
> - Eating haylage has no direct effect on the pH of the hind gut.
>   - Haylage is not acidic.
>   - Chewing haylage produces copious amounts of alkaline saliva. The bolus of haylage will be less acidic compared with the lower stomach; and it then passes through the alkaline small intestine.

producing the same organic acids, which lowers the pH (increased acidity). The lowering of the pH eventually kills the bacteria and stops the plant enzymes. This can take from 7 to 30 days and the haylage is at that point stable and able to be fed (Table 4.7).

If pH does not drop enough in wetter haylages, then aerobic bacteria such as *Listeria* sp. will proliferate and yeasts might grow.

You should not advise feeding haylage that is contaminated with soil or any bales that have been exposed to air for more than 4 days. Once the grass is exposed to oxygen the preservation is no longer intact and secondary fermentation will occur after a few days, which produces undesirable by-products.

Haylage can be stored outside, preferably off the ground, but clients need to check that there is no damage to the wrapping on a regular basis. Once the haylage is exposed to oxygen, it is no longer stable, and the forage will start to deteriorate. Haylage will vary in nutritional value in the same way that the original grass crop will be variable. The time of cutting and whether it is taken from a first or second cut will also affect the feed value (Table 4.8) (Ragnarsson and Lindberg, 2008).

Table 4.7 Stages of fermentation in preserving grass as haylage

1st stage	**2nd stage**	**3rd stage**	**4th stage**	**5th stage**
Respiration	Early fermentation	Lactic acid fermentation	Temperature drops	Stabilisation
The cut grass is still respiring and will use up the oxygen that was incorporated when the grass was baled and wrapped. The temperature will rise	Aerobic bacteria at this stage grow and produce acetic acid and other organic acids. pH starts to drop, oxygen used up. Plant enzymes continue to respire	Anaerobic bacteria (mainly lactic acid) ferment the sugars-starts 3–5 days after baling and acetic acid production drops. Plant enzymes stop	Lactic acid production continues for around 2 weeks. The bale's temperature drops to match the weather	Acid drops which in turn kills the bacteria, fungi and moulds. This takes around 20 days and at this stage the haylage is stable and can be fed
Finished product-after stabilisation, the haylage is available in various wrappings and sizes				
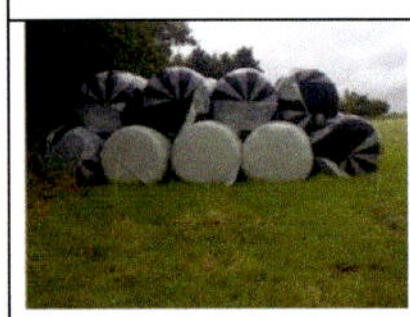	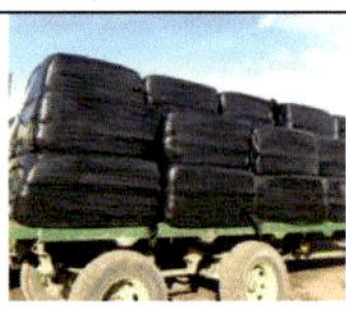	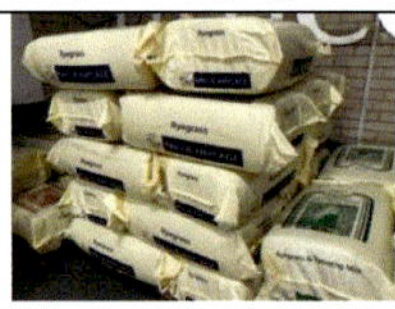	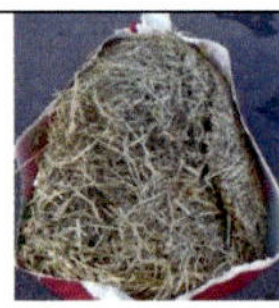	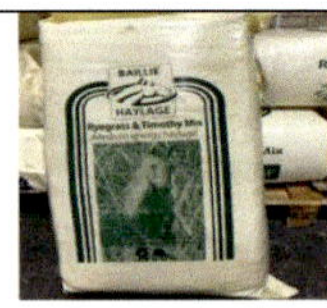
Tonne round bales	Tonne square bales	20 kg small bales	Longer and drier compared to silage	Small 20kg bale

Table 4.8 The effect of time of cutting on the nutritional value of haylage (g/kg DM) (adapted from Ragnarsson and Lindberg, 2008)

	CUT 1	CUT 2	CUT 3	CUT 4
Dry matter	469	501	430	447
Organic matter	918	940	946	937
Crude protein	175	132	102	93
Crude fibre	256	318	352	347
Ether extract	41	33	29	28
Sugars[a]	62	62	28	26
Neutral detergent fibre	503	593	639	615
	Fermentative characteristics			
pH	5.6	4.7	5.1	5.0
Lactic acid	4.2	7.5	11.1	10.2
Acetic acid	1.6	1.3	3.6	3.4
Butyric acid	< 0.1	< 0.1	1.2	< 0.1
Propionic acid	< 0.2	< 0.2	< 0.2	< 0.2

[a]Glucose + (fructose+sucrose+fructans)

Top tip

- Do familiarise yourself with the different haylages available.
- Be able to recognise:
  - the seed heads in the bales; and
  - good haylage versus haylage that has started to deteriorate.
  - The smell is a good indicator.
    - If it smells of cheesy feet, this is a sign that it is high in butyrate and indicates that the fermentation is incomplete –
    - usually because the grass was too wet or because the grass wasn't packed well enough and did not exclude all the oxygen.
- Lactic acid provides that sweet smell of a well fermented haylage and is considered the 'tasty' organic acid.

Preferences, Digestibility and Intake Comparisons of Common Forages Fed to Horses

Clients will have different views on which forage their horse prefers and the potential impact on gut health and behaviour. Some of these views will be based on research but it is important to note that many of the researchers compared forages with quite different analysis and this would confound the results. A useful comparison can be made by using the results from a sward of grass that was cut at the same maturity and botanical composition and made into hay, 2 types of haylage and silage (Table 4.9).

When horses were fed these forages, they chose to eat silage in preference to the other forages – 85% of the time they ate the silage more quickly, consuming more, and hay was the least preferred of all the forages (Muller and Uden, 2007). The silage was balage and not clamp silage with a fermentation profile closer to haylage; clamp silage is often higher in acetic acid and may have a lower pH, making it less palatable for horses. The completeness of fermentation might also affect palatability: the less sugar in the final product, the more complete is the fermentation. These factors are worth considering when advising forages to support weight gain or fat loss.

It is important that owners have a good understanding of the differences in the fibre sources available for feeding to their horses (Table 4.10) to help them choose the most appropriate grass replacement as well as ensuring that the correct amount of forage is fed to prevent any disease associated with a reduction in fibre intake.

Other fibre sources

Do remember you can discuss and advise other fibre sources, especially as climate change continues to impact on the availability of grass and straw. In fact, when horses are given a choice of fibre sources (leafy hazel twigs, fibre cubes, large swedes and carrots, ryegrass haylage, ryegrass/timothy haylage, heat-dried grass chaff, molassed oat straw chaff and molassed alfalfa chaff) they prefer all of them compared with hay (Goodwin *et al.*, 2002). Providing multiple fibre sources also encourages foraging behaviour (see Chapter 9: 'Allowing horses to exhibit foraging behaviour'); a grass shortage should not mean the fibre intake of horses is compromised.

Chaffs

Any forage can be dried and then chopped typically to 2–3 cm to produce a chaff; common examples are alfalfa (lucerne), grass, straw (Fig. 4.7) and mixed in various ratios to provide different levels of calories and protein. Some manufacturers will add extra ingredients to chaff to provide a balanced bucket feed. Do check to see if the forages are grown in the UK, preferably close to the drying plants, improving their environmental credentials.

Alfalfa

Alfalfa is grown specifically for cutting and high-temperature drying for horse. It is usually cut pre-flower and retains its green colour due to the rapid

Table 4.9 Effect of conservation (hay, haylage or silage) of the same grass sward on its nutrient composition (adapted from Muller and Uden, 2007)

Analysis *g/kg DM unless stated FM (fresh mass)*	Hay (*n* = 4)	High dry matter haylage (*n* = 5)	Low dry matter haylage (*n* = 5)	Silage (*n* = 9)
Dry matter (g/kg)	884	684	577	309
Ash	64	68	66	66
Crude protein	108	116	110	113
Estimated digestible crude protein	70	77	72	74
Neutral detergent fibre	605	607	608	585
Water-soluble carbohydrates	101	71	69	26
Lactic acid	na	0.3	2.6	31.8
Acetic acid	na	0.6	1.4	6.6
Butyric acid	na	< 0.4	< 0.4	1.0
pH	na	5.81	5.63	4.94
Ammonia-N	na	0.2	0.3	0.7
Lactic acid bacteria (×10^3 CFU/g FM)	na	35	1900	8000
Clostridia (×10^3 CFU/g FM)	nd	0.054	0.29	90
Enterobacteria (×10^3 CFU/g FM)	260	nd	0.65	nd
Yeasts (×10^3 CFU/g FM)	0.47	170	340	160
Moulds (×10^3 CFU/g FM)	0.23	nd	nd	0.055 b

Table 4.10 The differences between hay, haylage and straw

	Hay	Haylage	Straw (barley and oat)
When harvested (cut)	Usually just after seeding (dependent upon weather, typically by mid/late July)	Usually after flowering but before seeding (dependent upon weather, typically by early July)	After the cereal crop has been harvested
How cut/processed	Full length, left to wilt until loses 85% of its water content. Turned frequently	Full length, left to wilt until loses 50–70% of its water	Full length, normally dry when cut – should not be fed if left in field for > 2 weeks after grain harvest
How preserved	Baled when dry	Wrapped in plastic to form bales to maintain water content and exclude oxygen. Fermentation until sugar used up and pH dropped, which kills bacteria and stops the fermentation, resulting in a stable product in about 20 days	Baled when dried
How stored	In barns/under cover to keep dry	Stacked as bales, can be left outside as long as no danger of puncturing plastic	In barns/under cover to keep dry
Nutrient analysis (per kg as fed)	Moisture content 15% Protein 7–10% Water-soluble carbohydrates 8% Calories 7–9 MJ DE	Moisture content 25–50% Protein 4–7% Water-soluble carbohydrates 2–5% Calories 4–6 MJ DE	Moisture content 12% Protein 3–6% Water-soluble carbohydrates 0–2% Calories 3–5 MJ DE

and controlled drying conditions (Fig. 4.8), making it easy to recognise.

Alfalfa leaf is the most nutritious part of the plant (the leaf helps distinguish it from grass chaff, which has less leaf) but tends to be friable, so it is mixed with molasses or oil before packaging in a plastic-wrapped bale to ensure even distribution throughout the bale. Alfalfa is an excellent source

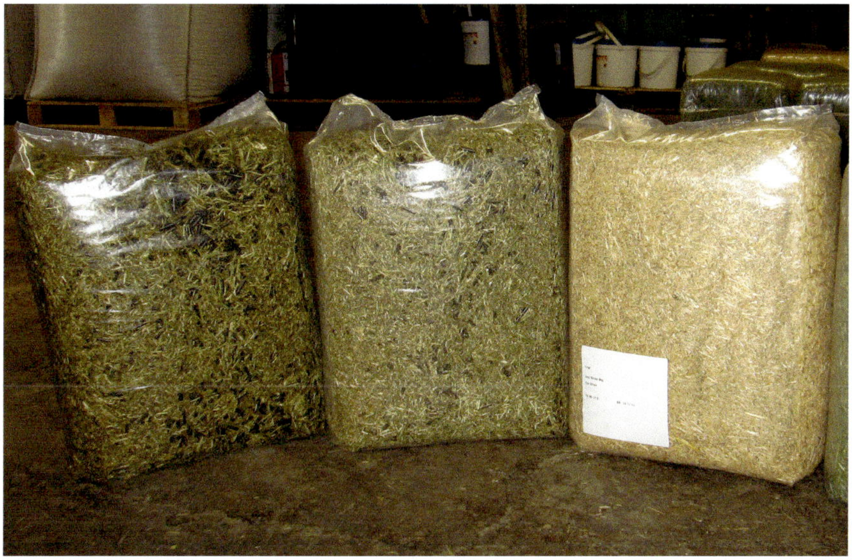

Fig. 4.7 Examples of chaffs.

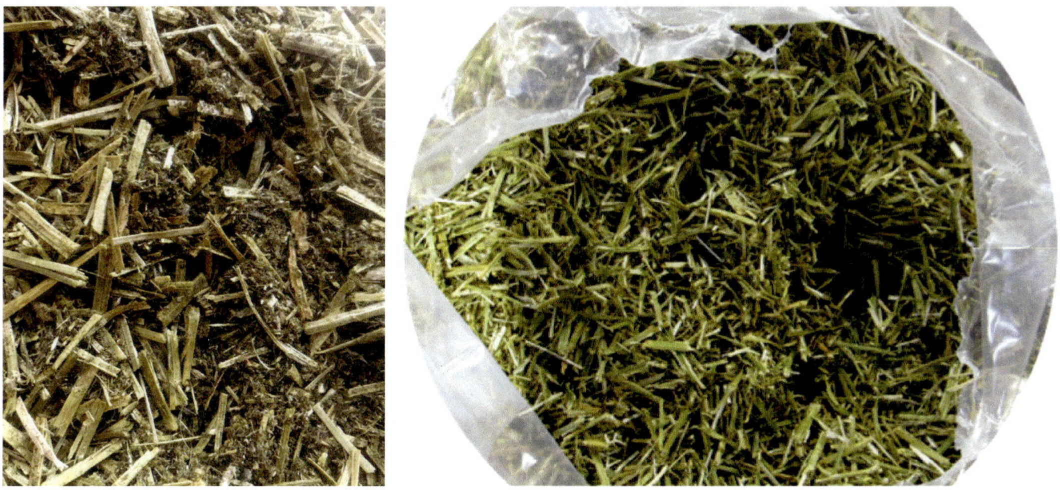

Fig. 4.8 Alfalfa chaff.

of quality protein (16%) and calcium (Cuddeford *et al.*, 1990) and has a similar digestible energy (10 MJ DE/kg as fed) to oats (Cuddeford *et al.*, 1992), making it ideal for the performance horse or the old horse losing weight/muscle.

Grass chaff

Sometimes but not always specifically grown for making chaff, the stage of growth and species can vary and thus so does the nutrient value: the greener the grass chaff, the better is the nutrient value (Fig. 4.9). Grass is also available as pellets, which provide fibre but needs 1200 chews/kg as opposed to 4600 chews/kg chaff.

Straw chaffs

These should be barley or oat straw. Some manufacturers will state cereal straw to allow them to include different straws according to availability. Straw chaffs are ideal as low-calorie chaffs (Fig. 4.10) to

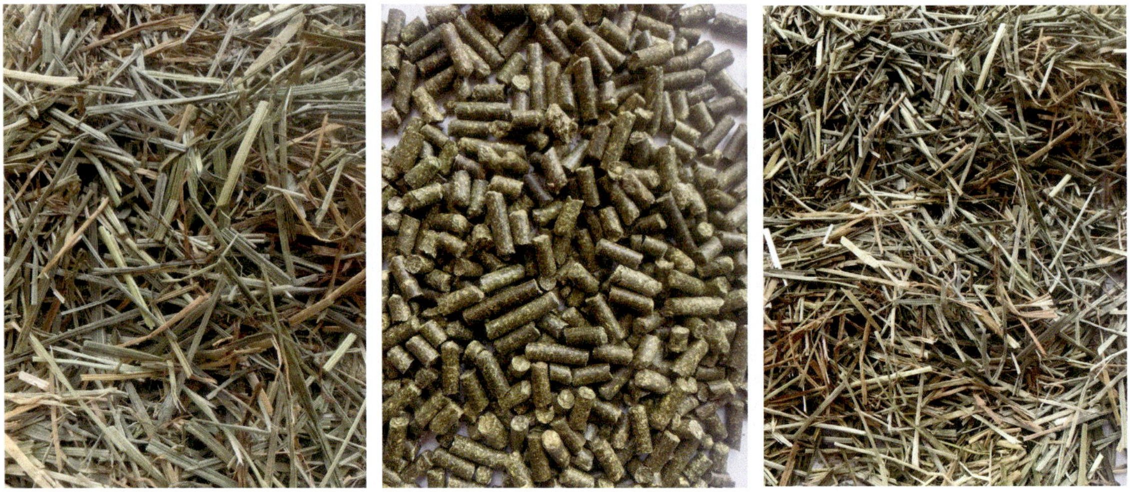

Fig. 4.9 Grass chaff.

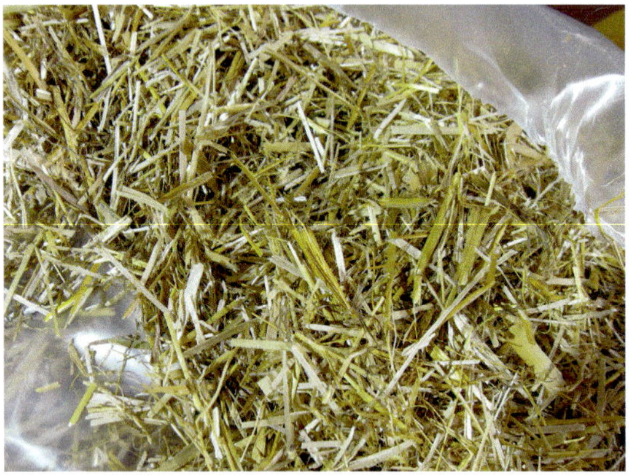

Fig. 4.10 Straw chaff.

add to a balancer (see Chapter 5) for overweight horses, unless large quantities of molasses are added. The addition of up to 40% molasses changes the value of a straw chaff and can be likened to empty calories obtained from cakes for ourselves.

Sugar beet

Sugar beet is a root vegetable grown in East Anglia within 30 miles of the drying plant to produce sugar for the food industry; sugar beet shreds and pellets are a by-product of that process, thus reducing food waste. The by-product is a high-fibre feedstuff which is low in sugar and protein. The fibre is predominantly fermented (63%) in the hind gut of the horse, but up to 16% of the sugar beet fibre is soluble enough to be absorbed from the small intestine (Moore-Colyer *et al.*, 2002; Hyslop, 2006). Sugar beet fermentation maintains a healthy pH in the hind gut, similar to that in hay-fed ponies, with the researchers concluding that sugar beet offers an alternative to hay (Moore-Colyer *et al.*, 2000) to provide the fibre component of the diet.

Feeding sugar beet improves the health of the hind gut compared with hay alone.

- It increases the number of cellulytic bacteria and VFA production (Grimm *et al.*, 2021) because it is better feed source for the bacteria, which also means that the bacteria ferment the hay more, increasing its feed value.
- It removes ammonia from the hind gut, resulting in faecal rather than renal excretion of nitrogen, which results in a lower load for the liver (Olsman *et al.*, 2004).

Sugar beet is available as pellets or chaff (Fig. 4.11) and as molassed or unmolassed, with the molassed being higher in calories. Pellets, whilst providing fibre, will not meet the horse's psychological need to chew compared with shreds.

Remember that sugar beet must be soaked overnight if pellets, and for 6 h if shreds, in twice its volume of water, making it invaluable as a succulent and relatively low-calorie fibre in proportion to the volume fed for clients wanting to feed their horse 'something' (Fig. 4.12).

Fortunately, clients have a large choice of fibre for their horses. If you are advising clients for competition

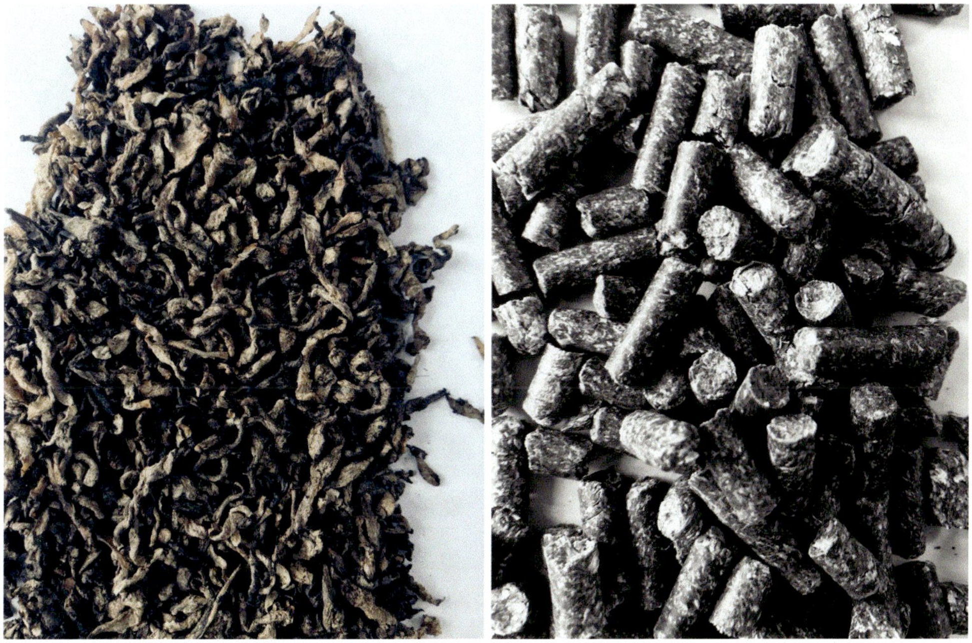

Fig. 4.11 Sugar beet pellets and shreds.

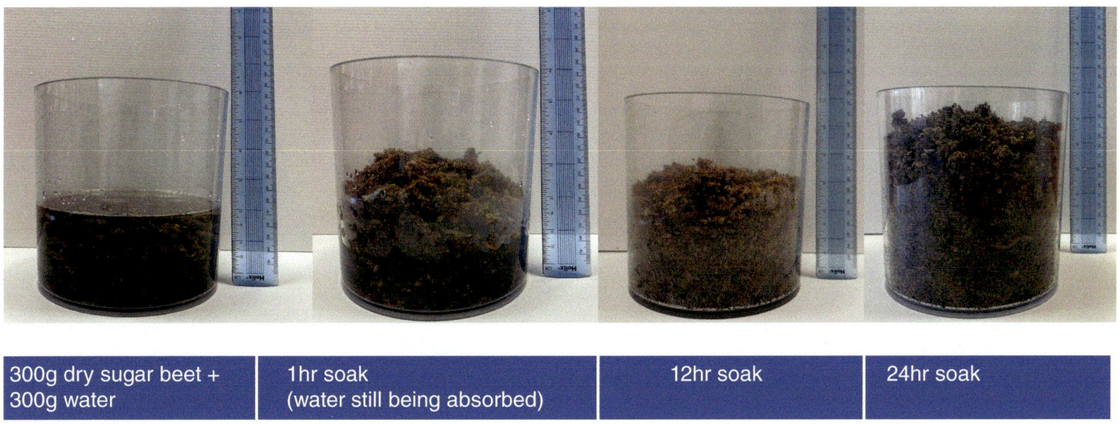

Fig. 4.12 Sugar beet needs soaking in the same weight of water before being fed.

or clinically comprised horses, then you should consider taking a forage sample for analysis.

Taking a Forage Sample

A simple way for clients to check the availability of grass is the supermarket bag grab (see Chapter 11: 'Controlling and monitoring grass intake'). Professional yards need to take a more quantitative approach.

How to measure grass quantity and quality

On large studs or commercial operations, you should work out the grass dry matter availability by using quadrats.

- Cut and collect the grass from the grazing area using randomly thrown quadrats of known area (note how many), following a W and collecting from the top and bottom of the W.

- Weigh the collected grass, dry[i] and calculate the mean dry matter in a square metre.
- Find the acreage of the field from google maps and then calculate the amount of grass dry matter in the field.
- A similar W sampling pattern should be used to collect grass for analysis, which should be sealed in a plastic bag and sent immediately to the lab, or stored in a cold box until back at the practice.

Grass availability should be based on accurate sampling and not an assumption of season. Despite an excess of grass (Table 4.11), ponies were fed extra hay in the field and the hay was not soaked at night, resulting in a 3% increase in BW in field B with subsequent increases in fat score. It is important to support clients in objective measurements: perception can prejudice health.

Sampling hay or haylage for analysis

As you might appreciate, taking a handful of hay from one bale is not representative and thus multiple samples need to be taken and then a subsample (see Chapter 7, Fig. 7.9: 'How to subsample') sent to the laboratory.

For hay sampling: split open bales across the front, middle and back of stack to take grab samples. If the yard objects to this idea, then using a drill or corer is more appropriate and you would need to use a corer for haylage and then reseal the holes. To minimise bias, use the same W pattern as you did for grazing.

What you need

Corer, bucket or plastic sheet, gloves, plastic bags, waterproof marker pens, cold box.

Table 4.11 Changes in grass dry matter availability in early winter as measured by quadrat sampling

	Calculated grass availability (kg DM/field)[a]		
Field	October	November[b]	Change in grass DM (kg/field)
A	1191	1160	–39
B	1399	1690	+280
C	2543	2493	–49

[a]Calculated from field hectares × DM in sampled quadrats; e.g. field A = 93 g DM grass; field B = 300 g DM grass
[b]Hay was provided because it was winter; horses were gaining 3% BW/week in field B in November and their fat scores increased

What to do

Take a grab sample at each point of the W at different depths of the bales across the stack or use a corer (essential if doing haylage; remember to tape up the hole afterwards).

- Put the samples into your bucket/sheet.
  - Mix thoroughly.
  - Subsample until you have around 0.5–1 kg.
- Put into your plastic freezer bag.
  - Remove the air.
  - Seal.
  - Label clearly with yard, type of forage and which cut/season if you know.
  - Don't forget contact details.
- Try not to sample on a Friday, as moisture loss will affect your results.
- Store in your cold box, but send to the lab as soon as possible.
- Make sure you have paid the lab.

The lab will send you an analytical report, which you should explain to the client (see Chapter 9: 'Interpreting forage analysis') and this will aid in advising how much to feed and what else is needed to balance the diet.

Summary: Fibre First and Foremost

- Forage should be the foundation of the diet to reduce the risks of gastric ulcers, colic, stereotypies and endotoxaemia.
- Anything else is fed to balance the deficiencies of the forage, whether that is in terms of calories (energy) or micronutrients.
- All horses should be fed as close to 2.5% of their bodyweight as possible (dry matter).
  - If you are advising an owner of a leisure horse, then this will be 90%+ forage.
  - If a competition horse, then this could vary from 80% to 50% forage and 20–50% concentrates by weight (see Chapter 5, Table 5.12: 'Advising the correct type of energy relative to the horse's workload and client's perception of character').
  - As the workload of the horse increases, the amount of forage is generally decreased. But forage for competition horses should never be fed at less than 50% of dry matter intake by weight.
- The feed value of the forage should be a key determinant in your advice.
- You must adjust for the water and calorie content of any forages you advise.

    - Haylage fed must meet the dry matter requirements of the horse.
    - High-calorie forages might need soaking or replacing with lower-calorie alternatives
- Ideally the horse should always have access to forage. If this is not feasible, encourage owners to consider ways of slowing down consumption (see Chapter 9: 'Replicating natural eating time budgets').

Forages and the fibre they contain are of vital importance for the health of the horse. Please remind clients on a regular basis about the five Fs: fibre first and foremost is a fundamental fact.

Note

[i] https://cropwatch.unl.edu/using-microwave-oven-test-moisture-content-forage-unl-cropwatch-aug-9-2012

Bibliography

Adams, K., Schulz-Kornas, E., Arzi, B., Failing, K., Vogelsberg, J. *et al.* (2016) Functional anatomy of the equine temporomandibular joint: collagen fiber texture of the articular surfaces. *The Veterinary Journal* 217, 58–64.

Armstrong, H.M. (1993) The MLURI hill grazing model using a computer to help set stocking rates. *ENACT* 1(4), 7–9.

Bailey, C. and Balch, C. (1961) Saliva secretion and its relation to feeding in cattle: 1. The composition and rate of secretion of parotid saliva in a small steer. *British Journal of Nutrition* 15(3), 371–382. doi: 10.1079/BJN19610047.

Borgia, L., Valberg, S., McCue, M., Watts, K. and Pagan, J. (2011) Glycaemic and insulinaemic responses to feeding hay with different non-structural carbohydrate content in control and polysaccharide storage myopathy-affected horses. *Journal of Animal Physiology and Animal Nutrition* 95, 798–807.

Coenen, M., Mösseler, A. and Vervuert, I. (2006) Fermentative gases in breath indicate that inulin and starch start to be degraded by microbial fermentation in the stomach and small intestine of the horse in contrast to pectin and cellulose. *The Journal of Nutrition* 136(7 Suppl.), 2108S–2110S.

Collins, M. (1988) Composition and fibre digestion in morphological components of an alfalfa-timothy sward. *Animal Feed Science and Technology* 19, 135–143.

Cuddeford, D., Woodhead, A. and Muirhead, R. (1990) Potential of alfalfa as a source of calcium for calcium deficient horses. *The Veterinary Record* 126(17), 425–429.

Cuddeford, D., Woodhead, A. and Muirhead, R. (1992) A comparison between the nutritive value of short-cutting cycle, high temperature-dried alfalfa and timothy hay for horses. *Equine Veterinary Journal* 24(2), 84–89.

Cuddeford, D., Pearson, R.A., Archibald R.F. and Muirhead, R.H. (1995) Digestibility and gastro-intestinal transit time of diets containing different proportions of alfalfa and oat straw given to Thoroughbreds, Shetland ponies, Highland ponies and donkeys. *Animal Science* 61, 407–417.

Cymbaluk, N.F. and Christensen, D.A. (1986) Nutrient utilization of pelleted and unpelleted forages by ponies. *Canadian Journal of Animal Science* 66, 237–244.

Dyer, J., Fernandez-Castaño Merediz, E., Salmon, K.S., Proudman, C.J., Edwards, G.B. *et al.* (2002) Molecular characterisation of carbohydrate digestion and absorption in equine small intestine. *Equine Veterinary Journal* 34(4), 349–358.

Edouard, N., Duncan, P., Dumont, B., Baumont, R. and Fleurance, G. (2010) Foraging in a heterogeneous environment—An experimental study of the trade-off between intake rate and diet quality. *Applied Animal Behaviour Science* 126, 27–36.

Forage and Grazing Terminology Committee (1991) *Terminology for Grazing Lands and Grazing Animals*. Pocahontas Press, Blacksburg, Virginia.

Glatter, M., Borewicz, K., van den Bogert, B., Wensch-Dorendorf, M., Bochnia, M. *et al.* (2019) Modification of the equine gastrointestinal microbiota by Jerusalem artichoke meal supplementation. *PLoS ONE* 14(8), e0220553. doi: 10.1371/journal.pone.0220553.

Goodwin, D., Davidson, H.P.B. and Harris, P. (2002). Foraging enrichment for stabled horses: effects on behaviour and selection. *Equine Veterinary Journal* 34, 686–691.

Gordon, I.J. (1989) Vegetation community selection by ungulates on the Isle of Rhum III. Determinants of vegetation community selection. *Journal of Applied Ecology* 26, 65–79.

Grimm, P., Julliand, V. and Julliand, S. (2021) 67 Partial substitution of cereals with sugar beet pulp and hindgut health in horses. *Journal of Equine Veterinary Science* 100, 103530.

Healey, M. and Jenkins, A. (2000) Kolb's experiential learning theory and its application in geography in higher education. *Journal of Geography* 99(5), 185–195. doi: 10.1080/00221340008978967.

Houston, K., Tucker, H.K., Matthew, R., Chowdhury, J., Shirley, N. *et al.* (2016) The plant cell wall: a complex and dynamic structure as revealed by the responses of genes under stress conditions. *Frontiers in Plant Science* 7, 984-1–18. doi: 10.3389/fpls.2016.00984.

Hyslop, J.J. (2006) *In situ* and mobile bag methodology to measure the degradation profile of processed feeds in different segments of the equine digestive tract. *Livestock Science* 100, 18–32.

Hyslop, J. and Cuddeford, D. (1999) Soaked unmolassed sugar beet pulp as a partial forage replacer in equine diets when ponies are offered grass hay ad libitum. *Proceedings of the British Society of Animal Science* 1999, 140. doi: 10.1017/S1752756200002957.

Lee, J.M., Donaghy, D.J., Sathish, P. and Roche, J.R. (2009) Interaction between water-soluble carbohydrate reserves and defoliation severity on the regrowth of perennial ryegrass (*Lolium perenne* L.)-dominant swards. *Grass and Forage Science* 64, 266–275.

Lee, J.M., Donaghy, D.J., Sathish, P. and Roche, J.R. (2010) Perennial ryegrass regrowth after defoliation – physiological and molecular changes. *Proceedings of the New Zealand Grassland Association* 72, 127–134.

Leng, J., McNally, S., Walton, G., Swann, J., Proudman, C. *et al.* (2021) Hay vs haylage: forage type influences the equine urinary metabonome and faecal microbiota. *Equine Veterinary Journal* 54, 614–625. doi: 10.1111/evj.13456.

Martinson, K., Allen, B., Jung, H. and Sheaffer, C. (2010) *Seasonal Forage Quality Variation of Twelve Cool Season Grass Species Used for Pasture*. Final Research report to Midwest Forage Association, Shoreview, Minnesota.

McCartney, D.H., Block, H.C., Dubeski, P.L. and Ohama, A.J. (2006) Review: the composition and availability of straw and chaff from small grain cereals for beef cattle in western Canada. *Canadian Journal of Animal Science* 86, 443–455.

Moore-Colyer, M.J.S., Hyslop, J.J., Longland, A.C. and Cuddeford, D. (2000) Intra-caecal fermentation parameters in ponies fed botanically diverse fibre-based diets. *Animal Feed Science and Technology* 84(3–4), 183–197.

Moore-Colyer, M.J.S., Hyslop, J.J., Longland, A.C. and Cuddeford, D. (2002) The mobile bag technique as a method for determining the degradation of four botanically diverse fibrous feedstuffs in the small intestine and total digestive tract of ponies. *British Journal of Nutrition* 88, 729–740.

Mueller, S.C. and Orloff, S.B. (1994) Environmental factors affecting forage quality. In: *Proceedings of 24th California Alfalfa Conference*, pp. 94–56.

Müller, C.E. and Udén, P. (2007) Preference of horses for grass conserved as hay, haylage or silage. *Animal Feed Science and Technology* 132, 66–78.

Murray, M.J., Schusser, G.F., Pipers, F.S. and Gross, S.J. (1996) Factors associated with gastric lesions in Thoroughbred racehorses. *Equine Veterinary Journal* 28(5), 368–374.

Murray, J.A., Longland, A. and Moore-Colyer, M. (2006) *In vitro* fermentation of different ratios of high-temperature dried lucerne and sugar beet pulp incubated with an equine faecal inoculum. *Animal Feed Science and Technology* 129. doi: 10.1016/j.anifeedsci.2005.12.00.

Naujeck, A. and Hill, J. (2003) Influence of sward height on bite dimensions of horses. *Animal Science* 77(1), 95–100.

Naujeck, A., Hill, J. and Gibb, M.J. (2005) Influence of sward height on diet selection by horses. *Applied Animal Behaviour Science* 90(1), 49–63.

Oelberg, K. (1956) Factors affecting the nutritive value of range forage. *Journal of Range Management Archives* 9, 220-225.

Olsman, A.F.S., Huurdeman, C.M., Jansen, W.L., Haaksma, J., van Oldruitenborgh-Oosterbaan, M.M.S. *et al.* (2004) Macronutrient digestibility, nitrogen balance, plasma indicators of protein metabolism and mineral absorption in horses fed a ration rich in sugar beet pulp. *Journal of Animal Physiology and Animal Nutrition* 88, 321–331.

Pearson, R.A., Archibald, R.F. and Muirhead, R.H. (2001) The effect of forage quality and level of feeding on digestibility and gastrointestinal transit time of oat straw and alfalfa given to ponies and donkeys. *British Journal of Nutrition*, 85, 599–606.

Pérez-Barbería, F.J. and Gordon, I.J. (1999) The functional relationship between feeding type and jaw and cranial morphology in ungulates. *Oecologia* 118(2), 157–165.

Pinchbeck, G.L., French, N.P., Proudman, C.J. and Archer, D.C. (2008) Risk factors for epiploic foramen entrapment colic in a UK horse population: a prospective case-control study. *Equine Veterinary Journal* 40(4), 405–410.

Ragnarsson, S. and Lindberg, J. (2008) Nutritional value of timothy haylage in Icelandic horses. *Livestock Science* 113(2–3), 202–208.

Ravosa, M.J., Scott, J.E., McAbee, K.R., Veit, A.J. and Fling, A.L. (2015) Chewed out: an experimental link between food material properties and repetitive loading of the masticatory apparatus in mammals. *PeerJ* 3, e1345. doi: 10.7717/peerj.1345.

Respondek, F., Goachet, A.G. and Julliand, V. (2008) Effects of dietary short-chain fructooligosaccharides on the intestinal microflora of horses subjected to a sudden change in diet. *Journal of Animal Science* 86, 316–323. doi: 10.2527/jas.2006-782.

Rotz, C.A. and Muck, R.E. (1994) Changes in forage quality during harvest and storage. In: Fahey, G.C. Jr (ed.) *Forage Quality, Evaluation, and Utilization*. American Society of Agronomy, Madison, Wisconsin, pp. 828–868.

Salem, S.E., Maddox, T.W., Berg, A., Antczak, P., Ketley, J.M. *et al.* (2018) Variation in faecal microbiota in a group of horses managed at pasture over a 12-month period. *Scientific Reports* 8(1), 8510. doi: 10.1038/s41598-018-26930-3.

Sawicki, C.M., Livingston, K.A., Obin, M., Roberts, S.B., Chung, M. *et al.* (2017) Dietary fiber and the human gut microbiota: application of evidence mapping methodology. *Nutrients* 9(2), 125.

Siciliano, P.D. (2015) Effect of sward height on grazing preference and pasture NSC concentration. *Journal of Equine Veterinary Science* 35, 435.

Siciliano, P.D., Gill, J.C. and Bowman, M.A. (2017) Effect of sward height on pasture nonstructural carbohydrate concentrations and blood glucose/insulin profiles in grazing horses. *Journal of Equine Veterinary Science* 57, 29–34.
Smith, L.W., Goering, H.K. and Gordon, C.H. (1972) Relationships of forage compositions with rates of cell wall digestion and indigestibility of cell walls. *Journal of Dairy Science* 55, 1140–1147.
SRUC (2018) *Straw and Forage Study. A Review commissioned under the Scottish Government RESAS Policy Underpinning: Special Economic Studies – 2017/18* (prepared by SRUC Julian Bell, Gillian Inman, Mary McDowell and regional SAC Consultants). Scotland's Rural College, Penicuik, UK
Trowell, H., Southgate, D.A., Wolever, T.M., Leeds, A.R., Gassull, M.A. *et al*. (1976) Letter: dietary fibre refined. *Lancet* 1, 967.
Van Soest, P.J. and Wine, R.H. (1967) Use of detergents in the analysis of fibrous feeds. Determination of plant cell-wall constituents. *Journal of the Association of Official Analytical Chemists* 50, 50–55.
Van Weyenberg, S., Sales, J. and Janssens, G.P.J. (2006) Passage rate of digesta through the equine gastrointestinal tract: a review. *Livestock Science* 99, 3–12.
Verma, L. and Nelson, B.D. (1983) Changes in round bales during storage. *Transactions of the ASAE* 26, 328–332.
Vervuert, I., Brussow, N., Hollands, T., Cuddeford, D. and Coenen, M. (2010) Electromyographic evaluation of masseter muscle activity in horses fed different types of roughage. In: Ellis, A.D., Longland, A.A., Coenen, M. and Miraglia, N. (eds) *The Impact of Nutrition on the Health and Welfare of Horses. 5th European Association of Animal Production, EAAP pub no 128*. Wageningen Academic Publishers, Netherlands, pp. 75–77.
Waite, R. and Boyd, J. (1953) The water-soluble carbohydrates in grasses 1. Changes occurring during the normal life cycle. *Journal of the Science of Food and Agriculture* 4, 197–200.
Waters, A.J., Nicol, C.J. and French, N.P. (2002) Factors influencing the development of stereotypic and redirected behaviours in young horses: findings of a four-year prospective epidemiological study. *Equine Veterinary Journal* 34(6), 572–579.
Weijs, W.A. and Dantuma, R. (1980) Functional anatomy of the masticatory apparatus in the rabbit (*Oryctolagus cuniculus* L.). *Netherlands Journal of Zoology* 31, 99–147.
Whittaker, A.G., Hughes, K.J., Parkin, T.D.H. and Love, S. (2009) Concentrations of dust and endotoxin in equine stabling. *Veterinary Record* 165, 293–295.
Wilkins, R.J. (2000) Forages and their role in animal systems. In: Givens, D.I., Owen, C., Axford, R.F.E. and Omed, H.M. (eds) *Forage Evaluation in Ruminant Nutrition*. CABI, Wallingford, UK, p. 1–14.
Williams, C.A., Kenny, L.B. and Burk, A.O. (2019) Effects of grazing system, season, and forage carbohydrates on glucose and insulin dynamics of the grazing horse. *Journal of Animal Science* 97(6), 2541–2554. doi: 10.1093/jas/skz103.

5 Diet Details: What Are Cereals and Complementary Feeds? The Importance of Energy Sources in the Horse's Diet

TERESA HOLLANDS AND LIZZIE DRURY

School of Veterinary Medicine, University of Surrey; Saracen Horse Feeds, Aylesford

Learning Objectives

LO1 Recognise the differences between compound feeds.
LO2 Recognise cereals and describe their nutrient value.
LO3 Explain factors that maximise digestibility of cereals and ensure safe starch feeding.
LO4 Explain the role of fat as an energy source in the equine diet.
LO5 Establish the most appropriate time of feeding different energy sources in relation to exercise.
LO6 Distinguish between the effect of cereal/compound feeding on feeding behaviour and temperament of the horses.
LO7 Choose and advise the most appropriate compound feeds to maintain the health and welfare of the horse.

At the end of this chapter, you will be able to provide evidence-based advice on the appropriateness of feed and feeding management relative to the horse's workload to maintain the health and welfare of the horse.

Introduction

It goes without saying that the fibre is the foundation of all horse's diets and most leisure horses can maintain or indeed gain bodyweight and fat on pasture and hay alone. But a high-forage/fibre diet is not a balanced ration: even well managed spring and summer pastures cannot provide enough vitamins and minerals (Jones *et al.*, 2005 a, b) to meet maintenance requirements; protein quality is also very variable in pasture (Särkijärvi *et al.*, 2012). These imbalances are exacerbated when the horses are being fed conserved forages (see Chapter 10, Fig. 10.9: 'How to recommend a diet for a horse eating ad lib conserved forage') and thus the diet needs to be balanced. As the workload of horses increases, then intake of conserved forages inevitably decreases alongside a reduction in pasture, resulting in an additional deficiency in protein as well as calories/energy for work.

Ambulatory nutritionists know that it is challenging to balance the diet of a successful 3-day-event horse, grand prix showjumper or racehorse on grass and forage alone, notwithstanding the client's scepticism.

Thus, all horses' diets require a level of intervention (compound feed) to provide a balanced ration. The key to successfully advising the correct feed to balance the fibre is aided by recognising and advising suitable energy sources to elicit the appropriate physiological response relative to the work type whilst at the same time maintaining gut health and replicating the horse's natural eating behaviour as closely as possible.

DOI: 10.1079/9781789245134.0005

What is a Compound Feed?

The term compound feed is constrained by Feed Legislation (REGULATION (EC) No 767/2009, Article 3)[i] and is defined as a feed made up of more than two ingredients, which may or may not contain additives (vitamins and minerals). Horse feeds fall into a subdivision of compound feeds described as complementary because they are formulated to complement the deficiencies in forage.

Complementary feeds are formulated: (i) to provide an optimum balance of essential nutrients to balance the deficiencies in forages; (ii) to meet specific life-stage requirements (young, growing, old, brood mares); and (iii) to take into account different workloads when fed at recommended intakes. It is often helpful to describe a formulation as a recipe and the final product as a cake: whilst the ingredients might vary in composition, manufacturers are able to ensure that the 'cake' is always the same if the same recipe is followed.

Commercially compound feeds have different descriptors (Table 5.1) based predominantly on their physical form, calorie content and recommended intakes. Formulations will vary within each physical group of feed type and encompass low to high calorie intakes (and varying protein intakes) to meet different lifestyles, but all will meet recommended vitamin/mineral intakes when fed correctly.

Composition of Compound Feeds

Unlike those for ruminants or pets, only a small number of ingredients (Table 5.2) are used to formulate horse feeds and by using different inclusion rates it is possible to provide formulations with differing fibre, protein oil and energy. Use the packaging (see Chapter 7) to identify the main nutrient source. Each ingredient provides several nutrients but it is common practice to group them according to their main provision – that of fibre, protein or energy. All have advantages and disadvantages which can be mostly mitigated if their feeding management is adjusted to maximise gut health and feeding behaviour.

Cereals

Cereals are edible seeds of specific grasses that over the years have been bred to increase the starch content of their grains. They belong to the gramineous family and are grown for food and feed. They store their energy as starch, providing the principal energy source for performance horses (Vervuert *et al.*, 2009b); they are not normally used for formulating leisure feeds.

You should be able to recognise the common cereals used in compound feeds (Table 5.3).

Cereals do not meet the nutritional requirements for lysine, threonine and methionine, or calcium content of < 0.1% DM (NRC, 2001, 2007), but they contain high levels of phosphorus (> 0.4% DM) (NRC, 2001). Phytic acid, a food inhibitor which chelates micronutrients, is the major storage form of phosphorus in cereals, reducing the availability of calcium, zinc and probably magnesium in the intestinal tract (Gupta *et al.*, 2015). If cereals are being fed alone or added to a balanced ration, then further adjustment to the diet will be needed. The main nutritional contribution of cereals to compound feeds is starch energy.

Safe starch solutions

Top tip

- Many of the health risks associated with the feeding of starch are simply due to inappropriate choice of feeds.
- It is unclear why horses prone to laminitis, obesity, EMS and PPID would be fed starch-based feeds.
- For horses in work, if feeding management is considered, starch is a safe energy source, needlessly maligned.

Starch digestion in the horse

It is often hypothesised that the horse is a poor digestor of starch, because low amylytic activity was measured in the foregut of horses (Alexander and Hickson, 1970). Horses have considerably lower estimated α-amylase activity in the jejunum between 10 and 50 U/g (Meyer *et al.*, 1993) and in pancreatic tissue (85–909 U/g of tissue) (Kienzle *et al.*, 1994) when compared with the pig (3500 U/g on average) (Roberts, 1974; Frape, 1986). Whilst the seed heads of modern grains contain a more concentrated source of starch compared with the original uncultivated grasses, clearly starch has always been part of the equine diet.

Contrary to popular belief, the horse is efficient at digesting starch, with 95% of starch digested over the total tract (Cuddeford, 2001). Starch fermentation in the stomach results in the disappearance of 95.9–97.9% oat starch, 65.6–70.7% barley starch

Table 5.1 Commercially categorised compound horse feeds available in the UK formulated to balance forages for horses

Feed form	Cubes/pellets	Sweet feed, coarse mixes and muesli	Balancers	Straights	Supplements (see Chapter 6)	Treats
Visual appearance	6 mm diameter pellets – can be pressed or extruded	Mixtures of flakes or other processed cereals, pellets and other ingredients coated in a molasses or oil-type coating	3 mm pellets containing quality protein, vitamins and minerals, low in calories	Single ingredients in unprocessed or processed form, e.g. rolled oats, sugar beet shreds	Mixtures of additives in powder, liquid or granular form Low-dose functional extras to the diet	Extruded pellet, baked biscuits
Typical feed rate	200–1200 g/100 kg BW	200–1200 g/100 kg BW	100 g/100 kg BW	100–1000 g/100 kg BW (depending on whether adjunct or main ingredient in ration)	1–25 g/100 kg BW	1–2 g/100 kg BW
Typical shelf life	3–6 months	3–6 months	3–6 months	3–6 months	6–12 months	6–12 months
Packaging	Plastic or paper sack or bag	Plastic or paper sack or bag	Plastic or paper sack or bag	Plastic or paper sack or bag	Plastic tubs	Plastic bag or tub
Typical examples	Saracen Super Fibre Cubes, Spillers Horse & Pony Cubes	Dodson and Horrell Pasture Mix	Saracen Essential Balancer Spillers Balancer range	Oats, maize and barley	NAF Super flex	Saracen Munchies

Table 5.2 Nutritional value of typical energy ingredients used in the formulation of horse feeds (kg DM)

Ingredient	Starch g/kg (%)	Estimated digestible energy (MJ DE/kg)	Fibre g/kg (%)	Protein g/kg (%)	Oil g/kg (%)	Typical inclusion rates (%)	
						Light work	**Hard work**
	High energy						
Oil	0	40.5	0	0	98.7	1–2%	2–6%
Maize	73.4	18.7	2.5	9.4	4.3	3–5%	8–17%
Wheat	69.1	18.2	2.6	12.6	1.7		
Barley	59.7	14.5	5.2	11.8	2.0	20–25%	9–14%
Oats	40.6	19.5	13.9	11.0	5.4		15–40%
Molasses	0	14.7	0.1	5.5	1.0	5–7%	6–9 %
	Low energy						
Nutritionally improved straw (NIS)	1.0	4.0	45.0	4.0	1.3		
Soya hulls	5.2	18.2	38.9	13.1	2.2	14	14
Wheat feed	27.5	11.5	9.0	17.5	4.0		
Oat feed	7.5	5.0	29.5	5.0	2.0	20–50%	
Dried grass	1.5	8.5	24.0	17.0	4.0		
Beet pulp (molassed)	0.5	17.1	20.8	8.7	0.5	4–16%	2–16%
Beet pulp unmolassed							
	Protein						
Soya bean meal	6.3	19.7	4.4	55.2	1.7		
Alfalfa	3.3	18.0	28.6	18.3	2.7	10–30%	10–20%
Peas	51.3	18.3	6.0	23.9	1.2	3–5%	2–12%
Sunflower meal	1.5	19.4	27.9	32.4	2.2		
	Vitamins and minerals						
Premix	0	0	0	0	1.0	2.5–3%	3%
Limestone	0	0	0	0	0		
Salt	0	0	0	0	0		0.3%

and 23.9–27.2% maize starch, with an increase in lactate and volatile fatty acids (VFAs) (de Fombelle *et al.*, 2003). The remainder of the starch is hydrolysed by enzymes (maltases, glucosidases, amylase, glucoamylase and sucrases) (Frape, 1986) in the small intestine to glucose, (Longland, 2001) and stored as liver and muscle glycogen (Newsholme and Dimitriadis 2001) with any excess stored as fat (Lawrence, 1990; Newsholme and Dimitriadis, 2001). Maintaining blood glucose levels during exercise is fundamental to the central nervous system. Cereals vary in their starch and fibre content, impacting digestibility. The rate and extent of starch digestion is determined by the differences in the starch granules contained within the cereal grains. Oat starch is partially fermented in the small intestine, similar to inulin (a fructan) (Coenen *et al.*, 2006).

Top tip

The key to successful, healthy feeding of starch is maintaining normal digestive physiological responses in both upper and lower guts by:

- advising low starch meals;
- maximising small intestine digestion; and
- minimising any undigested starch reaching the gut.

This can be achieved by a combination of factors:

- processing;
- meal size; and
- feeding relative to other components of the diet.

Table 5.3 Common cereals used in compound horse feeds

Cereal	Growing crop	Whole grain	Micronised grain
Oats	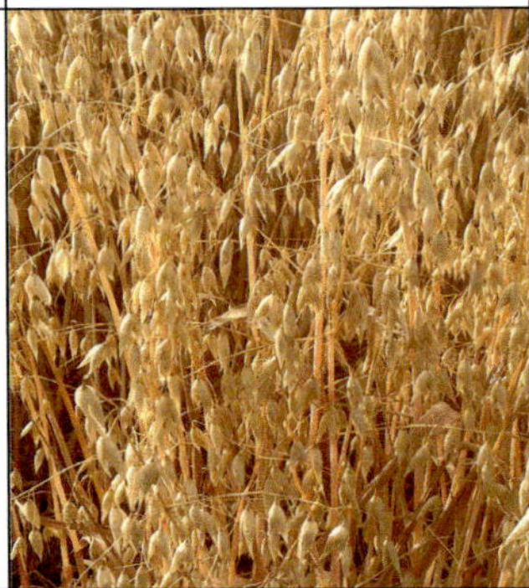	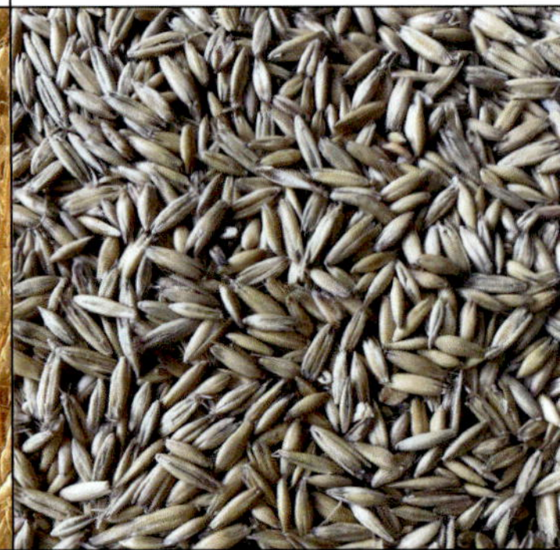	Oats are not fed micronised
Maize	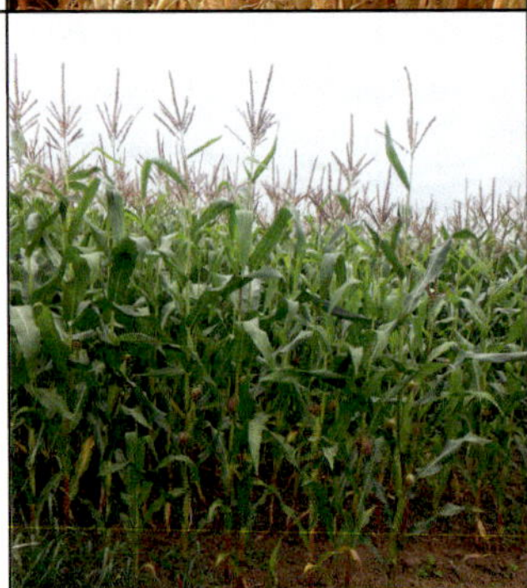	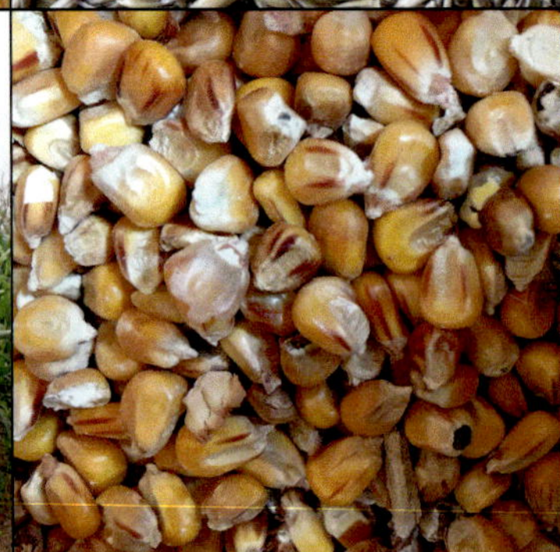	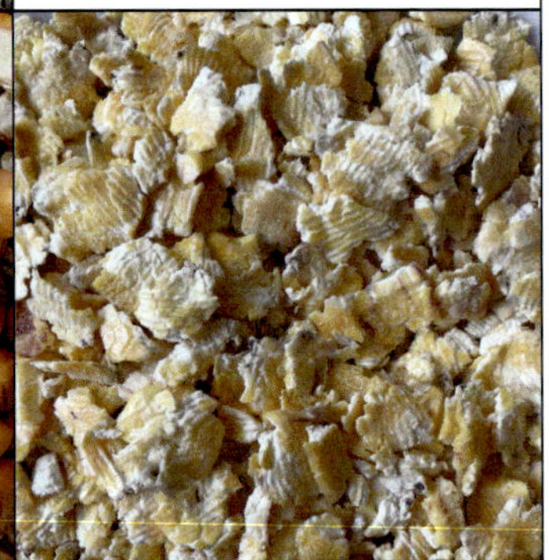
Barley	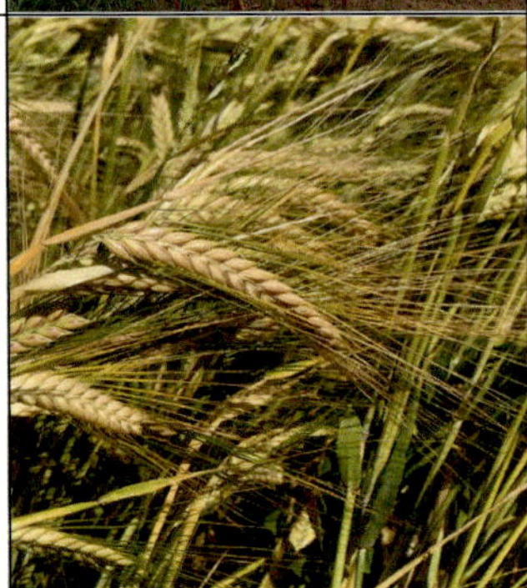	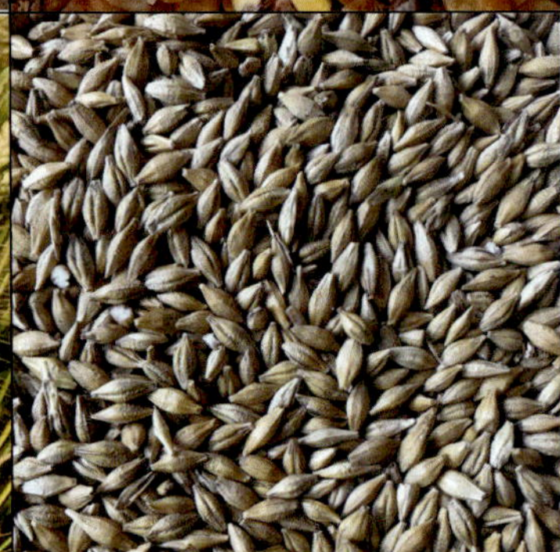	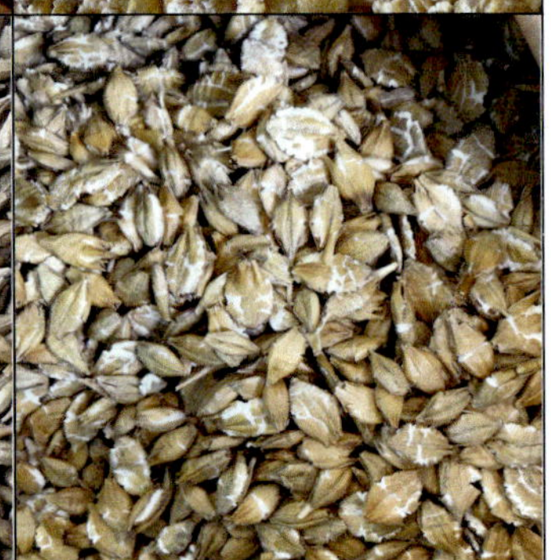
Wheat	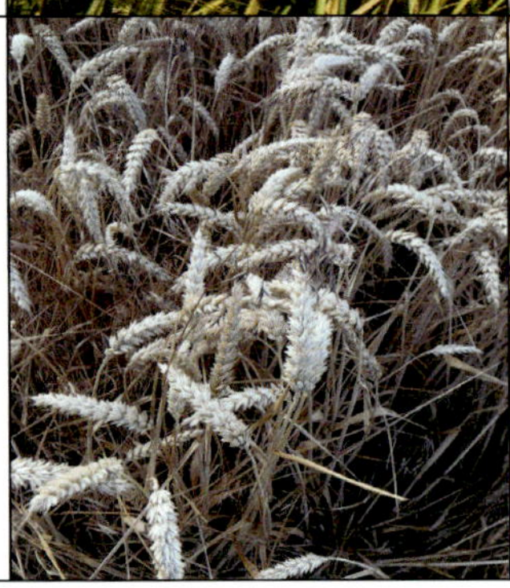	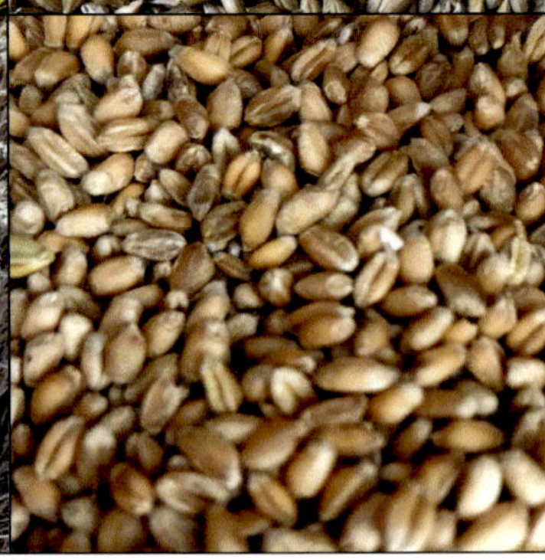	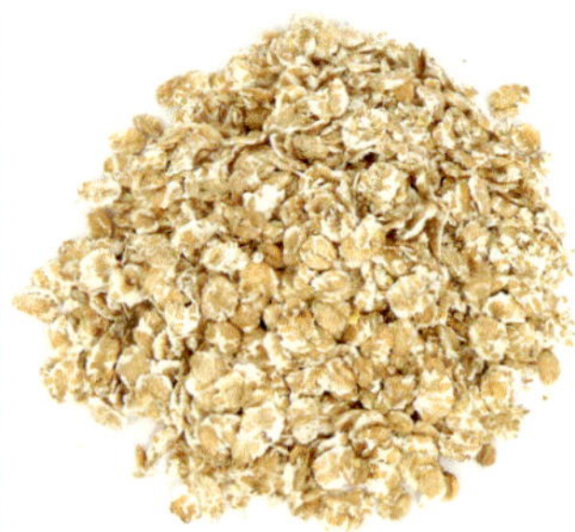

Processing

Physical or heat processing improves the horse's ability to digest most cereals (Juilliard *et al.*, 2006). Cereals such as barley and maize have hard seed coats, so need to be physically processed or cooked; whereas cereals such as oats that have a soft seed coat are easily chewed by the horse.

Physical and mechanical processing

Processes such as rolling or crushing break open the cereal kernel, exposing the starch-rich endosperm to digestive enzymes and increasing the potential for oxidation of fats and any vitamins.

Top tip

- Your clients expect to buy rolled or cracked oats, because they see 'whole' oats in their horse's droppings.
- On close inspection you will find these are the fibre coat which has not undergone hind gut fermentation
    - Or they have fed too large a meal, reducing SI digestion so whole oats pass through

Rolling, crushing or grinding of oats does not significantly improve starch digestibility (Kienzle *et al.*,1992) or that of maize (Meyer *et al.*, 1993). This makes sense, because horses already chew their food to 1.6 mm or less before swallowing (mean excreted food particle size of the faeces, 1.36 mm, range 1.15–1.72 mm; food particle size in stomach 1.29 mm, range, 0.69–1.76 mm (Carmalt and Allen, 2008)), sufficient to improve small intestinal starch digestibility of maize (maize does need processing, due to its very hard seed coat) (Kienzle *et al.*, 1992; Meyer *et al.*, 1993). In fact, grinding might be detrimental as smaller particles pass through the SI more rapidly, reducing digestibility (McLean *et al.*, 1999b).

Heat processing, cooking

Processing techniques such as cooking, e.g. micronising and steam flaking (Table 5.4) (which could be described to your clients as being like microwaving), significantly improve pre-caecal starch digestion of maize (Meyer *et al.*, 1993) and barley (McLean *et al.*, 2000; Vervuert *et al.*, 2008). Cooking (micronising and extrusion) improves the SI digestion of starch (barley: 2 g starch/kg BW fed 50:50 with forage) to the extent that there was no difference in starch concentration in the hind gut compared with ponies fed just a forage diet, whereas physically processed barley resulted in large increases in caecal lactate (McLean *et al.*, 2000).

Cooking cereals gelatinises the starch, stretching the normally globular starch molecule and increasing the surface area for enzymic digestion, improving digestibility and thus glycaemic response (Fig. 5.1), in the same way as cooking potatoes does for yourself. Alongside measuring the horse's glycaemic

Table 5.4 A summary of cooking processes used by manufacturers of horse feed

	Similar to	Preparation	Cooking process	Physical process
Micronising	Microwaving	Steeped in water for 4–12 h to swell starch granule	Infrared lamps 1.8–3.4 microns at 50 kw (102–200°C for 20 min) to gelatinise the starch	Cereal grain rolled to physically maintain the stretched starch molecule
Steam flaking	Steaming	'Temper' for 1–24 h prior to steaming and flaking, 18% moisture to swell starch granule	Min. 100°C	Cereal grain rolled to physically maintain the stretched starch molecule
Extrusion	Popcorn/ pressure cooking	Ground to < 1.2 mm and mixed with other ground ingredients and vitamins and minerals	Cooked at 125°C with added water (23–28%) to sterilise the product under 34–37 atm	Pushed under pressure through nozzle that, as the cooked feed moves through and pressure released, expand to the shape of the nozzle. Cooled and coated with fat
Pelleting	Baking	Ground to 3–6 mm in length, mixed with other ground ingredients and vitamins and minerals	Made into pellets by compressing with water at 90–120°C to sterilise the ingredients	Different-size pellets produced (both in length and in diameter)

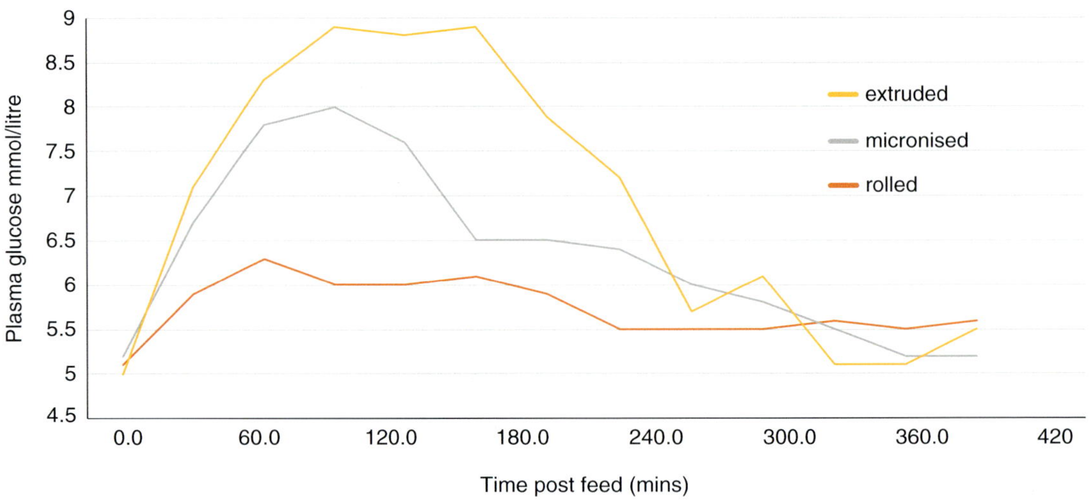

Fig. 5.1 The effect of cooking barley (2 g starch/kg BW) on small intestinal digestion of starch in the horse as measured by glycaemic response. (From Vervuert *et al.*, 2008, with permission.)

response to cooked versus raw starch, Vervuert *et al.* (2008) measured breath hydrogen and methane, which are by-products of starch fermentation; both were higher when rolled barley was consumed, suggesting that the starch had escaped enzymic digestion and was being fermented. Feeding uncooked starch results in a low glycaemic response because little or no starch has been digested in the small intestine.

> **Top tip**
>
> Advising cooked starch:
>
> - minimises undigested starch reaching the horse's hind gut; and
> - maximises SI absorption of glucose.

Meal size

As well as advising cooked starch, you need to check how much the client is feeding in one meal.

The larger the meal the client feeds, the bigger are the glycaemic response and risk of exceeding the normal physiological capacity of starch digestion (Fig. 5.2), which in turn could lead to a decrease in insulin sensitivity. Horses eat small meals at the same rate as larger ones, but remember that large meals of compound feeds leave the stomach more quickly compared with smaller meals (Métayer *et al.*, 2004); importantly, starch digestion is proportional to the time it stays in the small intestine (McLean *et al.*, 1999a,b,c,).

Amount of starch per meal

Whilst meal size is important, the amount of starch per meal (g starch/kg BW/meal) is the key to gut

> **Top tip**
>
> You should always advise 1 g starch/kg BW/meal or less – which keeps the gut healthy by:
>
> - maximising small intestine digestion (Vervuert *et al.*, 2008);
> - maintaining glycaemic and subsequent insulinaemic response within normal physiological parameters (Vervuert *et al.*, 2009b);
> - minimising undigested starch reaching the hind gut (McLean *et al.*, 2000); and
> - ensuring efficient glycogen replenishment in the hard-working horse.
> - There is 2.4 decrease in the risk of horses needing treatment for clinically squamous ulceration when fed < 1 g starch/kg BW (Lutherson *et al.*, 2009).
> - Always check the starch content of the feed and work out the amount of starch the horse is eating /kg BW/meal.

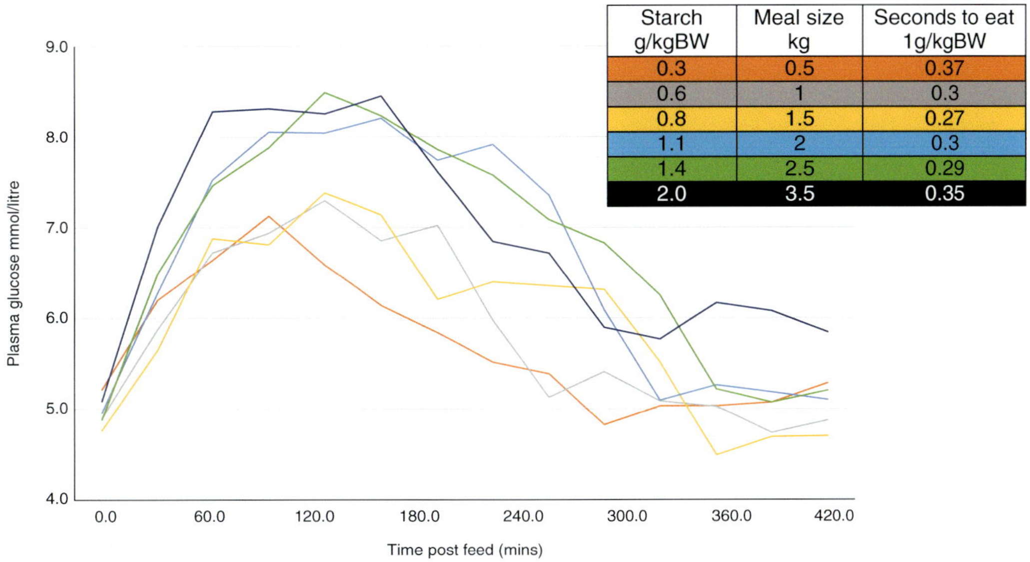
Starch g/kgBW
Meal size kg
Seconds to eat 1g/kgBW
0.3 0.5 0.37
0.6 1 0.3
0.8 1.5 0.27
1.1 2 0.3
1.4 2.5 0.29
2.0 3.5 0.35
Plasma glucose mmol/litre
9.0
8.0
7.0
6.0
5.0
4.0
0.0
60.0
120.0
180.0
240.0
300.0
360.0
420.0
Time post feed (mins)

Fig. 5.2 The effect of meal size and starch intake on the glycaemic response of horses.

health. There was no significant difference in caecum pH when a feed (starch 157 g/kg DM) was fed in one large meal to cannulated horses (mean BW 500 kg) rather than split into smaller meals (2 × 1.36 kg/meal or 3 × 0.91 kg/meal), despite an increase in caecum *Streptococcus bovis* (Venable *et al.*, 2016). The large meal only contained 0.8 g starch/kg BW/meal.

Diet composition and feeding management will impact upon starch digestion; to make sure the above is not in vain, you must check the feeding management of the whole diet.

Timing of feeding starch relative to fibre

Pre-feeding fibre

Feeding alfalfa chaff before starch increases small-intestine digestion of starch measured by glycaemic, insulinaemic response and breath hydrogen, so reducing the risk of starch overflow to the hind gut (Fig. 5.3) (Vervuert *et al.*, 2009a).

When oats were fed first or mixed with alfalfa, an increase in starch fermentation (as opposed to enzymic digestion) was recorded in the stomach/small intestine, possibly due to a rapid rate of passage through the gut (Vervuert *et al.*, 2009a). An increase in plasma concentration of interleukin-1β (IL-1β) because of rapid bacterial fermentation of starches and sugars in the digestive tract has been recorded an hour after feeding a high-starch meal (Suagee-Bedore *et al.*, 2020).

Feeding concentrates before forage

It is not just chaff that needs considering. Do not advise feeding hay after a compound, because the fibre content and saliva produced increases bolus size, pushing the starch through the SI, reducing enzymic digestion, with undigested starch fermented in the hind gut increasing acidity.

- Feeding barley 2 h before feeding hay results in a drop in the pH of the caecum (Philippeau *et al.*, 2009), as does feeding oats before forage (Zeyner *et al.*, 2004).
- Advising feeding concentrates 2 h before hay will significantly lower caecal pH 6 h after feeding (Sadet-Bourgeteau *et al.*, 2017).
- Feeding concentrates mixed with hay (measured with fistulated horses fed at 1.8 kg DM/100 kg BW in two equal meals) significantly lowered caecal pH 6 h after feeding and increased propionate in the colon and caecum (Sadet-Bourgeteau *et al.*, 2017).

Increases in propionate in all species is associated with a drop in pH.

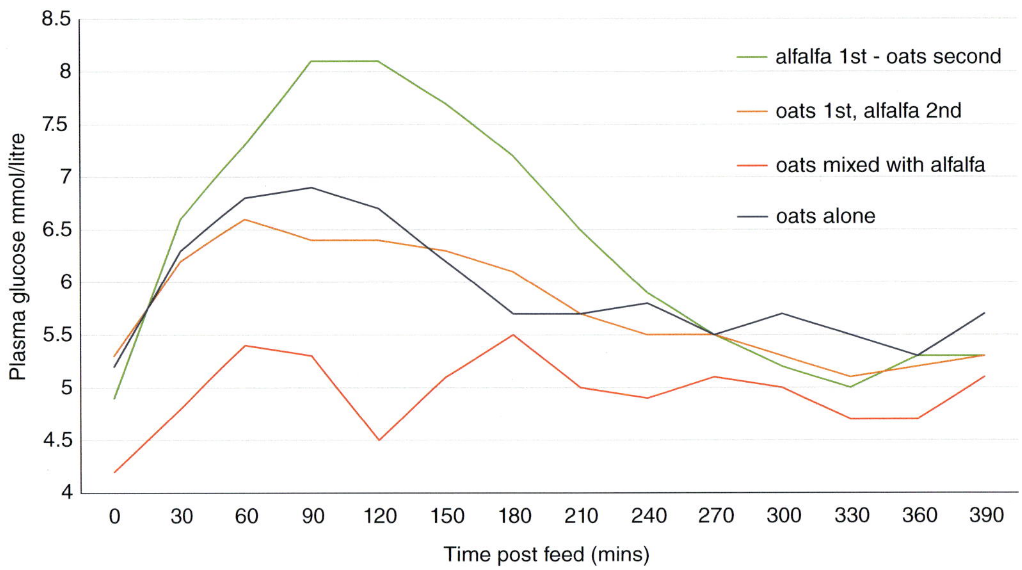

Fig. 5.3 The glycaemic response to time of feeding oat starch relative to fibre (alfalfa). The glycaemic response did not elicit an insulinaemic response outside of normal physiological parameters. Low glycaemic response indicates limited starch digestion in the small intestine and subsequent fermentation of starch in the hind gut. Oats provided 2 g starch/kg BW.

Top tip

- Make sure that your client's horse eats and finishes a small fibre meal (0.9 kg) of hay/chaff before eating a meal containing a moderate amount of starch or sugar.
- Replicate natural feeding, ensuring that starch is digested in the small intestine, stopping the inflammatory response to dietary concentrates (*Suagee-Bedore et al.,* 2020).
- If it is not possible to provide horses with a small amount of fibre before a meal, advise free access to hay, at least a few hours before a concentrate feed, to slow intake of concentrate feed.
- Remind clients that slowing intake slows digestive passage and increases starch digestion in the small intestine.

Other factors affecting starch digestion in the small intestine

Age

Ageing decreases the effectiveness of most biological process, including digestion (Fig. 5.4).

Always advise feeds with a high digestibility for older horses, if they are needed in addition to forages (see Chapter 16, Table 16.7: 'A comparison of lysine content of difference complementary horse feeds and the effect of recommended intake on daily intake of lysine for horses').

Individual variation

As you know, all preventative medicine is based on a cohort of animals with the mean and median used to establish dose or intakes. Nutrition is no exception and there is tacit acknowledgement that you will adjust advice according to the horse in front of you. Starch digestion of the same feedstuff can vary between and within horses from day to day, resulting in large individual insulinaemic response (Vervuert *et al.*, 2004).

Top tip

- Always make sure that a high-starch diet is fed as low-starch meals.
- Be reassured that advising < 1 g starch/kg BW/meal maintains insulin within normal physiological limits in healthy, exercising horses (Fig. 5.5); similar to peak insulinaemic responses to hay at 19–59 µU/ml (Borgia *et al.*, 2011).

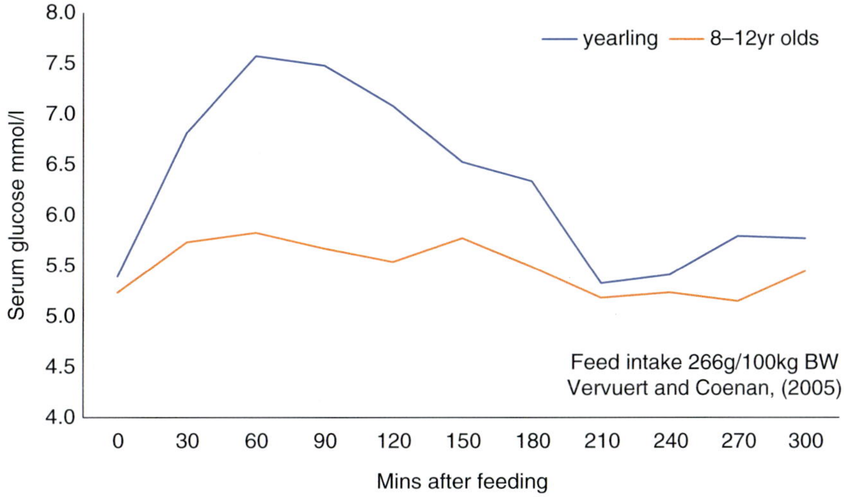

Fig. 5.4 A comparison of the effect of age on the digestion of starch in the small intestine of horses as measured by glycaemic response. Feed intake 266 g/100 kg BW. (With permission from Professor Dr Vervuert, University of Leipzig.)

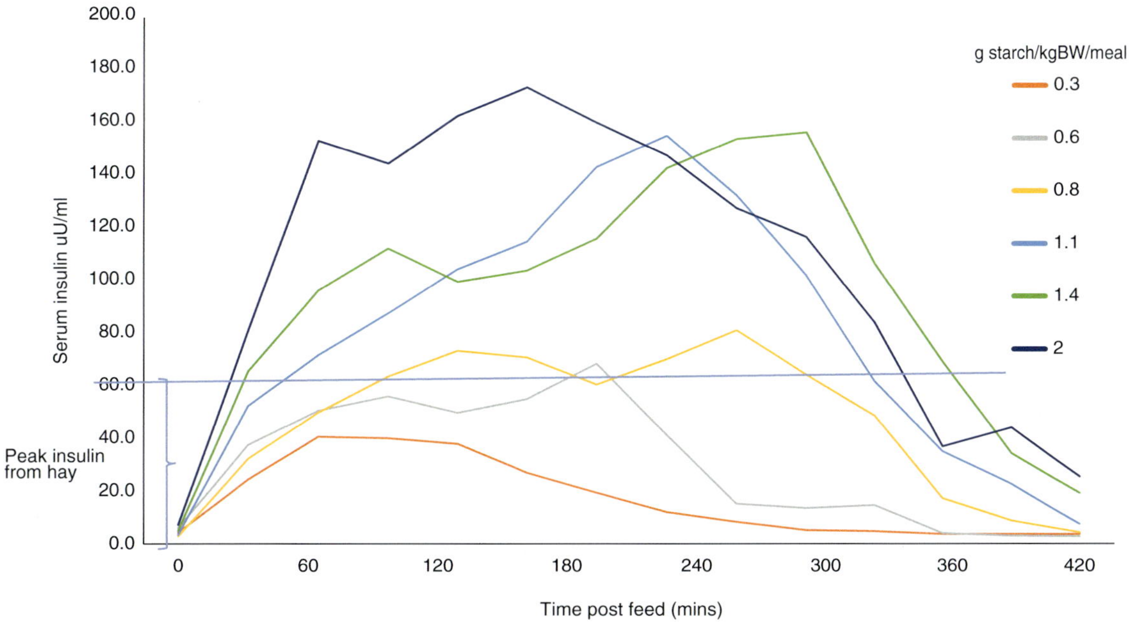

Fig. 5.5 The effect of starch intake on the insulinaemic response of healthy horses.

The energy from starch, as you might have noted from the glycaemic response graphs, is available to the horse 2 h after eating and is ideal for horses working anaerobically. Horses that need a slower energy release because they are working aerobically are often fed fat/oil.

Fat and Oils

There is a perception that horses do not consume large quantities of fat in the wild, but all cereal grains contain 2–4% oil or fat. Fats contain about 2.25× more energy/kg than carbohydrates, are highly digestible (Hollands and Cuddeford, 1992) and are absorbed as free fatty acids in the small intestine. Oil did not affect the digestibility of the overall diet or individual nutrients when 240 kg ponies were fed 100 g top-dressed corn oil/day (41.6 g oil/100 kg BW) or when 549 kg horses were fed between 310 g and 750 g of soya oil/day (56.4 g – 136.6 g/100 kg BW); the highest intake of fat had a 78% digestibility (Bush *et al.*, 2001). Diets with up to 230g fat/kg DM of concentrates (corn oil, peanut oil, animal vegetable fat blends and tallow) had no effect on the digestion of other nutrients (Kronfeld *et al.*, 2004). However, digestion of fibre and protein was reduced by 0.9% and 0.7% with every 10 g oil added to 1 kg DM (Jansen *et al.*, 2001); similarly, adding 86.6 g crude fat/kg DM to provide 37% of net energy decreased apparent total tract digestibility of crude fibre by 8% (Jansen, *et al.*, 2000). The NRC (2007) suggested that soyabean oil should be limited to 0.7g/kg BW/day, despite performance horses being fed diets containing up to 130 g oil/kg DM (Jansen *et al.*, 2000). Inclusion rate might be limited due to palatability issues.

Oil palatability

Corn oil, when compared with ten different types of fat (all 15% by weight) in cafeteria-style preference tests, was the most palatable (Bowman *et al.*, 1979). Highly unsaturated (soya) or saturated (coconut) oil is palatable over the long term (16 months) (Harris *et al.*, 1999), although, prolonged use of soya oil has been reported to lead to monotony (author observation) and of course should be discouraged from a sustainability perspective. Several sources of oil are fed to horses (Table 5.5).

Table 5.5 Characteristics of fats and oils fed to horses

Oil source	Fat content (% DM)	Advantages and disadvantages
Soya	100	Commonly used as the oil source of commercially formulated complete feeds; due to sustainability issues often substituted by rapeseed/canola oil.
Full-fat soya	18–20	Used in finished feed formulations as a source of oil.
Corn/maize		Preference tests have shown horses prefer corn oil over other oils or fat sources (Bowman *et al.*, 1979)
Canola/rapeseed	100	Frequently grown as a winter 'break-crop' in the UK. Rapeseed oil is replacing soya oil as UK grown and more sustainable
Linseed		Linseed oil is often fed to horses because it is high in omega 3 fatty acids. The linseed itself is around 37% oil
Fish	100	Superior source of omega 3 Must be deodorized for palatability
High-oil commercial feeds	8–15	Palatable and easy method of providing calorie-dense meals. Fully balanced when fed at the manufacturer's recommended feeding level. May be prone to rancidity and so should be stored correctly and used within the recommended shelf life. Manufacturers tend to counteract feed deterioration by adding additional natural or artificial antioxidants
Supplements	20–40	Come in powdered or pelleted form. Palatable and practical method of increasing the energy density of a feed ration. Check that they are balanced for vitamin E and Ca:P ratios. In pelleted form and usually fed at 0.5–1.0 kg daily (@16 MJ/kg).

> **Top tip**
>
> - Storage affects palatability.
> - Liquid oils are susceptible to oxidation and rancidity.
>   - They must be stored in the cool and the dark.
>   - Avoid introduction of air bubbles by frequent shaking.
> - Check the smell before feeding.
> - Advise minimum of 100 iu vitamin E per 100 ml oil (Harris, 1999).

The effect of fat feeding on the physiology of the horse

As with all nutritional trials, there is mixed evidence as to the effect of fat on the exercise physiology of the horse, partially dependent upon type and duration of exercise and the other feedstuffs fed in the diet.

The addition of fat to the equine diet as an energy supply has the perceived benefits of being sparing of glucose with less lactate accumulation, which in turn could delay the onset of fatigue. The addition of fat to the diet and digestive adaption increases the activity of lipoprotein lipase, accompanied by an increased uptake of non-esterified fatty acids from circulating triacylglycerol (Orme *et al.*, 1997; Geelen *et al.*, 2001).

Aerobic exercise

Horses adapted to high-fat diets (1 g fat/kg BW – 20% DE) show metabolic adaptions to digest and utilise fat as the primary energy source during aerobic exercise approximately 21 days after being fed a high-fat diet (Hughes *et al.*, 1995; Orme *et al.*, 1997). After 5–10 weeks of fat supplementation (10% fat – 29% DE), mature Arabian horses used 30% less glucose and muscle glycogen during an endurance exercise test (Pagan *et al.*, 2002).

Evidence to support these metabolic changes includes a decrease in the resting plasma triacylglycerol concentration and an increase in plasma cholesterol concentration (Orme *et al.*, 1997). Increases in enzyme activity, lipoprotein lipase, may also indicate an improved ability of the skeletal muscle to increase the uptake of non-esterified fatty acids (NEFAs) from the circulating triacylglycerol and this together with a lower respiratory exchange ratio suggests that the capacity to use NEFA for oxidation and energy production is increased (Dunnett *et al.*, 2002, Pagan *et al.*, 2002).

Exercising horses perform better when fed a high-fat diet (Potter *et al.*, 1992), particularly horses participating in more prolonged, submaximal activities such as endurance riding and eventing, with an increase in stamina because of altered substrate use. Carbohydrate utilisation is preserved, exerting a glycogen-sparing effect (Kronfeld, 1996; Kronfeld *et al.*, 1988). Other studies have contradicted these findings, reporting no change in performance (Topliff *et al.*, 1983; Pagan *et al.*, 1987).

It appears that the adaption to fat added to the diet is not the same for all horses and that there are some individual differences between horses in their ability to be able to use fat as an energy source during exercise, which may in part be due to exercise levels

Anaerobic exercise

Higher workloads have less reliance on fatty acid oxidation, suggesting that sprint-based exercise relies more upon the provision of carbohydrate energy, although supramaximal exercise does induce changes in specific plasma lipids in Thoroughbred (TB) racehorses, increasing citrate synthase and triglyceride lipase activity (Dunnett *et al.*, 2002). While the biological significance of these findings remains to be determined, these results provide baseline information for future studies in lipidomics but further research is warranted to better understand the role of lipids on energy metabolism in TB racehorses, (Nolazco Sassot *et al.*, 2019).

Diets that are supplemented with fat in place of starch may compromise the horse's ability to maintain optimum resting glycogen levels, increasing recovery times post-exercise. Muscle and liver glycogen reserves are important to delay the onset of early fatigue and must be restored post-training and competition. Some studies have reported an increase in resting muscle glycogen concentrations in horses fed diets that are high in fat (Harking *et al.*, 1992; Julen *et al.*, 1995; Hughes *et al.*, 1995), whereas in comparison, non-trained ponies showed a decrease in muscle glycogen in various muscle types when a high-fat diet was fed (Geelen *et al.*, 2001), or no change or a slight decrease in resting muscle glycogen (Orme *et al.*, 1997; Pagan *et al.*, 1987).

A glycogen-sparing effect of high-fat diets is seen only with simultaneous exercise. The mobilisation of glycogen during anaerobic exercise was increased in fat-supplemented horses (Julen *et al.*, 1995; Hughes *et al.*, 1995; Geelen *et al.*, 2001) but the rate of glycogen utilisation was not increased in horses performing a 1600 m race (Harking *et al.*, 1992).

There was no effect of fat feeding on blood lactate concentrations when horses completed either a simulated cutting test (Julen *et al.*, 1995) or a 1600 m race (Harking *et al.*, 1992). Standardbred horses performing a standardised sub-maximal exercise test fed a high-fat (11.8% in the dietary dry matter) instead of a low-fat (1.5% fat) diet showed lower blood lactate accumulation after 4 weeks of adaption (Sloet van Oldruitenborgh-Oosterbaan *et al.*, 2002). In comparison, standardbred horses fed a high-fat diet (39 g/kg DM in the total diet) for 21 days exercised sub-maximally had increases in plasma lactate levels during and after exercise (Lindberg *et al.*, 2006), maybe due to differences in total daily fat intake or duration of adaptation

Other considerations

- Replacing starch with dietary fat decreases water intake and available water in the intestine, possibly impacting on mineral balance, irrespective of fibre intake.
- High fat intake may reduce fibre digestibility, decreasing the water-binding and reservoir capacity in the hind gut (Zeyner *et al.*, 2002).
- Endurance horses need a water reservoir in the large intestine (Meyer, 1987) but the decrease in concentrate DMI could be replaced by forage, which may negate the reduction in digestibility.
- Supplementation of fat with a lower but higher-quality protein diet during sprint-based exercise reduces acidogenic effects (Graham Thiers *et al.*, 2001).
- The addition of extra fat increases the energy density of feeds, which is advantageous for horses with high-energy requirements (Kane and Baker, 1977; Snyder *et al.*, 1981; Kronfeld, 1996), allowing for a reduction in total concentrate feed intake (Hintz *et al.*, 1978).
- The lower weight of gastrointestinal contents might be beneficial to the performance horse, due to an improved power-to-weight ratio as a result of reduced DM intake and bowel ballast (Kronfeld, 1996; Kronfeld *et al.*, 1998).

Effect on thermal load

High ambient heat and humidity affect athletic performance over middle and long distances (Meyer, 1987) and excess heat must be dissipated to maintain normal body temperature. Any reduction in metabolic heat generated during exercise is particularly important for horses that are competing in hotter climates (Kronfeld, 1996; Kronfeld *et al.*, 1998). Substituting fat for soluble carbohydrate lowers heat increment and thermal load (Kronfeld *et al.*, 1994). This may be reduced still further when combined with a low-fibre diet, to reduce heat produced through fermentation (Kronfeld, 1996). It must be noted, however, that feeding low-fibre diets is not recommended, as this will compromise digestive health (Table 5.6).

Adaption to fat will result in small improvements in performance but evidence on exercise capacity is mixed; further work is needed. Many studies used small horse populations and exercise was simulated on treadmills to replicate exercise, which may distort the true effects. Total diet information was limited and, in some situations, horses were not being fed isocalorific diets or had inappropriate forage-to-concentrate allowances. Further studies of larger sample size, breed type and work rate are needed.

There is an increasing trend to feed forage and fibre-based diets with a lower reliance on cereals and starch, but the availability of glucose and rate of glycogen replenishment with such diets may compromise performance (Jansson and Lindberg, 2012).

Based on the evidence from research, current commercial feed formulations and practical advice and horse performance, you should consider the following.

- Horse breed
- The type of exercise being done (duration and intensity)
- Relative contribution of lipids and carbohydrates to muscle contraction
- Greater use of fat in Arabian versus Thoroughbred horses performing endurance-like exercise, due to a lower proportion of type I and type IIa muscle fibres in the latter
    - Diets of 80–100 g oil/kg DM intake (up to 20–25% of total DE intake) are used successfully in the field
- The proportional contributions of fat and carbohydrate to the energy expenditures associated with supramaximal exercise in Thoroughbreds is unknown
    - Diets of 50–60 g oil/kg DM intake (10–15% of total DE intake) are used successfully in the field
- Further research is required to establish the performance benefits of advising fat for horses performing supramaximal exercise.

Table 5.6 How to advise the feeding of oil to endurance horses competing in high temperatures

Horse signalment	450 kg BFS 4.5/9 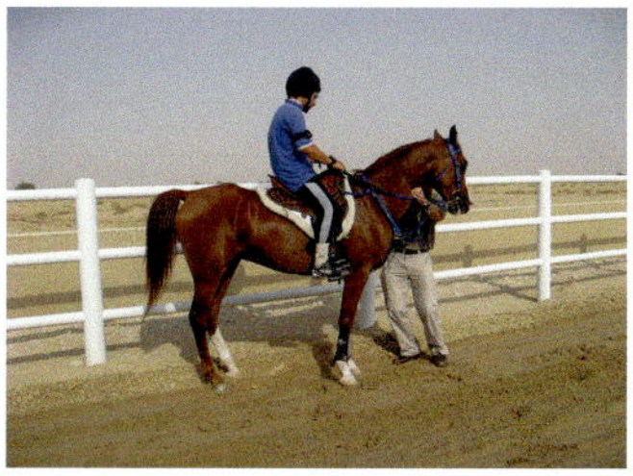
Horse history	• Good appetite. • Maintains condition well.

Workload	• Carrying a combined weight of rider and tack of 75 kg.
	• Early training work:
	  ◦ training in the sand in a warm environment 1.5–2.0 h/day;
	  ◦ slow trot/intermittent canter.
	Daily energy requirements (ME_m 57–68 MJ/day (NRC, 2007) plus ME work 42 MJ DE) = 99–110 MJ DE

Diet	• 1.5% BW forage • 7 kg of 9% protein hay = 52.1 MJ DE • 10% fat endurance concentrate feed: 3.5 kg = 45.1 MJ DE • 450 ml vegetable oil = 14.8 MJ DE • DE from oil = 19 MJ – 17–19% of DE from oil.

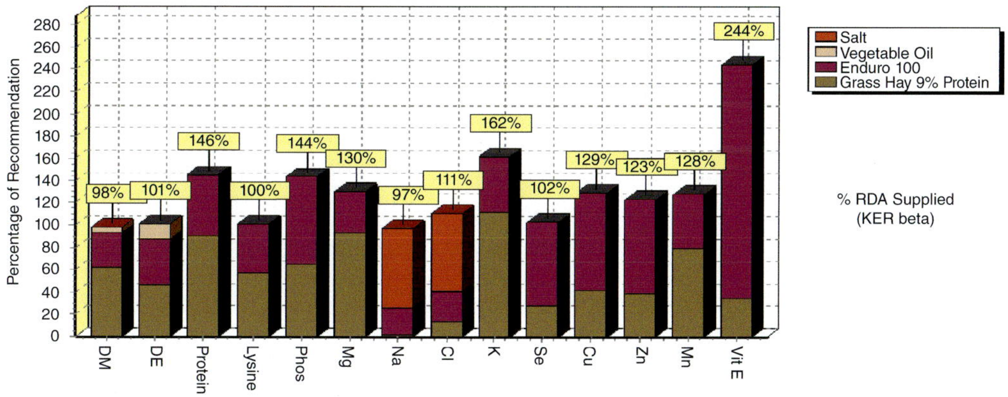

Top tips and considerations for advising oil

1. **High-oil performance feeds**
   - Often the preferred option
     - Balanced with respect to the protein, vitamins and minerals intake when fed with forage.
2. **Supplemental vegetable oils such as corn oil or soya oil**
   - Often added to high-oil or starch-based performance feeds
     - Not balanced in vitamins or minerals (contains none)
   - Advise volumes of up to 90 ml/day to start
     - Increase to 90 ml 2×/day after 12 days
     - Further 10–14 days to increase to 240 ml in morning and evening feeds
   - Advise a minimum of 100 iu vitamin E/100 ml of vegetable oil (Harris, 1999)
   - Oils are susceptible to oxidation or rancidity during storage and use.
     - Horses will reduce their intake if the oil tastes or smells rancid.
     - Advise:
       - sealing containers well and storing in a cool and dark place; and
       - avoiding shaking the oil, as this will create air bubbles, increasing rate of rancidity.

Continued

3. **Some horses dislike taste of rations that contain > 240 ml of oil**
   - Advise a high-fat supplement such as rice bran (22% fat):
     - more palatable;
     - check calcium to phosphorus ratios.
4. **Fat is a useful source of essential fatty acids (see Table 5.7).**

Essential fatty acids

Omega-3 fatty acids are long-chain polyunsaturated fatty acids (PUFAs), which help provide structure to cell membranes in tissues across the body.

In equine nutrition the use of specifically added PUFAs improves exercise parameters (King *et al.*, 2008), lowers heart rate (Woodward *et al.*, 2007), increases sperm production in breeding stallions, improves immune response (Hall *et al.*, 2004a,b), potentially improves insulin sensitivity (Hess *et al.*, 2013), has anti-inflammatory effects (Hess *et al.*, 2013) and increases stride length in arthritic horses (Manhart *et al.*, 2009).

Horses, in common with other herbivores, have a limited ability to convert α-linolenic acid (ALA), docosahexaenoic acid (DHA) and eicosapentaenoic acid (EPA). ALA-supplemented equine diets do not increase DHA or EPA levels in blood or plasma (Vineyard *et al.*, 2010). But when a basal diet of hay and barley was supplemented with 38 g of algal/fish unsaturated fatty acid oil ALA for 90 days, the horses' muscle and red blood EPA and DHA increased (Hess *et al.*, 2013). Requirements for α-linolenic acid are 0.1% total DMI, which can be met by advising rapeseed oil; for example, 120 ml of rapeseed oil (Table 5.7) fed to a 500 kg horse provides 10 g α-linolenic acid/day (Vitec, 1987).

Most compound feeds should have added omega-3 fats to balance the deficiencies in conserved forages. If the horse has unlimited access to fresh pasture, the essential fatty acid requirement can easily be met (Table 5.7).

However, many overweight horses have limited or no access to pasture and are often not fed a balancer. Advise supplementation of ALA and/or EPA/DHA to these horses or check the levels in the balancer.

Timing of Feeding Relative to Exercise

A frequently asked question by clients is when to feed the horse before a competition. Feeding should be timed so that all the nutrients from a meal have been digested, absorbed and stored before starting exercise, but not so long before that the horse begins to mobilise fuels.

Your advice should prioritise the digestion and absorption of concentrate feeds on blood glucose and insulin levels and how this will affect energy production during exercise.

Glucose and insulin

Most research efforts have concentrated on the time of feeding prior to a relatively short bout of exercise. A diet is typically fed at a given time prior to exercise and blood indicators of metabolism and stress are monitored throughout the exercise protocol. Changes in plasma glucose and plasma insulin prior to and during exercise relative to feeding time have been demonstrated (Pagan *et al.*, 1998).

There is a drop in plasma glucose related to the peak insulin post-feeding when horses are exercised within 3 h of feeding, promoting fuel storage in the working muscle, inhibiting lipolysis and the mobilisation of fatty acids (Pagan and Harris, 1999). This will decrease the time to fatigue and have a detrimental effect on performance. After a cereal-based concentrate meal (< 1 g starch/kg meal) insulin levels increase, peaking between 120 and 180 min, and return to baseline usually within 4–7 h post-feeding (Vervuert *et al.*, 2009b).

Cardiovascular effects

Top tip

- Pre-exercise feeding should be completed at least 3–4 h before the start of exercise.
- Do not advise more than 1 g starch/kg per meal.

The size and volume of a pre-exercise meal also requires thought, as feeding large meals of hay, or hay together with concentrates, may result in a decrease of plasma volume due to fluid shifts to the gastrointestinal tract (Clarke *et al.*, 1990). This increase in blood flow to the gastrointestinal tract, away from working muscles and other tissues, together with an increase in bodyweight, may be detrimental to performance. The effect appears to be relative to workload, because when horses were fed and exercised at 75% of maximum heart rate, the increase in heart rate and cardiac output met the demands of performance and the digestive tract (Duren *et al.*, 1992).

Although feeding forage is associated with reduced plasma volume and increased gut fill, this

Table 5.7. A comparison of dietary sources of omega-3 and 6 fatty acids

Source	Notes	Omega-3:6 ratio Concentration of Omega 3:Omega 6 g/kg DM or litre
Pasture	The oil level of fresh grass will depend upon its maturity, species and growing conditions; it is between 3% and 5% A 500 kg horse will consume around 200–264 g of omega-3 per day in the form of α-linolenic acid, when grazing in the spring and summer. Total PUFA and PUFA n-3 are 35.6% greater in fresh pasture compared with hay (Dervishi *et al.*, 2012)	4:1 20.9 g 5.2 g
Hay	Lower levels compared with grass, depends upon preservation (Glasswera *et al.*, 2013). Harvesting reduces total FA by over 50% with a greater loss of linolenic acid (C18:3 n-3) (Vavlo *et al.*, 2005) A high proportion (50-75%) of total fatty acids are the omega-3's (α-linolenic acid (C18:3 n-3) and 18-35% of the fat in hay.	3:1 0.25 g:0.075 g
Canola/ rapeseed[a]	Has the highest omega-3 fatty acid content of the vegetable oils, although it is still significantly lower than its omega-6 level (of its total fat content, 11% is omega-3 fatty acids versus 21% omega-6 fatty acids).	1:2 89 g omega-3 0.6 g alpha-linolenic acid per 100 g
Soya	Extracted from whole soybeans; second to canola as a vegetable oil source of omega-3s. It has a total fat content that is 8% omega-3 fatty acids versus 54% omega-6 fatty acids.	1:6 8 g:540 g
Flaxseed	Commonly confused with linseed. Nutritionally similar but flax is grown for linen. On average, flaxseed is 40% fat with about 58% of the total fat coming from omega-3s. Horses can consume flaxseed oil or whole flaxseed, but to obtain its nutrients they should eat it ground (due to the seed's hard outer coating).	1:0.24 58 g:13.9g
Corn	Corn oil contains 50 times more omega-6 fatty acids than omega-3 fatty acids.	2:28 10 g:550 g
Fish	Mainly derived from cold-water oily fish such as menhaden, herring, cod, or salmon, which serve as rich sources of omega-3 fatty acids. Research conducted at the University of Kentucky showed that adding fish oil to exercising horses' diets resulted in lower heart rates, plasma glycerol, free fatty acids and cholesterol during an exercise test than adding corn oil, a source of omega-6 fatty acids (O'Connor *et al.*, 2004).	6:1 25 g:2 g
Linseed *Linum usitatissimum*	Nutritionally similar to flaxseed but grown specifically for oil as the seed is bigger. 1.0 g/kg was effective in reducing the response to intradermal *Culicoides* allergen (O'Neill *et al.*, 2002; Pearson-O'Neill *et al.*, 2002). At this dose rate issues of palatability, cost and obesity are found (Rendle, 2013).	1:0.23 Linoleic acid C18:2 15% of the fatty acids Linolenic acid C18:3 55% of the fatty acids

[a]https://www.fediol.eu/data/FEDIOL%20Factsheet%20on%20rapeseed%20oil%20-%20June%202020.pdf

disadvantage is more than outweighed by the potential benefit to the horse's long-term health and wellbeing. Feeding only forage before competition does not appear to interfere with FFA availability.

Evidence suggests that the time of feeding is not as important for horses participating in intense exercise of short duration such as racing, but there is still insufficient information to provide clear recommendations for the feed management of racehorses.

Top tip

- Advise feeding up to the time of competition either a small haynet, or hand grazing.
- Completely withholding forage may lead to stomach ulcers (Pagan, 1997).
- Small forage meals encourage chewing and saliva production to help buffer the upper stomach and prevent a drop in pH (Merritt, 2003) (see Chapter 12: 'Forage "meal" size').

Top tip

- Pre-race meals should be kept to < 1 kg.
- Allow access to at least 1 kg of forage in the time between the last concentrate feed and the race.

Feeding after exercise

There are mixed results in the literature in terms of whether diet can enhance glycogen replacement after exercise in the horse (see Chapter 12: 'Muscle glycogen depletion').

The Effect of Feed Type on the Feeding Behaviour of the Horse

The aim of any feeding programme is to maintain as closely as possible the natural eating behaviour of the horse: trickle feeding for 16–18/24 h; moving to find forage – browsing and grazing. Horses will stay stationary while they bite the forage and then spend time chewing until the feed has been broken down to < 1.6 mm before swallowing. There is a seasonal difference in eating time: feral Welsh ponies spend less than 40% of their time eating in late summer compared with nearly 75% of their time in February/March (Morel *et al.*, 2006).

Horses are very effective at selective grazing, utilising their incisors to nibble forages as short as 2 mm. Get clients to think how their horse's premolars and molars meet along the length of the jaw and are highly specialised, with a flattened surface area which is further increased by ridges to provide a very effective grinding surface. Remind them that grazing at floor level allows their horse's lower jaw to drop and execute a wide lateral movement, which is more constrained when feeding from head-high haynets. Show them how the jawbone is hinged above the plane of the teeth and how the wide angle of the mandible provides a broad area of attachment for the well-developed masseter and ptyerygoid muscles (Fig. 5.6).

There is clear evidence that feeding management will change the feeding behaviour of a horse; inevitably, clients will talk to you about the effect that feed has on their horse's behaviour but whether feeding can change a horse's character and temperament is open to debate.

Chewing behaviour and speed of eating

Horses are very effective chewers. Horses produce smaller ingesta particles for their body mass compared with other hind gut fermenters (Fritz *et al.*, 2009), a reflection of their complex and adapted dental morphology (Jernvall and Selänne, 1999).

Top tip

Listening to a horse chewing hay in the quiet of the evening must be one of life's more relaxing activities – do recommend it for your client. Counting the number of chews is as therapeutic as counting sheep to fall asleep.

Concentrates are eaten more quickly than forages (Table 5.8) and forages better replicate the horse's natural chewing behaviour (see Chapter 9, Tables 9.3 and 9.8) compared with concentrates.

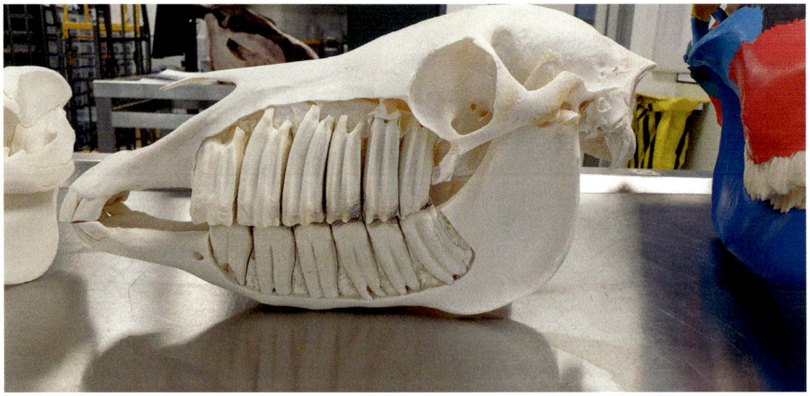

Fig. 5.6 The anatomy of the horse's jaw is specialised for cropping and grinding high-fibre plants. (Used with permission from Dr Ilknur Atkan, University of Surrey.)

Table 5.8 A comparison of effects of different feedstuffs on horse's eating behaviour. (Compiled using data from Janis *et al.*, 2010)

Feed type	Seconds to eat 1 g DM	Chews/second	Chews/kg DM
Straw	2.9–8		
Hay	1.8–4.8		
Haylage	1.7–1.8		
Concentrates	0.5–0.9	1.15	800–2000
Pellets[a] (as fed)	0.31–0.46	1.15	367–565
Oats as fed[b]	1[c]–1.66[d]		
Alfalfa hay	1.57–2	1.23	1889
Timothy hay	2.46–3	1	2540
Mixed hay	2.8–3.5	1.13	3160–3400
Fresh grass	3.9–5.1	1.2	4610

[a]Ellis *et al.* (2005)
[b]Campbell *et al.* (2020)
[c]Clydesdales
[d]Standardbreds and TBs 1.16

The time the horse spends eating concentrates varies according to the type of compound feed (Table 5.9). The size of meal and ingredients impact on consumption rate.

Because concentrates are chewed less, the horse produces less saliva (1 ml saliva/chew) (Houpt, 2012), increasing the risk of choke, which can be mitigated if forage is fed before concentrates.

As workload increases, the amount of forage decreases with a concurrent increase in concentrates, (Table 5.10), thus the client needs to be savvy and manage the diet to mitigate the decrease in feeding times.

Slowing intake

It is possible to double the time it takes a horse to eat hard feed if the horse wears a grazing muzzle (Venable *et al.*, 2016), or advise using novel feeding containers to increase hard-feed eating time (by 61% compared with feeding from buckets) (Carter *et al.*, 2012). A device that enables the horse to trickle-feed concentrates (Mazzola *et al.*, 2016) means clients can replicate feeding forage more closely from a time budget perspective.

When a waffle or balls were added to a concentrate meal, horses took longer to eat and peak insulin (62 μU/ml) was half that of the control meal (112 μU/ml), (Kutzner-Mulligan *et al.*, 2013).

Feeding small meals more frequently spreads eating time and saliva production over a longer period, better replicating trickle feeding. A high-starch diet fed in low-starch meals maximises small intestine digestion of carbohydrates, keeping the glycaemic response within normal physiological limits, and ensures minimal starch into the hind gut (Vervuert *et al.*, 2009b) even for competition horses whose forage intake is reduced.

Table 5.9 Feeding behaviour of horses and ponies fed different compounds and cereals. (Compiled using data from Bochnia *et al.*, 2019.)

Feed type	Mean chews/second: Horses Ponies	Mean chews/kg DM	Average number of minutes to eat 1 kg DM
Oats	1.14	1215	14.4
	1.28	1163	15.4
Muesli mix	1.4	1106	13
	1.43	1163	13.6
Pelleted high-fibre feed (5 mm)	1.45	899	10.3
	1.43	1154	13.5

How to advise feeding concentrates to replicate trickle feeding

As well as management tools for increasing the time it takes the horse to eat its forage (see Chapter 9: 'Replicating natural eating time budgets'), clients can slow the intake of concentrates as follows.

- Add succulents to concentrate feed.
- Feed small quantity of forage/chaff before the hard feed.
- Add chaff to hard feed (unless feeding > 1–1.5 g starch/kg BW).
- Put smooth round stones in the manger to reduce bite size.
- Split daily concentrate ration into small meals.
- Consider the use of feed balls and other devices to slow intake of concentrates.

The way the client manages their horse's diet will change their intake behaviour, with implications for gut health as well as behaviours linked to feeding behaviour, e.g. stereotypies.

The Effect of Feed on the Horse's Behaviour

Stereotypies

Horses fed on low-forage diets spend significantly more time chewing wood (Waters *et al.*, 2002),

Table 5.10 Effect of forage:concentrate ratios on feeding budgets and saliva production in a 500 kg horse

Horse workload	Forage[a] No. of chews (kg)	Concentrates[b] No. of chews (kg)	Total no. of chews	Litres of saliva[c]	Hours eating[d]
Leisure	57,000 (12.5)	0	57,000	5.7	16
Competition	36,800 (8)	4800 (4)	41,600	4.1	11.5
Racehorse	13,800 (3)	8400 (7)	22,200	2.2	6.1

[a]4600 chews/kg hay
[b]1200 chews/kg coarse mix
[c]1 ml saliva/chew
[d]1 chew/second

probably because their satiety feedback mechanism is not met, so they are still motivated to seek food or satisfy their need to chew (McGreevy *et al.*, 1995). When racehorses are fed less than 6.8 kg hay and bedded on materials other than straw, oral stereotypies increase, whereas if chaff is fed or if forage is fed > 3 times/day, oral stereotypies are reduced, (McGreevey *et al.*, 1995). Straw bedding reduces the risk of oral stereotypies, as does grazing (Christie *et al.*, 2006).

The odds of a horse developing oral stereotypies is reduced by 0.94 for every hour of grazing, so if a horse can graze for 12 h then the risk of stereotypy is reduced by 50% (Christie *et al.*, 2006). An increase in movement stereotypies has also been corelated with feeding less forage; the link is less clear but appears to be a result of frustration or 'boredom' (Mason *et al.*, 2007).

Remind clients that stereotypies develop due to frustration and are more likely to develop because of confinement (Mason *et al.*, 2007), isolation or inability to see other horses (Cooper *et al.*, 2000) and food deprivation (Christie *et al.*, 2006), even if enough calories are being fed.

Horses on high-starch diets fed in high-starch meals had higher propionate:acetate ratios in their hind gut compared with when they were just fed hay (measured in fistulated horses). The amount of time spent chewing wood was significantly correlated with the higher caecal propionate (Willard *et al.*, 1977).

Temperament

The horse world (notably the single horse owner) is unique in some of the terminology used to describe the perceived effect of feed on an individual horse's temperament. The type of vocabulary you might come across during a conversation with a client includes 'fizzy', 'laid back', 'heating' and 'non-heating'. The first two relate to their horse's character, the second two to the feed they might want to avoid.

Fizzy

'Fizzy' is used to describe horses with a natural enthusiasm for life with quick reactions; typically breeds that have been bred for speed, such as thoroughbreds, Arabs and thoroughbred crosses and some finely bred (light) pony types. It is worth keeping at the back of your mind that racing thoroughbreds and endurance Arabs are rarely described as fizzy, despite being fed large amounts of concentrates, although some fillies might be perceived as easily stressed.

Laid back

This term is used to describe horses that tend to be lazy or slow and maintain their body fat cover easily – typically breeds that were bred to work long hours at slow paces such as cobs, draughts and heavier breeds.

Heating

This term is rather unique to the UK used in the context of feeding oats, which are considered high in fast-release energy and so 'heats' up a horse. In the USA, horses are described as being 'ditzo' or/ 'ditzy'. Should such a horse react to too many calories in their diet, they are taken off corn and fed oats and their energy intake is reduced (Table 5.11).

Table 5.11 A comparison of the starch, fibre and energy levels of cereals commonly fed to horses

Cereal	DE MJ/kg	Starch %	Fibre %
Maize	14	71	2.4
Wheat	13	70	2.6
Barley	12	60	5.6
Oats	10	48	12.5

Non-heating

This is used to describe fats and fibre that are considered not to affect a horse's temperament, also leisure feeds using terms such as 'contains no oats'.

Evidence

The challenge with all of the above is that, despite common opinion, there is limited evidence to support the effect of oats on a horse's behaviour and indeed that feed per se can change a horse's character. In children, there is little evidence that specific nutrients increase agitation, whereas a lack of concentration is correlated with a poor or unbalanced diet (Bellisle, 2004).

Eating foods (oats) that have a low glycaemic index (Tosh and Chu, 2015) for breakfast increases attention in children, (Benton *et al.*, 2007), reducing insulin response due to the dampening effect of β-gluten (Lan-Pidhainy *et al.*, 2007).

A temporary increase in blood glucose is associated with an increase in alertness and concentration in people (Bellisle *et al.*, 1998), although an increase in plasma glucose did not increase time to fatigue in Standardbred horses (Farris *et al.*, 1998).

Contrary to your client's thoughts, high-carbohydrate meals in people promote drowsiness, sleepiness and calmness (Benton *et al.*, 2022; Spring *et al.*, 1987), due to tryptophan's effects on the brain and of course the subsequent drop in glucose. Similarly, Standardbred horses tire quicker when administrated tryptophan (Farris *et al.*, 1998).

A horse fed high-starch meals rather than low-starch meals will have higher peak insulin. Insulin induces muscle uptake of large amino acids, reducing plasma levels (except Trp) so more Trp is available for the brain because there is less competitiveness for Trp uptake.

High levels of tryptophan (Trp) needed to produce serotonin (5-hydroxytryptamine, 5-HT – a neurotransmitter) are associated with calmness in most species, (Gazzano *et al.*, 2018). Large amino acids compete with Trp uptake to the brain; if the horse is eating a properly balanced diet, then less Trp is taken up by the brain in relation to the other amino acids.

In all mammals, an increase in Trp reduces aggressive behaviour and post-stress plasma cortisol concentrations (Höglund *et al.*, 2019); similarly, an increase in serotonin decreases hostility and aggression in people (van der Mast and Fekkes, 2000; Nantel-Vivier *et al.*, 2011). Remember it is not just diet; stress, physical activity and immune system activation all affect plasma Trp concentrations and brain Trp availability.

It is not always appropriate to extrapolate human studies to horses, because human studies focus on emotional responses rather than a measure of heart rate or activity. People with reduced Trp and serotonin (5-HT) (due to low CHO diets) are more aggressive and restless but researchers caution that 'The magnitude of the effect varies greatly depending on the susceptibility of the subject to lowered mood or aggressivity' (Young and Leyton, 2002).

Individuality might explain the apparent lack of agreement of a diet's effects on a horse's behaviour. Timing of measurements in relation to feeding and improved reactions is likely to be time sensitive – the initial increase in blood glucose provides energy for the brain but later induces a calming effect. Other factors that lead to conflicting results include:

- not feeding isoenergetic diets;
- feeding more than 1g starch/kg BW/meal;
- overemphasising non-significant differences;
- feeding 'isocalorific' diets at the same intake to different bodyweight horses, introducing a variation in nutrient intake/kg BW;
- not acknowledging the impact of ration on individual nutrients;
- correlating physiological changes due to exercise and fitness to diet; and
- over-interpretation of data to fit common perceptions or marketing of feeds.

Increased cortisol is used to confirm 'behavioural stress' in many of the trials, but it is important to consider that the increase might be in response to physiological stress. In rats the overflow of undigested carbohydrates into the hind gut is linked to increased anxiety and aggression (Hanstock *et al.*, 2004).

Horses fed high-starch meals have a higher risk of stereotypies, but this was reduced by dietary supplementation with virginiamycin, an antibiotic that altered faecal pH (Johnson *et al.*, 1998).

You can mitigate that physiological stress by advising that a high-starch diet is fed as low-starch meals.

Low starch meals do **NOT**:

- increase the risk of EGUS;
- overwhelm the capacity of the stomach and small intestine;
- increase glycaemic and insulinaemic responses above normal physiological levels;
- increase transit rates of digesta;
- result in hydrolysable carbohydrate fermentation in the hindgut; nor
- lower pH.

In most of the studies comparing reactivity of horses to starch versus fat diets, it is important to note that 'fearfulness and investigative behaviour is only affected in challenging situations, whereas few differences occur in the normal behavioural profiles of horses at pasture' (Hothersall and Nicol, 2009).

You will have experienced this conflict of experience. Some clients can feed 'buckets' of oats to their cob or racing TB with no change in character, whereas others swear their horse only needs to sniff the oats for it to be unhandlable.

Perception is reinforced by the inclusion of oats in performance feeds but not lower energy feeds; when in fact oats are lower in calories compared with all the other cereals (Table 5.11). Take the time to understand what the client expects from the feed and use evidence base to explain the terminology.

Explaining Feed and Marketing Terminology by Relating to Gut Physiology

Energy versus calories

These terms are used to describe the same scientific value but have different meanings in everyday life (see Chapter 11: 'How to advise the correct compound feed'). As well as using scientific terms in everyday language, emotive adjectives further add to the confusion.

Heating versus non-heating

Heating

Heating is defined in the dictionary as the process of warming. Fermentation of fibre produces heat; this is measurable digestion, i.e. heat increment (HI). It is possible to quantify the heat increment of feed ingredients, although a relative comparison provides a stronger message for clients (Table 5.12).

Horses fed fat and hay had a 6% lower HI compared with horses fed hay and oats (17% less HI compared with just hay); the effect of the reduced HI was estimated to decrease water requirement by 6 kg/day, faecal water output by 4 kg and evaporative water losses by 2 kg (Kronfeld, 1996).

If a client wants a heating feed, then recommend high fibre, which is fermented in the hind gut, taking up to 65 h (often described as slow release) after eating before the volatile fatty acids are absorbed and incorporated as propionate into the Krebs cycle. Rectal temperatures can crudely monitor this 'heating effect' (Ellis *et al.*, 2002).

Non-heating

Ingredients that contain starch are digested by mammalian enzymes in the small intestine (no fermentation is involved) producing negligible heat increment. Their speed of digestion can be measured by the glycaemic response (Fig. 5.7); feeds containing these types of ingredients can be described as fast-releasing as the glucose is available 2 h after feeding.

The consequence of this misunderstanding results in the laid-back horse being fed more food to provide more energy (so gets fatter) and the active horse that burns off calories is fed less energy to 'keep it calm' (so loses weight).

Table 5.12 A comparison of relative heat increments (heat of digestion) of common feeds fed to horses.

Heat increment/ heat of digestion	Feeds
High	Hay, Straw, Alfalfa, Chaffs
Medium	Fibre Cubes, Oats, Soya, Molasses
Low	Oil, Maize, Wheat, Barley

> **Top tip**
>
> - Rather than using words that cannot be quantified, do consider describing diets as low calorie or high calorie.
> - Then relate how the energy is released – fast or slow releasing.

Which Feed – What to Advise

Despite all the academic evidence, you will know that most of your clients feed complementary feeds and not straights. Choose from an appropriate range comparable with the workload and from a brand that is reputable (see Chapter 8).

These feeds inevitably contain a mixture of ingredients to meet the nutritional specification on the bag and can meet the client's need for different energy sources which are underpinned by exercise physiology and muscle metabolism (Fig. 5.8).

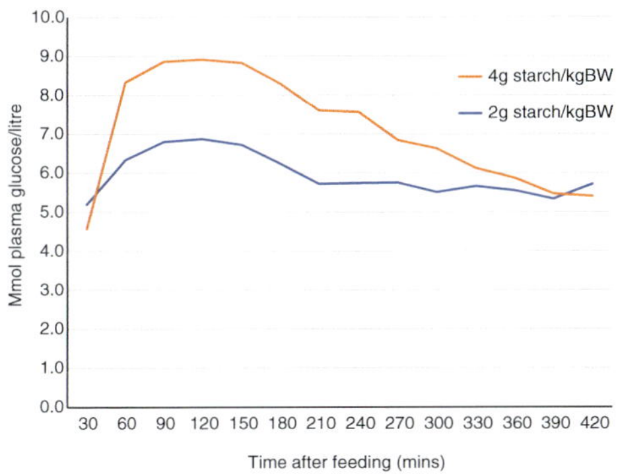

Fig. 5.7 A simplified summary of starch digestion in the horse.

- Check if the horse needs a high-calorie feed (usually a performance horse) or a low-calorie feed (normally a balancer for leisure).
- If the horse is in work, decide the type of work they are doing.
    - Fast work: the ingredients should be fast-releasing.
    - Slow work: consider slow-releasing energy ingredients.
- Quite often, the horse needs a mix of both. Whilst many of the queries will be about the 'problem' horses, it is important to appreciate that most horses fed appropriately just need a complementary feed to increase the calories they need for work.
- Advise 2.5% BW intake as kg DMI. Manipulate forage to concentrate ratios to meet calorie requirements.
- Please do not allow your clients to feed a handful of a mix to their horse in light work.
    - The likelihood is that the horse has a fat score over 3.5 on at least two parts of its body.
    - The only 'feed' they need is a balancer (see Chapter 11, Table 11.4: 'The difference in calorie intakes from a selection of leisure horse feeds formulated to be fed at different intakes but all providing vitamin/mineral and protein requirements when fed with forage').
    - Regardless of which feed you are advising, the key to a healthy gut is maintaining a dry matter intake of 2.5% BW and to manipulate the forage:concentrates ratio (Table 5.13).

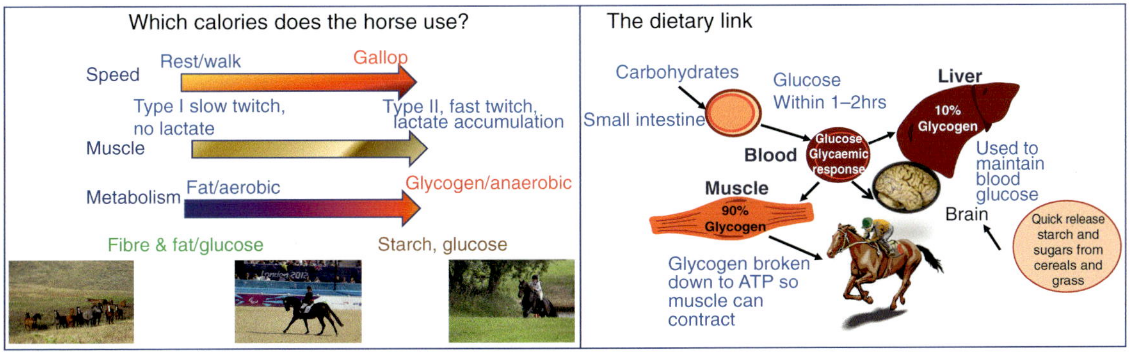

Fig. 5.8 The relationship between exercise types and energy metabolism in the horse. (Adapted from D Marlin/T Hollands, Cheltenham)

Table 5.13 Advising the correct type of energy relative to the horse's workload and client's perception of character

Horse	Character	'Type' of feed	Contribution to energy (%) by feed type	Ration
rising 4; 17.1; warmblood gelding; workload is light Dressage 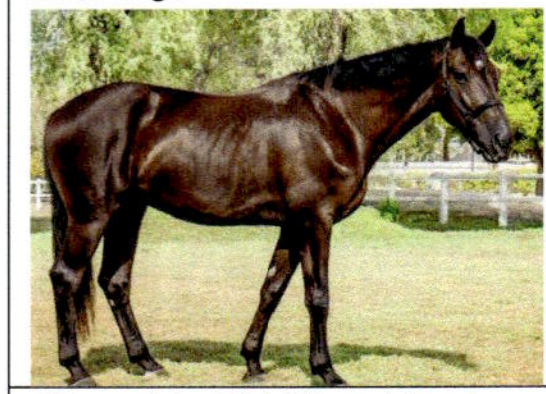	Fizzy & excitable *a horse which just loves life; his sheer exuberance will be fantastic for his future career as a top dressage horse but at the moment it is a little difficult to control* *he needs a lot of energy (calories) in his diet, because he burns so much off just simply being him.* *if I fed him less food, the horse would still be exuberant, but he might love life less and become grumpy.*	slow release, high calorie	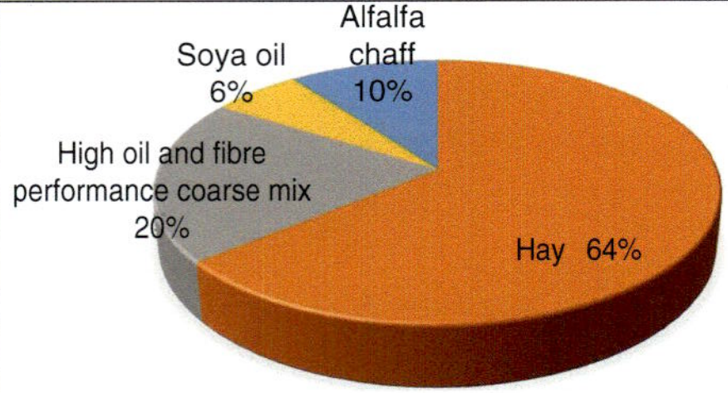	Total calorie intake 144 MJ DE/day 21.8 MJDE/100 kgBW Approx. 17.5 MJ forage, 1 MJ starch, 2.1 MJ 'fibre', 1.5 MJ oil/ 100 kgBW
12yrs old, 17.1 Warmblood gelding; Medium work Prix St George 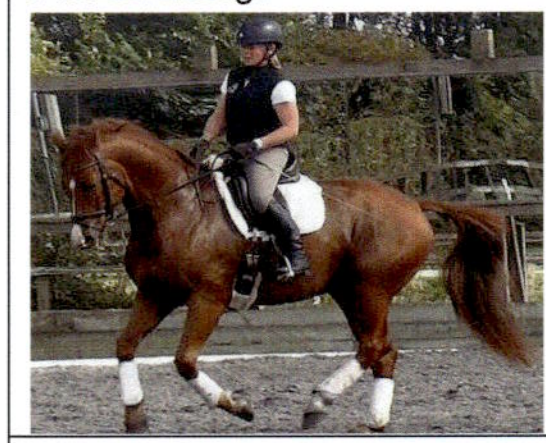	Laid back *I do not need to feed him lots of energy. It is very important with this horse to realise that it is sometimes a lack of motivation not a lack of energy which holds him back.'* *an internal worrier, he implodes when stressed, you could compare him to a human deep thinker. When he is stressed, he freezes and acts really dead*	Fast release, low calorie	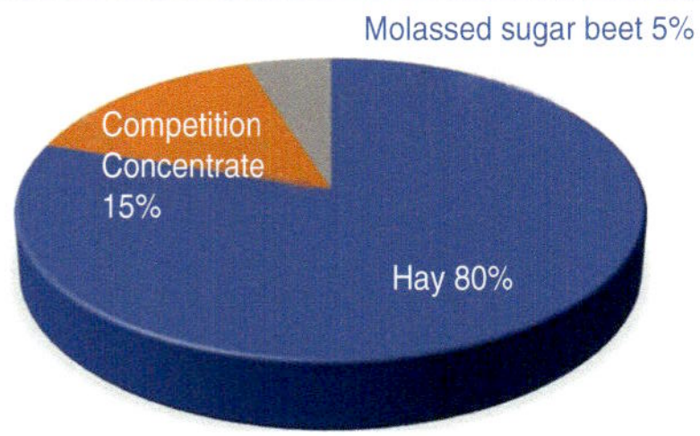	Total calorie intake 122.8 MJ DE/day 19.7 MJ DE/100 kgBW Approx. 14MJ forage, 3 MJ starch, 2.1 MJ 'fibre', 0.1 MJ oil/100 kgBW
6yr old TB Gelding 16.2hh National Hunt	Normal *needs enough energy to maintain his winning streak* 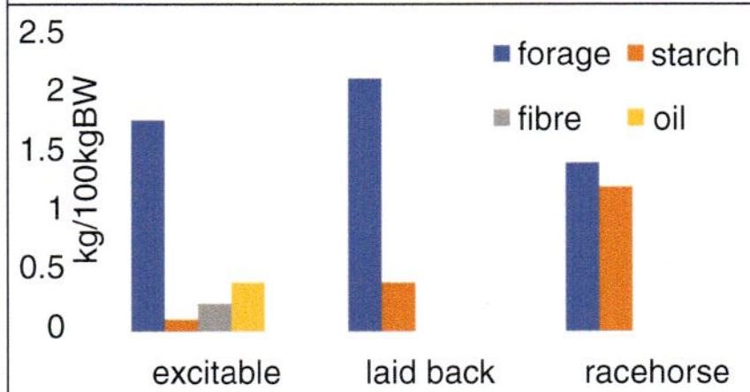	fast release high calorie	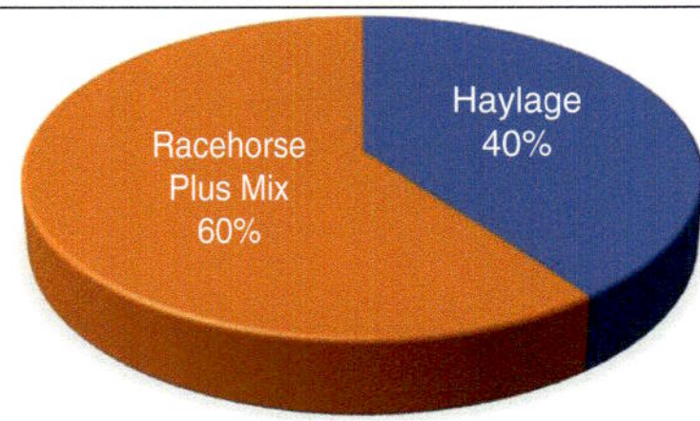	Total Calorie intake 130 MJ/day 25.8 MJ DE/100 kgBW Approx 11 MJ forage, 15 MJ starch/100 kgBW

Summary

Feeding performance horses is a delicate balance between art and science and their diets need to provide soluble carbohydrates, protein, fibre and fat to meet their nutritional requirements. Concentrate feeds formulated for performance horses are high in carbohydrates and fats to meet the energy demands for high-intensity work as well as ensuring muscle development.

The health, welfare and performance of the horse is best supported when feeding management and diet match the horse's workload and natural feeding behaviour – which is achievable in even the hardest working horses. Feeding a high-starch ration should be managed as small starch meals – split into small but frequent feeds throughout the day. Forage intake should not be compromised.

A balanced diet can be achieved by advising the correct feed for the correct need, ensuring micronutrient intakes and applying the evidence to encourage the science of rationing supports the art of feeding. Leisure horses rarely need extra calories over and above their forage, but will require some form of vitamin, mineral and protein balancer.

Note

[i] https://www.legislation.gov.uk/eur/2009/767/adopted#:~:text=was%20originally%20adopted).-,REGULATION%20(EC)%20No%20767/2009%20OF%20THE%20EUROPEAN%20PARLIAMENT%20AND,of%2013%20July%202009,-on%20the%20placing

Bibliography

Alexander, F. and Hickson, J. (1970) The salivary and pancreatic secretions of the horse. In: Philipson, A.T. (ed.) *Physiology of Digestion and Metabolism in the Ruminant*. Oriel Press, Newcastle, pp. 375–380.

Bellisle, F. (2004) Effects of diet on behaviour and cognition in children. *British Journal of Nutrition* 92 (suppl. 2), S227–S232. doi: 10.1079/bjn20041171.

Bellisle, F., Blundell, J., Dye, L., Fantiono, M., Fern, E. *et al*. (1998) Functional food science and behaviour and psychological functions. *British Journal of Nutrition* 80(S1), S173–S193. doi: 10.1079/BJN19980109.

Benton, D., Maconie, A. and Williams, C. (2007) The influence of the glycaemic loads of breakfast on the behaviour of children in school. *Physiology and Behaviour* 92, 717–724.

Benton, D., Bloxham, A., Gaylor, C., Brennan, A. and Young, H.A. (2022) Carbohydrate and sleep: an evaluation of putative mechanisms. *Frontiers in Nutrition* 9, 933898. do: 10.3389/fnut.2022.933898.

Bochnia, M., Goetz, F., Wensch-Dorendorf, M., Koelin, M. and Zeyner, A. (2019) Chewing patterns in horses during the intake of variable quantities of two pelleted compound feeds differing in their physical characteristics only. *Research in Veterinary Science* 125, 189–194.

Borgia, L., Valberg, S., McCue, M., Watts, K. and Pagan, J. (2011) Glycaemic and insulinaemic responses to feeding hay with different non-structural carbohydrate content in control and polysaccharide storage myopathy-affected horses. *Journal of Animal Physiology and Animal Nutrition* 95, 798–807.

Bowman, V.A., Fontenot, J.P., Meacham, T.N. and Webb, K.E.J.R. (1979) Acceptability and digestibility of animal vegetable and blended fats by equine. In: *Proceedings of the 6th Equine Nutrition and Physiology Society Symposium*, Texas A and M University, Equine Nutrition and Physiology Society, USA.

Bulmer, L.S., Murray, J.A., Burns, N.M., Garber, A., Wemelsfelder, F. *et al*. (2019) High-starch diets alter equine faecal microbiota and increase behavioural reactivity. *Scientific Reports* 9(1), 1–11.

Bush, J.A., Freeman, D.E., Kline, K.H., Merchen, N.R. and Fahey Jr, G.C. (2001) Dietary fat supplementation effects on in vitro nutrient disappearance and *in vivo* nutrient intake and total tract digestibility by horses. *Journal of Animal Science* 79(1), 232–239.

Campbell, T.E., Doughty, H., Harris, P.A., de Laat, M.A. and Sillence, M.N. (2020) Factors affecting the rate and measurement of feed intake for a cereal-based meal in horses. *Journal of Equine Veterinary Science* 84, 102869.

Cargile, J.L., Burrow, J.A., Kim, I., Cohen, N.D. and Merritt, A.M. (2004) Effect of dietary corn oil supplementation on equine gastric fluid acid, sodium, and prostaglandin E2 content before and during pentagastrin infusion. *Journal of Veterinary Internal Medicine* 18(4), 545–549.

Carmalt, J.L. and Allen, A. (2008) The relationship between cheek tooth occlusal morphology, apparent digestibility, and ingesta particle size reduction in horses. *Journal of the American Veterinary Medical Association* 233(3), 452–455. doi: 10.2460/javma.233.3.452.

Carter, M.J., Friend, T.H., Coverdale, J., Garey, S.M., Adams, A.L. *et al*. (2012) A comparison of three conventional horse feeders with the Pre-Vent feeder. *Journal of Equine Veterinary Science* 32(4), 252–255.

Christie, J.L., Hewson, C.J., Riley, C.B., McNiven, M.A., Dohoo, I.R. and Bates, L.A. (2006) Management factors affecting stereotypies and body condition score in nonracing horses in Prince Edward Island. *Canadian Veterinary Journal – La revue veterinaire canadienne* 47(2), 136–143.

Clarke, L.L., Roberts, M.C. and Argenzio, R.A. (1990) Feeding and digestive problems in horses: physiologic responses to a concentrated meal. *Veterinary*

Clinics of North America: Equine Practice 6(2), 433–450.
Coenen, M., Moesseler, A. and Vervuert, I. (2006) Fermentative gases in breath indicate that inulin and starch to be degraded by microbial fermentation in the stomach and small intestine of the horse in contrast to pectin and cellulose. *Journal of Nutrition* 136, 2108S–2110S.
Cohen, N.D. and Peloso, J.G. (1996) Risk factors for history of previous colic and for chronic, intermittent colic in a population of horses. *Journal of the American Veterinary Medical Association* 208, 697–703.
Cohen, N.D., Gibbs, P.G. and Woods, A.M. (1999) Dietary and other management factors associated with equine colic. *Journal of the American Veterinary Medical Association* 215, 53–60.
Cooper, J.L., McDonald, L. and Mills, D.S. (2000) The effect of increasing visual horizons on stereotypic weaving: implications for the social housing of stabled horses. *Applied Animal Behaviour Science* 69(1), 67–83.
Craig, D.R., Shivy, D.R., Pankowski, R.L. and Erb, H.N. (1990) Esophageal disorders in 61 horses: results of nonsurgical and surgical management. *Veterinary Surgery* 18(6).
Cuddeford, D. (1996) *Equine Nutrition*. Crowood Press.
Cuddeford, D. (2001) Starch digestion in the horse. In: Pagan, J.D. and Geor, J. (eds) *Advances in Equine Nutrition II*. Nottingham University Press, Thrumpton, UK, pp. 95–103.
De Fombelle, A., Goachet, A.G., Varloud, M., Boisot, P. and Julliand, V. (2003) Effects of diet on prececal digestion of different starches in the horse measured with the nylon bag technique. In: *Proceedings 18th Equine Nutrition and Physiology Society Symposium*, East Lansing, Michigan, pp. 115–116.
Dervishi, E., Joy, M., Sanz, A. *et al.* (2012). Forage preservation (grazing vs. hay) fed to ewes affects the fatty acid profile of milk and *CPT1B* gene expression in the sheep mammary gland. *BMC Veterinary Research* 8, 106.
Dunnett, C.E., Marlin, D. and Harris, R.C. (2002) Effect of dietary lipid on response to exercise: relationship to metabolic adaptation. *Equine Veterinary Journal* (34), 75–80. doi: 10.1111/j.2042-3306.2002.tb05395.x.
Duren, S.E., Manohar, M., Sikkes, B., Jackson, S. and Baker, J. (1992) Influence of feeding and exercise on the distribution of intestinal and muscle blood flow in ponies. *Pferdeheilkunde* 1, 24–28.
Duren, S.E., Pagan, J.D., Harris, P.A. and Crandall, K.G. (1999) Time of feeding and fat supplementation affect plasma concentrations of insulin and metabolites during exercise. *Equine Veterinary Journal* 31(S30), 479–484.
Eaton, M.D., Hodgson, D.R., Evans, D.L., Bryden, W.L. and Ross, M.W. (1995) Effect of a diet containing supplementary fat on the capacity for high intensity exercise. *Equine Veterinary Journal* (Suppl. 18), 353–356.
Ellis, J.M., Hollands, T. and Allen, D. (2002) Effect of forage intake on bodyweight and performance. *Equine Veterinary Journal* 34 (Suppl. 6), 66–70.
Ellis, A.D., Thomas, S., Arkell, K. and Harris, P. (2005) Adding chopped straw to concentrate feed: the effect of inclusion rate and particle length on intake behaviour of horses. *Pferdeheilkunde* 21.
Farris, J.W., Hinchcliff, K.W., McKeever, K.H., Lamb, D.R. and Thompson, D.L. (1998) Effect of tryptophan and of glucose on exercise capacity of horses. *Journal of Applied Physiology* 85(3), 807–816.
Frank, N., Andrews, F.M. and Elliot, S.B. (2005) Effects of dietary oils on the development of gastric ulcers in mares. *American Journal Veterinary Research* 66, 2006–2011.
Frape, D. (1986) *Equine Nutrition and Feeding.* 1st edn. Longman Scientific, Harlow, UK.
Fritz, J., Hummel, J., Kienzle, E., Arnold, C., Nunn, C. and Clauss, M. (2009) Comparative chewing efficiency in mammalian herbivores. *Oikos* 118(11), 1623–1632. doi: 10.1111/j.1600-0706.2009.17807.x.
Gazzano, A., Ogi, A., Torracca, B., Mariti, C. and Casini, I. (2018) Plasma tryptophan/large neutral amino acids ratio in domestic dogs is affected by a single meal with high carbohydrates level. *Animals* 8(5), 63. doi: 10.3390/ani8050063.
Geelen, S.N., Jansen, W.L., van Oldruitenborgh-Oosterbaan, M.M.S, Breukink, H.J. and Beynen, A.C. (2001) Fat feeding increases equine heparin-released lipoprotein lipase activity. *Journal of Veterinary Internal Medicine* 15(5), 478–481.
Glassera, F., Doreaua, M., Maxina G. and Baumonta, R. (2013) Fat and fatty acid content and composition of forages: A meta-analysis. *Animal Feed Science and Technology* 185, 19–34.
Graham-Thiers, P.M., Kronfeld, D.S., Kline, K.A. and Sklan, D.J. (2001) Dietary protein restriction and fat supplementation diminish the acidogenic effect of exercise during repeated sprints in horses. *The Journal of Nutrition* 131(7), 1959–1964.
Gupta, R.K., Gangoliya, S.S. and Singh, N.K. (2015) Reduction of phytic acid and enhancement of bioavailable micronutrients in food grains. *Journal of Food Science and Technology* 52(2), 676–684. doi: 10.1007/s13197-013-0978-y.
Hall, J.A., Van Saun, R.J. and Wander, R.C. (2004a) Dietary (n-3) fatty acids from menhaden fish oil alter plasma fatty acids and leukotrienes b synthesis in healthy horses. *Journal of Veterinary Internal Medicine* 18, 871–879.
Hall, J.A., Van Saun, R.J., Tornquist, S.J., Gradin, J.L., Pearson, E.G. *et al.* (2004b) Effect of type of dietary polyunsaturated fatty acid supplement (corn oil or fish oil) in immune response in healthy horses. *Journal of Veterinary Internal Medicine* 18, 880–886.
Hambleton, P.L., Slade, L.M., Hamar, D.W., Kienholz, E.W. and Lewis, L.D. (1990) Dietary fat and exercise

conditioning effect on metabolic parameters in the horse. *Journal of Animal Science* 51(6), 1330–1339. doi: 10.2527/jas1981.5161330x.

Hanstock, T.L., Clayton, E.H., Li, K.M. and Mallet, P.E. (2004) Anxiety and aggression associated with the fermentation of carbohydrates in the hindgut of rats. *Physiology & Behavior* 82, 357–368. doi: 10.1016/j.physbeh.2004.04.00.

Harking, J.D., Morris, G.S., Tulley, R.T., Nelson, A.G. and Kamerling, S.G. (1992) Effect of added dietary fat on racing performance in Thoroughbred horses. *Journal of Equine Veterinary Science* 12(2), 123–129.

Harris, P.A. (1999) *Feeding and management advice for tying up*. In: *Proceedings of the British Equine Veterinary Association Specialist Meeting on Nutrition and Behaviour*, pp. 100–104.

Harris, P.A. (2007) How should we feed horses - and how many times a day? *Veterinary Journal* 173(2), 252–253.

Harris, P.A., Pagan, J.D., Crandell, K.G. and Duren, S.E. (1999) Effect of feeding thoroughbred horses a high unsaturated or saturated vegetable oil supplemented diet for 6 months following a 10 month fat acclimation. *Equine Veterinary Journal* (Suppl. 30), 468–474.

Hess, T. and Ross-Jones, T. (2014) Omega-3 fatty acid supplementation in horses. *Revista Brasileira de Zootecnia* 43(12), 677–683.

Hess, T.M., Rexford, J., Hansen, D.K., Ahrens, N.S., Harris, M. *et al.* (2013) Effects of Ω-3 (n-3) fatty acid supplementation on insulin sensitivity in horses. *Journal of Equine Veterinary Science* 33(6), 446–453.

Hillyer, M.H., Taylor, F.G., Proudman, C.J., Edwards, G.B., Smith, J.E. *et al.* (2002) Case control study to identify risk factors for simple colonic obstruction and distention colic in horses. *Equine Veterinary Journal* 34, 455–463.

Hintz, H.F., Ross, M.W., Lesser, F.R., Leids, P.F., White, K.K. *et al.* (1978) The value of dietary fat for working horses. *I. Biochemical and Hematological Evaluations* 2, 483–488.

Hoffman, R.M. (2009) Carbohydrate metabolism and metabolic disorders in horses. *Revista Brasileira de Zootecnia* 38, 270–276.

Hoglund, E., Øverli, Ø. and Winberg, S. (2019) Tryptophan metabolic pathways and brain serotonergic activity: a comparative review. *Frontiers in Endocrinology* 10, 158.

Holden, R.J. (1995) Schizophrenia, suicide and the serotonin story. *Medical Hypotheses* 44(5), 379–391.

Holland, J.L., Kronfield, D.S. and Hoffman, R.M. (1996a) Weaning stress is affected by nutrition and weaning methods. *Pferdeheilkunde* 12, 257–260.

Holland, J.L., Kronfeld, D.S. and Meacham, T.N. (1996b) Behaviour of horses is affected by soy lecithin and corn oil in the diet. *Journal of Animal Science* 74, 1252–1255.

Hollands, T. and Cuddeford, D. (1992) Effect of supplementary soya oil on the digestibility of nutrients contained in a 40:60 roughage/concentrate diet fed to horses. In: *Europaische Konferenz uber die Ernahrung des Pferdes* 8, 128–132.

Hothersall, B. and Nicol, C. (2009) Role of diet and feeding in normal and stereotypic behaviors in horses. *Veterinary Clinics of North America: Equine Practice* 25(1), 167–181.

Houpt, K.A. (2012) A preliminary answer to the question of whether cribbing causes salivary secretion. *Journal of Veterinary Behavior* 7(6), 322–324.

Hughes, S.J., Potter, G.D., Greene, L.W., Odom, T.W. and Murray-Gerzik, M. (1995) Adaptation of thoroughbred horses in training to a fat supplemented diet. *Equine Veterinary Journal* 27(S18), 349–352.

Hyyppa, S., Saastamoinen, M. and Poso, A.R. (1999) Effect of a post exercise fat-supplemented diet on muscle glycogen repletion. *Equine Veterinary Journal* (Suppl.) 475–493.

Janis, C.M., Constable, E.C., Houpt, K.A., Streich, W.J. and Clauss, M. (2010) Comparative ingestive mastication in domestic horses and cattle: a pilot investigation. *Journal of Animal Physiology and Animal Nutrition* 94(6), e402–e409. doi: 10.1111/j.1439-0396.2010.01030.x

Jansen, W.L., Van der Kuilen, J., Geelen, S.N. and Beynen, A.C. (2001) The apparent digestibility of fibre in trotters when dietary soybean oil is substituted for an iso-energetic amount of glucose. *Archives of Animal Nutrition* 54(4), 297–304.

Jansen, W.L., Van der Kuilen, J., Geelen, S.N.J. and Beynen, A.C. (2000) The effect of replacing nonstructural carbohydrates with soybean oil on the digestibility of fibre in trotting horses. *Equine Veterinary Journal* 32(1), 27–30.

Jansson, A. and Lindberg, J.E. (2012) A forage-only diet alters the metabolic response of horses in training. *Animal* 6(12), 1939–1946.

Jernvall, J. and Selänne, L. (1999) Laser confocal microscopy and geographic information systems in the study of dental morphology. *Palaeontologia electronica* 2(1), 18.

Johnson, K.G., Tyrrell, J.B., Roqe, J.B. and Pethick, D.W. (1998) Behavioural changes in stabled horses given nontherapeutic levels of virginiamycin. *Equine Veterinary Journal* 30, 139–143.

Jones, L., Lax, J. and Hollands, T. (2005a)Analysis of the mineral content of spring summer grazing used for thoroughbred breeding stock in the UK. In: Proceedings of 44th BEVA Congress, Harrogate, p. 368.

Jones, L., Lax, J. and Hollands, T. (2005b) *The Mineral Content of Spring and Summer Pasture Grazed by Young Growing Thoroughbreds in the UK*. Short communication ENUCO, Hanover, Germany.

Jose-Cunilleras, E., Hinchcliff, K.W., Sams, R.A., Devor, S.T. and Linderman, J.K. (2002) Glycemic index of a meal fed before exercise alters substrate use and glucose flux in exercising horses. *Journal of Applied Physiology* 92(1), 117–128.

Julen, T.R., Potter, G.D., Greene, L.W. and Stott, G.G. (1995) Adaptation to a fat-supplemented diet by cutting horses. *Journal of Equine Veterinary Science* 15(10), 436–440.

Julliand, V., de Fombelle, A. and Varloud, M. (2006) Starch digestion in horses: the impact of feed processing. *Livestock Science* 100, 44–52. doi: 10.1016/j.livprodsci.2005.11.001.

Kane, E. and Baker, J.P. (1977) Utilization of a corn oil supplemented diet by the horse. *Proceedings of the Equine Nutrition and Physiology Society* 5, 41.

Kienzle, E., Radicke, S., Wilke, S., Landes, E., Meyer, H. (1992) Praeileale Sta¨rkeverdauung in Abha¨ngigkeit von Sta¨rkeart undzubereitung: 1. Europa¨ische Konferenz u¨ber die Erna¨hrung des Pferdes. Pferdeheilkunde, Hannover, Germany, pp. 103–105.

Kienzle, E., Radicke, S., Landes, E., Kleffken, D., Illenseer, M. *et al.* (1994) Activity of amylase in the gastrointestinal tract of the horse. *Journal of Animal Physiology and Animal Nutrition* 72, 234–241.

King, S.S., AbuGhazaleh, A.A., Webel, S.K. and Jones, K.L. (2008) Circulating fatty acid profiles in response to three levels of dietary omega-3 fatty acid supplementation in horses. *Journal of Animal Science* 86(5), 1114–1123. doi: 10.2527/jas.2007-0682.

Kronfeld, D.S. (1996) Dietary fat affects heat production and other variables of equine performance under hot and humid conditions. *Equine Veterinary Journal* (Suppl. 22), 22–34.

Kronfeld, D.S. and Harris, P.A. (2003) Equine grain-associated disorders. *Compendium* 25(12), 974–983.

Kronfeld, D.S., Ferrante, P.L. and Grandjean, D. (1994) Optimal nutrition for athletic performance, with emphasis on fat adaptation in dogs and horses. *The Journal of Nutrition* 124(Suppl. 12), 2745S–2753S.

Kronfeld, D.S., Custalow, S.E., Ferrante, P.L., Taylor, L.E., Wilson, J.A. and Tiegs, W. (1998) Acid–base responses of fat-adapted horses: relevance to hard work in the heat. *Applied Animal Behaviour Science* 59(1–3), 61–72.

Kronfeld, D.S., Holland, J.L., Rich, G.A., Custalow, S.E., Fontenot, J.P. *et al.* (2001) Digestibility of fat. In: Proceedings 17th Equine Nutrition and Physiology Society Symposium, pp. 156–158.

Kronfeld, D.S., Holland, J.L., Rich, G.A., Meacham, T.N., Fontenot, J.P. *et al.* (2004) Fat digestibility in *Equus caballus* follows increasing first-order kinetics. *Journal of Animal Science* 82(6), 1773–1780.

Kutzner-Mulligan, J., Eisemann, J., Siciliano, P., Smith, J., Hewitt, K., Sharlette, J. and Pratt-Phillips, S. (2013) The effect of different feed delivery methods on time to consume feed and the resulting changes in postprandial metabolite concentrations in horses. *Journal of Animal Science* 91(8), 3772–3779. doi: 10.2527/jas.2012-5727.

Lacombe, V.A., Hinchcliff, K.W., Kohn, C.W., Devor, S.T. and Taylor, L.E. (2004) Effects of feeding meals with various soluble-carbohydrate content on muscle glycogen synthesis after exercise in horses. *American Journal of Veterinary Research* 65(7), 916–923.

Lan-Pidhainy, X., Brummer, Y., Tosh, S.M., Wolever, T.M. and Wood, P.J. (2007) Reducing beta-glucan solubility in oat bran muffins by freeze-thaw treatment attenuates its hypoglycemic effect. *Cereal Chemistry* 84, 512–517. doi: 10.1094/CCHEM-84-5-0512.

Lawrence, L.M. (1990) Nutrition and fuel utilization in the athletic horse. *The Veterinary Clinics of North America. Equine Practice* 6(2), 393–418. doi: 10.1016/s0749-0739(17)30548-5.

Lawrence, L., Soderholm, L.V., Roberts, A., Williams, J. and Hintz, H. (1993) Feeding status affects glucose metabolism in exercising horses. *The Journal of Nutrition* 123(12), 2152–2157. doi: 10.1093/jn/123.12.2152.

Lindberg, J.E., Essen-Gustavsson, B., Dahlborn, K., Gottlieb-Vedi, M. and Jansson, A. (2006) Exercise response, metabolism at rest and digestibility in athletic horses fed high-fat oats. *Equine Veterinary Journal* 38(S36), 626–630.

Longland, A.C. (2001) Plant carbohydrates: analytical methods and nutritional implications for equines. In: *Proceedings 17th Equine Nutrition and Physiology Society Symposium*, Lexington, Kentucky, pp. 174–176.

Lutherson, N., Hou Neilson, K. and Harris, P. (2009) Risk factors associated with gastric ulceration syndrome in 201 horses in Denmark. *Equine Veterinary Journal* 41, 625–630.

Manhart, D.R., Scott, B.D., Gibbs, P.G., Coverdale, J.A., Eller, E.M. *et al.* (2009) Markers of inflammation in arthritic horses fed omega-3 fatty acids. *The Professional Animal Scientist* 25(2), 155–160.

Mason, G., Clubb, R., Latham, N. and Vickery, S. (2007) Why and how should we use environmental enrichment to tackle stereotypic behaviour. *Applied Animal Behaviour Science* 102, 163–188. doi: 10.1016'j.applanim.2006.05.041.

Mazzola, S., Palestrini, C., Cannas, S., Fè, E., Bagnato, G.L. *et al.* (2016) Efficacy of a feed dispenser for horses in decreasing cribbing behaviour. *Veterinary Medicine International* 2016, 4698602–4698606. doi: 10.1155/2016/4698602.

McDonald, P., Edwards, R.A., Greenhalgh, J.F.D. and Morgan, C.A. (1995) *Animal Nutrition*, 5th edn. Addison Wesley Longman, Singapore.

McGreevy, P.D., Cripps, P.J., French, N.P., Green, L.E. and Nicol, C.J. (1995) Management factors associated with stereotypic and redirected behaviour in the thoroughbred horse. *Equine Veterinary Journal* 27(2), 86–91. doi: 10.1111/j.2042-3306.1995.tb03041.

McLean, B.M.L., Hyslop, J.J., Longland, A.C., Cuddeford, D. and Hollands, T. (1999a) Development of the mobile bag technique to determine the degradation kinetics of purified starch sources in the pre-caecal

segment of the equine digestive tract. *Proceedings of the British Society of Animal Science* 1999, 138.
McLean, B.M.L., Hyslop, J.J., Longland, A.C., Cuddeford, D. and Hollands, T. (1999b) Effect of physical processing on *in situ* degradation of maize and peas in the caecum of ponies. *Proceedings of the British Society of Animal Science* 1999, 134.
McLean, B.M.L., Hyslop, J.J., Longland, A.C., Cuddeford, D. and Hollands, T. (1999c) Effect of screen diameter on particle size and water holding capacity of 15 starch based on equine feedstuffs ground through a 1.0 mm or 0.5 mm screen. *Proceedings of the British Society of Animal Science* 1999, 136.
McLean, B.M.L., Hyslop, J.J., Longland, A.C., Cuddeford, D. and Hollands, T. (1999d) *In vivo* apparent digestibility in ponies given rolled micronized or extruded barley. *In: BSAS (ed.) Proceedings of the British Society of Animal Science* 1999, 133.
McLean, B.M.L., Hyslop, J.J., Longland, A.C., Cuddeford, D. and Hollands, T. (2000) Physical processing of barley and its effects on intra-caecal fermentation parameters in ponies. *Animal Feed Science and Technology* 85, 79–87.
Merritt, A.M. (2003) The equine stomach: a personal perspective (1963–2003). *American Association of Equine Practitioners Proceedings* 49, 75–102.
Métayer, N., Lhôte, M., Bahr, A., Cohen, N.D., Kim, I., Roussel, A.J. and Jullian, V. (2004) Meal size and starch content affect gastric emptying in horses. *Equine Veterinary Journal* 36, 436–440. doi: 10.2746/0425164044868468.
Meyer, H. (1987) Nutrition of the equine athlete. In: Gillespie, J.R. and Robinson, N.E. (eds) *Equine Exercise Physiology 2*. ICEEP Publishing, Davis, California, pp. 644–673.
Meyer, H., Flothow, C. and Radicke, S. (1997) Preileal digestibility of coconut fat and soybean oil in horses and their influence on metabolites of microbial origin of the proximal digestive tract. *Archives of Animal Nutrition* 50, 63–74.
Meyer, H., Radicke, A., Kienzle, E., Wile, S. and Kleffken, D. (1993) *Investigations of preileal digestion of oats, corn and barley starch in relation to grain processing. In: Proceedings 13th Equine Nutrition and Physiology Society Symposium*, Gainsville, Florida, p. 92.
Morel, M.D., McBride, S.D., Chiam, R.S., McKay, A. and Ely, E. (2006) Seasonal variations in physiological and behavioural parameters in a bachelor group of stallion ponies (*Equus caballus*). *Animal Science* 82(5), 581–590.
Murray, M.J. and Grodinsky, C. (1989) Regional gastric pH measurement in horses and foals. *Equine Veterinary Journal* 7(Suppl.), 73–76
Nantel-Vivier, A., Pihl, R.O., Young, S.N., Parent, S., Bélanger, S.A. *et al.* (2011) Serotonergic contribution to boys' behavioral regulation. *PLoS ONE* 6(6), e20304.
Newsholme, E.A. and Dimitriadis, G. (2001) Integration of biochemical and physiologic effects of insulin on glucose metabolism. *Experimental and Clinical Endocrinology & Diabetes* 109, S122–S134.
Nolazco Sassot, L., Villarino, N.F., Dasgupta, N., Morrison, J.J., Bayly, W.M. *et al.* (2019) The lipidome of Thoroughbred racehorses before and after supramaximal exercise. *Equine Veterinary Journal* 51(5), 696–700.
NRC (National Research Council) (2001) *Nutrient Requirements of Dairy Cattle: Seventh Revised Edition*. The National Academies Press, Washington, DC. doi: 10.17226/9825.
NRC (National Research Council) (2007) *Nutrient Requirements of Horses: Sixth Revised Edition*. The National Academies Press, Washington, DC. doi: 10.17226/11653.
O'Connor, C.I., Lawrence, L.M., St. Lawrence, A.C., Janicki, K.M., Warren, L.K. *et al.* (2004) The effect of dietary fish oil supplementation on exercising horses. *Journal of Animal Science* 82(10), 2978–2984.
O'Neill, W., McKee, S. and Clarke, A.F. (2002) Flaxseed (*Linum usitatissimum*) supplementation associated with reduced skin test lesional area in horses with *Culicoides* hypersensitivity. *Canadian Journal Veterinary Research* 66(4), 272–277.
Orme, C.E., Harris, R.C., Marlin, D.J. and Hurley, J. (1997) Metabolic adaptation to a fat-supplemented diet by the Thoroughbred horse. *British Journal of Nutrition* 78, 443–458.
Pagan, J.D. (1997) Gastric ulcers in horses: a widespread but manageable disease. *World Equine Veterinary Review* 2, 28–30.
Pagan, J. (1998) Energy and the performance horse. *Liver* 90, 220.
Pagan, J.D. and Harris, P.A. (1999) The effects of timing and amount of forage and grain on exercise response in thoroughbred horses. *Equine Veterinary Journal* 31(S30), 451–457.
Pagan, J.D., Essen-Gustavsson, B., Lindholm, A. and Thornton, J. (1987) The effect of dietary energy source on exercise performance in Standardbred horses. In: Gillespie, J.R. and Robinson, N.E. (eds) *Equine Exercise Physiology: Proceedings 2nd International Conference*. ICEEP Publications, Davis, California, pp. 686–700.
Pagan, J.D., Burger, I. and Jackson, S.G. (1995) The long term effects of feeding fat to 2-year-old Thoroughbreds in training. *Equine Veterinary Journal* 27, 343–348. doi: 10.1111/j.2042-3306.1995.tb04949.x.
Pagan, J.D., Jackson, S.G. and Caddel, S. (1996) A summary of growth rates of Thoroughbreds in Kentucky. *Pferdeheilkunde* 12, 285–289.
Pagan, J.D., Burger, I. and Jackson, S.G. (1998) The influence of time of feeding on exercise response in Thoroughbreds fed a fat-supplemented or high-carbohydrate diet. In: Pagan, J.D. (ed.) *Advances in Equine Nutrition*. Nottingham University Press, Nottingham, UK, pp. 289–291.

Pagan, J.D., Harris, P.A., Kennedy, M.A.P., Davidson, N., Hoekstra, K.E. (1999) Feed type and intake affects glycemic response in Thoroughbred horses. In: *Proceedings 13th Equine Nutrition and Physiology Society Symposium*, pp. 149–150.

Pagan, J.D., Geor, R.J., Caddel, S.E., Pryor, P.B. and Hoekstra, K.E. (2001) The relationship between glycemic response and the incidence of OCD in Thoroughbred Weanlings: A Field Study. *Proceedings of the American Association of Equine Practitioners* 47, 322–325.

Pagan, J.D., Geor, R.J., Harris, P.A., Hoekstra, K., Gardner, S., Hudson, C. and Prince, A. (2002) Effects of fat adaptation on glucose kinetics and substrate oxidation during low-intensity exercise. *Equine Veterinary Journal* 34(S34), 33–38. doi: 10.1111/j.2042-3306.2002.tb05388.x.

Pearson-O'Neill, W., McKee, S. and Clarke, A.F. (2002) Flaxseed as a potential treatment for allergic skin disease in horses. Available at: http://equiworld.com/uk/horsecare/erc/flaxseed.htm (accessed 10 May 2022).

Philippeau, C., Faubladier, C., Goachet, A.G. and Julliand, V. (2009) Is there an impact of feeding concentrate before or after forage on colonic pH and redox potential in horses. In: *Applied Equine Nutrition and Training. Equine Nutrition Training Conference (ENUTRACO).* Wageningen Academic Publishing, Madrid, Spain, pp. 203–208.

Potter, G.D., Hughes, S.L., Julen, T.R. and Swinney, D.L. (1992) A review of research on digestion and utilization of fat by the equine. *Pferdeheilkunde Sonderausgabe* 119–123.

Proudman, C. (2012) Feeding the performance horse without increasing the risk of colic. Winning Ways, 16 & 17 June, 2012. *Training, Health, Nutrition, Biomechanics and Physiotherapy of the Performance Horse. Veterinary proceedings, Aintree Racecourse*, Liverpool, UK, p. 2–4.

Ralston, S.L. (1995) Postprandial hyperglycemia/hyperinsulinemia in young horses with osteochondritis dessicans. *Journal of Animal Science* 73, 184.

Reeves, M.J., Salman, M.D. and Smith, G. (1996) Risk factors for equine acute abdominal disease (colic): results from a multi-centre-case-control study. *Preventative Veterinary Medicine* 26, 285–301.

Rendle, D. (2013) Insect bite hypersensitivity: prevention and management. *Veterinary Times* 43(11), 8–12.

Roberts, M.C. (1974) Amylase activity in the small intestine of the horse. *Research in Veterinary Science* 17, 400–401.

Ross-Jones, T., Hess, T., Rexford, J., Ahrens, N., Engle, T. and Hansen, D.K. (2014) Effects of omega-3 long chain polyunsaturated fatty acid supplementation on equine synovial fluid fatty acid composition and prostaglandin E2. *Journal of Equine Veterinary Science* 34(6), 779–783.

Sadet-Bourgeteau, S., Philippeau, C. and Julliand, V. (2017) Effect of concentrate feeding sequence on equine hindgut fermentation parameters. *Animal* 11(7), 1146–1152.

Särkijärvi, S., Niemeläinen, O., Sormunen-Cristian, R. and Saastamoinen, M. (2012) Changes in chemical composition of different grass species and mixtures in equine pasture during grazing season. In: *Forages and Grazing in Horse Nutrition*. Wageningen Academic Publishers, Wageningen, Netherlands, pp. 45–48.

Scott, B.D., Potter, G.D., Greene, L.W., Hargis, E.S. and Anderson, J.G. (1992) Efficacy of a fat-supplemented diet on muscle glycogen concentrations in exercising Thoroughbred horses maintained in varying body conditions. *Journal of Equine Veterinary Science* 12(2), 109–113.

Sloet van Oldruitenborgh-Oosterbaan, M.M., Annee, M.P., Verdegaal, E.J.M.M., Lemmens, A.G. and Beynen, A.C. (2002) Blood metabolic profile in exercising horses fed either a low-or high-fat diet. *Equine Veterinary Journal* 34, 29–32.

Snyder, J.L., Meacham, T.N., Fontenot, J.P. and Webb, K.E. Jr (1981) Heat production in pony geldings fed fat supplemented diets. In: *Proceedings of the 7th Equine Nutrition and Physiology Society Symposium*, pp. 144–148.

Spring, B., Chiodo, J. and Bowen, D.J. (1987) Carbohydrates, tryptophan, and behavior: a methodological review. *Psychological Bulletin* 102(2), 234–256.

Stull, C.L. and Rodiek, A.V. (1995) Effects of postprandial interval and feed components on stress parameters in exercising Thoroughbreds. In: *Proceedings of the 14th Equine Nutrition and Physiology Society Symposium*, p. 17.

Suagee-Bedore, J.K., Linden, D.R., Bennett-Wimbush, K. and Splan, R.K. (2020) Feeding grass hay before concentrate mitigates the effect of grain-based concentrates on postprandial plasma interleukin-1β. *Journal of Equine Veterinary Science* 86, 102899.

Taylor, L.E., Ferrante, P.L., Kronfeld, D.S. and Meacham, T.N. (1995) Acid-base variables during incremental exercise in sprint-trained horses fed a high-fat diet. *Journal of Animal Science* 73(7), 2009–2018.

Tinker, M.K., White, N.A., Lessard, P., Thatcher, C.D., Pelzer, K.D. *et al.* (1997) A prospective study of equine colic risk factors. *Equine Veterinary Journal* 29, 454–458.

Topliff, D.R., Potter, G.D., Dutson, T.R., Kreider, J.L. and Jessup, G.T. (1983) Diet manipulation and muscle glycogen in the equine. In: *Proceedings 8th Equine Nutrition and Physiology Society Symposium*, pp. 224–229.

Tosh, S.M. and Chu, Y. (2015) Systematic review of the effect of processing of whole-grain oat cereals on glycaemic response. *British Journal of Nutrition* 114(8),1256–1262. doi: 10.1017/S0007114515

Traub-Duragatz, J.L., Kopral, C.A., Seitzinger, A.H., Graber, L.P., Forde, K. *et al.* (2001) Estimate of the national incidence of and operational-level risk factors for colic among horses in the United States, spring 1998 to spring 1999. *Journal of the American Veterinary Medical Association* 219, 67–71.

Treiber, K.H., Geor, R.J., Boston, R.C., Hess, T.M., Harris, P.A. *et al.* (2008) Dietary energy source affects glucose kinetics in trained Arabian geldings at rest and during endurance exercise. *The Journal of Nutrition* 138(5), 964–970.

Valberg, S.J. (2010) Review of muscle disease in sports horses. In: *Proceedings of the Veterinary Sports Horse Symposium*. American Association of Equine Practise, Lexington, Kentucky, pp. 107–120.

Valvo, M.A., Lanza, M., Bella, M., Fasone, V., Scerra, M. *et al.* (2005) Effect of ewe feeding system (grass v. concentrate) on intramuscular fatty acids of lambs raised exclusively on maternal milk. *Animal Science* 81, 431–436.

van der Mast, R.C. and Fekkes, D. (2000) Serotonin and amino acids: partners in delirium pathophysiology? *Seminars in Clinical Neuropsychiatry* 5(2), 125–131.

Venable, E.B., Bland, S.S., Holscher, H., Liu, T.W. and Swanson, K.S. (2016) Effects of meal size and frequency on the equine cecal microbiota. *Journal of Animal Science* 94(Suppl. 5), 395–395.

Vervuert, I., Coenen, M. and Bothe, C. (2004) Effects of corn processing on the glycaemic and insulinaemic responses in horses. *Journal of Animal Physiology and Animal Nutrition* 88, 348–355.

Vervuert, I., Voigt, K., Hollands, T., Cuddeford, D. and Coenen, M. (2008) Effects of processing barley on its digestion by horses. *Veterinary Record* 162, 684–688. doi: 10.1136/vr.162.21.684.

Vervuert, I., Voigt, K., Hollands, T., Cuddeford, D. and Coenen, M. (2009a) The effect of mixing and changing the order of feeding oats and chopped alfalfa to horses on: glycaemic and insulinaemic responses, and breath hydrogen and methane production. *Journal of Animal Physiology and Animal Nutrition* 93(5), 631–638.

Vervuert, I., Voigt, K., Hollands, T., Cuddeford, D. and Coenen, M. (2009b) Effect of feeding increasing quantities of starch on glycaemic and insulinaemic responses in healthy horses. *The Veterinary Journal* 182(1), 67–72. doi: 10.1016/j.tvjl.2008.04.011.

Vincze, A., Szabó, C., Bakos, Z., Szabó, V., Veres, S. *et al.* (2016) Effect of dietary energy source on the plasma parameters of equine athletes trained in a deep water aqua treadmill. *Italian Journal of Animal Science* 15(1), 137–143.

Vineyard, K.R., Warren, L.K. and Kivipelto, J. (2010) Effect of dietary omega-3 fatty acid source on plasma and red blood cell membrane composition and immune function in yearling horses. *Journal of Animal Science* 88(1), 248–257.

Vitec (1987) Omega 3 Fatty Acids, *Roche Report*: A5, 1–5.

Waters, A.J., Nicol, C.J. and French, N.P. (2002) Factors influencing the development of stereotypic and redirected behaviours in young horses: findings of a four year prospective epidemiological study. *Equine Veterinary Journal* 34(6), 572–579. doi: 10.2746/0425 16402776180241.

Willard, J.G., Willard, J.C., Wolfram, S.A. and Baker, J.P. (1977) Effect of diet on cecal pH and feeding behavior of horses. *Journal of Animal Science* 45(1), 87–93. doi: 10.2527/jas1977.45187x.

Williams, C.A., Kronfeld, D.S., Staniar, W.B. and Harris, P.A. (2001) Plasma glucose and insulin responses of Thoroughbred mares fed a meal high in starch and sugar or fat and fiber. *Journal of Animal Science* 79, 2196–2201.

Woodward, A.D., Nielsen, B.D., O'Connor, C.I., Skelly, C.D., Webel, S.K. *et al.* (2007) Supplementation of dietary long-chain polyunsaturated omega-3 fatty acids high in docosahexaenoic acid (DHA) increases plasma DHA concentration and may increase trot stride length in horses. *Equine and Comparative Exercise Physiology* 4, 71–78.

Wolever, T.M.S., Jones, P.J.H., Jenkins, A.L. *et al.* (2019) Glycaemic and insulinaemic impact of oats soaked overnight in milk vs. cream of rice with and without sugar, nuts, and seeds: a randomized, controlled trial. *European Journal of Clinical Nutrition* 73, 86–93.

Young, S.N. and Leyton, M. (2002) The role of serotonin in human mood and social interaction: insight from altered tryptophan levels. *Pharmacology Biochemistry and Behavior* 71(4), 857–865.

Zeyner, A. Bessert, J. and Gropp, J.M. (2002) Effects of feeding exercised horses on high-starch or high-fat diets for 390 days. *Equine Veterinary Journal* (Suppl.34), 50–57.

Zeyner, A., Geißler, C. and Dittrich, A. (2004) Effects of hay intake and feeding sequence on variables in faeces and faecal water (dry matter, pH value, organic acids, ammonia, buffering capacity) of horses. *Journal of Animal Physiology and Animal Nutrition* 88(1–2), 7–19.

Zeyner, A., Romanowski, K., Orgis, A., Vernunft, A. Gottschalk, J. *et al.* (2017) Feed intake patterns and immediate glycaemic and insulinaemic responses of horses following ingestion of different quantities of starch from oat, barley and grains. *The Open Nutrition Journal* 11(1), 39–51.

6 What Are Supplements? The Importance of Micronutrients in the Horse's Diet

BRIONY WITHEROW

Practical Equine Nutrition, Cambridge; Writtle University College, Essex

Learning Objectives

LO1 List the basic micronutrients and provide a simple explanation of their role in the body.
LO2 Compare and contrast typical feeding regimes where vitamins and minerals are likely to be deficient (high-forage diets, less-than-recommended levels of compound feeds, etc.)
LO3 Recognise the difference between nutraceuticals versus nutrients.
LO4 Describe steps taken before advising supplements.

At the end of this chapter, you should be able to: identify the main micronutrients needed for the health of the horses; list the more common scenarios when you might need to advise supplementing; and appraise and critique the evidence base behind the more common supplements fed to horses.

Introduction

Forage, which forms the basis of your client's horse's diet, will not provide adequate vitamins and minerals, and even well-managed spring and summer grazing has been shown to be inadequate (Jones *et al.*, 2005; Longland, 2012; Saastamoinen and Hellämäki, 2012; Zhao and Müller, 2015). A large percentage of horses in the UK are malnourished, being overfed with calories and inadequate vitamins and minerals (Jansson *et al.*, 2012; Longland, 2012) not dissimilar to human nutrition, where micronutrient deficiency and its association with obesity is viewed as an emerging public health concern (Miller *et al.*, 2016; Poli *et al.*, 2017). Key functions and sources of vitamins and minerals can be easily looked up, but what is important is recognising common management and feeding practices and clinical issues that may impact upon requirement and provision, so that you can provide suitable advice.

While requirements can provide a guideline to intake, be aware that many of these are not definitive. The horse itself and a thorough history (see Chapter 2: 'Diet history') should be considered. Remember that all manufactured horse feeds contain 'supplements' /premixes (see Chapter 7: 'Vitamins and minerals') which, if fed at manufacturer's recommended intake, provide the horse with its daily requirements for vitamins and minerals. You would normally only need to recommend a supplement if the horse is being fed less than recommended amounts or has a specific need to balance its vitamin and mineral requirements.

You will find that your client's understanding of a supplement is based on human nutrition, so it is important that you discuss that 'supplements' are not legally recognised in the feeding-stuff regulations (see Chapter 8). Horses will obtain their micronutrients

 Evidence-based Equine Nutrition: A Practical Approach for Professionals (T. Hollands and L. Drury)
DOI: 10.1079/9781789245134.0006

either as part of a formulated compound feed (intake between 100 g and 1.2 kg /100 kg BW) or separately (12–40 g/100 kg BW), usually as a powder or pellet. All vitamins and minerals that are sold separately from a feed *must* be labelled as a complementary feed (see Chapter 7); and if they are not, then you should not be recommending them.

Supplements

The use of supplements in the UK continues to grow (BETA, 2019), representing an estimated £91 million in 2019. Reliance on supplementation as a first resort or 'quick fix' is ill-advised, particularly where the overall balance of the diet is not considered.

But supplementation to balance micronutrients can often resolve many issues, whether these be due to high performance demands or specific clinical concerns, providing a more tailored, individual approach.

In equine nutrition, EU law classifies a supplement as a compound feed, the main difference being the quantity fed (Table 6.1); it should be labelled as a 'complementary' feedstuff.

Supplements are available in powders, pellets, liquids and pastes and are categorised into two specific groups, depending on their principal purpose:

- **Nutrients**: designed to balance the ration, ensuring nutrient requirements are met. Examples include general-purpose broad-spectrum vitamin and mineral supplements, hoof supplements, antioxidants and electrolytes (see Chapter 13).
- **Nutraceuticals**: designed to provide specific benefit beyond regular nutritional requirements (not including legally defined drugs). Used for supportive effects on health, performance and/or behaviour, not to balance the diet; e.g. joint and digestive supplements.

Nutrients

Broad-spectrum vitamins and minerals and specific micronutrient supplementation

These can be grouped as:

- supplementation of a broad spectrum of vitamins and minerals;
- specific minerals in isolation (commonly calcium, phosphorus, copper, selenium); and
- specific vitamins in isolation (commonly vitamins C and E).

These forms of supplementation are widely used as an alternative or addition to an unbalanced concentrate diet. But you should not advise multiple products, particularly where single mineral supplements are used. The complex interaction of minerals makes the addition of single minerals over prolonged periods of time hazardous, particularly where narrow safety margins exist (such as selenium).

Vitamins

Vitamins are categorised according to solubility, as either fat-soluble (vitamins A, E, D and K) or water-soluble (C and B complex vitamins). While they are only required by the body in small quantities, they serve a fundamental role in physiological function.

Vitamin requirements can vary with age and workload (Tables 6.2 and 6.3) with requirement tending to increase with physiological stress. Naturally occurring vitamins within feedstuffs vary hugely and will decrease during the conservation of forages, manufacturing processes and storage.

Supplementation of all vitamins is usually achieved by feeding the appropriate feed at recommended amounts for size and workload or, if the horse is receiving adequate calories from the forage, then as a 'supplement'. Risk of toxicity is typically low, but research has documented incidences where vitamin provision in the ration far exceeds requirement (Harris, 2000; Williams *et al.*, 2009).

Table 6.1 Quantity fed and cost per day of compound feed versus vitamin and mineral supplement to provide a balanced ration of vitamins and minerals for a 500 kg horse

Product type	Recommended amount for rest to light work	Percentage of total intake (DM)	Cost per day
Cube or mix	2–2.5 kg (400–500 g/100 kg BW)	20–25%	£1.20–£1.50
Balancer	0.5 kg (100 g/100 kg BW)	5%	£0.70
Vitamin and mineral supplement	45–100 g (9–20 g/100 kg BW)	< 1%	£0.37–£0.83

Table 6.2. Fat-soluble vitamins: key functions and requirements. (Modified from NRC, 2007; Zeyner and Harris, 2013.)

Vitamin	Key functions	Requirement at maintenance	Key sources	Feed management or clinical status which may increase requirement (NRC, 2007)	Risk of excess intake/toxicity
Vitamin A (retinol)	Immune response, fertility, vision, gene expression, bone and tissue integrity and development, metabolism of fats and carbohydrates	[a]30 IU/kg BW (150 IU/kg BW $^{0.75}$)	Leafy plant matter (grass or legume), carrots and fish oils. Commonly provided in complementary feed	Mares during late gestation and lactation and growing youngstock have elevated requirements (60 IU/kg BW and 45 IU/kg BW, respectively). It should be noted that those with no access to fresh forage will be more reliant on vitamin A from supplementary feed (Griewe-Crandell *et al.*, 1995; Donoghue *et al.*, 1981).Deficiency is rare in horses (NRC, 2007).	Potentially excess (complementary feeds often contain high levels vitamin A), toxicity levels are yet to be reported in horses (NRC, 2007).
Vitamin D (calciferol)	Regulation of absorption of calcium and phosphorus	[b]6.6 IU/kg BW 30 IU/kg BW$^{0.75}$	Produced by the horse, within skin, in the presence of sunlight, fish oils, grasses and naturally conserved forages and colostrum. Commonly provided in complementary feed.	Requirement assumed to be met from exposure to sunlight (NRC, 2007). Liver or kidney disease, which may inhibit metabolism. Deficiency and excess rare in horses (NRC, 2007).	Complementary feeds often contain vitamin D; excess is more likely to be an issue than deficiency. While vitamin D_2 (ergocalciferol) is not readily stored in any great quantity, D_3 (cholecalciferol) can be. Excess supply of D_3 can be cause for concern (Harmeyer and Schlumbohm, 2004). The safe upper limit provided by the NRC (1987) for vitamin D is 44 IU/kg BW per day.
Vitamin E (tocopherol)	Antioxidant properties, muscle development and function, immune function and fertility	1 IU/kg BW (5 mg/kg BW$^{0.75}$)	Fresh forage (grass or legume) and cereal germs. Commonly provided in complementary feed	Horses in moderate to hard work (White-Springer *et al.*, 2021), gestation, lactation and growth or on a fat-enriched diet have elevated requirements of 10 mg/kg BW$^{0.75}$ per day, increasing further to 20 mg/kg BW$^{0.75}$ per day for those in intense training (Williams, and Carlucci, 2006) and those susceptible to ERS. Many high oil feeds and supplements may account for additional vitamin E requirements in their formulation, but check	Excess is not common in the horse and even with high intakes, toxicity has not been reported (NRC, 2007)

Vitamin K (menaquinone)	Blood coagulation, protein synthesis, bone formation and neural function	[c]NA	Primarily synthesised by the microbial population in the hind gut	Low forage intake over a prolonged period Ingestion/administration of substances that impair blood clotting (Tanand Lee, 2021) or severe and prolonged hind gut disruption Deficiency rare (NRC,2007)	There is no known toxicity for the natural forms of vitamin K, K_1 (phylloquinone) and K_2 (menaquinones) (NRC, 2007); furthermore, dietary K_2 and K_3 (a synthetic form known as menadione) are thought to have low toxicity; proposal of at least 1000 times dietary requirement (NRC, 2007)

[a]Limited evidence-based information to inform requirements.
[b]This recommendation is for horses without or with limited access to sunlight; requirements of horses with access to sunlight have yet to be determined, but metabolic requirement is assumed to be met by this.
[c]The amount in a typical diet/horse's own synthesis is thought to meet needs without additional supplementation

Table 6.3. Water-soluble vitamins: key functions and requirements. (Modified from NRC, 2007; Zeyner and Harris, 2013)

Vitamin	Key functions	Requirement at maintenance	Key sources	Feed management or clinical status which may increase requirement (NRC, 2007)	Risk of excess intake/ toxicity
Vitamin C (ascorbic acid)	Antioxidant properties, formation of cartilage and bone, immune function	NA	Synthesised in the horse's liver from glucose	Elevated levels during stress (illness/infections, heavy/intense exercise and respiratory compromise) 30 mg/kg BW/day recommended Deficiency not described in the horse	Vitamin C toxicity has not been described in the horse (Snow *et al.*, 1987)
Vitamin B1 (thiamine)	Energy production (more specifically carbohydrate metabolism) and nervous system component	0.06 mg/kg BW/day (0.3 mg/kg $BW^{0.75}$/day)	Cereal grains and grain by-products, brewers' yeast and synthesised by the microbial population in the hind gut	Working horses or those on a high-starch, low-forage diets Iincrease requirements to 0.11–0.13 mg/kg BW (NRC, 2007)	Excess in B vitamins has not been described in horses (NRC, 2007)
Vitamin B2 (riboflavin)	Metabolism of macronutrients, formation of enzymes involved in energy production, growth and development	0.04 mg/kg BW/day (0.2 mg/kg $BW^{0.75}$/day)	Synthesised by the microbial population in the hind gut. Also found naturally in legumes and grass (fresh and conserved)	Low forage intake over a prolonged period	
Biotin	Constituent of many different enzymes and subsequently metabolism of key nutrients and gene expression	[b]NA	Synthesised by the microbial population in the hind gut and dietary sources such as fresh alfalfa	3–4 mg/100 kg BW/day recommended for horses with poor hoof quality (Wintzer, 1986); overall balance of macro and micronutrients must be considered	
Vitamin B6 (pyridoxine)	Metabolism of macronutrients, enzyme function and the production of red blood cells	[b]NA	Grass and fresh plant matter		

Vitamin B3 (nicotinic acid or niacin)	Metabolic processes, skin health and enzyme function	[ab]NA		Synthesised from the amino acid tryptophan by the microbial population in the hind gut. Cereal grains		
Pantothenic acid	Metabolism of macronutrients and immune function (formation of antibodies)	[ab]NA		Oats, barley, brewer's yeast, molasses		
Folic acid (folacin)	Production of red blood cells	[b]NA		Fresh plant matter. Synthesised by the microbial population in the hind gut	Low forage intake over a prolonged period.	
Vitamin B12 (cobalamin)	Appetite stimulation, formation of red blood cells, utilisation of protein, metabolism of micronutrients	[ab]NA		Synthesised by microbial population in the hind gut (in the presence of cobalt, which B12 contains). Oats and brewer's yeast		
Choline	Transportation of fats, nerve transmission, cell membrane structure	[b]NA		Oats, barley, sugar beet, linseed, molasses		Excess has not been described in horses (NRC, 2007)

[a]Limited evidence-based information to inform requirements.
[b]The amount in a typical diet/horse's own synthesis is thought to meet needs without additional supplementation.

> **Top tip**
>
> Remember that you would only see a limited number of vitamins declared either on a label or brochure (see Chapter 7). This is not a true reflection of the premix that is incorporated into feed and if you need more details (because you are wanting to compare the micronutrients in the feed with a 'supplement') then contact a nutritionist or the feed company.

Minerals

Minerals are only required in small amounts but are essential to many key functions in the horse's body. Minerals can be categorised into major or macro minerals, which are required in grams per day, and trace or micro, required in milligrams per day.

Due to complex mineral interactions, supply and balance of minerals should be considered as a whole and are rarely supplemented in isolation.

Requirements should be provided per kilogram (kg) of bodyweight (BW) or per kg dry matter in the diet (Tables 6.4 and 6.5). The upper limits for trace elements within feeds (complete diet at 88% DM) are tightly regulated by EU legislation: e.g. zinc (120 mg/kg), copper (25 mg/kg) and selenium (0.5 mg/kg)

Deficiency should be considered in terms of both direct and indirect causes. Often clients unwittingly cause a deficiency or imbalance in one micronutrient by overfeeding single nutrients that they add to the diet, e.g. copper (Table 6.5).

Assessment of the Diet for Micronutrient Balance

Assessment of the ration and horse is essential to determine requirements (see Chapter 2).

Points to consider when assessing the ration for micronutrient balance

- Daily forage intake.
- Daily intake of concentrate feed (for soaked feeds, measure the quantity of dry food).
- Daily intake of supplements.
- Beware of any single mineral supplementation.

If significant micronutrient imbalance is suspected, the forage source should be analysed.

- Input the data into a rationing programme (see Chapter10). Where forage analysis is not available, this can be done using typical values. While this is not likely to be as accurate, it can serve as a useful illustration.
  - Remember, forage alone cannot guarantee a balanced diet, particularly as nutrient levels fluctuate throughout the year (Table 6.6). Many horses at rest or in light work may not show any signs of ill health without additional micronutrient supplementation in the short term; effects for those undergoing increased physiological stress are likely to be apparent sooner.

What to check: typical situations when supplements are needed

When assessing the diet, do some quick checks.

- Is the feed type appropriate for the workload and reproductive status?
- Is the owner feeding the recommended quantities?
  - Concentrate feeds, fed at the recommended feeding amount for the size and workload of the horse, meet micronutrient requirements based on average forage analysis
- Is your owner mixing and matching multiple fortified concentrate feeds?
- Is the horse kept in a typical situation where requirements are not met (Table 6.7)?

Advising supplements to balance single or narrow range of vitamins and minerals

Frequently clients use a more targeted vitamin or mineral supplement, such as salt.

Salt supplementation

Even horses fed their full complement of concentrate feed are likely to require additional salt.

- Forage alone is low in sodium.
- Compound feeds need an element of flexibility, because daily requirements are dependent upon electrolytes lost during exercise (as sweat).
- Salt has the potential to degrade other nutrients when included in a compound feed. *Continued p. 119.*

Table 6.4 Major minerals. Key functions and requirements. (Modified from NRC, 2007.)

	Function	Requirement[a]	Key natural sources[b]	Feed management or clinical status which may increase requirement (NRC, 2007)	Risk of excess intake/toxicity
Calcium (Ca)	Bone formation, nerve and muscle function, blood clotting (required for prothrombin to form thrombin), enzyme activation	0.04 g/kg BW or 2.4–6.8 g/kg DM	Grass forage, legumes (alfalfa (5:1 ratio), clover), root vegetables (incl. sugar beet)	Elevated requirement for exercising horses (1.5 times maintenance), breeding and youngstock Higher risk of deficiency when sole nutrient reliance is on poorly managed pastures (Laan *et al*., 2000, Swartzman *et al*., 1978; James and Butcher, 1972; Panciera *et al*., 1990), straight cereal diets, high magnesium intake (Pagan *et al*., 2020)	Calcium in excess, and low phosphorus is thought to cause skeletal abnormalities (Toribio, 2011). Maximum tolerable level for calcium at 2% of the diet, provided adequate phosphorus is met (NRC, 2007)
		Ratio of 1.5–2:1 (Ca:P) optimal (1:1 acceptable in mature horse diets)			
Phosphorus (P)	Bone mineralisation and development, energy production, protein synthesis, enzyme formation; cofactor for many enzymes and activates B-complex vitamins	0.028 g/kg BW or 1.7–3.8 g/kg DM	Leafy forages, cereal grain, cereal by-products	Elevated requirement for breeding (2.2–2.8-fold increase), and youngstock (1.7-fold increase)	Excess phosphorus in the diet can cause calcium deficiency and an inverse calcium to phosphorus ratio Maximum tolerable level for phosphorus at 1% of the diet, provided an adequate calcium to phosphorus ratio is maintained (NRC, 2007)
Magnesium (Mg)	Regulation of calcium to phosphorus ratio, bone integrity, energy production, nerve and muscle function, cell metabolism, enzyme activation, required for normal insulin sensitivity	0.015 g/kg BW or 0.9–1.2 g/kg DM	Leafy forages, sugar beet, molasses, notably, wheat bran and rice bran and seeds high in protein	Gestation and lactation increase requirement. High cereal grain, low forage diets may pose risk of deficiency, but this is rare	Maximum tolerable level estimated at 0.8%. Absence of data on magnesium toxicity (NRC, 2007)

Continued

Table 6.4. Continued.

	Function	Requirement[a]	Key natural sources[b]	Feed management or clinical status which may increase requirement (NRC, 2007)	Risk of excess intake/ toxicity
Sodium (Na)	Regulates fluid balance, a major electrolyte maintaining acid–base balance, nerve transmission, essential for the absorption of glucose and amino acids, muscle function	0.02 g/kg BW or 1–3 g/kg DM	Sodium chloride or salt main source of sodium in the diet; forage and cereals are poor sources	Increased requirement seen with chronic diarrhoea and exercise Low sodium intake common under typical feed management	Sodium excess is rare provided there is access to fresh water, maximum tolerable level of 6% of intake (NRC, 2007)
Potassium (K)	Regulation of body fluids, nerve and muscle function, metabolic uptake of carbohydrates	0.05 g/kg BW or 3 g/kg DM	Leaves of plant matter, molasses, soya bean meal	Increased requirement with chronic diarrhoea and exercise Risk of deficiency increased where forage is restricted	Evidence of toxicity is low. Estimates of maximum tolerable levels (1% of intake (NRC, 2007)) are conservative given its relative abundance in forage. Excessive dietary potassium should be avoided for horses suffering with hyperkalaemic periodic paralysis (HYPP) (Reynolds *et al.*, 1998)
Chlorine (Cl)	Regulation of body fluids, a major electrolyte maintaining acid–base balance. A component of hydrochloric acid and activation of digestive enzymes	0.08 g/kg BW [c]	Common salt (NaCl). Found in many feeds, notably legumes and molasses	Increased requirement seen with chronic diarrhoea and exercise Risk of deficiency increased where forage is restricted	Toxicity not documented but anecdotally tolerated well, provided adequate access to water (NRC, 2007)

[a]Where a range is provided, the requirement level will be influenced by age, physiological state/workload, bioavailability, nutrient interactions and stress
[b]Level of mineral within crops/forages dependent on soil factors, plant species and environmental factors at point of harvest.
[c]Limited evidence-based information to inform requirements.

Table 6.5 Trace minerals. Key functions and requirements. (Modified from NRC, 2007.)

	Function	Requirement[a]	Key natural sources[b]	Feed management or clinical status which may increase requirement	Risk of excess intake/toxicity
Sulphur (S)	Synthesis of amino acids, hoof growth, enzyme activation, a constituent of insulin	1.5 g/kg DM[c]	Legumes, linseed meal, maize, molasses	Increased requirement for exercising horses Deficiency likely where straw is the main forage source or in periods of forage restriction	Extrapolation from other species suggests maximum tolerable levels to be at 0.5% of intake (NRC, 2007); data is lacking in horses
Zinc (Zn)	Essential for the metabolism of carbohydrate and lipids, antioxidant properties being an essential component of antioxidant enzymes (superoxide dismutase). Also essential for skin, bones and hair	40–50 mg/kg DM	Legumes, oil seed meals and cereal grains	Risk of deficiency increased where forage is restricted if no complementary feed provided (Wichert *et al*., 2002)	Oversupply through supplementation unlikely to result in toxicity, industrially contaminated pasture with zinc has been associated with DOD in foals (Campbell-Beggs *et al*., 1994; Eamens *et al*., 1984) (indirectly causing copper deficiency). A legal upper limit of 120mg/kg complete feed[e]
			Ratio of 3–4:1 (Zn:Cu) required		
Copper (Cu)	A component or essential for many enzymes. Necessary for bone, collagen, elastin and connective tissues, synthesis of haemoglobin and myoglobin. Essential component of keratinisation of hair and involved in melanin synthesis (coat colour)	0.172 mg/kg BW or 10–30 mg/kg DM	Growing grass, legumes and early-cut conserved forages	Elevated requirement for breeding, youngstock and exercising horses (Gee *et al*., 2000) Forage alone unlikely to meet requirements even for maintenance without concentrate supplementation Excess zinc or iron may indirectly cause deficiency	Largely unknown but data exist to suggest that excess is well tolerated (Cymbaluk *et al*., 1981).

Continued

Table 6.5. Continued.

	Function	Requirement[a]	Key natural sources[b]	Feed management or clinical status which may increase requirement	Risk of excess intake/toxicity
Selenium (Se)	Antioxidant properties as a component of the enzyme glutathione peroxidase	0.1 mg/kg DM[c]	Selenium-concentrating plants and plant matter/ cereals grown from high selenium soils		Toxicity at relatively low intake (from ten times requirement) with a maximum tolerable concentration of 2 mg/ kg DM. An upper limit (defined legally by the EU) of 1 mg/100 kg BW or 0.5 mg/kg (DMI 88%) exists. The most common cause of oversupply is through provision of multiple supplements or overfeeding supplements or through forage. Where soil selenium content is high or pasture contains selenium concentrating plants, toxicity can occur (Davis *et al.*, 2012). Chronic selenium excess reduces utilisation of sulphur in the formation of keratin; high intakes causing hair loss and hoof lesions. Milder symptoms frog horn and persistent thrush with moderate selenium intakes (Kempson, 2005)
Manganese (Mn)	Healthy development of bone, skin, hair and horn and more specifically cartilage (the formation of chondroitin sulphate)	0.76–0.99 mg/kg BW or 40–50 mg/kg DM[c]	Fresh grass, legumes, rice bran and wheat bran	No evidence of increased requirements	Risk of excess low, with minimal evidence to substantiate maximum tolerable level (NRC, 2007)

Iron (Fe)	Production of red blood cells and formation of haemoglobin, nervous system function, enzyme activation	4–50mg/kg DM[d]	Forage and oilseeds	Requirements slightly elevated in exercising horses and youngstock (typically met by increased DM intake) Deficiency rare Provision of iron-rich supplements in addition to a concentrate ration is not recommended	Maximum tolerance estimated at 500 mg/kg ration, risk of excess moderate (primarily due to its presence in forage); reports of toxicity from common dietary sources is low (NRC, 2007)
Cobalt (Co)	Component of the B12 vitamin, promotes bacterial activity necessary for B12 synthesis	0.05 mg/kg DM[d]	Fresh plant matter, particularly legumes	Deficiency rare	Excess rare and maximum tolerable level extrapolated from other species set at 25 mg/kg DM intake (NRC, 2007)
Iodine (I)	Formation of thyroxin and therefore metabolic function, growth and development	0.1 mg/kg DM	Limited knowledge on grass content. Seaweed	Requirement increases during gestation; maternal oversupply is of concernExcess and deficiency are considered rare	Excess is thought to be more prevalent than deficiency, with toxicity reported from 40 mg per day (Schryver, 1990). Excessive intakes by pregnant mares derived from compound feed, single or multiple concurrent supplements has been implicated in foals born with goitre (enlargement of the thyroid gland) (Doige and McLaughlin, 1981; Eroksuz *et al*., 2004)
Molybdenum (Mo)	Enzyme reactor	[c]	Grass, conserved forage and legumes		Limited evidence available

[a]Where a range is provided, the requirement level will be influenced by age, physiological state/workload, bioavailability, nutrient interactions, and stress
[b]Level of mineral within crops/forages dependant on soil factors, plant species and environmental factors at point of harvest.
[c]Limited evidence-based information to inform requirements; as such, any requirements stated are provisional.
[d]The amount in a typical diet is thought to meet needs without additional supplementation.
[e]https://www.legislation.gov.uk/eur/2016/1095/body

Table 6.6. Typical micronutrient levels of USA forage (per kg DM). Based on Equi-Analytical Laboratory Services data, 2000–2018 (Equi-Analytical, 2020; NRC 2001, 2007)

Micronutrient	Daily requirement 500 kg horse at rest	Grass pasture average (range)	No. of samples	Grass hay average (range)	No. of samples
Calcium (g)	~20	5.2 (2.7–7.7)	15,387	4.9 (2.7–7.1)	99,095
Phosphorus (g)	~14	3.1 (0–7.0)	15,383	2.4 (1.5–3.3)	99,344
Magnesium (g)	7.5	2.4 (1.4–3.5)	14,179	2.1 (1.3–2.9)	91,966
Potassium (g)	25	20.6 (9.2 –32.0)	14,193	18.5 (12.0–24.9)	92,722
Sodium (g)	10[a]	0.96 (0–3.7)	11,399	0.7 (0–2.1)	49,620
Iron (mg)	400	334.6 (0–915.8)	11,408	197.8 (0–486.9)	49,272
Zinc (mg)	400[a]	35.2 (0–88.0)	11,402	30.3 (0–1084.6)	29,193
Copper (mg)	100[a]	9.3 (3.9–14.7)	11,407	8.5 (0–17.4)	49,232
Manganese (mg)	400	92.7 (8.7–176.7)	11,401	83.1 (16.2–150.0)	49,182
Molybdenum (mg)		1.1 (0–3.3)	11,407	1.2 (0–2.8)	49,131
Cobalt (mg)	0.5	0.6 (0–1.2)	682	0.6 (0–1.9)	2533
Sulphur (g)	15	2.3 (1.3–3.4)	9720	1.7 (1.1–2.5)	60,031
Chloride (g)	40	8.2 (2.0–14.4)	6374	6 (1.7–10.3)	48,902

[a]Minerals deficient at maintenance when fed 2% bodyweight dry matter (10 kg) of grass-based forage as sole dietary intake based on average nutrient levels.

Table 6.7. Typical management when a broad-spectrum vitamin and mineral supplement might be advised

Practical feeding scenario	Micronutrients likely to be lacking and why/Comments	Possible solutions
	Leisure	
Forage-only diets	Forage-only diets unlikely to meet micronutrient requirement, notably deficient in copper, zinc and sodium (see Chapter 10: Figs 10.8 and 10.9)	Advise recommended amount of a compound feed or broad-spectrum vitamin and mineral supplement
Weight loss/restrictive diets	Restricted forage (particularly if soaked) or where dry matter is not considered – reduced dry matter intake that will impact micronutrient intake	
Soaking hay for purposes of reducing respirable particles (10–30 min)	Significant losses of sodium (36–43%), potassium (27–40%), phosphorus (14%), copper (27–30%) and magnesium (14–15%) (Moore-Colyer, 1996; Blackman and Moore-Colyer, 1998) even in 10–30 min of soaking	If forage analysis is available, typical losses can be taken into account when rationing (hay with an initial high mineral content may still meet requirements) Or advise elevated levels of compound feed or broad-spectrum vitamin and mineral supplement Steaming hay has not been shown to result in a decrease in micronutrients (Moore-Colyer *et al.*, 2016)
Soaking hay for purposes of reducing water-soluble carbohydrates (> 3 h)	Micronutrients decreased: sodium (20–60%); potassium (58–61%); phosphorus (35–43%); magnesium (19%) (Moore-Colyer, 1996; Blackman and Moore-Colyer, 1998; Argo *et al.*, 2015)	

Continued

Table 6.7. Continued.

Practical feeding scenario	Micronutrients likely to be lacking and why/Comments	Possible solutions
Relying on naturally occurring micronutrients	Many fibre-based concentrate diets are not fortified with additional vitamins and minerals, resulting in variable micronutrient intake; not ideal as the sole source of micronutrients for those where deficiencies may impact clinical or performance issues	Provide an additional source of micronutrients or the recommended amount of a compound feed or broad-spectrum vitamin and mineral supplement
Feeding an inappropriate type of concentrate feed	Feeds are formulated to meet workload/reproductive requirements. Feeds for maintenance/light work, fed at elevated rates, are unlikely to meet micronutrient requirements for moderate and hard levels of work	Select a feed suitable for the workload/reproductive status of the horse and feed at the manufacturer's recommended rates
Low intakes of compound feeds	A product appropriate for workload, not fed at the correct quantity for size and workload, micronutrient requirements are unlikely to be met Underfeeding of compound feeds is common with soaked feeds, where the dry matter content is often not considered, and with fortified chaff diets, where a large volume often results in underfeeding	Ensure compound feeds are fed to the rates recommended by the manufacturer for the horse's bodyweight and workload. If this provides too much energy or calories, the horse is on the wrong feed
Lengthy and/or poor storage conditions of concentrate feed	The vitamin content of feed will decrease over time when stored	Check that storage conditions of concentrate feed are optimal and best-before dates of feeds (see Chapter 8)
Group feeding and reliance on field/stable licks for provision of micronutrients	Intake cannot be guaranteed; micronutrients are commonly deficient	Where a daily individual feed cannot be provided, group feeding or mineral licks are an option
	Performance	
Restricting forage or underfeeding haylage	Restricted forage ration (dry matter is not considered) puts greater reliance on the concentrate ration	If minimum fibre intake is met, increase compound feed or advise general vitamin/mineral supplement
Feeding straight cereals	Cereals have an inverted calcium:phosphorus ration. Feeding straight cereals in the absence of an appropriate balancer or vitamin and mineral supplement imbalances ration	Balance the ration with an appropriate vitamin and mineral source; many Oat Balancer products are widely available to complement straight cereal rations

For horses at rest or in light work on a high forage ration:

- Advise that 30 g (a heaped tablespoon) of table salt/day provides 12 g of sodium (sufficient for a 500 kg horse meeting the minimum requirements of 0.02 g Na/kg BW).
- The other electrolytes are provided by forage and the recommended amount of a concentrate ration (Coenen and Meyer, 1987; Coenen, 2013).

Horses in moderate to hard work need:

- 2–4 tablespoons of table salt/day; and
- an appropriate electrolyte supplement (see Chapter 13: 'Maintaining electrolyte balance').

How to advise adding salt

- Salt can be mixed in with the concentrate feed, offered as loose salt in a bucket, or introduced to the diet gradually and divided over concentrate feeds where possible.
- Salt blocks can be provided to meet requirements for rest or light work. This relies on the horse consuming adequate and consistent quantities (which need to be monitored).

Self-regulation of salt consumption varies, and sufficient intake is not guaranteed (Jansson *et al.*, 1996; Jansson and Dahlborn, 1999).

Other factors to consider

Several other factors need considering when single or a reduced spectrum of vitamins and minerals are fed (more common with performance horses and youngstock) (Table 6.8).

Advising a hoof health nutrient supplement

Typical ingredients in hoof supplements include amino acids (methionine, lysine, cystine, glycine), minerals (calcium, zinc, sulphur, copper), vitamins (biotin, vitamin C), omega-3 fatty acids and MSM. While some have been identified as key constituents of the hoof wall (most notably amino acids), not all have been studied for their effects on horn growth and quality.

> **Top tip**
>
> Your first step should be to check the overall nutrient and protein intake of the ration. Frequently, poor hoof quality is associated with high forage diets and a specific supplement will not provide a balanced diet.

Daily intake of biotin

Dietary intake of 3–4 mg biotin/100 kg BW per day (15–20 mg per day for a 500 kg horse (Wintzer, 1986); higher intakes of up to 30mg have also been suggested (Comben *et al.*, 1984; NRC, 2007) for therapeutic effects on horn quality. When fed for more than 6 months, biotin has been shown to improve the structure and strength of horn and improve growth rate (Kempson, 1987; Buffa *et al.*,

Table 6.8 Factors to consider when advising targeted vitamin or mineral supplements

Product type	Key ingredients	Factors contributing to perceived problem	Practical considerations when supplementing
		Nutrients	
Hoof	Biotin, calcium, zinc, methionine	Poor management and trimming	Supplementation should be in addition to an already balanced diet for therapeutic results. Due to horn growth rate, supplementation needs to be long-term for therapeutic effects
Antioxidants	Vitamins E and C, selenium, flavonoids	Diet unbalanced in macro- and micronutrients	Duration of treatment must be sufficient – a supplementation period of at least 1 month is required (Kirschvink *et al.*, 2008). A combination of high-quality antioxidants is recommended. Selenium is toxic at 2 mg/kg DM (NRC, 2007) with levels in excess of 0.5 mg/kg DM rarely justified. As such, care must be taken if multiple supplements are being added to hard feed. If client adding further straight oil to the diet (more than 100 ml) advise 100–150 IU of vitamin E for every additional 100 ml of oil added (Harris, 2009)
Blood tonics	Iron, copper, zinc, pyridoxine, B12 and folic acid		Very limited research to support this practice. Iron deficiency occurs very rarely in the horse under normal feeding conditions. Horses very rarely get anaemia due to iron deficiency; however, copper deficiency (copper being intrinsic in iron metabolism) or excess can cause indirect deficiency

1992; Josseck *et al.*, 1995; Zenker *et al.*, 1995; Reilly *et al.*, 1998). Subsequently when supplementation has been reduced or removed completely after long-term supplementation, hoof health has declined. Different forms of biotin exist, D-biotin being the form that is active as a co-enzyme (McDowell 1989).

The hoof wall grows at a rate of 8–10 mm per month, so it will take at least 9–12 months for the hoof wall to be replaced. Therapeutic doses need to be fed long term, combined with regular trimming to maintain hoof balance.

Advising antioxidant nutrient supplements

The horse's body contains some natural endogenous defences against oxidative stress in the form of antioxidant enzymes (glutathione peroxidases (GPX) and superoxide dismutase (SOD)). These natural enzymatic defences improve with training and decrease with age (Ememe *et al.*, 2015; Smarsh and Williams, 2017).

Some vitamins (e.g. vitamins A, C and E) and minerals (e.g. selenium) have direct antioxidant properties; others (e.g. copper, manganese and zinc) are crucial co-factors for antioxidant enzymes.

'Alternative' ingredients with antioxidant properties (e.g flavonoids such as grape polyphenol) are used in some rations instead of, or alongside, vitamin E; their efficacy in horses is conflicted (Kirschvink *et al.*, 2008). Oxidative stress can cause irreversible damage and therefore prevention should be sought. Antioxidant supplementation has been associated with increasing antioxidant status (de Moffarts *et al.*, 2005). There is still some controversy over the correct form and quantity of supplement required to provide sufficient antioxidant effect (Velazquez-Canton *et al.*, 2018) and it is clear there is scope for further research to determine optimal levels of supplementation (Williams *et al.*, 2005).

The routine use of antioxidants for exercising horses and antioxidant therapy for the treatment of certain conditions (such as tying up or Respiratory airway obstruction (RAO)) (Kirschvink *et al.*, 2008; Deaton *et al.*, 2004) can be beneficial but should be part of a holistic approach.

Dietary advice: feeding multiple supplements

It is important to calculate the intake of micronutrients against requirements when horses are being fed multiple supplements. For example a 12-year-old (500 kg) advanced eventer mid-season was being fed multiple supplements, all containing vitamin E, D and A and selenium. Daily provision from the concentrate ration and supplements was calculated (forage levels are hard to ascertain, due to vitamin degradation in storage). Micronutrients are exceeded by the concentrate ration alone (Table 6.9). Discuss with the client to evaluate why the client is feeding multiple supplements.

Table 6.9. Effect of eventer being fed multiple supplements on nutrient requirements[a]

Supplement	Feeding rate per day	Vitamin E (IU)	Vitamin D (IU)	Vitamin A (IU)	Selenium (mg)
Baileys No. 4 Top Line Conditioning Cubes	6.3 kg	1890	9450	78750	3.15
NAF Vitamin E and Selenium Plus	30 g	1326	–	–	0.326
NAF M Power	30 g	468	1833	1281	0.0048
Science Supplements ImmunAid	49 g	1500	6000	–	2 mg
Daily provision		5184	17283	789131	5.48
NRC requirement (NRC, 2007)		1000	3300	22500	1.25
Percentage of NRC requirement		502%	524%	350%	438%
Toxicity		Not reported	Safe upper limit (NRC, 2007) 44 IU/kg BW/day (22000 IU)	Not reported	Exceeds upper limit of 1 mg/100 kg BW (5 mg). Can cause toxicity from 10× requirement (12.5 mg)

[a]Nutrient provision correct as of March 2020, sourced from manufacturer's website or directly from product labelling.

Dietary advice: increasing Ca intake for bone development

Adding extra nutrients to a young horse's ration is very common. A typical example might be a 6-month-old PRE (Andalusian) gelding (anticipated mature bodyweight of 500 kg) aimed at showing in the short term and low-level competition in the long term.

- Limestone flour was added to ration to support healthy growth and development.
- Copper supplement to help enhance coat colour.
- Growth rate and appetite in this horse were decreased.

Pasture analysis showed high calcium and copper levels, resulting in high intakes of copper and calcium and 1.2:1 zinc to copper and 3.66:1 calcium to phosphorus ratio (Table 6.10).

Client was made aware that high intakes of calcium and copper can reduce the absorption of zinc contributing factors for the signs shown. Always highlight the dangers of individual mineral supplementation and the importance of forage analysis.

As well as mixing single nutrient supplements, clients often choose 'supplements' with high levels of single or multiple nutrients for which there are no minimum requirements for health; these nutrients are decribed as nutraceuticals.

Nutraceuticals

The term nutraceutical, from *nutr*ient and pharm*aceutical*, is used to describe a wide range of dietary supplements. The term originates from human nutrition and lacks a regulatory definition; often exploited as a marketing term, it can be somewhat confusing, and even misleading for horse owners. Products marketed as veterinary nutraceuticals generally aim to support normal body structure and function, with a focus on improving animal health.

Horse owners use nutraceuticals to 'treat' joint issues (Agar *et al.*, 2016), hoof issues, colic or digestive issues but usage varies between recreational and competition riders (Swirsley *et al.*, 2017).

- Joint, hoof, general (vitamin/mineral, garlic) and digestive supplements are widely fed to the general horse population (Burk and Williams, 2008)
- Electrolytes, salt, antioxidants, gastrointestinal protectives and joint supplements are fed to competition horses (Agar *et al.*, 2016; Pratt-Phillips, 2016; Kaya-Karasu *et al.*, 2018).
- Joint and vitamin/mineral supplements are fed to senior horses (Hoffman *et al.*, 2009; McGowan *et al.*, 2010; Bushell and Murray, 2016).

Scientific evidence for the efficacy of the most widely used nutraceuticals is scarce because of small sample size, sensitivity in the methods employed to detect effects, dosage and timing, study design, exercise conditions and assessment of performance and product variability. When it comes to evaluating the evidence behind nutraceuticals, the findings can often be inconclusive and contradictory.

Veterinary advice regarding supplements is highly sought, being the strongest influencing factor in several studies (Hoffman *et al.* 2009; Agar *et al.*, 2016; Gemmill *et al.*, 2016; Swirsley *et al.*, 2017).

> **Top tip**
>
> Any orally administered products claiming to be involved in the treatment or prevention of disease should be classified as a drug and therefore subject to different regulation and approval. If these are positioned as a nutraceutical, the manufacturer is breaking the law and you should consider carefully whether you should advise them.

Table 6.10. Effect of calcium supplementation for youngstock on their micronutrient requirement

Supplement	Feeding rate per day (DM)	Zinc (mg)	Copper (mg)	Calcium (g)	Phosphorus (g)
Spillers Grow-N-Win	1 kg	450	175	30	15
Pasture analysis values	5.5 kg	66	55	44	8.25
Equine-America-Copper-Plus Powder	20 g	2	200	–	–
NAF Limestone Flour	70 g	–	–	26.6	4.2
Daily provision		518	430	100.6	27.5
NRC requirement (NRC, 2007)		215.9	54	39	21
Percentage of NRC requirement		240%	796%	258%	131%

Clearly, you should take a holistic approach to health, behaviour and performance-related issues rather than using supplementation as an easy 'go-to' option for the client, which is not always the best solution, when applied in isolation.

What and when to advise

There is a huge number of nutraceuticals. Recognising key ingredients, compounding issues and practical considerations is helpful (Table 6.11). Some nutraceuticals are fed to support general health, others (including herbs) are used to target specific 'problems'. For complex issues or support when making recommendations, it can be useful to align yourself with a nutritionist practising in your area (see Chapter 8: 'Suitably qualified nutritionists').

Advising a joint nutraceutical

Joint supplements are commonly fed (Ireland *et al.*, 2011; Oke and McIlwraith, 2010; Agar *et al.*, 2016; Murray *et al.*, 2018) to old and performance horses.

As well as the key active ingredients (Table 6.12) the supplement might include collagen, avocado soy unsaponified (ASU), zinc, various herbs (notably Devil's claw, Boswellia and yucca), vitamin C, polyunsaturated fatty acids (PUFAs) and, more recently, green lipped muscle, shark cartilage and turmeric (curcumin; the efficacy and absorption are still not confirmed).

Several studies have raised questions as to the disparity between label claims of active ingredients and actual contents (Ramey *et al.*, 2002; Oke *et al.*, 2006).

Evidence as to the efficacy of nutraceuticals on clinical signs of pain and lameness is weak (Vandeweerd *et al.*, 2012). Some studies have indicated some positive effect (Pearson *et al.*, 2009; Murray *et al.* 2014; Murray *et al.*, 2017) of supplements containing a combination of ingredients but do not discern which specific constituents contribute to the positive effect. The methodology often employed to research joint supplements, including self-report, subjective measures or indirect indications of joint movement (such as stride length), may not in itself offer a definitive answer.

Recent studies indicate beneficial effects of glucosamine and chondroitin (Gupta *et al.*, 2009).

Glucosamine is included within horse joint supplements in two forms: either glucosamine hydrochloride or glucosamine sulphate. The overall bioavailability of glucosamine is low and there is some controversy over whether bioavailability varies significantly between the two forms (Block *et al.*, 2010)

From the current research, it is apparent that the molecular weight/size of the active ingredient, the inflammatory status of the horse and the dosage are all contributing factors in the efficacy of joint supplements (Murray *et al.*, 2017).

Advising a behaviour nutraceutical

Products aimed at modifying behaviour contain magnesium, tryptophan, B vitamins, valerian (Ross and Roberts, 2018) along with other herbal supplements (notably vervain, *Withania somnifera*, chamomile, lemon balm and hops), often provided in combination. It is also increasingly commonplace for these supplements to contain ingredients that aim to optimise digestive function.

> **Top tip**
>
> Be aware that many nutraceuticals are banned substances under NOPS (see Chapter 8: 'Prohibitive substances – Naturally occurring substance (NOPS)').
>
> Discuss with clients how behaviour and temperament can be assessed reliably across a number of individual horses in a way that enables the impact of a product or ingredient to be evaluated.
>
> Often a placebo effect proves effective, so do not dismiss the supplement due to a lack of evidence base.
>
> Caution should be exercised when recommending calmers as shortcuts before addressing underlying issues such as training, stable confinement, reduced socialisation and feed management.

Clients use calmers to manage behaviours encountered in daily management and care, particularly if they are inexperienced in training and behaviour (Harris, 2005; Roberts and Murray, 2014; Murray *et al.*, 2018).

There is limited evidence of the efficacy of behavioural supplements (Freire *et al.*, 2008; Noble *et al.*, 2008; McCall, 2009; Talbot *et al.*, 2013), with evidence often being anecdotal or extrapolated from other species (Table 6.13).

Table 6.11 Summary of common scenarios when nutraceuticals are fed: practical considerations.

Clinical issue	Key ingredients	Factors contributing to perceived problem	Practical considerations when supplementing
Joint	Glucosamine, chondroitin sulphate, hyaluronic acid, collagen, MSM, polyunsaturated fatty acids (PUFAs), various herbs (Devil's claw, Boswellia and yucca), rosehips, vitamin C	Carrying excessive weight and condition.	Devil's claw (harpagoside) is on the FEI prohibited substance list
Behaviour	Magnesium, tryptophan, valerian, other herbal ingredients (vervain, *Withania somnifera*, chamomile, lemon balm and hops)	A base ration that is high in starch and sugar, providing energy in excess of requirement. Management which restricts movement, with inadequate exercise.	Valerian (valerenic acid) is on the FEI prohibited substance list
Digestive: Maintaining function	Pre- and probiotics	Frequent or rapid changes to the diet (particularly of the forage ration).	Probiotics[a] have no proven benefit in horses with healthy microbial populations and therefore are better fed short term, while prebiotics can be fed longer term.
Digestive: Gastric ulcers	Beta-glucans, pectins and gum arabics along with liquorice, glutamin and antacids	Use of ingredients that are known to have a higher acid-binding capacity such as beet and alfalfa (Lybbert *et al.*, 2007) and avoidance/reduced use of cereals, which have poor acid-buffering capacity. Adapt management practices to increase saliva production and ensure access to forage prior to exercise.	The effect of antacids is thought to be short-lived, making practical application challenging. Research on soluble fibres (beta-glucans, pectins, gum arabics etc) is limited in the horse and therefore effective feeding rates are largely unknown.
Muscle builders/ amino acids	Branch chain amino acids (BCAAs), lysine, beta-alanine	Not providing a balance of macro nutrients, in particular quality protein and inadequate energy. Inadequate exercise.	Quality protein can be delivered in the main ration and provide sufficient amino acids, so do not require additional supplementation. Addressing the quality of protein in the base ration should therefore be the starting point.
Respiratory	Vitamin E, C, selenium, herbs, garlic	Management of the environment, including forage sources, is key to reduce respirable particles.	Many products available, but only a few blends with scientific evidence of efficacy. No definitive evidence base for garlic; however, problems can be caused with excessive supplementation (> 0.4 g/kg BW per day).

[a]need to be authorised for use under feed additive regulations EU

Table 6.12 Comparison of joint supplements and their active ingredients when fed at the recommended amount for a 500 kg horse.

Common joint supplements[a]	Glucosamine *Glucosamine sulphate (GS)/ Glucosamine hydrochloride (GHCl)*	Chondroitin sulphate	MSM	Hyaluronic acid	Other active ingredients
Minimum quantities indicated by research for a 500 kg horse (per kg BW)	10 g (0.02 g/kg BW GHCl (Laverty *et al.* 2005) In combination, 5.5 g glucosamine HCl and 2 g of chondroitin sulphate	2 g (Forsyth *et al.*, 2006)	4 g (0.008 g/kg BW) (Maranon *et al.*, 2008)	100 mg (as an oral hyaluronic gel) (Bergin *et al.*, 2006)	
Active ingredient delivery when fed at recommended maintenance for 500 kg horse (loading/elevated rates where applicable)					
NAF Superflex	5 g (10 g (GS))	0.012 g (0.024 g)	5 g (10 g)	11.5 mg (23 mg)	Antioxidants (botanical)
NAF Superflex Liquid	5 g (10 g (GS))	0.16 g (0.32 g)	2.75 g (5.5 g)	9 mg (18 mg)	Antioxidants (botanical)
NAF Superflex Senior	7.2 g (14.4 g (GS))	0.085 g (0.17 g)	7.19 g (14.38 g)	42.5 mg (85 mg)	Omega-3, antioxidants
NAF Glucosamine 1000 Plus with MSM	5.5 g (11 g (GS))	–	1.1 g (2.2 g)	–	–
TopSpec 10:10 Joint Support	5 g (10 g)	–	5 g (10 g)		Vitamin C, E, beta-carotene
Feedmark Best-Flex HA	17 g (GHCL)	6.5 g	17 g	1100 mg	Vitamin C. Omega-3, *Boswellia serrata*
Feedmark Extra-Flex HA	6.25 g (12.5 g (GHCL))	0.5 g (1 g)	5 g (10 g)	200 mg (400 mg)	Rosehips
Feedmark Flexamine 10:10	6.25 g (12.5 g (GHCL))	–	5 g (10 g)	–	–
Equine America Cortaflex HA Regular Solution	–	–	2.5 g	30 mg	Collagen (450 mg), silicon (10 mg), manganese, vitamin B6, copper
Science Supplements FlexAbility Plus	10 g (20 g (GHCL))	4.1 g (8.2 g)	6.5 g (13 g)	150 mg (300 mg)	Vitamin C, Omega 3
Lintbells YuMOVE Horse Active	5 g	-	4 g	125 mg	Green lipped mussel, vitamins C and E
Aviform Suppleaze Gold	11 g (GHCL)	4 g	10 g	200 mg	Vitamin C
Nutravet Nutraquin+	2.6 g (15.3 g (GHCL))	1.1 g (6.3 g)	–	–	Vitamin C, zinc, Boswellia.
Protexin Cosequine Equine	2.7 g (5.4 g (GHCL))	0.9 g (1.8 g)	–	–	Vitamin E, manganese
Vet Plus Synequin	2.5 g (15 g (GHCL))	1 g (6 g)	–	–	Vitamin C, zinc
Plus Vital Flex Supp	5 g	1 g	5 g	100 mg	Rosehip, selenium, algae
Audevard Ekyflex Arthro	6.8 g (13.6 g)	0.55 g (1.1 g)	4.5 g (9 g)	–	Collagen (5.5–11 g), turmeric, black pepper

[a]Active ingredients taken from manufacturers' websites or product labels correct as of February 2020. Products may contain other important/active ingredients not listed in the table above

Advising a digestive nutraceutical

Supplements that maintain or enhance digestive fall into two categories:

- maintenance and optimisation of digestive function, (e.g. pre- and probiotics); or
- support for particular clinical issues (e.g. gastric ulcers).

Probiotics

Probiotics are live microbes with the potential (when provided in adequate quantities) to enhance the health of the digestive tract, and in doing so, potentially the health of the recipient (Schoster *et al.*, 2014; FAO/WHO, 2002)

> **Top tip**
>
> Probiotics are typically lactobacilli and are not legally recognised in the feedstuffs regulations. There are no live bacteria products registered for use in equine feed or supplements in the UK and Europe.
> Note: A legisltaion is not static, please check latest authorisations at https://www.food.gov.uk/business-guidance/animal-feed-additivesa

Originally probiotics were used after digestive upset to 're-establish' the bacterial flora of the small intestine and stomach to exclude pathogens such as *Escherichia coli* and *Salmonella* . However, the term probiotics is often used loosely for supplements containing live yeast in the equine market

Yeast

There are four strains of live yeast (*Saccharomyces cerevisiae*) permitted for use in the EU: *Saccharomyces cerevisiae* CBS 493.94; *Saccharomyces cerevisiae* CNCM I-4407; *Saccharomyces cerevisiae* CNCM I-1077; *Saccharomyces cerevisiae* MUCL 39885 (EU Commission[i], 2021).

Live yeast can be recommended in the short term after any event that has disturbed the hind gut's bacterial population. Live yeast supplementation helps create a more favourable hind gut environment to repopulate the hind gut with beneficial fibre-digesting microbes (Medina *et al.*, 2002; Jouany *et al.*, 2009; Agazzi *et al.*, 2009), indirectly improving fibre digestion (Morgan *et al.*, 2007; Jouany *et al.*, 2009). However, there is no evidence that providing yeast to animals with a healthy microbial population will have any further beneficial effect (Mackenthun *et al.*, 2013).

Prebiotics

Prebiotics are non-living feed ingredients that help to encourage the proliferation of existing useful bacteria and can help support the microbial population during changes in feed and management; dead yeast is included in this definition.

Prebiotics can be fed for longer periods of time, commonly recommended before and during stressful events/periods that may impact the gut and used as a preventative measure for those that show particular sensitivity during seasonal changes (Respondek *et al.*, 2008).

Examples of prebiotics include fructooligosaccharides (scFOS) / fructans and mannan-oligosaccharides (MOS). While evidence of efficacy is not abundant, scFOS supplementation has been shown to be effective at reducing disruption of the microbial population in the hind gut when horses were fed high-starch rations (Respondek *et al.*, 2008).

Antacids and equine gastric ulcers

There is some evidence to suggest that, as a preventative, feeds high in calcium carbonate, such as alfalfa, improve non-glandular gastric ulcer scores (Andrews *et al.*, 2006). Antacids (aluminium or magnesium hydroxide or calcium carbonate) have a short-lived effect on horses, and while they may be used as a preventative, there is not sufficient evidence for their exclusive use in ulcer treatment (Zavoshti and Andrews, 2017). Ingredients such as beta-glucans, sea buckthorn berries, pectins, liquorice, antacids and gum Arabic (Table 6.14) have been shown to provide benefits for squamous ulcers (Andrews *et al.*, 2016; Kerbyson *et al.*, 2016) such as acid buffering, regulation of passage rate and protection of the stomach lining. More research is required to determine to what extent they are beneficial, and to highlight optimum feeding rates (Murray and Grady, 2002; Huff *et al.*, 2012; Woodward *et al.*, 2014; Luca *et al.*, 2017).

Clients often feed gastric ulcer supplements alongside veterinary treatments; compared with the buffering effect of saliva, they are rather inconsequential and use in isolation as an alternative to

Table 6.13 Common ingredients included in equine calming supplements

Ingredient	Evidence-based research	Equine research	Known effective dosage	FEI prohibited substance	Practical considerations and example products
Magnesium	Reported to have calming effects in other species (Poleszak *et al.*, 2004; Kaplan *et al.*, 2007; Cardoso *et al.*, 2009) but no conclusive data available for horses. Magnesium deficiency in mice has been shown to affect an increase in anxiety; however, magnesium deficiency is rare in horses. High levels of bioavailable magnesium were thought to decrease reaction speed in horses (Dodd *et al.*, 2015) but more recently a further study has questioned the mechanisms behind this finding.	Some	No	No	Magnesium supplementation can interfere with calcium balance, leading to an increased risk of orthopaedic problems. NAF Magic*, Feedmark Steady Up*, Blue Chip Karma*
Valerian	Used in humans to treat sleeping disorders (Williams and Lamprecht, 2008) and a sedative effect has been shown in other animals (pigs, rats). No published studies on calming effect in horses.	None	No	Yes	The use of valerian has been associated with side effects such as diarrhoea and colic and interaction with other medications (enhancing the effect of anaesthetics). Avoid use in horses with kidney compromise. Hilton Herb's Calm and Collected*, Wendals Calmer for horses*, Gold Label Equikalm*
Tryptophan	Has been shown to have sedative and anti-anxiety effects in pigs (Peeters *et al.*, 2004). However, very few studies exist in horses; subsequently, there is a lack of evidence for safe and effective dosage (Grimmett and Sillence, 2005; Harris, 2005). Effects are thought to be species dependent and possibly influenced by other factors such as diet, exercise and age. Several studies have reported commercial doses of tryptophan as ineffective in mediating behaviour parameter (Grimmett and Sillence, 2005; Malmkvist and Christensen, 2007).	Some	No	No	Low doses have been reported to cause excitement as opposed to calming (Bagshaw *et al.*, 1994; Noble *et al.*, 2016) and while there is some evidence of short-term desired effect there is indication that long-term provision may be detrimental to performance (Davis *et al.*, 2017). TopSpec Calmer*, Blue Chip Karma*, So-Kalm*, B Kalm*

omeprazole is not yet warranted (Huff *et al.*, 2012; Andrews *et al.*, 2016; Kerbyson *et al.*, 2016; Luca *et al.*, 2017).

Diet and management should be addressed first, as saliva is one of the best antacids you can 'prescribe'.

Herbs and other functional ingredients

Herbs (Table 6.15) and other functional ingredients (including botanicals) are added for perceived functional effect and/or as a flavouring (Williams and Lamprecht, 2008; Elghandour *et al.*, 2018). Many can be fed either in isolation (garlic, for example) or in combination with other ingredients as part of a supplement (rosehips are commonly found in joint supplements, for example) or compound feed.

Despite a perception of these supplements being 'natural', owners should be advised that this does not automatically confer safety (Williams and Lamprecht, 2008; Elghandour *et al.*, 2018); evidence of efficacy and safety for the horse is minimal, as is the potential for interaction with other drugs (Poppenga, 2001; Posadzki *et al.*, 2012; Awortwe *et al.*, 2018) and the risk of prohibited substances.

Practical Steps for Supplement Selection

Following a clinical approach to advising supplements will result in a happy client (Fig. 6.1).

Working out the amount of active ingredient in a dose

Where supplement labels are lacking transparency, you could argue that you should not advise them.

The first step is to help clients work out the actual content of active ingredient in a daily dose. Units of measurements can vary and over-reliance on percentage or concentration can mislead horse owners and make product comparison challenging (Table 6.16).

Checking the advice for duration of supplementation

Do check how long the client will need to feed the supplement. Clearly a 'result' will not be instant and sometimes supplements are not given time to have an impact on the physiological process (Table 6.17).

Table 6.14. Common ingredients in equine gastric ulcer supplements

Supplement ingredient	Description and common sources	Mode of action	Equine-specific research
Antacids	Aluminium hydroxide, magnesium hydroxide, magnesium oxide, calcium carbonate	Buffering of stomach contents to aid in recovery of tissue exposed to stomach acid.	Yes, but mainly in combination with other ingredients (Clark *et al.*, 1996; Woodward *et al.*, 2014).
Beta glucans	Soluble fibre (non-starch polysaccharide) found in the cell walls of cereals and yeast	Forms a gel in the stomach of other species forming a protective coating for the stomach lining. Some indication that it may decrease passage rate through the digestive tract in other species (Schop *et al.*, 2020).	Very minimal in horses
Pectin	Soluble fibre (non-starch polysaccharide), found in the cell walls of fruits and sugar beet	Forms a gel when exposed to acidic environment (in combination with lecithin, is thought to form a hydrophobic barrier protecting the stomach lining) and is thought to bind bile acids (Zavoshti and Andrews, 2017)	Yes, but primarily in combination with other ingredients (most commonly pectin–lecithin complex) (Venner *et al.*, 1999; Sanz *et al.*, 2014; Sykes *et al.*, 2015; Woodward *et al.*, 2014)

Table 6.15. Typical herbs fed to horses

Common name	Formal name	Claims[a]	Equine-specific research
Aloe[c]	*Aloe vera*	Anti-inflammatory, antioxidant, cytoprotective, and mucus stimulatory.	Andrews *et al.*, 2016; Luca *et al.*, 2017; Bush *et al.*, 2018
Boswellia serrata[c]	Indian frankincense	Anti-inflammatory	Limited. Fusini *et al.*, 2016; EFSA *et al.*, 2022
Chamomile	*Matricaria recutita* or *Matricaria chamomilla*	Antioxidant, anti-inflammatory, healing, calmative	Limited. Alsaadi and Aljobory, 2016
Chaste tree berry[c]	*Vitex agnus castus*	Antioxidant and dopaminergic action (proposed to increase dopaminergic activity in the equine pituitary)	Beech *et al.*, 2002; Jones and Larkins, 2009; Bradaric *et al.*, 2013
Cinnamon[cd]		Antioxidant, insulin receptor activator, flavouring	NR
Devil's claw[bc]	*Harpagophytum procumbens*	Anti-inflammatory, anorexigenic effect (potential to limit feed intake)	Pearson *et al.*, 2000; Axmann *et al.*, 2019
Echinacea[c]	*Echinacea angustifolia*/*purpurea*	Anti-inflammatory, antioxidant and immunomodulator	Some. O'Neill *et al.*, 2002; Bagno *et al.*, 2018
Fenugreek[cd]	*Trigonella foenum-graecum*	Antioxidant, appetite stimulant, flavouring and to slow carbohydrate absorption	NR
Garlic	*Allium sativum*	Antioxidant, anti-inflammatory, antiparasitic, insect repellent, expectorant and immunostimulant Chronic feeding has been shown to cause toxicity (anaemia and gastric irritation) when fed in large quantities (> 0.2 mg/kg BW per day) (Pearson *et al.*, 2005)	YesPearson, 2003; Pearson *et al.*, 2005; Williams and Lamprecht, 2008; Chmelikova *et al.*, 2018; Buono *et al.*, 2019
Ginger	*Zingiber officinale*	Anti-inflammatory, antioxidant and some indication for increasing recovery rate from cardiovascular exercise	Some. Liburt, 2005; Smarsh *et al.*, 2010
Ginseng[c]	*Panax ginseng*	Antioxidant, anti-inflammatory and antilipidemic properties	Limited. Pearson *et al.*, 2007
Flaxseed		Anti-inflammatory and antioxidant	Harman, 2002; O'Neill *et al.*, 2002; Ross-Jones *et al.*, 2014
Liquorice	*Glycyrrhiza glabra*	Anti-inflammatory, cytoprotective and mucus-stimulatory effects	Limited. Stucchi *et al.*, 2017; Ahmadnejad *et al.*, 2022
Milk thistle	*Silibum marianum*	Anti-inflammatory, antioxidant and hepatoprotective.	Limited. Reisinger *et al.*, 2014; Gugliandolo *et al.*, 2020; Dockalova *et al.*, 2021
Rose hips		Antioxidant and anti-inflammatory properties.	Limited. Winther *et al.*, 2010, 2012
Turmeric[c]	*Curcumin*	Antioxidant, anti-inflammatory	Limited. Thorne Research, 2001; Horohov, 2012; Fusini *et al.*, 2016
Valerian[b]	*Valeriana officinalis*	Sedative	NR
Vervain	Common verbena	Sedative	NR
Yucca	*Yucca shidigera*	Anti-inflammatory and antioxidant	NR

NR = No references available
[a]Information compiled from Bergero and Valle, 2006; Williams and Lamprecht, 2008; Tinworth *et al.*, 2010 and Elghandour *et al.*, 2018
[b]Prohibited under FEI rules
[c]Human studies indicate interaction with synthetic drugs (Posadzki *et al.*, 2012; Awortwe *et al.*, 2018)
[d]Safety has not been evaluated in horses

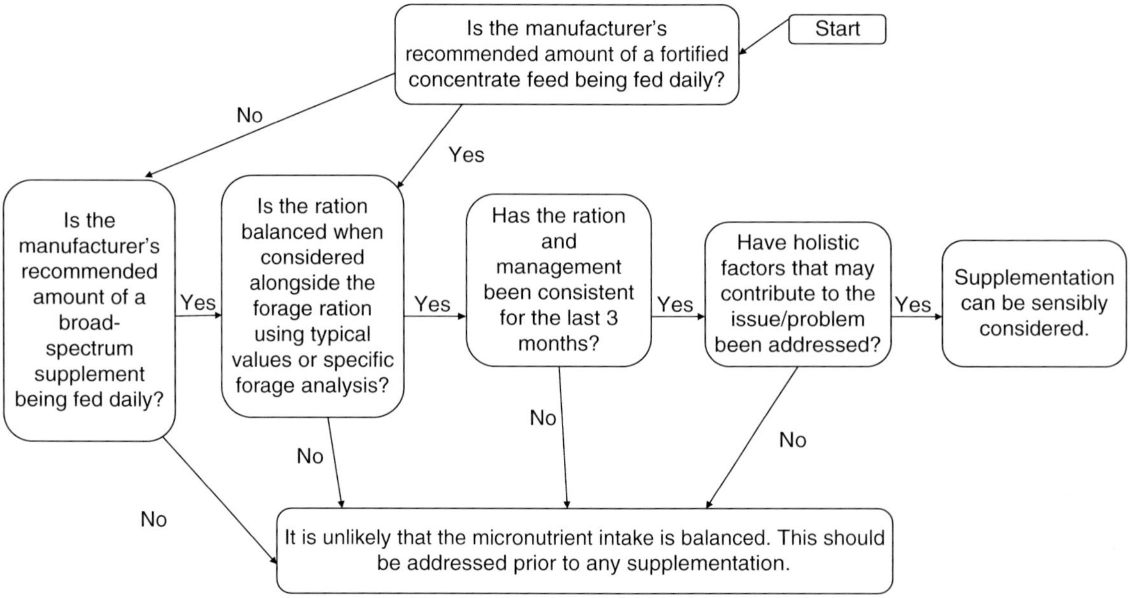

Fig. 6.1 Summary of steps for assessment of micronutrient balance.

Table 6.16 Daily intake of glucosamine (GU) for a 500 kg horse from variously labelled joint supplements[a]

Product	Label	Glucosamine in supplement (g/kg)	Feeding rate for 500 kg horse (g/day)	GU daily intake (g)	GU daily intake (mg)
A	No fillers, 100% glucosamine	1000	10	10	10,000
B	50% Glucosamine	500	12	6	6000
C	40% Glucosamine	400	13	5.2	5200
D	20% Glucosamine	200	90	18	18,000
E	Glucosamine 40,000 mg/kg	40	40	1.6	1600

[a]Be sure to make the distinction between scoop size and actual amount fed. For example, a 50 ml scoop may contain only 30 g of supplement.

Table 6.17 Diet advice for horse presenting with poor hoof quality and growth.

Horse history	The owner had tried various hoof supplements previously, to no avail Initial assessment thorough history and appraisal of current management and diet	Poor hoof quality and growth (brittle horn and consistently losing shoes)
Current diet	The feeding history suggested previous hoof supplements had been tried, but owner had only persisted for 1–2 months at a time	Diet was meeting macro- and micronutrient requirements; quality (amino acid content) of the protein provided was good
Advice	Add a biotin supplement (providing 20 mg of biotin per day) alongside the current diet and management (including routine farriery) Client was advised that, as it takes 9–12 months for the horn to grow down from the coronet band, the supplement would need to be provided for the long term in order to provide therapeutic benefits	Owner was recommended to monitor using photos taken prior to supplementation to provide objective appraisal of change in horn quality and growth, and then once every 3 months going forward; keeping a diary of shoeing intervals and lost shoes and feedback from the farrier

Supporting clients to monitor progress

Encourage owners to objectively appraise the use of the supplement by:

- recording behaviour;
- checking faeces;
- checking skin or hoof condition over time;
- using videos, photos or training 'apps'; and
- also seeking more objective opinions from paraprofessionals.

Where possible, dietary changes should be made one at a time. This helps to attribute any changes to a particular product. Making multiple supplement changes can lead to micronutrient imbalance as well as increased costs.

Summary

- Micronutrient provision and overall balance is key to supporting health and performance in the horse.
  - Knowledge of key roles and requirements of specific micronutrients emphasises the importance of a holistic approach and informs a sensible approach to supplementation.
  - Check the base ration first.
  - Knowledge of key practical scenarios where micronutrient balance may be compromised is essential to inform assessment protocol and interpretation.
- Have a clear idea of what supplementation aims to achieve.
- Beware claims but also keep an open mind: in some situations, supplements may be beneficial, whether as a placebo or otherwise.
  - Read the label to check daily intake (not declarations).
- Evaluate the evidence but be aware of the difficulty in demonstrating the efficacy of certain supplement types.
  - When assessing supplement efficacy, remain objective.
  - Encourage clients to use videos or pictures where possible and assess effects over the long-term.
- Make one change at a time, so any impact can be isolated and attributed to that specific change.
- Remember that no benefit is achieved with hypernutrition – more is not necessarily better.

Note

[i] https://eur-lex.europa.eu/eli/reg_impl/2014/11-0

Bibliography

Agar, C., Gemmil, L.R., Hollands, T. and Freeman, S.L. (2016) The use of nutritional supplements in dressage and eventing horses. *Vet Record* 3, 1–7.

Agazzi, A., Invernizzi, G., Ferroni, M., Fanelli, A. and Savoini, G. (2009) Effect of live yeast (*Saccharomyces cerevisiae*) administration on apparent digestibility of horses. *Italian Journal of Animal Science* 8(2), 685–687.

Ahmadnejad, M., Jalilzadeh-Amin, G. and Sykes, B.W. (2022) Prophylactic effects of Glycyrrhiza glabra root extract on phenylbutazone-induced Equine Glandular Gastric Disease (EGGD). *Journal of Equine Veterinary Science* 118, 104088.

Alsaadi, S.A.R.A. and Aljobory, A.M.I.S. (2016) Study the variation in biochemical parameters of post colic surgical horses which treated with chamomile flowers. *Imperial Journal of Interdisciplinary Research* 2, 1964–1968.

Andrews, F.M., Buchanan, B.R. and Smith S.H. (2006) *In vitro* effects of hydrochloric acid and various concentrations of acetic, propionic, butyric, or valeric acids on bioelectric properties of equine gastric squamous mucosa. *American Journal of Veterinary Research* 67(11), 1873–1882.

Andrews, F.M., Camacho-Luna, P., Loftin, P.G., Gaymon, G., Garza Jr, F., Keowen, M.L. and Kearney, M.T. (2016) Effect of a pelleted supplement fed during and after omeprazole treatment on nonglandular gastric ulcer scores and gastric juice pH in horses. *Equine Veterinary Education*, 28(4), 196-202.

Argo, C.M., Dugdale, A.H.A. and McGowen, C.M. (2015) Considerations for the use of restricted, soaked grass hay diets to promote weight loss in the management of equine metabolic syndrome and obesity. *The Veterinary Journal* 206(2), 170–177.

Awortwe, C., Makiwane, M., Reuter, H., Muller, C., Louw, J and Rosenkranz, B. (2018) Critical evaluation of causality assessment of herb-drug interactions in patients. *British Journal of Clinical Pharmacology* 84, 679–693.

Axmann, S., Hummel, K., Nöbauer, K., Razzazi-Fazeli, E. and Zitterl-Eglseer, K. (2019) Pharmacokinetics of harpagoside in horses after intragastric administration of a Devil's claw (*Harpagophytum procumbens*) extract. *Journal of Veterinary Pharmacology and Therapeutics* 42(1), 37–44. doi: 10.1111/jvp.1271

Bagshaw, C.S., Ralston, S.L. and Fisher, H. (1994) Behavioural and physiological effect of orally administered tryptophan on horses subjected to acute isolation stress. *Applied Animal Behaviour Science* 40(1), 1–12.

Bagno, O.A., Shevchenko, S.A., Shevchenko, A.O. and Dyadichkina, T.V. (2018) Influence of phytobiotic feed additive from echinacea purpurea and sedimin preparation on growth and development of young horses. *Achievements of Science and Technology in Agro-Industrial Complex* 8, 62–65.

Beech, J., Donaldson, M.T. and Lindborg, S. (2002) Comparison of Vitec agnus castus extract and pergolide in treatment of equine Cushing's syndrome. *AAEP Proceedings* 48, 175–177.

Bergero, D. and Valle, E. (2006) A critical analysis on the use of herbs and herbal extracts in feeding sport horses. *Pferdeheilkunde* 22(4), 550–557.

Bergin, B.J., Pierce, S.W., Bramlage, L.R. and Stromberg, A. (2006) Oral hyaluronan gel reduces post operative tarsocrural effusion in the yearling thoroughbred. *Equine Veterinary Journal* 38(4), 375–378.

BETA (British Equestrian Trade Association) (2019) *The National Equestrian Survey*. British Equestrian Trade Association.

Blackman, M. and Moore-Colyer, M.J.S. (1998) Hay for horses: the effects of three different wetting treatments on dust and nutrient content. *Animal Science* 66, 745–750.

Block, J.A., Oegema, T.R., Sandy, J.D. and Plaas, A. (2010) The effects of oral glucosamine on joint health: is a change in research approach needed? *Osteoarthritis and Cartilage* 18, 5–11.

Bradaric, Z., May, A. and Gehlen, H. (2013) Use of the chasteberry preparation Corticosal for the treatment of pituitary pars intermedia dysfunction in horses. *Pferdeheilkunde* 29(6), 721–728.

Brosnahan, M.M. and Paradis, M.R. (2003) Demographic and clinical characteristics of geriatric horses: 467 cases (1989–1999). *Journal of the American Veterinary Medical Association* 223(1), 93–98.

Buffa, E.A., Van Den Berg, S.S., Berstraete, F.J. and Swart, N.G. (1992) Effect of dietary biotin supplement on equine hoof horn growth rate and hardness. *Equine Veterinary Journal* 24(6), 472–474.

Buono, F., Pacifico, L., Piantedosi, D., Sgroi, G., Neola, B., Roncoroni, C., Genovese, A., Rufrano, D. and Veneziano, V. (2019) Preliminary observations of the effect of garlic on egg shedding in horses naturally infected by intestinal Strongyles. *Journal of Equine Veterinary Science* 72, 79–83.

Burk, A.O. and Williams, C.A. (2008) Feeding management practices and supplement use in top-level event horses. *Comparative Exercise Physiology* 5.

Bush, J., van den Boom, R. and Franklin, S. (2018) Comparison of aloe vera and omeprazole in the treatment of equine gastric ulcer syndrome. *Equine Veterinary Journal* 50(1), 34–40. doi: 10.1111/evj.12706

Bushell, R. and Murray, J. (2016) A survey of senior equine management: owner practices and confidence. *Livestock Science* 186, 69–77.

Campbell-Beggs, C.L., Johnson, P., Messer, N.T., Latimer, J.C., Johnson, G.C. and Casteel, S.W. (1994) Osteochondritis dissecans in an Appaloosa foal associated with zinc toxicosis. *Journal of Equine Veterinary Science* 14, 546–550.

Cardoso, C.C., Lobato, K.R., Binfare, R.W., Ferreira, P.K., Rosa, A.O. *et al.* (2009) Evidence for the involvement of the monoaminergic system in the antidepressant-like effect of magnesium. *Progress in Neuro-Psychopharmacology and Biological Psychiatry* 33, 235–242.

Chmelikova, E., Nemecek, D., Dvorakova, M., Heroutova, I. and Sedmikova, M. (2018) Organo-sulphur garlic compounds influence viability of mammalian cells: a review. *Scientia Agriculturae Bohemica* 49, 9–16.

Clark, C.K., Merritt, A.M., Burrow, J.A. and Steible, C.K. (1996) Effect of aluminum hydroxide/magnesium hydroxide antacid and bismuth subsalicylate on gastric pH in horses. *Journal of the American Veterinary Medical Association* 208(10), 1687–1691.

Coenen, M. (2013) Macro and trace elements in equine nutrition. In: Geor, R., Harris, P. and Coenen, M. (eds) *Equine Applied and Clinical Nutrition*. Saunders Elsevier, China, pp. 191–228.

Coenen, M. and Meyer, H. (1987) Water and electrolyte content of the equine gastrointestinal tract in dependence of the ration type. In: *Proceedings of the Equine Nutrition and Physiology Symposium 10*, pp. 531–536. The Fort Collins Marriott, Colorado State University.

Comben, N., Clarke, R.J. and Sutherland, D.J. (1984) Clinical observations on the response of equine hoof defects to dietary supplementation with biotin. *Veterinary Record* 25–26, 642–645.

Conover, A.L., Shultz, A.M. and Wagner, A.L. (2015) Effects of GastroTech on equine gastric ulcer syndrome (EGUS). *Journal of Equine Veterinary Science* 35, 418–436.

Cymbaluk, N.F., Schryver, H.F. and Hintz, H.F. (1981) Copper metabolism and requirement in mature ponies. *The Journal of Nutrition* 111(1), 87–95. doi: 10.1093/jn/111.1.87.

Davis, B.P., Engle, T.E., Ransom, J.I. and Grandin, T. (2017) Preliminary evaluation on the effectiveness of varying doses of supplemental tryptophan as a calmative in horses. *Applied Animal Behaviour Science* 188, 34–41.

Davis, T.Z., Stegelmeier, B.L., Panter, K.E., Cook, D., Gardner, D.R. and Hall, J.O. (2012) Toxicokinetics and pathology of plant-associated acute selenium toxicosis in steers. *Journal of Veterinary Diagnostic Investigation* 24(2), 319–327. doi: 10.1177/1040638711435407

Deaton, C.M., Marlin, D.J., Smith, N.C., Harris, P.A., Schroter, R. *et al.* (2004) Antioxidant supplementation in horses affected by recurrent airway obstruction. *The Journal of Nutrition* 134(8), 2065S–2067S.

de Moffarts, B., Kirschvink, N., Art, T., Pincemaik, J. and Lekeux, P. (2005) Effect of oral antioxidant supplementation on blood antioxidant status in trained thoroughbred horses. *The Veterinary Journal* 169(1), 65–74.

Dockalova, H., Zeman, L. and Horky, P. (2021) Influence of milk thistle (*Silybum marianum*) seed cakes on biochemical values of equine plasma subjected to physical exertion. *Animals* 11(1), 210.

Dodd, J., Doran, G., Harris, P. and Noble, G. (2015) Magnesium aspartate supplementation and reaction speed response in horses. *Journal of Equine Veterinary Science* 35(5), 401–402.

Doige, C.E. and McLaughlin, B.G. (1981) Hyperplastic goitre in newborn foals in Western Canada. *The Canadian Veterinary Journal* 22(2), 42.

Donoghue, S., Kronfeld, D.S, Berkowitz, S.J. and Copp, R.L. (1981) Vitamin A nutrition of the equine: Growth, serum biochemistry, and hematology. *The Journal of Nutrition* 111, 365.

Eamens, G.J., Macadam, J.F. and Laing, E.A. (1984) Skeletal abnormalities in young horses associated with zinc toxicity and hypocuprosis. *Australian Veterinary Journal* 61, 205–207. doi: 10.1111/j.1751-0813.1984.tb05989.x.

EFSA Panel on Additives and Products or Substances used in Animal Feed (FEEDAP), Bampidis, V., Azimonti, G., Bastos, M.D.L., Christensen, H., Fašmon Durjava, M. *et al.* (2022). Safety and efficacy of a feed additive consisting of an extract of olibanum from Boswellia serrata Roxb. ex Colebr. for use in dogs and horses (FEFANA asbl). *EFSA Journal* 20(3), e07158.

Elghandour, M.M.M.Y., Reddy, P.R.K., Salem, A.Z.M., Redyy, P.P.R., Hyder, I. *et al.* (2018) Plant bioactives and extracts as fed additives in horse nutrition. *Journal of Equine Veterinary Science* 69, 66–77.

Ememe, M.U., Mshelia, W.P. and Ayo, J.O. (2015) Ameliorative effects of resveratrol on oxidative stress biomarkers in horses. *Journal of Equine Veterinary Science* 35(6), 518–523.

Equi-Analytical Laboratory Services (2020) Common Feed Profiles. [Online]. Equi-Analytical Laboratory Services, Ithaca, New York. Available at: https://equi-analytical.com/common-feed-profiles/ (accessed 22 February 2020)

Eroksuz, H., Eroksuz, Y., Ozer, H., Ceribasi, A.O., Yaman, I. and Ilhan, N. (2004). Equine goiter associated with excess dietary iodine. *Veterinary and Human Toxicology* 46(3), 147–149.

FAO/WHO (2002) Food and Agricultural Organization of the United Nations and World Health Organization. Joint FAO/WHO working group report on drafting guidelines for the evaluation of probiotics in food. *Food and Agricultural Organization of the United Nations* [online], (2002).

Forsyth, R.K., Brigden, C.V. and Northrop, A.J. (2006) Double blind investigation of the effects of oral supplementation of combined glucosamine hydrochloride (GHCL) and chondroitin sulphate (CS) on stride characteristics of veteran horses. *Equine Veterinary Journal* 36, 622–625.

Freire, R., Clegg, H.A., Buckley, P., Friend, M.A. and Mcgreevy, P.D. (2008) Behavioural and physiological effects of virginiamycin in the diets of horses with stereotypies. *Veterinary Record* 163, 413–417.

Fusini, F., Bisicchia, S., Bottegoni, C., Gigante, A., Zanchini, F. and Busilacchi, A. (2016). Nutraceutical supplement in the management of tendinopathies: a systematic review. *Muscles, Ligaments and Tendons Journal* 6(1), 48–57.

Gee, E., Grace, N., Firth, E. and Fennessy, P. (2000) Changes in liver copper concentration of Thoroughbred foals from birth to 160 days of age and the effect of prenatal copper supplementation of their dams. *Australian Veterinary Journal* 78, 347–353. doi: 10.1111/j1751-0813.2000.tb11791.x.

Gemmill, R., Agar, C., Freeman, S.L. and Hollands, T. (2016) Factors affecting owners' choice of nutritional supplements for use in dressage and eventing horses. *Vet Record* 3(1).

Grace, N.D., Gee, E.K., Firth, E.C. and Shaw, H.L. (2002) Digestible energy intake, dry matter digestibility and mineral status of grazing New Zealand Thoroughbred yearlings. *New Zealand Veterinary Journal* 50, 63–69.

Greiwe-Crandell, K.M., Kronfeld, D.S., Gay, L.A. and Sklan, D. (1995) Seasonal vitamin A depletion in grazing horses is assessed better by the relative dose response test than by serum retinol concentration. *The Journal of Nutrition* 125(10), 2711–2716.

Grimmett, A. and Sillence, M.N. (2005) Calmatives for the excitable horse: a review of L-tryptophan. *The Veterinary Journal* 170(1), 24–32.

Gugliandolo, E., Crupi, R., Biondi, V., Licata, P., Cuzzocrea, S. and Passantino, A. (2020) Protective effect of silibinin on lipopolysaccharide-induced inflammatory responses in equine peripheral blood mononuclear cells, an in vitro study. *Animals* 10(11), 2022.

Gupta, R.C., Canerdy, T.D. and Skaggs, P. (2009) Therapeutic efficacy of undenatured type-II collagen (UC-II) in comparison to glucosamine and chondroitin in arthritic horses. *Journal of Veterinary Pharmacological Therapies* 32(6), 577–584.

Harman, J. (2002) The toxicology of herbs in equine practice. *Clinical Techniques in Equine Practice* 8, 74–80. doi: 10.1053/ctep.2002.34475

Harmeyer, J. and Schlumbohm, C. (2004), Effects of pharmacological doses of Vitamin D3 on mineral balance and profile of plasma and Vitamin D3 metabolites in horses. *Journal of Steroid Biochemistry and Molecular Biology* 89–90, 595–600.

Harris, P.A. (2000) Feeding practices in the UK and Germany. In: Pagan, J.D. (ed.) *Advances in Equine Nutrition II. Proceedings from the KER Equine Nutrition Conference*, pp. 429–452. Kentucky Equine Research (KER), Versailles, Kentucky.

Harris, P. (2005) Nutrition, behaviour and the role of supplements for calming horses: the veterinarian's dilemma. *The Veterinary Journal* 170, 10–11.

Harris, P. (2009) Feeding management of elite endurance horses. *The Veterinary Clinics of North America. Equine Practice* 25(1), 137–viii. doi: 10.1016/cveq.2009.01.005.

Hoffman, C.J., Costa, L.R. and Freeman, L.M. (2009) Survey of feeding practices, supplement use, and knowledge of equine nutrition among a subpopulation of horse owners in New England. *Journal of Equine Veterinary Science* 29(10), 719–724.

Horohov, D.S.S. (2012) The effect of exercise and nutritional supplementation on pro inflammatory cytokine expression in young racehorses during training. *Journal of Equine Veterinary Science* 32 (121), 805–815.

Huff, N.K., Auer, A.D., Garza, F., Keowen, M.L., Kearney, M.T. *et al.* (2012) Effect of sea buckthorn berries and pulp in a liquid emulsion on gastric ulcers scores and gastric juice pH in horses. *Journal of Veterinary Internal Medicine* 26, 1186–1191.

Ireland, J.L., Clegg, P.D., McGowan, C.M., McKane, S.A. and Pinchbeck, G.L. (2011) A cross-sectional study of geriatric horses in the United Kingdom. Part 1: Demographics and management practices. *Equine Veterinary Journal* 43(1), 30–36. doi: 10.1111/j.2042-3306.2010.00145.x

James, L.F. and Butcher, J.E. (1972) Halogeton poisoning of sheep: effect of high level oxalate intake. *Journal of Animal Science* 35, 1233–1238.

Jansson, A. and Dahlborn, K. (1999) Effects of feeding frequency and voluntary salt intake on fluid and electrolyte regulation in athletic horses. *Journal of Applied Physiology* 86, 1610–1616.

Jansson, A., Rytthammar, A. and Lindberg, J.E. (1996) Voluntary salt (NaCl) intake in Standardbred horses. *Pferdeheikunde* 12, 443–445.

Jansson, A., Saastamoinen, M. and Lindberg J.E. (2012) Forage feeding systems. In: Saastamoinen, M., Fradinho, M.J., Santos, A.S. and Miraglia, N. (eds) *Forages and Grazing in Horse Nutrition*, Vol. 132. Wageningen Academic Publishers, Wageningen, The Netherlands.

Jones, K.A. and Larkins, N.J. (2009) Field study into the efficacy of a medicinal plant based complex for management of Equine Cushings Syndrome in ageing horses. *Planta Medica* 75, 28.

Jones, L., Lax, J. and Hollands, T. (2005) Analysis of the mineral content of spring summer grazing used for thoroughbred breeding stock in the UK. In: *Proceedings of 44th BEVA Congress*, Harrogate, UK.

Josseck, H., Zenker. W. and Geyer, H. (1995) Hoof horn abnormalities in Lipizzaner horses and the effect of dietary biotin on macroscopic aspects of hoof horn quality. *Equine Veterinary Journal* 27(3), 175–182.

Jouany, J.P., Medina, B., Bertin, G. and Julliand, V. (2009) Effect of live yeast culture supplementation on hindgut microbial communities and their polysaccharidase and glycoside hydrolase activities in horses fed a high-fiber or high-starch diet. *Journal of Animal Science* 87(9), 2844–2852.

Kaplan, B.J., Crawford, S.G., Field, C.J. and Simpson, J.S. (2007) Vitamins, minerals and mood. *Psychological Bulletin* 133(5), 747–760.

Kaya-Karasu, G., Huntington, P., Iben, C. and Murray, J.A. (2018) Feeding and management practices for Racehorses in Turkey. *Journal of Equine Veterinary Science* 61, 108–113.

Kempson, S.A. (1987) Scanning electron microscope observations of hoof horn from horses with brittle feet. *Veterinary Record* 120(24), 568–570.

Kempson, S.A. (2005) Nutritional management of horses with hoof diseases. Applied equine nutrition. 1st Equine NUtrition COnference (ENUCO), Hannover, Germany, 1–2 October, 2005, pp. 105–112.

Kerbyson, N., Knottenbelt, D.K., Carslake, H.B., Conwell, R.C., Sutton, D.G.M. *et al.* (2016) A comparison between omeprazole and a dietary supplement for the management of squamous gastric ulceration in horses. *Journal of Equine Veterinary Science* 40, 94–101.

Kirschvink, N., de Moffarts, B. and Lekeux, P. (2008) The oxidant/antioxidant equilibrium in horses. *The Veterinary Journal* 177(2), 178–191.

Kuusela, E. (2006) Annual and seasonal changes in mineral contents (Ca, Mg, P, K and Na) of grazed clover-grass mixtures in organic farming. *Agricultural and Food Science* 15(1), 23–34.

Laan, T.T., Spoorenberg, J.F. and van der Kolk, J.H. (2000) Hypocalcemia in a four-week old foal. *Tijdschr Diergeneeskd* 125, 185–187.

Laverty, S., Sandy, J.D., Celeste, C., Vachon, O., Marier, J.F. *et al.* (2005) Synovial fluid levels and serum pharmacokinetics in a large animal model following treatment with oral glucosamine at clinically relevant doses. *Arthritis and Rheumatism* 52(1), 181–191.

Liburt, N.R. (2005) Effects of ginger and cranberry extracts on markers of inflammation and performance following intense exercise in horses. Master's Thesis. Rutgers, the State University of New Jersey.

Lindinger, M.I., MacNicol, J.M., Karrow, N. and Pearson, W. (2017) Effects of a novel dietary supplement on indices of muscle injury and articular GAG release in horse. *Journal of Equine Veterinary Science* 48, 52–60.

Longland, A.C. (2012) Nutritional Assessment of forage quality. In: Saastamoinen, M., Fradinho, M.J., Santos, A.S. and Miraglia, N. (eds) *Forages and Grazing in Horse Nutrition*, Vol. 132. Wageningen Academic Publishers, Wageningen, The Netherlands.

Luca, S., Enrica, Z., Alessia, S., Giovanni, S., Serena, C. *et al.* (2017) Efficacy of the administration of a natural feed supplement in the management of equine gastric ulcer syndrome in 7 sport horses: a field trial. *American Journal of Animal Veterinary Science* 12, 104–110.

Lybbert, T., Gibbs, P. and Cohen, N. (2007) Feeding alfalfa hay to exercising horses reduces the severity of gastric squamous ulceration. *Proceedings of 53rd American Association of Equine Practitioners Annual Convention*, Orlando, Florida, pp. 525–526.

Mackenthun, E., Coenen, M. and Vervuert, I. (2013) Effects of *Saccharomyces cerevisiae* supplementation on apparent total tract digestibility of nutrients and fermentation profile in healthy horses. *Journal of Animal Physiology and Animal Nutrition* 97, 115–120.

Malmkvist, J. and Christensen, J.W. (2007) A note on the effects of a commercial tryptophan product on horse reactivity. *Applied Animal Behaviour Science* 107(3), 361–366.

Maranon, G., Munoz-Esxassim B., Manley, W., Garcia,C., Cayado, P., de la Muela, M.S. *et al*. (2008) The effect of methyl sulphonyl methane supplementation on biomarkers of oxidative stress in sport horses following jumping exercise. *Acta Veterinaria Scandinavica* 7, 45–50.

McCall, C. (2009) Equine behaviour: a nutritional link? In: Al, P.E. (ed.) *Advances in Equine Nutrition IV*. Nottingham University Press, pp. 77–87.

McDowell, L.R. (1989) *Vitamins in Animal Nutrition*, 1st edn. Academic Press, New York.

McGowan, T.W., Pinchbeck, G., Philips, C.J.C., Perkins, N., Hodgson, D.R. *et al*. (2010) A survey of aged horses in Queensland, Australia. Part 1: management and preventative health care. *Australian Veterinary Journal* 88, 420–427.

Medina, B., Girard, I.D., Jacotot, E. and Julliand, V. (2002) Effect of a preparation of *Saccharomyces cerevisiae* on microbial profiles and fermentation patterns in the large intestine of horses fed a high fiber or a high starch diet. *Journal of Animal Science* 80(10), 2600–2609.

Miller, R., Spiro, A. and Stanner, S. (2016) Micronutrient status and intake in the UK – where might we be in 10 years' time? *Nutrition Bulletin* 41(1), 14–41.

Moore-Colyer, M.J.S. (1996) Effects of soaking hay fodder for horses on dust and mineral content. *Animal Science* 63, 337–342.

Moore-Colyer, M.J.S., Taylor, J.L.E. and James, R. (2016) The effect of steaming and soaking on the respirable particle, bacteria, mould and nutrient content in hay for horses. *Journal of Equine Veterinary Science* 39, 62–68.

Morgan, L.M., Coverdale, J.A., Froetschel, M.A. and Yoon, I. (2007) Effect of yeast culture supplementation on digestibility of varying forage quality in mature horses. *Journal of Equine Veterinary Science* 27(6), 260–265.

Murray, M.J. (1999) Pathophysiology of peptic disorders in foals and horses: a review. *Equine Veterinary Journal* 29, 14–18.

Murray, M.J. and Grady, T.C. (2002) The effect of a pectin-lecithin complex on prevention of gastric mucosal lesions induced by feed deprivation in ponies. *Equine Veterinary Journal* 34, 195–198.

Murray, J.M.D., Hanna, E. and Hastie, P. (2018) Equine dietary supplements: an insight into their use and perceptions in the Irish equine industry. *Irish Veterinary Journal* 71(4).

Murray, R., Walker, V., Tranquille, C., Adams, V. and Frost, R. (2014) Effect of an oral joint supplement on orthopaedic evaluation scores and limb kinematics. *Equine Veterinary Journal* 46(S46), 44.

Murray, R.C., Walker, V.A., Tranquille, C.A., Spear, J. and Adams, V. (2017) A randomised blinded crossover clinical trial to determine the effect of an oral joint supplement on equine limb kinematics, orthopedic, physiotherapy and handler evaluation scores. *Journal of Equine Veterinary Science* 50, 121–128.

Noble G.K., Brockwell Y.M., Munn K.J., Harris P.A., Davidson H.P.B. *et al*. (2008) Effects of a commercial dose of L-tryptophan on plasma tryptophan concentrations and behaviour in horses. *Equine Veterinary Journal* 40, 51–56.

Noble, G.K., Li, X., Xhang, D. and Sillence, M.N. (2016) Randomised clinical trial on the effect of a single oral administration of L-tryptophan, at three dose rates, on reaction speed, plasma concentration and haemolysis in horses. *Veterinary Journal* 213, 84–86.

NRC (2001) *Nutrient Requirements of Dairy Cattle*, 7th edn. National Academies Press, Washington, DC. doi: 10.17226/11653.

NRC (2007) *Nutrient Requirements of Horses*, 6th edn. National Academies Press, Washington, DC.

Oke, S.L. and McIlwraith, C.W. (2010) Review of the economic impact of osteoarthritis and oral joint-health supplements in horses. *AAEP Proceedings* 56, 12–16.

Oke, S., Aghazadeh-Habashi, A., Weese, J.S. and Jamali, F. (2006) Evaluation of glucosamine levels in commercial equine oral supplements for joints. *Equine Veterinary Journal* 38(1), 93–95.

Pagan, J.D., Petroski-Rose, L., Mann, A. and Hauss, A. (2020) Omeprazole reduces calcium digestibility in Thoroughbred horses. *Journal of Equine Veterinary Science* 86.

O'Neill, W., McKee, S. and Clarke, A.F. (2002) Immunological and haematinic consequences of feeding a standardized Echinacea (*Echinacea angustifolia*) extract to healthy horses. *Equine Veterinary Journal* 34, 222–227.

Panciera, R.J., Martin, T., Burrows, G.E., Taylor, D.S. and Rice, L.E. (1990) Acute oxalate poisoning attributable to ingestion of curly dock (*Rumex crispus*) in sheep. *Journal of the American Veterinary Medical Association* 196, 1981–1984.

Pearson, W. (2003) Ethnoveterinary medicine: the science of botanicals in equine health and disease. In: *Proceedings of the second annual European equine health and nutrition congress*. Lelystad, The Netherlands.

Pearson, W., McKee, S. and Clarke, A.F. (2000) Effect of a proprietary herbal produce on equine joint disease.

Journal of Nutraceuticals, Functional & Medical Foods 2(2), 31–46. doi: 10.1300/j133v02n0204.

Pearson, W., Boermans, H.J., Bettger, W.J., McBride, B.W. and Lindinger, M.I. (2005) Association of maximum voluntary dietary intake of freeze-dried garlic with Heinz body anaemia in horses. *American Journal of Veterinary Research* 66, 457–465.

Pearson, W., Omar, S. and Clarke, A.F. (2007) Low-dose ginseng (*Panax quinquefolium*) modulates the course and magnitude of the antibody response to vaccination against Equid herpesvirus 1 in horses. *Canadian Journal of Veterinary Research* 71, 213–217.

Pearson, W., Orth, M.W. and Lindinger, M.I. (2009) Evaluation of inflammatory responses induced via intra-articular injection of interleukin-1 in horses receiving a dietary nutraceutical and assessment of the clinical effects of long-term nutraceutical administration. *American Journal of Veterinary Research* 70(7), 848–861.

Peeters, E., Driessen, B., Steegmans, R., Henot, D. and Geers, R. (2004) Effect of supplemental tryptophan, vitamins E and a herbal product on responses by pigs to vibration. *Journal of Animal Science* 82(8), 2410–2420.

Poleszak, E., Szewczyk, B., Kedzierska, E., Wlaz, P., Pilc, A. *et al.* (2004) Antidepressant- and anxiolytic-like activity of magnesium in mice. *Pharmacology Biochemistry and Behaviour* 78(1), 7–12.

Poli, V.F.S., Sanches, R.B., Moraes, A.D.S., Fidalgo, J.P.N., Nascimento, M.A. *et al.* (2017) The excessive caloric intake and micronutrient deficiencies related to obesity after a long-term interdisciplinary therapy. *Nutrition* 38, 113–119.

Poppenga, R.H. (2001) Risks associated with the use of herbs and other dietary supplements. *Veterinary Clinics of North America: Equine Practice* 17(3), 455–477.

Posadzki, P., Watson, L. and Ernst, E. (2012) Herb-drug interactions: an overview of systemic reviews. *British Journal of Clinical Pharmacology* 75(3), 603–618.

Pratt-Phillips, S.E. (2016) Feeding practices and nutrient intakes among elite Show Jumpers. *Journal of Equine Veterinary Science* 43, 39–43.

Ramey, D.W., Eddington, N., Thonar, E. and Lee, M. (2002) An analysis of glucosamine and chondroitin sulfate content in oral joint supplement products. *Journal of Equine Veterinary Science* 22, 125–127.

Reilly, J.D., Cottrell, D.F., Martin, R.J. and Cuddeford, D.J. (1998) Effect of supplementary dietary biotin on hoof growth and hoof growth rate in ponies: a controlled trial. *Equine Veterinary Journal* (26), 51–57.

Reisinger, N., Schaumberger, S., Nagl, V., Hessenberger, S. and Schatzmayr, G. (2014) Milk thistle extract and silymarin inhibit lipopolysaccharide induced lamellar separation of hoof explants in vitro. *Toxins* 6(10), 2962–2970.

Respondek, F., Goachet, A.G. and Julliand, V. (2008) Effects of dietary short-chain fructooligosaccharides on the intestinal microflora of horses subjected to a sudden change in diet. *Journal of Animal Science* 86(2), 316–323.

Reynolds, J.A., Potter, G.D., Greene, L.W., Wu, G., Carter, G.K. *et al.* (1998) Genetic-diet interactions in the hyperkalemic periodic paralysis syndrome in Quarter Horses fed varying amounts of potassium: III. The relationship between plasma potassium concentration and HYPP symptoms. *Journal of Equine Veterinary Science* 18(11), 731–735.

Roberts, J.L. and Murray, J.A. (2014) Equine nutrition in the United States: a review of perceptions and practices of horse owners and veterinarians. *Journal of Equine Veterinary Science* 34, 854–859.

Ross, D.J. and Roberts, J.L. (2018) Equine calming products: a short survey into their use, effect and knowledge using a small sample of horse owners in North of Scotland, UK. *Journal of Equine Veterinary Science* 68, 63–67.

Rucker, R.B. (2007) Allometric scaling, metabolic body size and interspecies comparison of basal nutritional requirements. *Journal of Animal Physiology and Animal Nutrition* 91(3–4), 148–156.

Saastamoinen, M.T. and Hellämäki, M. (2012) Forage analyses as a base of feeding of horses. In: Saastamoinen, M., Fradinho, M.J., Santos, A.S. and Miraglia, N. (eds) *Forages and Grazing in Horse Nutrition*, vol. 132. Wageningen Academic Publishers, Wageningen, The Netherlands.

Sanz, M.G., Viljoen, A., Saulez, M.N., Olorunju, S. and Andrews, F.M. (2014) Efficacy of a pectin-lecithin complex for treatment and prevention of gastric ulcers in horses. *Veterinary Record* 175(6), 147.

Schop, M., Jansman, A.J.M., de Vries, S. and Gerrits, W.J.J. (2020) Increased diet viscosity by oat β-glucans decreases the passage rate of liquids in the stomach and affects digesta physicochemical properties in growing pigs. *Animal* 14(2), 269–276.

Schoster, A., Weese, J.S. and Guardabassi, L. (2014) Probiotic use in horses – what is the evidence for their clinical efficacy? *Journal of Veterinary Internal Medicine* 28(6), 1640–1652. doi: 10.1111/jvim.12451

Schryver, H.F. (1990) Mineral and vitamin intoxication in horses. *Veterinary Clinics of North America: Equine Practice* 6(2), 295–318.

Smarsh, D.N. and Williams, C.A. (2017) Oxidative stress and antioxidant status in standardbreds: effect of age and training in resting plasma and muscle. *Journal of Equine Veterinary Science* 48, 93–102.

Smarsh, D.N., Liburt, N., Streltsova, J., McKeever, K. and Williams, C.A. (2010) Oxidative stress and antioxidant status in intensely exercising horses administered nutraceutical extracts. *Equine Veterinary Journal Supplement* 38, 317–322.

Snow, D.H., Gash, S.P. and Cornelius, J. (1987) Oral administration of ascorbic acid to horses. *Equine Veterinary Journal* 19, 520–523. doi: 10.1111/j.2042-3306.1987.tb02664.x.

Stucchi, L., Zucca, E., Serra, A., Stancari, G., Ceriotti, S. *et al*. (2017) Efficacy of the administration of a natural feed supplement in the management of equine gastric ulcer syndrome in 7 sport horses: a field trial. *American Journal of Animal and Veterinary Sciences* 12(3), 104–110

Swartzman, J.A., Hintz, H.F. and Schryver, H.F. (1978) Inhibition of calcium absorption in ponies fed diets containing oxalic acid. *American Journal of Veterinary Research* 39, 1621–1623.

Swirsley, N., Spooner, H.S. and Hoffman, R.M. (2017) Supplement use and perceptions: a study of US horse owners. *Journal of Equine Veterinary Science* 59, 34–39.

Sykes, B. and Jokisalo, J.M. (2015). Rethinking equine gastric ulcer syndrome: Part 3–Equine glandular gastric ulcer syndrome (EGGUS). *Equine Veterinary Education* 27(7), 372–375.

Talbot, W.A., Pinchbeck, G.L., Knottenbelt, D.C., Graham, H. and Mckane, S.A. (2013) A randomised, blinded, crossover study to assess the efficacy of a feed supplement in alleviating the clinical signs of headshaking in 32 horses. *Equine Veterinary Journal* 45, 293–297.

Tan, C.S.S. and Lee, S.W.H. (2021) Warfarin and food, herbal or dietary supplement interactions: a systematic review. *British Journal of Clinical Pharmacology* 87, 352–374. doi: 10.1111/bcp.14404

Thorne Research (2001) Curcuma longa (tumeric). *Alternative Medicine Review* 6, 62–66.

Tinworth, K.D., Harris, P.A., Sillence, M.N. and Noble, G.K. (2010) Potential treatments for insulin resistance in the horse: a comparative multi-species review. *Veterinary Journal (London, England: 1997)* 186(3), 282–291. doi: 10..1016/j.tvjl.2009.08.032.

Toribio, R. (2011) Disorders of calcium and phosphate metabolism in horses. *The Veterinary Clinics of North America. Equine Practice* 27, 129–147. doi: 10.1016/j.cveq.2010.12.010.

Vandeweerd, J.M., Coisnon, C., Clegg, P., Cambier, C., Pierson, A. *et al*. (2012) Systematic review of efficacy of nutraceuticals to alleviate clinical signs of osteoarthritis. *Journal of Veterinary Internal Medicine* 26(3), 448–456.

Velazquez-Canton, E., de la Cruz-Rodriguez, N., Zarco, L., Rodriguez, A., Angeles-Hernandez, J.C. *et al*. (2018) Effect of selenium and vitamin E supplementation on lactate, cortisol, and malondialdehyde in horses undergoing moderate exercise in a polluted environment. *Journal of Equine Veterinary Science* 69, 136–144.

Venner, M., Lauffs, S. and Deegen, E. (1999) Treatment of gastric lesions in horses with pectin-lecithin complex. *Equine Veterinary Journal* 31(S29), 91–96.

White-Springer, S.H., Vineyard, K.R., Kivipelto, J. and Warren, L.K. (2021) Dietary omega-3 fatty acid supplementation does not impair vitamin E status or promote lipid peroxidation in growing horses. *Journal of Animal Science* 99(7), skab177. doi: 10.1093/jas/skab177.

Wichert, B., Frank, T. and Kienzle, E. (2002) Zinc, copper and selenium intake and status of horses in *Bavaria The Journal of Nutrition* 132(6), 1776S–1777S. https://doi.org/10.1093/jn/132.6.1776S

Williams, C.A. and Carlucci, S.A. (2006) Oral vitamin E supplementation on oxidative stress, vitamin and antioxidant status in intensely exercised horses. *Equine Veterinary Journal* 38, 617–621. doi: 10.1111/j.2042-3306.2006.tb05614.x

Williams, C.A. and Lamprecht, E.D. (2008) Some commonly fed herbs and other functional foods in equine nutrition: a review. *The Veterinary Journal* 178, 21–31. doi: 10.1016/j.tvjl.2007.06.004

Williams, C.A., Kronfeld, D.S., Hess, T.M., Saker, K.E., Waldron, J.E. *et al*. (2005) Vitamin E intake and systemic antioxidant status in competitive endurance horses. *Equine and Comparative Exercise Physiology* 2(3), 149–152.

Williams, C.A., Parise, B.A. and Burk, A.O. (2009) Elite three day event horses are over-supplemented during competition. *Journal of Animal Physiology and Animal Nutrition* 93(2), 146.

Winther, K., Kharazmi, A., Hansen, A.S.V. and Falk-Rønne, J. (2010) A randomised placebo controlled double-blind study on the effect of subspecies of rose-hip (*Rosa canina*) on the immune system, working capacity and behaviour of horses. In: Ellis, A.D., Longland, A.C., Coenen, M. and Miraglia, N. (eds) *The Impact of Nutrition on the Health and Welfare of Horses. EAAP* Vol. 128. Wageningen Academic Publishers, Wageningen, The Netherlands, pp. 283–287.

Winther, K., Kharazmi, A., Hansen, A.S.V. and Falk-Rønne, J. (2012) The absorption of natural vitamin C in horses and anti-oxidative capacity: a randomised, controlled study on trotters during a three-month intervention period. *Comparative Exercise Physiology* 8(3-4), 195–201.

Wintzer, H.J. (1986) The effect of vitamin H substitution on the growth and condition of hooves. *Tierarztliche Praxis* 14(4), 495–500.

Woodward, M.C., Huff, N.K., Garza, F., Keowen, M.L., Kearney, M.T. *et al*. (2014) Effect of pectin, lecithin, and antacid feed supplements (Egusin) on gastric ulcer scores, gastric fluid pH and blood gas values in horses. *BMC Veterinary Research* 10(Suppl. 1), S4.

Zavoshti, F.R. and Andrews, F.M. (2017) Therapeutics for equine gastric ulcer syndrome. *Veterinary Clinics of North America: Equine Practice* 33(1), 141–162.

Zenker, W., Josseck, H. and Geyer, H. (1995) Histological and physical assessment of poor hoof horn quality in Lipizzaner horses and a therapeutic trial with biotin and a placebo. *Equine Veterinary Journal* 27(3), 183–191.

Zeyner, A. and Harris, P. (2013) Vitamins. In: Geor, R.J., Harris, P.A. and Coenen, M. (eds) *Equine Applied and Clinical Nutrition*. Elsevier, London, pp. 168–189.

Zhao, X. and Müller, C.E. (2015) Macro- and micromineral content of wrapped forages for horses. *Grass and Forage Science* 71, 195–207.

7 Advising a Feed: How to Read a Label

Lizzie Drury and Teresa Hollands

Saracen Horse Feeds, Aylesford; School of Veterinary Medicine, University of Surrey

Learning Objectives

LO1 Explain the legal information that is contained within a statutory statement on a feed label.
LO2 Distinguish between a claim and nutritional information.
LO3 Interpret information provided outside the statutory statement, including symbols and logos.
LO4 Relate nutrient declarations to nutritional requirements.
LO5 Describe how to take a feed sample for analysis and comparison against what is declared on a label.
LO6 Evaluate and recommend a suitable feed based on a feed analysis and label information.

At the end of this chapter, you will be able to use the information on the back of the bag or label to evaluate the suitability of a feed whilst at the same time appreciating the limitation of the information.

Feed Labelling Demystified

The horse owner or manager has access to a multitude of sources of equine nutrition information.

Helping your clients navigate the wide variety of products in the feed and supplement market can be challenging. The interpretation of a feed label is a useful skill to have; knowing where to look and what the information means on a feed bag will enable you to advise your clients appropriately. Appropriate feed choices will reduce some of the main feed and management issues faced by today's veterinary surgeons and clients.

The front of a bag is usually eye catching and will show the product name. Whilst companies are not allowed to mislead, the information here is of limited use from a nutritional perspective.

The important information on the bag is constrained legally within the statutory statement: The Feed Regulations[i] govern the statutory statement and the description of the food. Claims and marketing information are constrained by Industry Codes of Practice[ii], The Feed Regulations[iii] and The Veterinary Medicines Directive[iv]. For horses the legal requirements currently are the same as for food-producing animals, differing slightly from that of petfood.

Additional legislation controls the labelling for feeds that have been formulated for specific nutritional purposes. The use of this category is more common in pets, simply due to the better evidence base, but there are some products for horses. Importantly there is useful information provided outside of the statutory statement; this too is legally constrained, meaning that the packaging information has limitations.

Statutory Statement

The main aim of the statutory statement for the product is to ensure food safety, suitability and traceability.

 Evidence-based Equine Nutrition: A Practical Approach for Professionals (T. Hollands and L. Drury)
DOI: 10.1079/9781789245134.0007

The manufacturer must not mislead the client in terms of 'intended use or characteristics of the feed, the nature, method of manufacture or production, properties, composition, quantity, durability, species or categories of animals for which it is intended nor by attributing to the feed effects or characteristics that it does not possess or by suggesting that it possesses special characteristics when in fact all similar feeds possess such characteristics'.[v]

Local authorities are responsible for the enforcement of the Feed Regulations 2015; in practice the work tends to be done by Trading Standards Departments at county level. Clearly as a professional you will only want to advise feeds that meet the legal requirements as well as checking their suitability. The information you need is commonly found printed on a bag or a sewn in label (Fig. 7.1).

From your perspective the statutory information can be grouped according to the following:

- Safety and traceability
  - Batch number
  - Establishment number
  - Manufacturer's name and address
  - Product code
- Nutritional appropriateness
  - Type of animal for which it is intended; guidelines as to whether it is complementary or complete (see Chapter 5: 'What is a compound feed?')
  - Composition
  - Analytical constituents
- Quality control
  - Best-before date
  - UFAS registration number
  - Net weight.

Safety and Traceability

Product name, individual bag number and batch number

Good manufacturing practice dictates that in the event of a query the product and its ingredients are traceable. This means that if a complaint is ever made against a product, the company will use this information to investigate how and if the issues arose within the manufacturing process. The information is sufficiently detailed that it is possible to trace the ingredients within the feed to the farmer's field, and is usually found in the bag gusset (Fig. 7.2).

Manufacturer's name and address

It is essential that you or the client can contact the establishment that is responsible for placing the feed on the market; the companies can be found by googling. If you have a query, their feed helplines are the best place to start.

Establishment number

The establishment number is a demonstration that the manufacturer is an authorised establishment and is committed to traceability, feed safety and quality control standards (see Chapter 8, Fig. 8. 1: 'Clarifying quality').

It is not unusual for the feed business which formulates and markets the feed to use a contract manufacturer to make their feed. The establishment number allows you to check who manufactures the feed.

It is enlightening that many brands are owned by and made by the same umbrella company; your clients will be totally unaware of this.

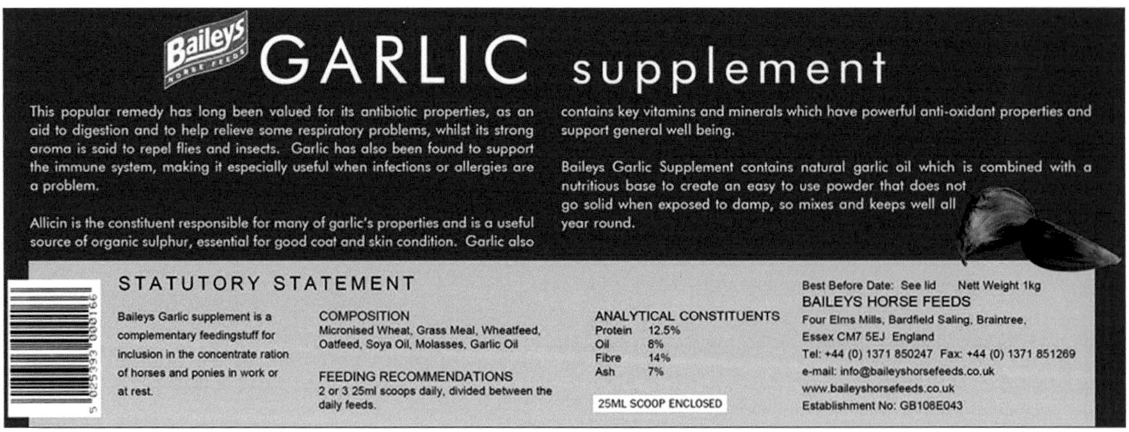

Fig. 7.1 A typical common statutory statement for an equine complementary feed.

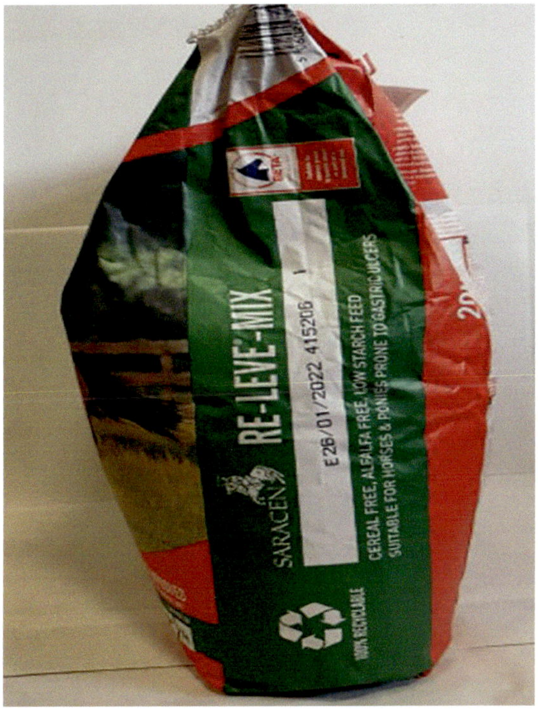

Fig. 7.2 Typical position of the batch number.

Nutritional Appropriateness

The packaging needs to identify if it is a complementary or complete feed, and the species of animal for which the feed is intended, and provide a brief description of how to feed. Animal feed of any kind should only be fed to the species for which it is intended.

Product name

The name that is given to the product identifies the intended use for that product and the suitability. However, do not be too quick to dismiss a product based on the name alone, especially if you are looking after clients with large numbers of horses on the same yard.

The key to successful feeding and optimum feed management is to avoid a large variety of different feeds in one feed room. Some feeds (e.g Veteran Mix) might be equally suitable for a younger horse that requires extra protein but lower calorie intake.

Description

The description or 'strap line' might be found on the front of a bag underneath the product name, providing a more detailed summary about product suitability. If it is on the front of the bag, it is not part of the statutory statement. Further detail may be provided on the back of the bag (Fig. 7.3), e.g. that it is suitable for weight gain, and giving clear guidance on suitable storage.

Composition (ingredients)

The ingredients list details the feed materials/ingredients used to make up the feed listed in descending order of inclusion (weight). The ingredients will be printed either on the label that is attached to the bag or directly on the packaging, meaning you can straight away identify if the feed is cereal- (see Chapter 5: 'Cereals') or fibre-based (see Chapter 4: 'What is forage?') (Fig. 7.4). The type of ingredient together with the feeding guide will provide an indication of whether the feed is high or low in energy/calories. Wheat feed and oat feed are by-products from the milling industry (the fibre coat of the cereal); if they are first on the list, it indicates that the feed is high in fibre.

If an ingredient has been described as part of the marketing information, then the % inclusion must be declared within the listing.

A full list of ingredients (some companies use categories) is helpful for clients with horses that have ingredient hypersensitivities or who need to manage or exaggerate individual temperaments or performance. Remember, good nutrition is more than one ingredient; you need to calculate the nutritional provision per kilogram of the diet, including forage type, and grazing time.

While the composition will tell you what is in that bag of feed, it does not tell you the analytical composition, i.e. the nutritional value. If your client has a horse that requires a low-sugar diet, do not instantly dismiss a bag of feed that contains molasses; the contribution of molasses to the water-soluble carbohydrate is low. The only way you can check the sugar intake is to read the analytical composition and the feeding guide.

Analytical composition

This is where you can find the nutritional value of 1 kg of feed. The analytical values of oil, crude protein, crude fibre, ash and sodium will be listed.

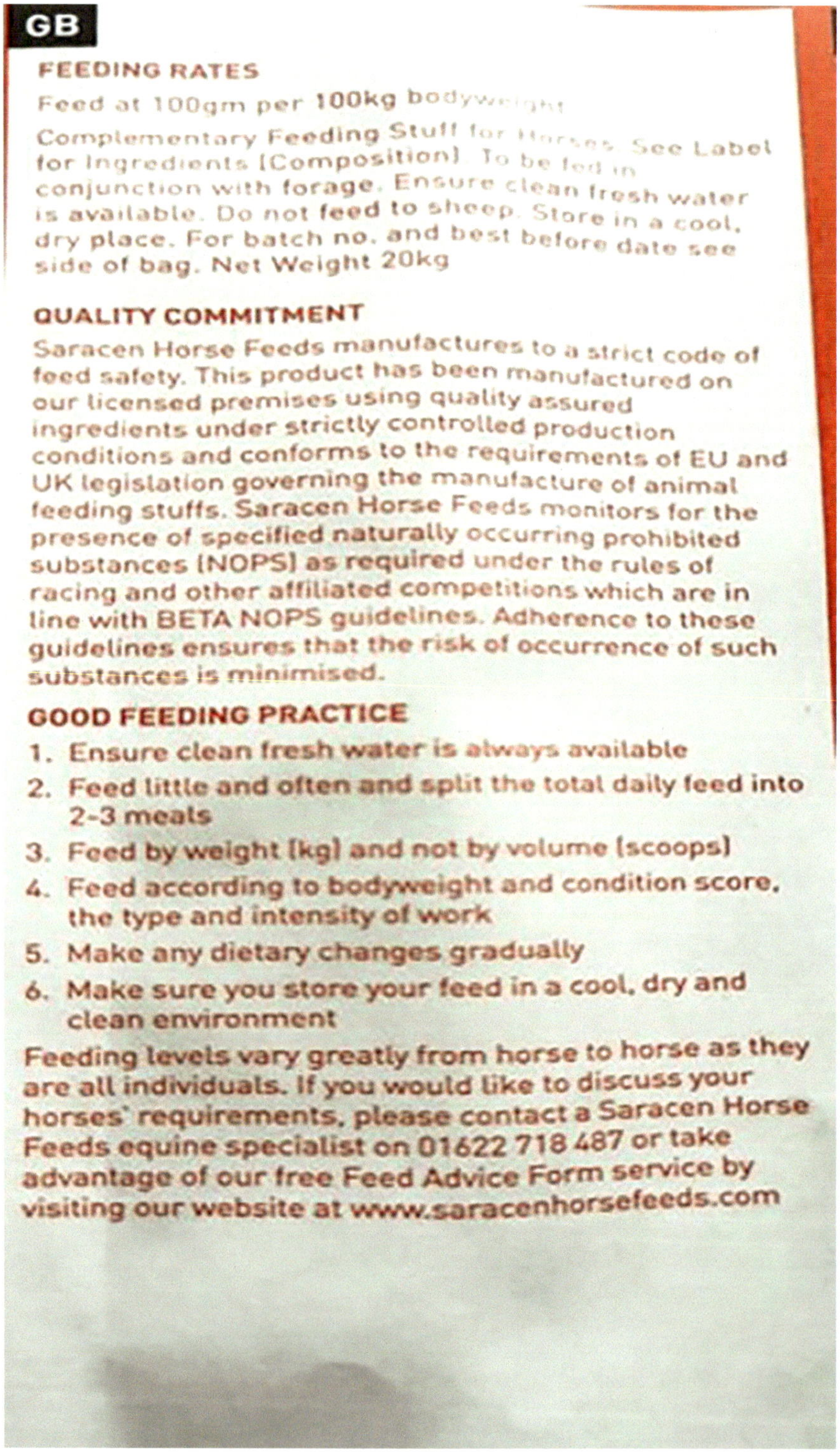

Fig. 7.3 Typical wording and position of the descriptive part of the statutory statement on a bag.

Protein

Declared as % crude protein, this is not an indication of protein quality. Manufacturers may add lysine to improve protein quality or simply declare the % as an indication of the quality. High-quality protein sources include soya, legumes, rapeseed or alfalfa, which contain good levels of essential amino acids.

Fibre

Fibre is declared as crude fibre, which provides no indication of digestibility. Examples of fibre are soya hulls, sugar beet pulp, alfalfa, the inclusion of short chopped forages and the seed coats of cereals such as oat feed and wheat feed. If the fibre ingredients are high on the composition label, then these feeds will be low in calories and the fibre declaration high (Table 7.1).

Ash

This refers to the inorganic material (anything that is not water, protein, oil, or carbohydrate) and is an indication of the total mineral content of the feed but is neither specific nor quantitative. This term is confusing for clients and ironically, contrary to common misapprehension, it is a sign of quality, not sweepings from the floor.

111555 – COMPETITION-FIT MIX

Complementary Feeding Stuff for Horses

ANALYTICAL CONSTITUENTS Crude Protein 13.5%, Crude Fibre 10.0%, Crude Fat 6.5%, Crude Ash 7.5%, Sodium 0.34%, Energy 13.0MJ/KG **C**

COMPOSITION Crushed Oats, Lucerne Pellets, Barley Flakes, Maize Flakes, Molasses, Soya Bean Meal*, Soya Flakes*, Vitamins & Minerals, Wheatfeed, Soya Oil*, Pea Flakes, Dried Sugar Beet Pulp, Calcium Carbonate, Sodium Chloride, Monocalcium Phosphate, Soya Hulls*, Sunflower seed meal, Sodium Chloride, Mixture of flavouring compounds **Genetically modified material*

ADDITIVES Vitamins Vitamin A (3a672) Retinyl acetate 15,000iu/kg, Vitamin D3 (3a671) Cholecalciferol 2,300iu/kg, Vitamin E (3a700) ALL-rac-alpha-tocopheryl-acetate 540iu/kg

Trace Elements 0.5mg of iodine from Calcium iodate anhydrous (3b202), 34.5mg of copper from Copper (II) sulphate pentahydrate (3b405), 3mg of copper from Copper (II) chelate of glycine hydrate (3b413), 52.4mg of manganese from Manganous sulphate monohydrate (3b503), 9.6mg of manganese from Manganese chelate of glycine hydrate (3b506), 100mg of zinc from Zinc sulphate monohydrate (3b605), 9.6mg of zinc from Zinc chelate of glycine hydrate (3b607), 0.33mg of selenium from coated granulated sodium selenite (3b802), 0.17mg of selenium from Selenised yeast, inactivated (3b810)

Zootechnical Additives 4b1710 *Saccharomyces cerevisiae* MUCL 39885 (Vistacell). Number of Colony Forming Units (CFU): Minimum 2.5 x 10^10 CFU/KG

Fig. 7.4 Typical composition declaration of a UK horse feed.

Table 7.1 Examples of feed types and typical percentage of crude fibre

	Low fibre	Medium fibre	High fibre
Percentage of fibre (as fed)	5–10%	11–15%	16–20%
Suitability	Competition and racing feeds formulated to support power and speed-based exercise	Feeds for veteran and breeding horses and some performance feeds formulated for stamina (see Chapter 12)	Feeds suitable for horses prone to EGUS or muscle myopathies (see Chapter 12) Low-energy leisure feeds (see Chapter 11)
Typical feeds	Competition Fit Mix Polo Cubes	Veteran Mix Enduro Performance 16 +	Re-Leve Ease and Excel Cubes Super Fibre Cubes

Oil

Veteran, conditioning and performance feeds will typically have higher oil levels compared with feeds that are formulated for resting or horses that are in light work.

Nutritional additives

Sensory additives, herbs and spices

These are usually added to help maintain optimum palatability, especially in horses that are fussy feeders. Herbal mixtures, such as garlic, mint, aniseed and fenugreek, and more innovative flavours, such as blackcurrant and cinnamon, are used. Clients will often associate a nutritional benefit to these herbs but the inclusion is rarely high enough to confer that benefit (see Chapter 6: 'Herbs and other functional ingredients').

Vitamins and minerals

These are declared as per kilogram and labelled only if there is a maximum tolerable level, to ensure that they are within acceptable minimum or maximum declarable levels (in any species, not just the horse). For example, the upper safe limit for vitamin E intake is 1000 mg/kg DM (NRC, 1987); for vitamin D, 44 iu/kg BW/day (NRC, 1987); and for vitamin A, 360 iu/kg BW/day (NRC, 2007). Many clients assume that these are the only micronutrients provided in the feed, but that is most definitely not the case.

> **Top tip**
>
> Feeding instructions provided on the bag indicate the minimum feeding levels that are required to ensure that the horse receives optimum levels of all the vitamins and minerals (and protein) to balance a typical intake of forage.

Quality Control

Weight

The product must state the weight of the goods. If this is not printed elsewhere on the tub or the bag, it must be stated within the statutory statement. Supplements generally have the information printed on the packaging.

UFAS registration

This identifies that the manufacturer is accredited under the Universal Feed Assurance Scheme, (UFAS). In the UK and Ireland, 95% of the commercially produced compound feeds are accredited. The scheme is audited and certified by an independent certification body, in accordance with the internationally recognised standard ISO 17065 (formerly Guide 65). ISO 17065 provides rules for organisations that certify products. The standards ensure that the resulting product certifications are impartial, consistent with international standards, and based on objective testing.

UFAS is based on Hazard Analysis and Critical Control Point (HACCP) principles (originally pioneered by the space agency NASA) forming the bedrock of EU Food and Feed legislation. The certification body is independently assessed every year to ensure that the standard is implemented and administered consistently and fairly. Consequently, local authorities now include participation in UFAS in their risk assessments of feed businesses.

'Best before' date

This confirms that if the feed is eaten by the stated date, it will provide the recommended intake of vitamins. Often the shelf life of the product exceeds this date, but there is no guarantee that the vitamins will still be adequate. Most horse feeds carry a shelf life of between 3 and 6 months and supplements 6 months to 1 year.

How Does the Labelling for Feeds with a Particular Nutritional Purpose Differ?

Some feeds are formulated to meet the specific nutritional needs of a horse whose process of assimilation, absorption or metabolism is, or could be, temporarily or irreversibly impaired and which can benefit from ingestion of the feed appropriate to their condition. These are categorised as 'Feedingstuffs for particular nutritional purpose', 'PARticular NUTritional purpose' (PARNUTs).

A feed manufacturer can only produce a PARNUT if the feed is for a defined purpose in terms of having a specific composition or method of production that can be distinguishable from ordinary feed or medicated feed. There are only limited PARNUTs approved for horses (Table 7.2).

Table 7.2 Descriptors for feed approved for particular nutritional purposes for horses (Commission Regulation (EU) 2020/354 of 4th March list of intended uses of feed intended for particular nutritional purposes)

Nutritional purpose	Essential nutritional characteristics	Labelling declarations	Recommended length of time	Other provisions
1. Support of renal function in case of chronic renal insufficiency	High density of energy with more than 8.8 MJ/kg feed with a moisture content of 12%. Highly digestible and highly palatable sources of starch. Restricted protein level: ≤ 106 g crude protein/kg feed with a moisture content of 12%. Level of sodium: 2 g/100 kg BW per day. High level of eicosapentaenoic acid and docosahexaenoic sum ≥ 0.2 g/kg $BW^{0.75}$ per day	• Protein and energy source(s) • Calcium • Phosphorus • Potassium • Magnesium • Sodium • Sum of eicosapentaenoic acid and docosahexaenoic acid	Initially up to 6 months Long term or until resolution of the issue	The feed shall be placed on the market as complementary feed Indicate on the labelling: • 'It is recommended that a veterinarian's opinion be sought before use or before extending the period of use.' • The complementary feed should not be used in case of hypernatraemia and hyperchloraemia. • The complementary feed should contribute to at least 10–20% of the daily energy supply (approximately 0.05 to 0.1 MJ/kg $BW^{0.75}$ per day). The ration should ensure an energy supply of > 0.62 MJ/kg $BW^{0.75}$ per day. The ration should not exceed 50 mg calcium/kg dry matter/day. Indicate in the instructions for proper use: 'Water should be available at all times.'
2. Support of liver function in the case of chronic liver insufficiency	Low level of protein but of high quality and highly digestible carbohydrates	• Protein and fibre sources • Highly digestible carbohydrates including their treatment, if appropriate • Methionine • Choline • Content of n-3 fatty acids (if added)	Initially up to 6 months	Indicate on the labelling: • 'It is recommended that a veterinarian's opinion be sought before use or before extending the period of use.' Guidance should be provided on the way the feed should be fed, including many small meals per day.
3. Support the regeneration of hooves, and skin	High level of zinc. The complementary feed may contain zinc in a concentration higher than 100 times the relevant fixed maximum content in complete feed.	• Zinc (total) • Methionine (total) • Biotin (if added)	Up to 8 weeks	The instructions for proper use for the feed shall ensure that the legal maximum contents of zinc for complete feed are respected.

Continued

Table 7.2 Continued.

Nutritional purpose	Essential nutritional characteristics	Labelling declarations	Recommended length of time	Other provisions
4. Support the preparation for and recovery from sport effort	High level of selenium and a minimum content of 50 mg vitamin E per kg complete feed with moisture content of 12%. The complementary feed may contain compounds of selenium in a concentration higher than 100 times the relevant fixed maximum content in complete feed.	• Vitamin E (total) • Selenium (total)	Up to 8 weeks before sport effort Up to 4 weeks after sport effort	The instructions for proper use for the feed shall ensure that the legal maximum contents of selenium for complete feed are respected.
5. Compensation of electrolyte loss in the cases of heavy sweating	Must contain sodium chloride and should contain potassium chloride. Low levels of magnesium, calcium and phosphorus The inclusion of other electrolyte salts is optional.	• Sodium • Chlorides • Potassium • Calcium • Magnesium • Phosphorus	One to three days after heavy sweating.	Guidance shall be provided on the situations in which the use of the feed is appropriate. The instructions for proper use must give administration guidelines based on the duration and intensity of exercise performed relevant to the formulation and presentation of the feed. Indicate on the labelling: • 'Water should be available at all times.' • In the case of the administration of electrolytes not mixed with water (e.g. in feed or in syringe format): 'Water must be available for at least 20 minutes or preferably for 1 hour post administration.' Furthermore, guidance must be given to monitor subsequent drinking, if insufficient water intake is observed veterinary advice should be sought. Guidance may optionally be given regarding the quantity of water (in litres) to be provided alongside in feed or syringed electrolytes.
6. Support of energy metabolism and of the muscle function in the case of rhabdomyolosis	Starch and sugar not more than 20 % of available energy. Crude fat more than 20 % of available energy Minimum of 350 IU Vitamin E/kg complete feed with a moisture content of 12 %	• Starch • Sugar • Crude fat • Vitamin E (total)	Initially for a minimum of 3 months	Guidance shall be provided on the situations in which the use of this feed is appropriate. The instructions for proper use shall contain guidance on the balance of the daily ration and the appropriate daily intake. Indicate on the labelling: 'It is recommended that a veterinarian's opinion be sought before use.'

7. Compensation for chronic digestive disorders of large intestine	• Starch content to provide < 1 g/kg BW/meal (< 0.5 g/kg BW/meal, if diarrhoea present) • Cereal grains processed via a hydrothermal treatment, such as extrusion, micronisation, expansion or flaking, to improve small intestinal starch digestion • Additional supply of water-soluble vitamins and adequate minerals/ electrolytes levels • Additional supply of oil if no diarrhoea	• Highly digestible feed materials including their processing, if appropriate. • Total sugar and starch • Protein sources	Long term or until resolution of the issue	Guidance shall be provided on • the precise situations in which the use of the feed is appropriate • meal size and forage intake. The instructions for proper use shall refer, depending on the oil content, to the potential gradual use and suggest a monitoring for diarrhoea.
8. Stabilisation of the physiological digestion	Feed additives of the functional group 'Gut flora stabiliser' as referred to in Annex I to Regulation (EC) No 1831/2003 or, pending the re-authorisation procedure as referred to in Article 10 of Regulation (EC) No 1831/2003, feed additives of the group 'micro-organisms'	• Name and added amount of the gut flora stabiliser or micro-organism	Up to 4 weeks	Indicate on the labelling: 'In case of risk of, during periods of, or recovery from digestive disturbance'. The instructions for proper use of the feed shall ensure that the legal maximum content of the gut flora stabiliser or micro-organism for complete feed is respected.

Information Provided Outside of the Statutory Statement

Some information is not legally required but the feed manufacturer may voluntarily list other nutrients to aid the use, understanding, marketing and sale of the product. This information can help you advise your clients to make the right choice for their individual horse.

Feeding guide

This explains how the product should be fed, including the recommended daily feeding, which is determined by bodyweight and workload to determine the amount of feed that is required to ensure an 'average' horse or pony receives a balanced diet. Some companies provide a range, some are more precise and provide intakes in terms of kg/100 kg BW, others do not include daily recommended feeding rates; you are advised to contact the company feed helpline for further advice.

Please remind clients that the feeding rate is just a guide, based on average forage analysis, intake and an average horse; you will need to adjust according to the horse in front of you, specifically taking into account the forage:concentrate ratio and the fat score of the horse, assuming they are on a suitable feed.

Digestible energy (DE)

Although this is not a legal requirement (there is limited research as to the DE of mixed ingredients for horses), estimated DE can be declared outside of the statutory statement. Estimated DE (MJ/kg) is calculated from ruminant metabolisable energy of the individual ingredients and an industry standard adjustment made. The DE will allow you to calculate the estimated calorie intake of the horse's daily ration of compound feed.

Clinically, body fat score/condition is the best indicator of whether any individual horse or pony is consuming the correct calories for their workload (Carter and Dugdale, 2013).

Starch

In response to the client's perceptions of the effects of sugar and starch and association with the risk of laminitis and equine metabolic syndrome (Geor and Harris, 2009), starch and sugar are often declared on the label or highlighted in the general information on the packaging.

Please take care in interpretation, because carbohydrates are simply a calorie source and will be very low in leisure feeds. Knowing the % (g/100 g feed) means you can calculate the intake to set the client's mind at rest.

If starch or any nutrient has been highlighted or brought to the attention of the 'user', the % has to be declared in the composition.

If the starch level is not declared you can look at the feed composition to categorise the approximate starch level; high-starch feeds will have the cereals listed as the first ingredients, low-starch feeds will have cereals that are further down the list or not listed at all (Fig. 7.5).

Processing

Chelated minerals

Many feed companies will list the minerals as 'chelated' or 'Bioplex' minerals, which are minerals that have been attached to other molecules to improve their bioavailability (Pagan *et al.*, 1999; Baker *et al.*, 2003); other forms of minerals include 'oxide' or 'sulphate' ('sulfate').

Micronising or cooking of cereals

The cooking of cereals is often highlighted because it increases small-intestine digestibility of starch by gelatinising the starch (Vervuert *et al.*, 2008). This improves glycogen replacement and minimises the risk of undigested starch reaching the hind gut (Vervuert *et al.*, 2009). Clearly you would expect micronised cereals to be low on the list for leisure feeds compared with performance feeds (Gater and Counsell, 2006).

Symbols and logos

Several logos or symbols provide useful information (Fig. 7.6) when advising an appropriate feed.

Marketing information and general descriptions

This might highlight the presence or the absence of an ingredient in the feed, or refer to a specific nutritional characteristic or a specific function. There are strict rules[vi], including the following.

HIGH STARCH

Complementary Feeding Stuff for Horses. ANALYTICAL CONSTITUENTS Crude Protein 13.5%, Crude Fibre 10.0%, Crude Fat 6.5%, Crude Ash 7.5%, Calcium 1.06%, Phosphorus 0.54%, Sodium 0.36%, Energy 13.0MJ/KG

COMPOSITION Oats, Lucerne Pellets, Maize Flakes, Barley Flakes, Molasses, Soya Flakes*, Soya Bean Meal*, Dried (Sugar) Beet Pulp, Wheatfeed, Pea Flakes, Vitamins, Soya Oil*, Soya Hulls*, Sunflower Extract, Minerals, Sodium Chloride, Calcium Carbonate, Yeast, Mixture of Flavouring Compounds **Genetically modified material*

ADDITIVES Vitamins Vitamin A (3a672a) Retinyl acetate 21,000iu/kg; Vitamin D3 (3a671) Cholecalciferol 3,450iu/kg; Vitamin E (3a700) All-rac-alpha-tocopheryl-acetate 285iu/kg Trace Elements Iron (3b103) 40mg/kg; Iodine (3b201) 0.50mg/kg; Copper (3b405) 35mg/kg, (3b406) 3mg/kg; Manganese (3b503) 52mg/kg, (3b504) 10mg/kg; Zinc (3b605) 100mg/kg, (3b612) 10mg/kg; Selenium (3b801) 0.33mg/kg, (3b8.10) 0.17mg/kg Zootechnical Additives 4b1710 Saccharomyces cerevisiae MUCL 39885 (Vistacell).

LOW STARCH

Complementary Feeding Stuff for Horses. ANALYTICAL CONSTITUENTS Crude Protein 13.0%, Crude Fibre 19.5%, Crude Fat 9.0%, Crude Ash 9.0%, Calcium 1.17%, Phosphorus 0.36%, Sodium 0.25%, Energy 12.9MJ/KG

COMPOSITION Lucerne Pellets, Dried Sugar Beet Pulp, Soya Hulls*, Pea Flakes, Soya Oil*, Molasses, Soya Flakes*, Vitamins, Soya Bean Meal*, Minerals, Mixture of Flavouring Compounds, Yeast **Genetically modified material*

ADDITIVES Vitamins Vitamin A (3a672) Retinyl acetate 11,000iu/kg; Vitamin D3 (3a671) Cholecalciferol 1,100iu/kg; Vitamin E (3a700) RRR-alpha-tocopheryl-acetate 35iu/kg; Vitamin E (3a700) ALL-rac-alpha-tocopheryl-acetate 325iu/kg Trace Elements Iron (3b103) 40mg/kg; Iodine (3b201) 0.5mg/kg; Copper (3b405) 30mg/kg, (3b406) 7.5mg/kg; Manganese (3b503) 50mg/kg, (3b504) 13mg/kg; Zinc (3b605) 88mg/kg, (3b606) 22mg/kg; Selenium (3b801) 0.34mg/kg, (3b8.11) 0.16mg/kg Zootechnical Additives 4b1710 Saccharomyces cerevisiae MUCL 39885 (Vistacell). Number of Colony Forming Units (CFU): Minimum 2.5×10^{10} CFU/KG

Fig. 7.5 A comparison between a cereal-free, low-sugar, low-starch performance ration and a high-starch ration fed to horses (fibre and cereals highlighted).

- The claim must be objective, verifiable and understandable (Fig. 7.7).
- On request, the person labelling the feed has to provide you (or the client) with scientific evidence of their claim. This can be specific published work or extrapolation of the claim, from publicly available scientific evidence or through documented company research.
- The feed can describe optimisation of the nutrition and support or protection of the physiological conditions (EU) 205/3281.[vii]
- But they cannot write that it will prevent, treat or cure a disease (VMD, 2020).[viii]
- Nor that it has a particular nutritional purpose, unless that purpose is in the permitted list and the feed is labelled properly (EU)2020/354 annex/ part B).[ix]

Label Declarations and Their Relevance to Nutritional Requirements

The limitations of reading the label

The label analysis has several limitations; legally it is restricted to provide only details to ensure that the feed is safe. There is provision (as with human food) for some tolerance which is tightly controlled around the declaration because of the natural analytical variation of ingredients used in the formulation; manufacturers will be fined for exceeding tolerances.

Protein

Protein is often erroneously confused with energy. Protein is used for cell renewal, tissue and muscle

Organisation	Logo	What it means	Extra information
BETA NOPS LOGO		feed is suitable for horses competing under FEI or BHA rules (ch 8) A list of participating companies can be found on the BETA website.	https://www.beta-uk.org/pages/feed-safety/beta-nops-scheme
BETA EGUS APPROVAL LOGO		product is suitable to be fed to those horses and ponies that are prone to gastric ulcers. These feeds have met a set of criteria around the level of sugar and starch that they contribute per meal and per day. Any additional claims that are made are supported by scientific evidence. These feeds will have been independently verified to provide customer confidence	https://www.beta-uk.org/pages/feed-safety/beta-feed-approval-mark-for-products-suitable-for-horses-prone-to-equine-gastric-ulcer-syndrome
THE LAMINITIS TRUST APPROVAL MARK –		The laminitis trust is a charitable organisation that supports laminitis research; the feeds approvedare formulated to be suitable for laminitics. Other feeds are also suitable to be fed to horses and ponies at risk of laminitis may have a hoof logo or similar. If in any doubt speak to a nutritionist for more advice	
THE VEGETARIAN SOCIETY APPROVAL		All horse feeds are vegetarian! But the Vegetarian Society checks if vitamins are covered in a pork gelatine coating. and only endorses products that are completely free from these products	https://www.vegsoc.org/vegetarian-and-vegan-trademarks/
Universal Feed assurance Scheme		Audited regularly With any of these logos please check what research is being done; and note that a trademark does not automatically confirm a UFAS approval	Chapter 8

Fig. 7.6 Commonly used logos on UK horse feeds.

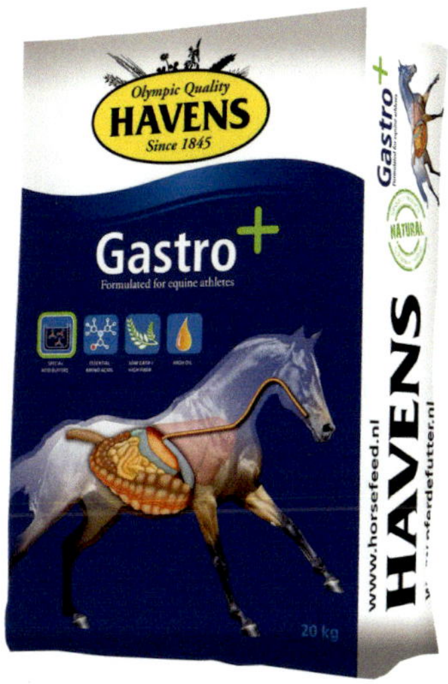

An example of a bag that does not mislead

Example of wording that is making medicinal claims	Wording that is on the edge of making medicinal claims	Legal wording
For horses and ponies that suffer from digestive problems or stomach ulcers	Supports normal stomach activity-contains special cocktail of x, y and z to neutralise acid and regenerate stomach lining	• For the maintenance of a healthy stomach environment. • Maintains normal stomach activity • Prone to gastric ulcers IF carries BETA certification

Example of misleading claim	Check ingredients	Why might be misleading
High content of alfalfa to promote chewing and saliva production	Must contain alfalfa chaff not just alfalfa pellets	Pellets are chewed around 800–1000 times/kg- chaffs are chewed around 5000–6000 times/kg. Horses swallow feed particles around 1.6mm-pelleted fibre is already ground

Fig. 7.7 A comparison of legal, medical and misleading terms on equine feed bags.

growth and repair, growth and development. Remind clients that protein is not the primary energy source for horses and it will not cause excitability (Williams *et al.*, 2001), laminitis (King and Mansmann, 2004) or muscular disorders (Harris and Rivero, 2017).

Because crude protein is declared, you can only guess the quality by referring to the composition list. The limiting amino acid for horse is lysine. The manufacturer will provide you with the lysine content of their feed if you ask. It is easy for clients to become focused on the % protein inclusion in a ration, when it is the intake of quality of the protein (and exercise) that is key for maintaining muscle and growth.

Fibre

Fibre is essential for maintaining digestive health and is a source of healthy, slow-release energy (see Chapters 4 and 9). There is no nutritional requirement for fibre, but forage should be advised at a minimum of 1.5% BW as dry matter for a performance horse to 2.5% for leisure horses.

Oil

Oil is added to feeds to help increase the energy density of the feed, reducing minimum feeding levels and reliance on cereals. Oil will also provide essential fatty acids for skin health and condition (see Chapter 5, Table 5.7: 'A comparison of dietary sources of omega-3 and 6 fatty acids'). Soya or rapeseed oil is commonly used; some feeds will contain high-fat supplements, e.g. pelleted rice bran. Feeds that are high in oil help to support stamina in horses that are doing endurance-based exercise and might be suitable for horses that suffer from muscle myopathies (see Chapter 12: 'Equine exertional rhabdomyolysis').

Ash

Feeds that are formulated to have a low daily intake, such as feed balancers, will be fortified with higher levels of the vitamin and mineral premix and therefore will have a higher ash level, e.g. Competition Fit Balancer (100 g/100 kg BW), ash 17.3%, versus All Round Competition Mix, 6.5%, which are fed at higher minimum feeding rates (200–1000 g/100 kg BW).

Nutritional additives

Only those additives that must be declared by law to ensure nutritional safety will be listed on the label or the bag.

Compound feeds and feed balancers all contain a 'full spectrum of vitamins and minerals' or will be 'fully fortified with vitamins and minerals', specific to that feed use. A stud and youngstock premix will be different to a premix that is formulated for a feed suitable for horses that are resting; do call the feed company for further information. Most companies work to the indicated minimum amounts needed to sustain normal health, production and performance of horses (NRC, 2007). Call the manufacture for a full specification of their minerals and vitamins or check for data sheets on their website (Fig. 7.8).

Checking the Nutrient Content of Feeds

For more accurate nutrient concentrations, detailed analysis should be obtained from the manufacturer

Ultimate Balancer is a complementary feedingstuff specifically for horses and ponies

Product Profile

Profile	
Protein	25%
Lysine	17g/kg
Methionine	4.5g/kg
Oil	5.75%
Fibre	5.5%
Ash	13.5%
Starch	10%
Sugar	6.5%
Est. DE	11.4MJ/kg

Vitamins	
Vitamin A	75,800iu/kg
Vitamin D	10,000iu/kg
Vitamin E	1,800mg/kg
Vitamin C	440mg/kg
B1	120mg/kg
B2	120mg/kg
B6	120mg/kg
B12	0.5mg/kg
Biotin	30mg/kg
Nicotinic Acid	150mg/kg
Folic Acid	100mg/kg

Macro Minerals	
Calcium	2.6%
Phosphorus	1%
Magnesium	0.4%
Sodium	0.4%
Chloride	0.8%
Potassium	1.4%

Micro Minerals	
Cobalt	4.5mg/kg
Copper	260mg/kg
Zinc	660mg/kg
Manganese	550mg/kg
Iron	330mg/kg
Iodine	5mg/kg
Selenium	3.2mg/kg

Statutory Information

Additives: Nutritional	
Vitamin A/3a672a	75,800iu/kg
Vitamin D/3a671	10,000iu/kg
Vitamin E/3a700	1,800mg/kg
Iron (Iron (II) Sulphate Monohydrate/3b103)	202mg/kg
Iodine (Calcium iodate, anhydrous/3b202)	5mg/kg
Cobalt (Coated granulated cobalt (II) carbonate/3b304)	5mg/kg
Copper (Copper (II) sulphate pentahydrate/3b405)	202mg/kg
Copper (Copper (II) chelate of glycine hydrate/3b413)	50mg/kg
Manganese (manganese (II) oxide/3b502)	404mg/kg
Manganese (Manganese chelate of glycine hydrate/3b506)	101mg/kg
Zinc (Zinc Oxide/3b603)	485mg/kg
Zinc (Zinc chelate of glycine hydrate/3b607)	121mg/kg
Selenium (Sodium selenite/3b801)	2mg/kg
Selenium (Selenised yeast, inactivated/3b810)	1mg/kg
L-lysine-monohydrochloride (3c322)	4.6g/kg
Additives: Antioxidants	
Vitamin C/3a300	440mg/kg
Mixed Tocopherols/1b306(i)	770mg/kg
Additives: Zootechnical	
Actisaf yeast (Saccharomyces cerevisiae NCYC Sc47/4b1702)	$2x10^{10}$ cfu/kg

Ultimate Balancer Composition

Wheatfeed; Soya (bean) meal, feed (GM Soya); Sunflower Seed Meal, Dehulled; Ricebran (Expeller); Vitamin Mineral Premix; Molasses; Fructo-oligosaccharides (1.6%); Dicalcium Phosphate; Rapeseed Oil; Calcium Carbonate; Sodium Chloride; MSM (0.8%); Lysine; Mixture of: Blackcurrant, Kale, Spinach, Beetroot, Rosemary, Rosehip, Pomegranate; Yeast; Vitamin Premix.

Feeding Rate

Feed 100g/100kg bodyweight per day in conjunction with free access to forage. Do not exceed 200g/100kg bodyweight per day in total. Divide into at least 2-3 meals per day.

Ensure a minimum intake of 2kg/100kg bodyweight of forage per day.

Fresh drinking water must be

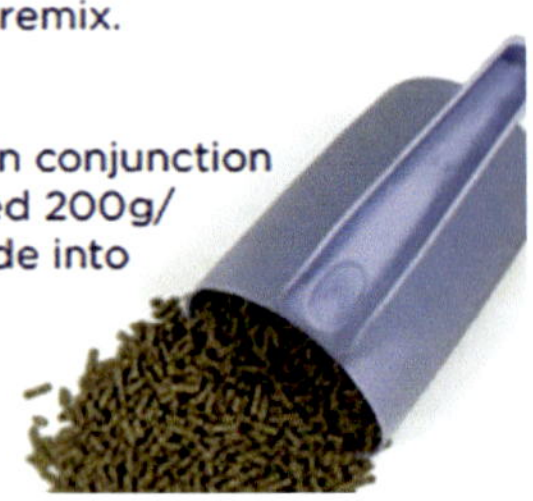

Fig. 7.8 An example of a full data sheet.

or a feed sample sent for analysis. Chemical analysis is only needed for a more in-depth ration evaluation to justify possible changes in performance or productivity levels or in cases of disease or illness.

Nutrient concentrations are determined by various wet chemistry/proximate analysis[x] or by near-infrared (NIR) reflectance analysis. When precise analysis is required for animals that are not performing as expected or for high performance rations, analysis should be undertaken as wet chemistry.

Wet chemistry

Proximate analysis provides a classification of water (moisture), ash, crude fat/oil (ether extract), crude protein and crude fibre. Nitrogen-free extract (NFE) is calculated by difference to provide an estimate of sugars and starches for legal declarations. Many companies use more nutritionally relevant analysis to provide a more precise classification of fibre, e.g. neutral detergent fibre (NDF) (see Chapters 4 and 9) and of water-soluble carbohydrates and starch (see Chapter 5).

NIR

NIR does not measure nutrients directly but provides calibrated measurements based on wet chemistry, providing an efficient and fast turnaround of results. Predicted values will be better than average tabular values but will only be as accurate as the calibrations with wet chemistry that have been used to train the machine.

NIR mineral results are routinely used by the feed industry for ration formulation.

Check that the lab is approved, that they participate in ring tests and update their calibrations regularly, which should be based on the typical feeds/forages from your country (feed values vary from country to country).

The chemical analysis of a feed is only as good as the sampling method used and if the feed sample is not representative then the analysis will have no value.

How to sample a feed

Repeatable and reproducible sampling is the crucial first step in the entire quality assurance programme. There is a standard protocol (ISO/TC 34/SC10) that states a 'minimum weight of 0.5 kg to get a homogeneous test sample (with minimum weight of 100 g) with the same constitution, with the same composition and without any contamination' (ISO 6498:1998)

Steps

1. Empty bag of feed into a clean feed bin (this is to ensure you are collecting a homogeneous sample and not just from the top of the bag).
- Alternatively, come prepared with a large polyethene sheet onto which you empty the bag.

2. Take random grab samples, wearing gloves to minimise risk of caffeine contamination etc., across the sample.
- Ideally you would sample around 2 kg, then subsample by quartering the sample, taking a sample from every other quarter (Fig. 7.9) and so on until you have enough feed to fill a large freezer bag (minimum 500 g, maximum 1 kg).

3. Label with batch number, name of product and establishment number and date, your name and contact details (Fig. 7.10).

4. Where possible, sample at the beginning of the week and send first class to minimise any deterioration.

It is important that you avoid the more common sampling errors (Table 7.3).

Feed companies follow strict sampling protocols as part of their QC process (EU, 2017/625/title11/ch IV; chapter 8).[xi]

Importance of feed evaluation

The equine industry is responding to environmental concerns and sustainability by investigating novel sources of safe, nutritious feed and feed ingredients to provide the products needed in the future. Providing horses with adequate, balanced diets, free of toxins and contaminants, optimises feed utilisation, which in turn decreases the level of excretion of feed nutrients, reducing environmental pollution.

Feed analysis confirms that the diet that the feed manufacturer produces, labels and markets meets its labelled declarations. Added benefits for the manufacturer include:

- generating reliable data on the chemical constituents;
- the most efficient use of raw materials in each diet; and

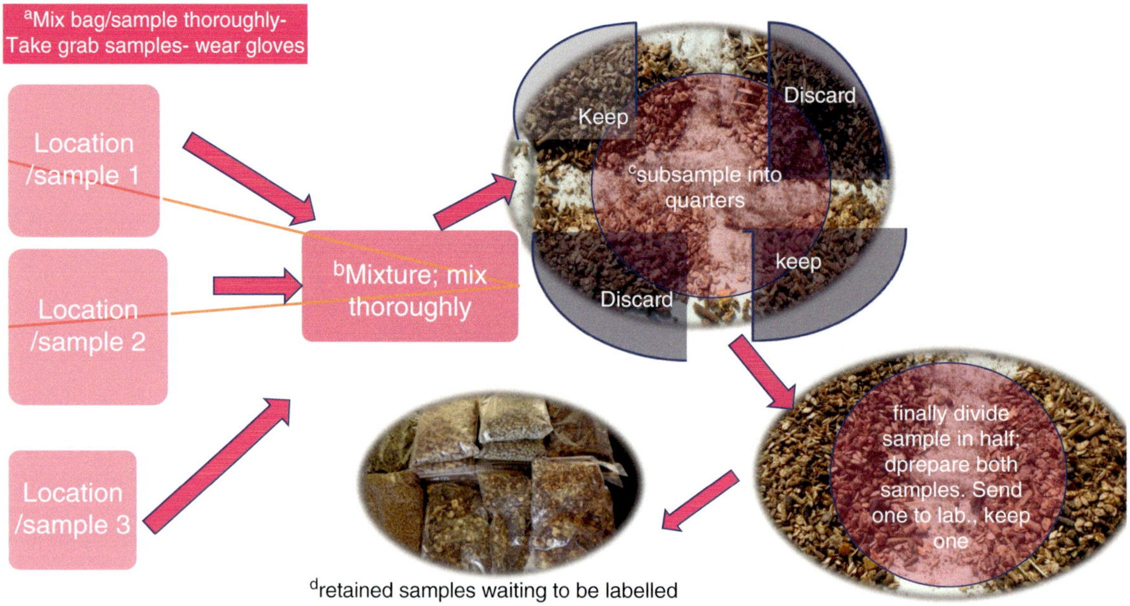

Fig. 7.9 How to subsample. **(a)** Carry a clean bucket or sheet for subsampling. **(b)** Combine samples from different locations to form a composite sample. **(c)** Divide original samples and keep or discard as shown. **(d)** Prepare 2 samples to retain and for laboratory analysis.

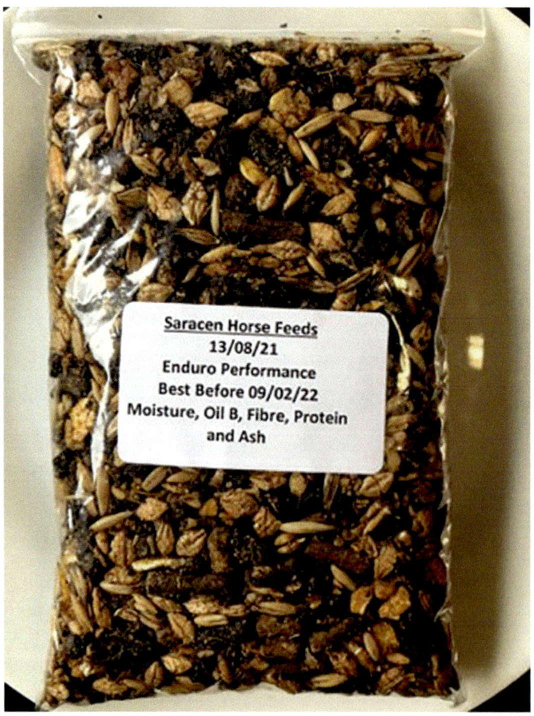

Fig. 7.10 A sample prepared for laboratory analysis.

Table 7.3 Common sampling errors

Source	Examples	Precautions
Feed sample identification	Poor labelling of samples	Maintenance of documentation throughout sampling and analytical process
Condition of sample	Insufficient quantity or quality of sample does not meet requirement for testing	Explicit instructions in sample requirements and appropriate training of staff
Transport and handling	Samples contaminated, degraded or depleted during transport or storage. Loss of samples	Protocol specifies conditions to be maintained. Efficient processing of sample

- identifying areas of the formulation where some raw material inclusion levels may be able to be reduced to meet sustainability targets while still meeting declared levels.

Using the Feed Label Information in Practical Feeding Scenarios

Using packaging information will help you to make informed decisions about which feed would be the most suitable to be fed to the horse.

Which feed provides the most protein?

You have advised a balancer for a horse that is fat score 4, 4, 4 being fed ad lib soaked hay and in light work, but the client is concerned that it is too high in protein (25.75%) and would rather feed a mix that is lower in protein (9.5%). You check the packaging (Fig. 7.11).

The numbers in Fig. 7.11 identify the information needed for each numbered point in the following list.

1. Check suitable for the horse.
2. Check % of protein and convert to g per 1 kg:
   - 25.75% × 10 = 257 g/kg feed
   - 9.5% × 10 = 95 g/kg feed
3. Calculate how many grams of protein the horse is eating per day from each ration:
   - Feed rate of balancer is 100 g/100 kg BW (horse is approx. 450 kg) so horse is consuming 257 g × 0.5 kg = 137.5 g protein.
   - Feed rate of mix is 500 g/100 kg BW so horse is consuming 2.5 (0.5 × 4.5) × 95 g = 237.5 g protein.

You can use the above to explain that horses do not eat % of protein but grams of protein and your client's horse will be eating less protein if fed the balancer.

Client feeding less or more than recommended intakes

A horse that is losing weight on a particular feed may not be consuming enough energy from the feed being fed; a horse that is gaining too much weight on a

Product [b]

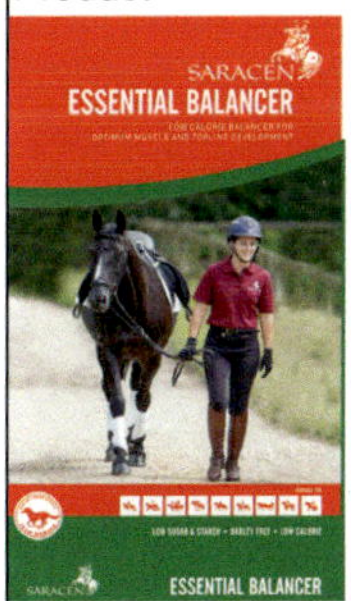

[1 & a] Suitable for

SUITABLE FOR

- Good-Doers requiring a low calorie diet
- Horses and ponies at rest and in light work
- Horse and ponies with natural energy
- Feeding alongside forage only rations

[c] Analytical Composition

2

Nutrient	Quantity
Oil	4.8%
Protein	26.0%
Fibre	6.5%
Digestible Energy	12.2 MJ/kg
Starch	6.0%
Sugar	9.0%
Biotin	30mg/kg
Vitamin A	65,000 iu/kg
Vitamin D	10,000 iu/kg
Vitamin E	2,000 iu/kg
Yeast	5 x 10^10 CFU/kg

3

Feed	Body Weight	Frequency
100g	Per 100kg	Daily

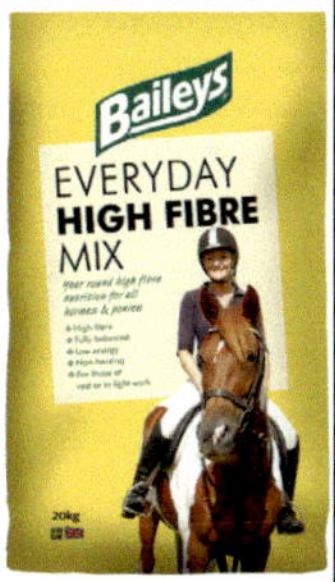

- Horses and ponies at rest or in light work
- Horses with low energy requirements needing to maintain condition
- Owners looking for consistency at a sensible price

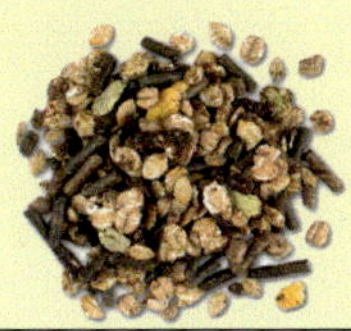

ANALYTICAL CONSTITUENTS

Digestible Energy 10MJ/kg

Protein[2]	9.5%
Starch	29%
Sugar	5%
Oil	4%
Fibre	16%
Ash	7.5%

[3] Feeding Guide 500g/100kgBW

[a] these feeds are both formulated for leisure horses but balance the forage in different ways.
[b] The balancer is formulated to be fed with a higher forage intake so the horses eats more protein from their forage portion compared to the horse eating the mix
[c] Feed companies can check the total protein intake vs requirements for you (ch 10).

Fig. 7.11 Information from the packaging to advise client on the protein intake from two different feeds.

particular feed even at the manufacturer's minimum recommended quantities is on the wrong product.

Intake below recommended intake and horse is overweight

If clients are feeding less than the recommended intakes, the horse's intake of vitamins and minerals will be compromised.

Using the feeds in Fig. 7.11, the client was feeding 0.5 scoop of Everyday mix twice a day (1.5 kg/day); she was aware the horse was 'a little chubby' so was feeding less than recommended quantities. This provides:

$$10\,\text{MJ DE} \times 1.5\,\text{kg} = 15\,\text{MJ DE/day but only } 66\% \text{ of vitamin/mineral and protein requirements (recommended intake} = 2.25\,\text{kg)}$$

- Recommended intake of balancer would provide 12.5 MJ × 0.5 = 6.25 MJ DE/day and 100% of vitamin/mineral and protein requirements

The feed balancer provides fewer calories; however, sometimes the client does not want to change. In this instance you can advise adding:

- vitamin and mineral supplement at 33% of the recommended intake; or
- 165 g of the balancer (33% of recommended intake).

Do insist that the horse loses some of the fat in the winter.

Intake above recommended intake and horse is losing weight

If the client has a horse that is struggling to maintain optimum body condition/fat score on their perception of the manufacturer's recommended feeding levels, check the points below before advising a higher energy/calorie feed.

- Check that the client knows how much in kilograms the horse is being fed for both compound feed and forage.
- Calculate how many calories the horse is eating from the compound feed (as per above) and the forage (using either analysis or mean ranges from Chapters 4 and 9).
- Compare with requirements (see Chapter 3).

A typical query you might encounter is the following:

'I am not keeping enough condition on my show pony (450 kg 13.2 hh). I need advice on what to feed. I am feeding 2 scoops/day of a conditioning feed (soaked as recommended by my feed merchant, by

Calm & Condition

Feeding Instructions:

DO NOT FEED DRY – THIS PRODUCT CONTAINS UNMOLASSED SUGAR BEET AND MUST BE SOAKED FOR 5-10 MINUTES BEFORE FEEDING.
Introduce a new feed gradually over 7 to 10 days building up to the amounts needed to maintain condition and energy levels (0.25 – 5.0kg depending on size, type, workload and condition).
Place feed in a shallow bucket, add twice as much water as feed, then stir. Wait for 5 to 10 minutes before feeding this product. Be sure the pellets have fully soaked and formed a nice soft mash, then feed. Unmolassed chaff or soaked Fast Fibre can be added after soaking, if adding unmolassed chaff, stir well before feeding.

ALLEN&PAGE
QUALITY HORSE FEEDS

Ideal for . . .

- Horses and ponies at rest to hard work
- Poor doers struggling to gain and/or maintain weight
- Horses and ponies requiring slow release, stamina giving energy
- Horses and ponies struggling to chew due to worn or missing teeth
- Horses with intolerances to barley, alfalfa and/or molasses

clients often do not read all the instructions

Calm & Condition

Feeding Recommendations:

1 Stubbs scoop holds 1.5kg of dry Calm & Condition. Please note, all feed amounts are in dry weight/per day.

Weight	Rest-light work	Medium work	Hard work
200kg	0.25 – 0.5kg	0.5 – 1.0kg	1.0 – 1.5kg
300kg	0.25 – 0.8kg	1.0 – 1.5kg	1.5 – 2.5kg
400kg	0.5 – 1.25kg	1.25 – 2.0kg	2.0 – 3.0kg
500kg	0.5 – 1.5kg	1.5 – 2.5kg	2.5 – 3.5kg
600kg	0.75 – 1.75kg	1.75 – 3.0kg	3.0 – 4.5kg
700kg	0.75 – 2.0kg	2.0 – 3.5kg	3.5 – 5.0kg

Fig. 7.12 Packing and marketing information for a conditioning feed.

adding twice the volume of water)' (Fig. 7.12). (We will ignore the rest of the diet just for this example.)

This one is relatively straight forward but relies on you asking the right questions and reading the extra marketing material provided online.

- What size/sort of scoop are you using?
- Is that two scoops of soaked feed, or did you measure out two scoops first and then soak them?

The scoop is a large coffee cup and the two scoops is after soaking – the owner is feeding 0.5 kg of the feed, so despite the perception, the pony is being fed less than recommended intakes.

Intake above recommended intake and horse is at ideal fat score

If the client is feeding more than the recommended quantities of a feed, check their feeding management and horse's fat score. If the horse is being fed multiple meals so < 1 g starch/kg BW/meal (see Chapter 5), is fat score 3, 3, 3 and is eating at least 50% of their dry matter intake as forage, then there is no reason to change the ration, assuming there are no issues.

If the client is unable to feed the product to ensure safe starch feeding, then they need to change to a higher-calorie product within the appropriate workload range.

Sometimes it is simply a case of checking the product descriptor and moving a competition horse off a product from the light work range to a competition product.

Comparing feeds within a specific range

Leisure range

Using information from outside the statutory statements (estimated DE) and feeding rates allows you to calculate the calorie contribution of individual feeds within a range (Table 7.4) and advise accordingly.

Performance feeds

It is a good idea to familiarise yourself with bags and labels (Fig. 7.13) so that you can use the ingredient list and the information within and outside the statutory statement to determine whether feeds are: (i) providing slow or fast energy release; and (ii) starch or fibre based. (Table 7.5) provides an example of two performance feeds that provdide

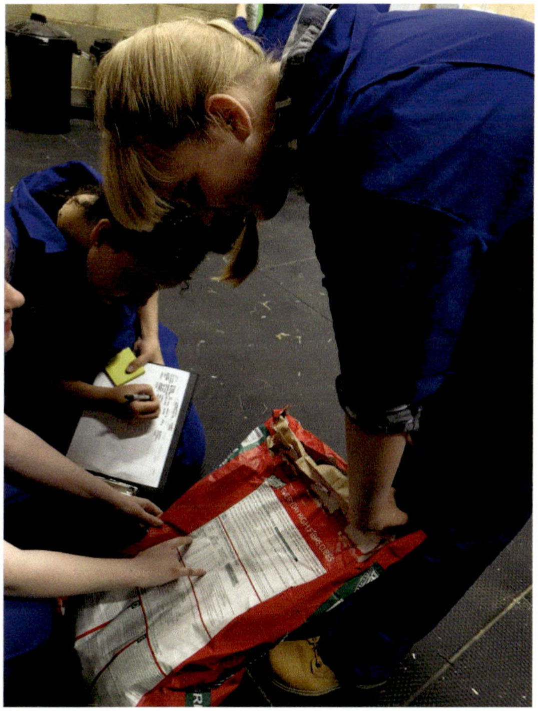

Fig. 7.13 Familiarise yourself with labels and packaging.

Table 7.4 The effect of different formulations on the calorie intake (MJDE) of leisure horses.

Product[b]	MJ/kg	Feed rate[a]	Scoops (Stubb)	Daily calorie intake	Main source of calories
Leisure Balancer	11.5	500 g	0.5	**5.75**	Minimal
Leisure Mix	10	1.5 kg	1.5	**15**	High fibre, cereal and cereal by-products
High-fibre balanced chaff mix	8.5	2.5 kg	5	**21**	Chopped fibre
High Fibre Nuts	9.5	1.5 kg	1	**14.25**	Fibre

[a]500 kg horse in light work fed to recommended intakes from packaging

[b]Remember all the feeds meet the vitamin/mineral and protein requirements for the horse in light work – what differs is the calorie intake.

Table 7.5 Two UK performance feeds providing the same calorie intake but from different feed ingredients to provide slow or fast releasing energy

	Performance feed 1	Performance feed 2
Description	High-energy balanced feed formulated to fulfil the nutritional needs of horses in medium to hard work	High-energy performance feed formulated to support performance horses that require a low starch ration
Ingredient listing (descending order)	Oats, alfalfa, oat feed, maize, barley, soya, beet pulp, vitamins and minerals	Soya hulls, alfalfa pellets, beet pulp, peas, soya, vitamins and minerals
Minimum recommended daily feeding rate	400 g/kg BW/day	400 g/kg BW/day
Energy level	13 MJ/kg	13 MJ/kg
Starch	26%	8%
Fibre	10%	18%
Oil	6.5%	9%

exactly the same amount of calories, but the energy supplied is either slow or fast release.

Cereal products are digested rapidly within the small intestine within 2–4 h after feeding, as measured by the horse's glycaemic response (Vervuert *et al.*, 2009). There is some suggestion in human performance sports that this rapidly absorbed glucose is used by the brain (Chambers *et al.*, 2009; Jeukendrup and Chambers, 2010; Robinson *et al.*, 2018) and thus Feed 1 in Table 7.5 might provide similar energy enhancement for the horse.

Feed 2 contains more ingredients (composition) that are high in fibre, which will be fermented in the large intestine and absorbed as volatile fatty acids before being incorporated into the Krebs cycle (Rechkemmer *et al.*, 1988). There will be a delay in the availability of glucose (up to 24–65 h after consumption); however, soluble fibre sources like these provide adequate calories for the performance horse (Brøkner *et al.*, 2016).

Most professional performance horses are considered 'normal' by their riders; feed is not considered as having an effect on their behaviour but is needed to maximise performance. It is perfectly acceptable to advise mixing compound feeds if they are fed in proportion ensuring vitamins/minerals and protein adequacy.

Summary

Understanding and recognising feed ingredients and using information on digestible energy level, protein, starch and fibre to calculate intake will help you and the client make decisions as to the most appropriate feed.

Use the packaging (or support the client in so doing) to do the following.

- Identify the company and perhaps research their websites or talk to a company nutritionist for advice and guidance.
- Note the feed description in the statutory statement rather than the marketing information on the front of the bag to identify suitability.
- Check the composition and analytical constituents to check that they reflect the description of the product.
- Reject any products that are making health claims (e.g. suitable to be fed to laminitics).
  - If it is a feed for a specific nutritional purpose, check the research/evidence to support these claims;
- Check the quality accreditations on the packaging and enquire as to the testing procedures specifically if you are advising performance horses, to ensure safe and low risk.
- Quantify the daily intake of the nutrients in the ration either by hand or using a feed ration programme (see Chapter 10).

Notes

[i] https://www.legislation.gov.uk/uksi/2010/2503/made

[ii] https://www.food.gov.uk/business-guidance/animal-feed-legislation

[iii] https://www.beta-uk.org/media/trade/download/Feed%20Code.pdf

[iv] https://www.gov.uk/government/organisations/veterinary-medicines-directorate

[v] Regulation (EC No 767/2009 Of The European Parliament And Of The Council, Chp 4 , article 11; available at: https://www.legislation.gov.uk/eur/2009/767

[vi] https://www.beta-uk.org/media/trade/download/Feed%20Code.pdf

[vii] https://www.legislation.gov.uk/uksi/2005/3281/contents/made

[viii] https://www.gov.uk/government/organisations/veterinary-medicines-directorate

[ix] https://www.legislation.gov.uk/eur/2020/354/annex/part/A

[x] http://www.fao.org/3/y4705e/y4705e12.htm

[xi] https://www.legislation.gov.uk/eur/2017/625/title/II/chapter/IV

Bibliography

Baker, L.A., Kearney-Moss, T., Pipkin, J.L., Bachman, R., Haliburton, J.T. and Veneklasen, G. (2003) The effect of supplemental inorganic and organic sources of copper and zinc on bone metabolism in exercised yearling geldings. In: *Proceedings of the 18th Equine Nutrition and Physiology Society Symposium*. Michigan State University, East Lansing, Michigan, pp. 100–105.

Brøkner, C., Austbø, D., Næsset, J., Blache, D., Bach Knudsen, K. *et al.* (2016) Metabolic response to dietary fibre composition in horses. *Animal* 10(7), 1155–1163. doi: 10.1017/S1751731115003006.

Carter, R.A. and Dugdale, A.H.A. (2013) Assessment of body condition and bodyweight. In: *Equine Applied and Clinical Nutrition*. Elsevier, Amsterdam, pp. 393–404.

Chambers, E.S., Bridge, M.W. and Jones, D.A. (2009) Carbohydrate sensing in the human mouth: effects on exercise performance and brain activity. *The Journal of Physiology* 587(Pt 8), 1779–1794. doi: 10.1113/jphysiol.2008.164285.

Gater, J. and Counsell, T. (2006) *A Comparative Study of Equine Compound Feeds for Leisure and Performance Horses*. BSAP Occasional Publication, Vol. 35: *Applying Equine Science: Research into Business*, pp. 179–182.

Geor, R.J. and Harris, P. (2009) Dietary management of obesity and insulin resistance: countering risk for laminitis. *Veterinary Clinics: Equine Practice* 25(1), 51–65.

Harris, P.A. and Rivero, J.L.L. (2017) Nutritional considerations for equine rhabdomyolysis syndrome. *Equine Veterinary Education* 29(8), 459–465.

ISO (International Organization for Standardization) (2012) ISO 6498, Animal feeding stuffs – Guidelines for sample preparation. Edition 3. Technical Committee ISO/TC 34/SC 10 Animal feeding stuffs. ICS (International Classification for Standards): 65.120. Available at: https://www.iso.org/standard/12874.html

Jeukendrup, A.E. and Chambers, E.S. (2010) Oral carbohydrate sensing and exercise performance. *Current Opinion in Clinical Nutrition & Metabolic Care* 13(4), 447–451.

King, C. and Mansmann, R.A. (2004) Preventing laminitis in horses: dietary strategies for horse owners. *Clinical Techniques in Equine Practice* 3(1), 96–102.

NRC (National Research Council) (1987) *Vitamin Tolerance of Animals*. National Academies Press, Washington, DC.

NRC (National Research Council) (2007) *Nutrient Requirements of Horses: Sixth Revised Edition*. National Academies Press, Washington, DC. doi: 10.17226/11653.

Pagan, J., Karnezos, P., Kennedy, M., Thomas, T. and Hoekstra, K. (1999) Effect of selenium source on selenium digestibility and retention in exercised Thoroughbreds. In: *Proceedings of the Equine Nutrition and Physiology Society Symposium*, pp. 135–140.

Rechkemmer, G., Rönnau, K. and Engelhardt, W.V. (1988) Fermentation of polysaccharides and absorption of short chain fatty acids in the mammalian hindgut. *Comparative Biochemistry and Physiology Part A: Physiology* 90(4), 563–568.

Robinson, M.M., Lowe, V.J. and Nair, K.S. (2018) Increased brain glucose uptake after 12 weeks of aerobic high-intensity interval training in young and older adults. *The Journal of Clinical Endocrinology & Metabolism* 103(1), 221–227.

Vervuert, I., Voigt, K., Hollands, T., Cuddeford, D. and Coenen, M. (2008) Effects of processing barley on its digestion by horses. *Veterinary Record* 162(21), 684–688.

Vervuert, I., Voigt, K., Hollands, T., Cuddeford, D. and Coenen, M. (2009) Effect of feeding increasing quantities of starch on glycaemic and insulinaemic responses in healthy horses. *The Veterinary Journal* 182(1), 67–72.

Williams, C.A., Kronfeld, D.S., Staniar, W.B. and Harris, P.A. (2001) Plasma glucose and insulin responses of Thoroughbred mares fed a meal high in starch and sugar or fat and fiber. *Journal of Animal Science*, 79(8), 2196–2201.

8 Which Feed? Advising a Quality Feed Formulation, Quality Control and Expertise Standards

LIZZIE DRURY AND TERESA HOLLANDS

Saracen Horse Feeds, Aylesford; School of Veterinary Medicine, University of Surrey

Learning Objectives

LO1 Describe the processes needed to produce quality, safe horse feed.
LO2 Identify the key legislation that manufacturers have to meet to produce quality horse feed.
LO3 Explain the importance and significance of naturally occurring substances in the production of quality horse feeds for performance horse feeds.
LO4 Identify the steps taken by producers of quality horse feed to provide traceability and accountability.
LO5 Discuss the importance and significance of auditing process – UFAS and BETA NOPS.
LO6 Describe the steps clients need to take to store and maintain the quality of their horse feed.
LO7 Identify suitably qualified nutritionists and their role in the manufacture of quality horse feeds.
LO8 Describe the steps taken by producers of quality horse feeds to increase sustainability and reduce environmental impact.
LO9 Identify product research supporting production of feed.
LO10 Identify if the company uses qualified equine nutritionists.

At the end of this chapter, you will be able to recognise a high-quality and fit-for-purpose safe feed.

Introduction

Clients perceive quality in different ways when choosing a feed; for some it is the nutrient content or the presence of certain ingredients, for others the consistent appearance, smell and physical form. For some it could be on recommendation from top riders, as well as the visual results of other horses and ponies; for others it is the assurance of the absence of undesirable substances.

Only a few of the above are evidence of a quality feed, so it falls to the vet/nutritionist to support the client in making a choice based on facts rather than emotion and forums.

The manufacturer's role is essentially to have a comprehensive system in place that ensures consistency and quality of their products, from harvest of the individual raw material through to its storage and transport, by adopting a quality system that is structured in a logical manner. The system needs to identify potential nutritional, microbial or physical hazards and apply controls to processes which might: (i) impact on finished product quality; (ii) affect the health or performance of horses; or (iii) affect the legal status of the feed. Accreditation from the Universal Feed Assurance Scheme (UFAS) indicates reputable production; it is critical that

 Evidence-based Equine Nutrition: A Practical Approach for Professionals (T. Hollands and L. Drury)
DOI: 10.1079/9781789245134.0008

any product used for performance horses conforms to the Naturally Occurring Prohibited Substances (NOPS)[i] feed code

It is illegal to knowingly manufacture feed that is: (i) not safe; (ii) not legally labelled; or (iii) without appropriate recommendations for storage and the use.

Adverse quality can result in physical harm to the horse and can seriously affect a feed business in several ways, including unwelcome media and social media interest, loss of business, irreversible damage to the brand and prosecution.

Global regulations and nutritional standards

Horse feed is regulated by governmental animal feed laws, which vary according to country but in all instances exist to ensure that manufacturers are responsible for making safe, nutritionally balanced feed that supports lifelong health, performance and wellbeing.

Organisations consisting of industry specialists and researchers, such as the Association of American Feed Control Officials (AAFCO)[ii] in the USA and the European Feed Manufacturers Federation (FEFAC)[iii] in the European Union (EU), help develop legally binding directives or work with local industry groups to produce codes of practice.

Horse feed is highly regulated, from the ingredients used, through to production, marketing and sales. An understanding of the regulations (Box 8.1) governing feed hygiene and safety, full testing and traceability will help identify high-quality horse feed that is fit for purpose and help your clients understand why cheaper is not always better. Not all feed companies invest equally in quality systems; identifying those that have quality assurance systems in place is part of your professional role (Fig. 8.1).

The Manufacturer's Quality Challenge

Manufacturers strive to:

- make products that consistently contain what they should and are free from what they should not contain; and
- maintain quality across variable mixes of feed forms, ingredients, feed rate, packaging and shelf life.

What drives feed assurance?

The primary driver of feed quality and assurance is a fundamental desire to ensure the consistency and quality of all horse feed (Box 8.2), maintaining both client (owner/feed purchaser) and consumer (the horse) satisfaction.

Box 8.1 Key EU animal feed legislation regulations

EC Regulation 178/2002: general principles and requirements of food law, establishes the European Food Safety Authority (EFSA) and lays down procedures in matters of food safety.

European Regulation on Feed Hygiene (Regulation EC183/2005): standards relating to the transport and storage of feed, maintenance of equipment, the training of personnel, and the keeping of records. It requires most businesses involved in the use, manufacture, or marketing of feeds to be approved or registered with their competent authority.

EC regulation 1831/2003 on Feed Additives: harmonised procedures for the authorisation and labelling of feed additives. This includes:

- vitamins
  - preservatives
  - binders and gelling agents
  - colourants
  - antioxidants
  - stabilisers
  - trace elements
  - enzymes
- micro-organisms – some of which are subject to maximum limits, target species of animal, and other conditions of use.

Such additives can only be used if they have undergone assessment for safety, quality and efficacy.

EC directive 2002/32 and Commission Regulation (EU) No. 744/2012: Undesirable Substances and Products, control of contaminants such as heavy metals, certain mycotoxins, cyanogenic glycosides and dioxins. In addition to listing maximum permitted levels for each substance, prohibits the blending down of contaminated feedstuffs with feeds of lower contaminated level.

https://www.food.gov.uk/business-guidance/animal-feed-legislation

https://www.europarl.europa.eu/factsheets/en/sheet/51/food-safety

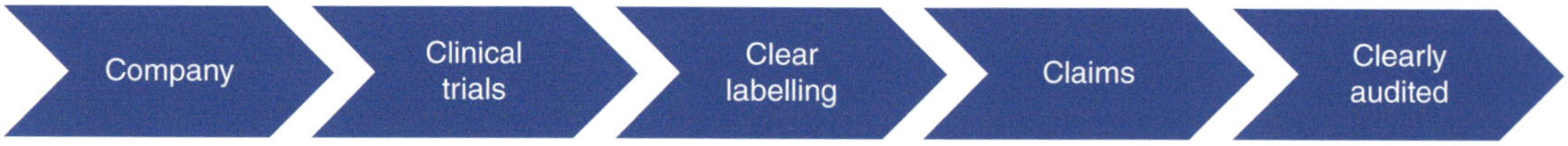

Company

- Do you recognise the company marketing the product and are they reputable?
- Look for indications of quality e.g. UFAS approval
- Are the manufacturer's contact details clearly given on the label
- Do they employ nutritionists

Clinical trials

- Has the product been fed independently for safety, efficacy, with formulation based on peer-review published results?

Clear labelling

- All ingredients should be listed on the label.
- Feeding instructions should be clear and based on the bodyweight of the horse
- It should be easy to calculate the amount of nutrients provided/day.

Claims

- Feeds are not medicines and therefore must not make any claims of medicinal benefits.
- Product literature or labelling must meet with feeding stuff legislation-if it sounds too good to be true it probably is

Clearly audited

- Is the company accountable for its competition feeds using BETA NOPS ensuring they are suitable for competing under BHA/FEI rules?.
- Look for indications of quality e.g. UFAS
- Do they adhere to an environmental audit

Fig. 8.1 Clarifying quality. BETA, British Equine Trade Association; BHA, British Horseracing Authority; FEI, Fédération Equestre Internationale (International Federation for Equestrian Sports); NOPS, naturally occurring prohibited substance; UFAS, Universal Feed Assurance Scheme.

Box 8.2 Key factors that govern the success of a company's commitment to quality

- **Leadership** – Clearly defined commitment to quality from director level and downwards.
  - **Culture** – Quality is embedded in the company ethos and is believed, lived and used each day by all the company personnel.
  - **Well invested** – People, equipment and expenditure are consistently resourced to deliver quality products.
- **Simple** – Easy-to-understand systems and controls that all involved are able to follow and a system that is reviewed regularly, involving people from different departments.

There are also strictly documented quality control procedures that need to be in place, monitored by external independent bodies as part of legislation requirements and expected and required industry standards; both approaches are needed to successfully produce quality feed (Box 8.3).

Box 8.3 Key points: drivers of quality are both internal and external

Internal:

- An individual company's desire to be able to do the best for its customers and to be able to demonstrate responsible behaviour.

External:

- Independent expert opinion, e.g. UFAS, NASC (US).
- Industry standards.
- Legislative requirements. For example:
  - EU: via 183 / 2005 – Feed hygiene regulations: EU 183 / 2003 Feed additives; EU 2002 / 32 – Undesirable substances
  - USA: via Federal Food Drug and Cosmetic Act (FFDCA), Food Safety and Modernization Act, GRAS, AAFCO Official Publication.

Regulatory requirements

An EU regulation is a legal act that applies directly at national level. Once approved at the EU level, it becomes directly and immediately applicable within the countries of the EU. Whilst we are no longer part of the EU, the UK has maintained the legal framework (classing the horse as a food-producing animal) (Box 8.1), designed to maximise food and feed safety throughout the food chain.

Feed hygiene and undesirable substances

Frameworks to recall harmful or undesirable substances (Box 8.4) that might enter an equine diet (such as microbiological contaminants, pesticides, dioxins, mycotoxins, heavy metals) are in place. There are US versus EU differences in maximum tolerance levels for contaminants such as mycotoxins.

There is also a further category of substances: those that are not considered harmful but are prohibited under the rules of racing and equestrian sport. The principle behind these rules is that all competition should be won or lost on the merits of the horse and rider and not enhanced by unfair means.

Prohibited substances – naturally occurring substances (NOPS)

What are NOPS?

NOPS are naturally occurring prohibited substances (Table 8.1) present naturally in certain ingredients or occurring due to accidental contamination before reaching the feed manufacturer. There is a code of conduct to reduce the risk of NOPS in equine feed and supplements (BETA NOPS, 2009).

Herbs

There are two categories of herbal supplements: (i) high-priority (Table 8.2) are completely banned from any horse supplement/feed; and (ii) low-priority (Table 8.3), which can be formulated into supplements and be clearly labelled on packaging and are permitted but limited to horses who are not competing. Both are banned from use in competition under FEI/BHA rules; if detected, the horse will be eliminated, with financial consequences.

Table 8.1 Main naturally occurring prohibited substances (NOPS) that are tested in the UK

Name	Source
Caffeine	Coffee and tea
Theobromine	Cocoa, tea
Theophylline	Tea, cocoa
Morphine	Opium poppies
Atropine	Nightshade plants
Lupanine	Lupins
Bufotenine	Reed canary grass
Cannabinoids	Cannabis

Box 8.4 Examples of adverse feed product recalls in the marketplace

- **Oct 2002, Jan 2003**: 43 horses, including 16 winners, tested positive for morphine in post-race samples in UK and Ireland. The source was identified as racehorse feed (BHA, 2004)[iv].
- **April 2009**: 21 polo ponies died of acute selenium toxicity, after receiving a supplement manufactured by a compounding laboratory in Florida. Selenium levels were found to be 10–15 times higher than normal in the horses' blood and a mathematical conversion error was blamed.
- **Feb 2019**: Voluntary recall of animal feed due to aflatoxin levels that exceeded FDA's action levels. Affected products were removed from retail shelves throughout February–April 2019, which was then extended back to October 2018. Livestock,
- **Oct 2020**: Cane molasses containing zilpaterol hydrochloride supplied into Ireland then also entered the UK and subsequently supplied to a few equine feed companies. Whilst posing no health risks to horses, it is prohibited for horses competing under rules. There were positives detected under the rules of racing in France from feed originating from one Irish company. It was further identified that the contaminated material had also affected other horse feed manufacturers, although contamination was at lower levels than was the case in Ireland. These companies were in direct contact with their known performance clients to advise on the situation and to provide any advice and instruction to those competing under rules. The Food Standards Agency in the UK took no further action, due to the very low concentrations in the finished feed, which were not considered significant in terms of food or feed safety and were not a risk to equine health or welfare. The level of zilpaterol that has been found in feed was less than 1 part per billion, well below the level that would trigger food or feed safety considerations.

How can contamination occur?

From being grown, harvested, stored, transported, processed, distributed, or stored at the destination, contamination of NOPS can occur at any stage. Risk assessments are carried out at various stages, ensuring traceability of a product if a problem were to occur.

Table 8.2 High-priority herbal NOPS

Name	Source
Digitoxin	Foxgloves
Synephrine	Bitter orange
Ephedrine, pseudophedrine	*Ephedra sinica*
Reserpine	Indian snakeroot
Cathinone, cathine	Khat

Table 8.3 Low-priority herbal NOPS

Name	Source
Valerenic acid	Valerian
Salicylic acid	Willow bark Meadowsweet
Harpagosides	Devil's claw
Yohimbine	Yohimbine tree

How to Achieve Quality: General Principles

The starting point for defining quality is the product specification that both describes and quantifies its desirable and undesirable characteristics. An individual company's quality assurance activities then act to ensure that the specification is continuously delivered. The general principles of assuring feed quality are:

- a coordinated and audited supply chain providing well-defined (via specification) ingredients and products;
- traceability from the point of origin of the ingredient through to the use of the product; and
- independently verified quality assurance activities (e.g. UFAS and BETA NOPS).

Common steps are taken by a feed manufacturer (Table 8.4) to ensure the quality, safety, traceability, specification and consistency of any products that they manufacture.

Table 8.4 Common steps taken to ensure the quality control of a horse feed

Action	Outcome
HACCP Plan	Assesses potential food safety hazards (chemical, microbiological and physical) and identifies official control points and monitoring systems for each
Insect and rodent traps	Monitor background levels of pests in the manufacturing facility Check to ensure that the system in place is working
Incoming raw material inspection and risk assessment: • supplier check • visual assessment • nutritional check • storage pests	Check against defined specification: are the supplier and haulier approved? Check no prohibited substances have been carried on previous loads Spear samples to check appearance, colour, grain or pellet size, absence of foreign bodies and objects Analysis of key nutrients checked against specifications
Finished product specification	Defines the parameters to be checked after manufacture, e.g. product appearance, nutrient profile, packaging quality.
Finished product assessment • visual assessment • nutritional check • undesirable substance check	Checks against defined specification Colour, pellet size, mix components present in exact proportions Key nutrients checked to ensure present at specified levels and to ensure legal conformance Monitoring checks for unwanted contaminants, such as naturally occurring prohibited substances and mycotoxins Refer to example of routine testing as part of the quality control plan Samples of each batch kept for auditing process
Work instructions, standard operating procedures	Define how to conduct key operational processes Personnel training records and performance indicators
Supplier and manufacturer audit	Paperwork, samples and manufacturing records will be checked against SOP, purchase and sales records; processes monitored

This approach is based on identification of the hazards, assessment of the risk associated with the hazard (its significance, severity and likelihood of occurrence) and estimate of the effectiveness of potential control measures, and is the basis of many modern food safety systems.

It should be noted that no risk management options will provide absolute safety (i.e., there will always be some risk), the objective being to assess and manage the risk accordingly.

How Is Feed Quality Demonstrated?

HACCP

The Hazard Analysis and Critical Control Points (HACCP) system is an internationally recognised methodology to help assure safe production for all foodstuffs. Essentially it provides a systematic approach to evaluation and reduction of risks (Fig. 8.2) and includes the following.

- The **identification** of hazards, determination of the severity of the hazard and an estimate of how likely it is that the hazard will occur.
- The **determination** of critical control points (CCPs) required to control a given hazard. A CCP can be a location, practice, procedure or process used to minimise or prevent unacceptable contamination, survival or growth of spoilage organisms or pathogens, or the introduction of unwanted chemical substances or foreign objects.
- The establishment and **implementation** of monitoring procedures to determine that each CCP is under control, with corrective actions defined for when a CCP results shows the system to be out of control.
- Good-quality feed also ensures a better-quality product and a cleaner, greener environment.
- The safety and quality of animal feed is also vital for preventing hazardous substances entering the food.

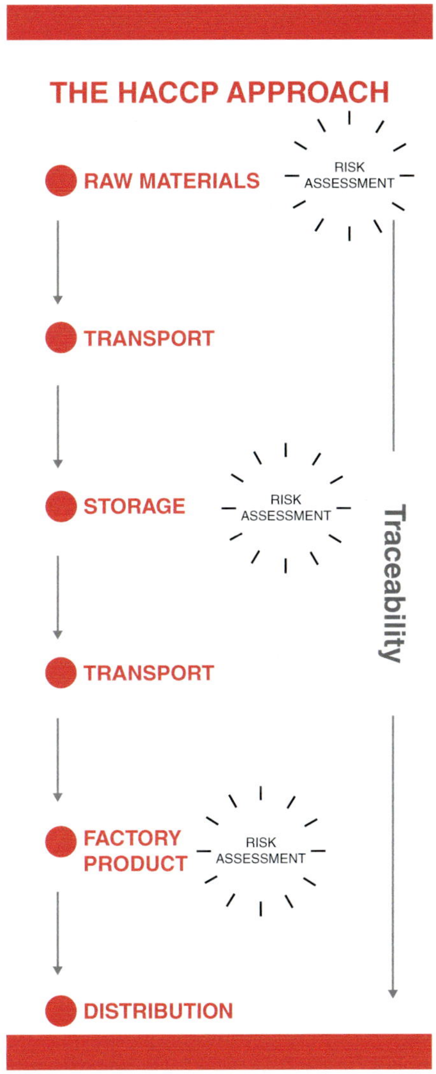

Fig. 8.2 The stages at which the protocols are carried out in the Hazard Analysis and Critical Control Points (HACCP) system.

Appropriate sampling and testing for risk

It is challenging to accurately sample bulk loads of feed ingredients; more than 60% of the error associated with sampling and testing has been attributed to sampling alone (Leung *et al.* 2006; Casado *et al.*, 2009) and requires a large number of samples (Whitaker, 2006).

Contamination is not consistent across the whole load. For example, the distribution of *Fusarium* mycotoxins might be nonuniform within a field, due to local climatic conditions and crop and soil factors (Casado *et al.*, 2009). Salmonella is similarly considered to be heterogeneously distributed (CAC, 1999; EFSA, 2009).

These pose problems to manufacturers because of: (i) the practicality of taking large numbers of samples; and (ii) the length of time required to turn around a test result for an incoming load before it can enter the factory.

Sampling is targeted in accordance with HACCP, which is more sensitive and cost-effective than traditional sampling of finished products and feed materials to verify a CCP.

Lack of equine data

The principles of HACCP require, per hazard identified, an assessment of its significance, its severity and the likelihood of occurrence.

However, there is often a lack of published data on both the normal concentrations of certain hazards in feed ingredients used in equine diets and the effect of certain hazards in relation to health and effect on performance; there is a need for more published assessments.

It is normal to report no observed adverse effect levels (NOAELs) or safe upper limits (SULs) for drugs and additives for food-producing animals but there is a lack of quality safety data in horses; this is particularly noticeable for some ingredients added to horse feed or indeed used in 'supplements' (Box 8.5).

In many situations, research from other species provides important information as to safe or hazardous levels but will not provide a guarantee of the same in equines.

Insect and rodent controls

Cleanliness and general housekeeping of stores and premises are paramount. Most manufacturers employ external consultancy services for specialised pest control to monitor pest infestations from rodents; clearly poisons are not used on site. Methods such as 'sticky boards' and monitoring rodent populations, movement and nesting are the main control measures. Cleanliness of the mill and the storage facility is the responsibility of the manufacturing team, and everyone has a role in ensuring that cleaning procedures are carried out, minimising the risk of insect infestations, which are monitored using insect traps and inspecting storage bins.

> **Box 8.5** Safety data on evening primrose oil for horses
>
> - The fatty acids in primrose oil could, theoretically, benefit equine skin, coat and hooves (Reilly *et al*., 1998).
> - Anecdotally, horse owners report that primrose oil helps treat sweet itch in horses, but no scientific studies have confirmed these observations.
> - In laboratory studies, primrose oil has been shown to have anti-inflammatory effects, with evidence of antioxidant activity in racehorses given primrose oil (Mikesova *et al*., 2014).
> - Large doses of primrose oil have been associated with stomach upset and diarrhoea in people and no dosing guidelines have been established for horses (Elghandour *et al*. (2018).

Sampling and testing (raw materials and final product)

Spear samples will be taken to check appearance, colour, grain, or pellet size, and absence of foreign bodies and objects before a load is accepted for intake to the manufacturing facility. Checks are also made to ensure that no prohibited substances have been carried on previous loads. Hauliers must provide details about the last three loads carried and cleaning procedures undertaken

Feed analysis laboratories are essential for ensuring accurate information on the composition of feed ingredients and determining the level of desirable and undesirable substances, enabling the production of safe, balanced diets for all livestock. However, testing for microbiological contaminants and mycotoxins is time consuming and often lacks sensitivity and specificity, and the levels of sampling routinely applied have a low probability of detecting defective lots if the proportion of defectives in the lot is low, according to the International Commission on Microbiological Specifications for Foods (ICMSF[v]). The ICMSF website gives details of its own books and relevant papers.

The same ingredient can vary from one supplier to another, and between seasons and years. For example, in drought years, cereals fill poorly and are therefore lower in nutrients.

Most importantly, if feeds are not evaluated, it is not possible to tell if the raw material or finished feed will be suitable for feeding to equines.

Final product specification and assessment

The final product specification defines the parameters post-manufacture, such as product appearance, nutrient testing, checks for unwanted contaminants, conformation to the intended product declarations, packaging and marketing quality, and evidence of supporting material required to support specific nutritional claims (see Chapter 7, Table 7.2: 'Descriptors for feed approved for particular nutritional purposes for horses'; Fig. 7.7: 'A comparison of legal, medical and misleading terms on equine feed bags').

Samples from each run of finished feed are collected and stored for the life of the product (best-before date). Random sampling will also be undertaken for in-house analysis and checking against analytical constituents' declarations. Most companies will also keep samples for visual comparisons to ensure consistency, as this is the first factor the client will notice.

Work instructions and standard operating procedures (SOPs)

You will be familiar with these concepts as they are standard practice in veterinary businesses. Clearly the aim of the documentation is to ensure that the business can continue regardless of which staff are in place; it also provides the basis for auditing.

External auditing

Just as veterinary practices are audited by the RCVS, so are companies externally audited to demonstrate a commitment to quality using an accepted auditing process for manufacturing. International Organisation for Standardisation (ISO) standard 9001:2008 (ISO 9001:2008) (Anonymous, 2008) is a generic, clearly defined set of processes that defines a commitment to creating products and services in accordance with pre-defined standards applicable to all manufacturing organisations, regardless of type, size and product provided.

Suppliers and hauliers are inspected annually to ensure that they meet their own required quality control (QC) standards. Some of these checks will be 'spot' checks, typically including the inspection of the cleanliness of the premises, up-to-date paperwork and records and staff training. If nonconformances are identified, these are recorded and timelines are set to provide evidence of correction.

In addition to the ISO standard, the animal feed sector internationally adopted voluntary independent assurance schemes, specifically designed to demonstrate feed safety. These are usually administered by feed trade associations in individual countries and either exceed or meet regulatory standards for hygiene and feed safety in their country, for example the Universal Feed Assurance Scheme (UFAS) and, more specific to the equine industry, BETA NOPS.

Feed industry assurance schemes

Universal Feed Assurance Scheme (UFAS)

UFAS accounts for more than 95% of the commercially produced compound feed in the UK and Ireland. The scheme is audited and certified by an independent certification body, in accordance with the internationally recognised standard EN45011 (previously ISO Guide 65).

The certification body is itself independently assessed every year to ensure that the standard is implemented and administered consistently and fairly; local authorities now include participation in UFAS in their risk assessments of feed businesses.

British Equestrian Trade Association naturally occurring prohibited substances scheme (BETA NOPS)

This is a feed assurance scheme, designed to minimise the risk of feed contamination with substances that can cause a disqualification from racing or competition.

Some substances occur naturally in feedstuffs. Clearly a zero-tolerance approach in blood or urine samples would be impractical, such as theobromine, salicylic acid and the heavy metal, arsenic.

The largest risk of feed contamination comes from theobromine, which is a metabolite of caffeine that is found in biscuit and coffee residues. Most manufacturers operate strict 'no caffeine' policies that range from supplier and haulier agreements, which stipulate that they must not handle caffeine-containing materials to no-caffeine-buying policies, together with positive release, so that no product is sold until the results of a negative caffeine and theobromine test have been received. Thus accidental contamination is rare.

UK and Irish companies following NOPS will state either their suitability 'for feeding to horses competing under Jockey Club or FEI rules' or that they are free from both caffeine and theobromine.

A 'prohibited substance' as defined by the Jockey Club and FEI is a substance that originates externally to a horse, whether or not it is endogenous to it, and which falls into any of the categories contained in a defined list. The definition applies to drugs in relation to illegal performance enhancement, but some naturally occurring substance in feeds (see Tables 8.1, 8.2 and 8.3, above) can potentially cause a dope test failure. The list of prohibited substances produced by the Jockey Club and FEI is unspecific (BHA, 2021)[vi] – an unprecedented challenge for manufacturers.

> **Top tip**
>
> You should assume that any medication or supplement (including herbal substances) that has, or claims to have, an effect on horses (or any other species) is prohibited unless you have specific advice from the BHA Equine Health and Welfare Department that states otherwise (BHA, 2021)[vii].

In some countries the absence of central regulation has meant that certain groups have developed their own standards, designed to generate industry credibility.

National Animal Supplement Council (NASC)

The NASC is a US supplement industry association, seeking to address the apparent lack of specific regulation for equine supplements by both setting quality standards for the animal supplement industry and providing a forum for all those involved in the supply of products, from manufacturers to legislators. In the UK, supplements fall under The Feed Regulations for Complementary Feeds (see Chapter 6).

The council and its members work cooperatively with state, federal and international government officials to create a legislative and regulatory environment to ensure ethical manufacturing and labelling practices are complied with throughout the industry. There are strict guidelines for product quality assurance in writing, consistent raw material sourcing and manufacturing standards, adverse event reporting, and labelling requirements that are within the guidelines provided by the regulatory agencies. These tasks are undertaken by BETA[viii] in the UK with Agricultural Industries Confederation (AIC[ix]) and Food Standards Agency (FSA[x]).

Feed Quality and Safety Throughout the Distribution Chain

The shelf life for equine feedstuffs can vary from 90 days to 2 years.

The risks to equine feed products principally arise through the poor handling and storage of a relatively bulky and perishable commodity negating all the undertakings of the manufacturer.

There are many elements of good practice to maintain feed quality post-manufacturing, applicable to both commercial stores and private feed rooms.

Feed storage

Failure to store feed and forage correctly significantly increases the risk of feed degradation, mould growth and contamination that could potentially harm horses and ponies.

Once the feed arrives at its destination it becomes the responsibility of your client to ensure continued feed safety.

To decrease the risks of decomposition and mould development, bagged feed should be stored in cool, dry environments, with containers tightly closed to seal out moisture, insects, or rodents.

Metal or hard plastic containers with secure lids reduce losses and spoilage (Fig. 8.3) as well as prevent contamination with pathogens that pests can introduce such as *Leptospira* sp. causing leptospirosis. Horses can contract leptospirosis by ingesting feed contaminated with the urine of infected mammals. Discard forage or cereals that have been soiled with pest urine or faeces. The best prevention is to store feed where rodents or other pests cannot access it.

Exposing cereals such as oats, barley and maize to high humidity or moisture can lead to mycotoxin production, with dangerous health consequences for horses. Mycotoxins are produced from fungi present at cereal harvest that proliferate in the presence of moisture or humidity during storage. In normal and healthy horses very small amounts of mycotoxins are unlikely to cause a problem but higher levels or exposure to horses that are sick or stressed can increase the risk of serious health issues (Table 8.5). Manufacturers ensure the safety of their feed by keeping mycotoxin levels in feeds below levels that would cause adverse effects in horses, set by feed legislation (Kamphues, 2013).

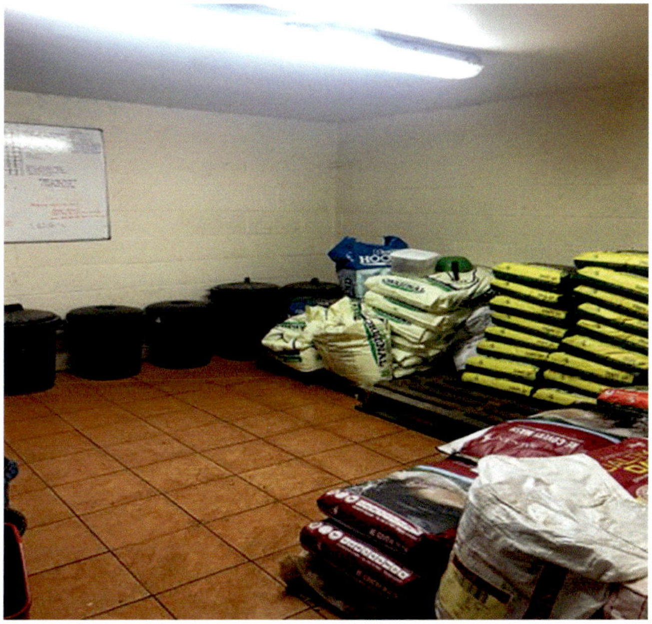

Fig. 8.3 Proper storage is essential for maintaining the quality of horse feed.

Early signs of a possible problem may include reduced feed intake (Diekman and Green, 1992; Akande *et al*., 2006); more serious effects can include abortion in broodmares (Newman and Raymond, 2005).

Moisture encourages not only mould growth but also insect proliferation within cereal grains. Insects such as grain mites eat cereals from the inside out, removing nutrients and in the process causing damage.

Top tip

A distinctive sweet smell is used to identify mites; there may also be a fine, brown dust coating on the outer bag.

Feed infested with mites and other insects should be immediately isolated from clean feed and destroyed. The area should be thoroughly cleaned and sanitised to reduce the risk of uncontaminated feed becoming a problem.

Storing feed with climate changes in mind

Feed bags should be stored on pallets and should not be stacked more than five high, especially in humid climates. Sealed bags last longer than open bags. If purchasing large volumes at one time, storage rooms should be air-conditioned. If feed is being stored in an environment that is considered hot or humid, then it is recommended that feed is stored in an air-conditioned unit maintaining temperature at no more than 15°C but ideally at 10°C.

Some feed manufacturers who are exporting feeds to countries with more challenging environmental conditions, such as the Middle East, will include fumigation of containers of feed to guarantee the

Table 8.5 Upper safe intakes of mycotoxin (with 88% DM) for horses[a]

Mycotoxin	Guidance value in mg/kg (ppm) relative to a feedstuff with a moisture content of 12%
Aflatoxin	Complementary 5 mg/kg
Fumonisins	Max. 5 mg/kg
Zearalenone	Max. 2–3 mg/kg
Deoxynivalenol (DON)	Cereals and cereal products except maize by-products (12 mg/kg) 8 mg/kg
	Complementary feeds 0.9 mg/kg
Ochratoxin A	Cereal and cereal products 2.5 mg/kg

[a]https://eur-lex.europa.eu/eli/reco/2006/576 (2006/576/EC)

feed to be free from any pest contamination prior to arriving at the destination. Working closely with shippers may also mean that containers can be shipped on board in the lower decks below sea level to help maintain cooler transportation conditions; water activity within the feed must be controlled.

Bagged feed longevity

Most horse feed companies designate expiration dates within 3–9 months after the product has been manufactured and include a mould inhibitor and a mycotoxin binder to help preserve shelf life. The processes that utilise natural preservatives, including antioxidants and low-oxygen-barrier packaging, can extend shelf life for up to as long as 2 years (Tavman *et al.*, 2019).

Feed preservatives and binders are declared on the feed labels (see Chapter 7) but these cannot prevent feed deterioration if the storage conditions are poor.

It is the responsibility of the client to carry out a certain amount of record keeping so that if a feed- or food-related problem occurs its origins can be quickly identified, and it can then be handled with minimal disruption to the yard or establishment.

Your client should be advised to keep a record of:

- the product name;
- the product batch details and best-before date;
- the date purchased; and
- where it was purchased.

Names of products and batch numbers can be found on product labels/bags and these labels or photos of the bags can be retained to help fulfil this record-keeping requirement.

Suitably Qualified Nutritionists

As in the human nutrition world, there are a plethora of people who describe themselves as nutritionists. Reputable companies will employ suitability qualified equine nutritionists who will also work alongside nutritionists from premix companies and formulation software experts to ensure the production of quality feed. Advanced education with an emphasis on equine nutrition, such as a master's degree or a doctorate, and day-to-day work in the field usually indicate a high degree of expertise, especially if a nutritionist regularly offers up ideas or products new to the industry based on published work. An appropriately qualified equine nutritionist will be registered with a professional body such as the Association for Nutrition (AfN) and use the letters RNutr (Animal) after their name. A register of qualified nutritionists is maintained at AfN[xi]; listing confirms that the individual has signed up to a professional code of conduct, including maintaining their expertise by recording regular approved Continuing Professional Development (CPD), and is renewable annually.

Qualified nutritionists also play a role in supporting the quality products, often by managing a team of advisors on a nutritional helpline with a mix of practical and technical expertise.

Sustainability and Environmental Policies

The production of quality horse feed cannot be at the expense of the environment; reputable manufacturers will be developing feeds that meet critical sustainability targets. Manufacturing's impact is determined by the raw materials, production, transport and packaging. Whilst horses are relatively small consumers of the feed industry, your clients should know that animal feed production requires 75% of arable land, 35% of world cereal crops and creates around 14.5% of greenhouse gas emissions (Shurson, 2020).

Look for manufacturers that have a clear sustainability charter on their websites, that use renewable energy or are researching the recycling of steam to drive machinery, reducing the reliance on fossil fuel. Businesses can incorporate a number of small steps (Table 8.6) towards sustainability.

Evidence-based Quality Formulations and Feeding Management

Many ingredients, including herbs (Carey and Lamprecht, 2008), and finished products have not been extensively tested on horses. Reasons for this include clients' active objection to testing on animals and the prohibitive costs of equine research which, unlike food-producing animals, has very limited government funding. Study design for equine nutrition studies is by necessity very specific and so cannot always be extrapolated to the wider population – unlike food-producing animals, the output is much less defined. Most equine nutrition research is privately funded by manufacturers or companies owned by the manufacturer (e.g Waltham Centre of Equine Studies[xii] and Spillers Horse Feed[xiii] are both owned by Mars Inc[xiv]) or by

Table 8.6 Steps that manufacturers can take to increase sustainability of quality horse feed

Action points	Solutions and initiatives
Raw materials	Local versus imported – most businesses source 70% of their crops within a close radius of production facilities
Novel ingredients: algae and insects	Algae could provide a major nutritionally rich biomass; they are already recognised as a prime source of omega-3 fatty acids (Coffey *et al.*, 2016) Entocycle[a], the UK's first large-scale farm breeding insects, is developing novel alternatives to soya for animal feed and pet food Start to familiarise your clients with idea of using insects as ingredient in horse feed for when the legislation catches up.
Sources of soya and rapeseed meal	Soya is the main source of vegetable protein in herbivore feeds and it has a huge carbon cost – many companies are starting to use rapeseed meal as UK-grown alternative If soya is used, is the company taking proportionate steps to ensure that it is not grown on deforested land? Are they part of the UK Sustainable Soya Sourcing?
By-products: Wheat/oat feed Soya hulls Sugar beet pulp	Incorporating by-products from human cereal and sugar manufacturing reduces food waste and provides very valuable fibre for horse feed – with the benefit that it was produced to human food grade
Reduced inputs	Oats compared with other cereals require much lower inputs of chemicals
Packaging	Check how sacks are made; for example, sacks are manufactured in a facility that is powered by their own on-site solar panels and the materials used in bags are 100% recyclable, including the oil resistant liners Are they members of Valpak[b]?
Transport	Are they moving towards using waste feed oil or ethanol in lorries and manufacturing plants
Climate Change Levy	Do they belong to the climate change discount levy? Are they investigating the use of biomass? (Nitsche *et al.*, 2017)
Premixes (vitamins and minerals)	Do they buy from premix companies that have a clear sustainability commitment?

[a]https://www.entocycle.com/; [b]https://www.valpak.co.uk/

partners that work alongside them (such as Saracen Horse Feeds[xv] and KER[xvi]).

The nutritional requirements to support a healthy horse have been researched extensively and manufacturers use this published research (NRC, 2007) to ensure that their formulations provide the recommended intake of nutrients for the horse at different life stages and workloads.

Look for evidence base for individual ingredients: for yeast (van Dorland *et al.*, 2019), Yea Sacc is approved by the EU for equine use based on extensive research; the digestible energy (DE) (Cuddeford *et al.*, 1992) and the digestibility of calcium in alfalfa compared with hay (Cuddeford *et al.*, 1990) has been established. Fructans (fructooligosaccharides, FOS) alongside soaking hay have been researched as an adjunct to improve insulin sensitivity in equine metabolic syndrome (EMS) horses (McGowan *et al.*, 2013). There is plenty of evidence base for the digestibility of certain cereals and their physiological effect in the horse (Jose-Cunilleras *et al.*, 2004; Vervuert *et al.*, 2003, 2004, 2007, 2008) as well as the implications of feeding management of ingredients and feeds (Vervuert *et al.*, 2009a,b).

Feeds formulated specifically as nutritional treatment or therapy must be evidence based[xvii] (see Chapter 7, Table 7.2: 'Descriptors for feed approved for particular nutritional purposes for horses'); if you request sight of that evidence, businesses must share that information with you. Whilst disorders of the small intestine are covered, there is no provision for gastric ulceration or laminitis. In the UK, BETA has developed a Code of Good Labelling practice in partnership with Veterinary Medicines Directive (for medicinal claims) and Food Standards Agency (for feed labelling). The code available from BETA permits claims for the nutritional support of horses and ponies prone to laminitis and gastric ulcers, if specific dietary specifications are met.

Every chapter in this book provides the backbone of evidence base on which equine nutritional advice and feed formulation are based.

Summary

The production of quality horse feed is an extremely controlled and monitored business, transparently audited – the result of nutritional, production, raw material investment backed with clear ethical intent.

The following checklist should guide you in picking a quality feed – accepting the fact that not all feeds are equal in terms of the below.

- Where are the feeds produced and manufactured?
  - Can this plant be visited?
- Who formulates the feeds? What are their credentials and does your nutritionist play an active role?
- Do they have an equine nutritionist? Are they available for consultation or questions?
  - What are their qualifications?
  - Do they support vets?
- What quality control measures are used to assure the consistency and quality of your feeds?
  - Are they independently audited?
  - Are they a member of UFAS and NOPS and BETA?
  - Do they follow the BETA Feed Code of Practice?
  - Are their feeds tested by nutrient analysis and do they carry out feed trials?
- Will the company provide you with a complete nutrient analysis or data sheet for the product you want to advise?
  - What is the estimated digestible energy of the feed?
    - How did they calculate it?
    - Does a rough estimate using the raw materials provide you with a similar ballpark figure?
- What research do they do and where are the results published?

The old adage of 'quality in equates to quality out' (QIQO) is very pertinent in the production of horse feed.

Notes

[i] https://www.beta-uk.org/pages/feed-safety/beta-nops-scheme.php
[ii] AAFCO: https://www.aafco.org
[iii] FEFAC: https://fefac.eu
[iv] BHA (2004): http://w.com/resources/about/whatwedo/disciplinary/disciplinaryDetail.asp?item=083611
[v] https://www.icmsf.org
[vi] BHA (2021): https://www.britishhorseracing.com/regulation/anti-doping-medication-control/prohibited-substances/
[vii] BHA (2021): https://www.britishhorseracing.com/regulation/anti-doping-medication-control/prohibited-substances/
[viii] BETA: https://www.beta-uk.org
[ix] AIC: https://www.agindustries.org.uk
[x] FSA: https://www.food.gov.uk
[xi] AfN: https://www.associationfornutrition.org/register/search-the-register
[xii] https://www.winergy.com/about-waltham
[xiii] https://www.spillers-feeds.com
[xiv] https://www.mars.com/
[xv] https://saracenhorsefeeds.com
[xvi] https://ker.com/
[xvii] https://www.legislation.gov.uk/eur/2020/354

Bibliography

Akande, K.E., Abubakar, M.M., Adegbola, T.A. and Bogoro, S.E. (2006) Nutritional and health implications of mycotoxins in animal feeds: a review. *Pakistan Journal of Nutrition* 5(5), 398–403.

Anonymous (2008) European Standard EN ISO 9001-2008 Quality Management Systems: Requirements (English version).

CAC (1999) *Codex Alimentarius Commission - Principles and Guidelines for the Conduct of a Microbiological Risk Assessment*. FAO, Rome. CAC/GL-30.

Carey, A. and Lambrecht, E.D. (2008) Some commonly fed herbs and other functional foods in equine nutrition: a review. *The Veterinary Journal* 178(1), 21–31. doi: 10.1016/j.tvjl.2007.06.004.

Casado, R.M., Parsons, D.J., Weightman, R.M., Magan, N. and Origgi, S. (2009) Modelling a two-dimensional spatial distribution of mycotoxin concentration in bulk commodities to design effective and efficient sample selection strategies. *Food Additives and Contaminants* 26(9), 1298–1305.

Coffey, D., Dawson, K., Ferket, P. and Connolly, A. (2016) Review of the feed industry from a historical perspective and implications for its future. *Journal of Applied Animal Nutrition* 4.

Cuddeford, D., Woodhead, A. and Muirhead, R. (1990) Potential of alfalfa as a source of calcium for calcium deficient horses. *The Veterinary Record* 126(17), 425–429.

Cuddeford, D., Woodhead, A. and Muirhead, R. (1992) A comparison nutritive value of short-cutting cycle, high temperature-dried alfalfa and timothy hay for horses. *Equine Veterinary Journal* 24(2), 84–89.

Diekman, M.A. and Green, M.L. (1992) Mycotoxins and reproduction in domestic livestock. *Journal of Animal Science* 70(5), 1615–1627.

EFSA (2009) Analysis of the baseline survey on the prevalence of Salmonella in holdings with breeding pigs in the EU, 2008 – Part A: salmonella prevalence estimates. *EFSA Journal* 7(12), 1277. doi: 10.2903/j.efsa.2009.1277

Elghandour, M.M., Reddy, P.R.K., Salem, A.Z., Reddy, P.P.R., Hyder, I. *et al.* (2018) Plant bioactives and extracts as feed additives in horse nutrition. *Journal of Equine Veterinary Science* 69, 66–77.

Jose-Cunilleras, E., Taylor, L.E. and Hinchcliff, K.W. (2004) Glycemic index of cracked corn, oat groats and rolled barley in horses. *Journal of Animal Science* 82, 2623–2629.

Kamphues, J., (2013) Feed hygiene and related disorders in horses. In: Geor, R.J., Harris, P.A. and Coenen, M. (eds) *Equine Applied and Clinical Nutrition*. Saunders, Philadelphia, Pennsylvania, pp. 367–380.

Leung, M.C., Díaz-Llano, G. and Smith, T.K. (2006) Mycotoxins in pet food: a review on worldwide prevalence and preventative strategies. *Journal of Agricultural and Food Chemistry* 54(26), 9623–9635.

McGowan, C.M., Dugdale, A.H., Pinchbeck, G.L. and Argo, C.M. (2013) Dietary restriction in combination with a nutraceutical supplement for the management of equine metabolic syndrome in horses. *The Veterinary Journal* 196(2), 153–159.

Mikešová, K., Härtlová, H., Zita, L., Chmelikova, E., Hůlková, M. *et al.* (2014) Effect of evening primrose oil on biochemical parameters of thoroughbred horses under maximal training conditions. *Czech Journal of Animal Science* 59(10), 488–493.

Newman, K.E. and Raymond, S.L. (2005) Effects of mycotoxins in horses. In: Diaz, D. (ed.) *The Mycotoxin Blue Book*. Nottingham University Press, pp. 57–76.

Nitsche, M., Hensgen, F. and Wachendorf, M. (2017) Energy generation from horse husbandry residues by anaerobic digestion, combustion, and an integrated approach. *Sustainability* 9(3), 358. doi: 10.3390/su9030358.

NRC (National Research Council) (2007) *Nutrient Requirements of Horses. Sixth Revised Edition*. National Academies Press, Washington, DC. doi: 10.17226/11653.

Reilly, J.D., Hopegood, L., Gould, L. and Devismes, L. (1998) Effect of a supplementary dietary evening primrose oil mixture on hoof growth, hoof growth rate and hoof lipid fractions in horses: a controlled and blinded trial. *Equine Veterinary Journal* 30(S26), 58–65.

Schulz, A.K., Kersten, S., Dänicke, S., Coenen, M. and Vervuert, I. (2015) Effects of deoxynivalenol in naturally contaminated wheat on feed intake and health status of horses. *Mycotoxin Research* 31(4), 209–216.

Shurson, G.C. (2020) What a waste. Can we improve sustainability of food animal production systems by recycling food waste streams into animal feed in an era of health, climate, and economic crises? Available at: https://blog-swine.extension.umn.edu/2020/11/what-waste-can-we-improve.html (accessed 10 May 2022)

Tavman, S., Otles, S., Glaue, S. and Gogus, N. (2019) Food preservation technologies. In: Galanakis, C.M. (ed.) *Saving Food: Production, Supply Chain, Food Waste and Food Consumption*. Academic Press, London, pp. 117–140.

van Dorland, A., Janett, F., Bruckmaier, R., Wach-Gygax, L., Jeannerat, E. *et al.* (2019) Herbal yeast product, Equi-Strath®, alters the antioxidant status of stallion semen. *Animal Reproduction Science* 208, 106119.

Vervuert, I., Coenen, M. and Bothe, C. (2003) Effects of oat processing on the glycaemic and insulin responses in horses. *Journal of Animal Physiology and Animal Nutrition* 87(3–4), 96–104.

Vervuert, I., Coenen, M. and Bothe, C. (2004) Effects of corn processing on the glycaemic and insulinaemic responses in horses. *Journal of Animal Physiology and Animal Nutrition* 88(9–10), 348–355.

Vervuert, I., Bothe, C. and Coenen, M. (2007) Glycaemic and insulinaemic responses to mechanical or thermal processed barley in horses. *Journal of Animal Physiology and Animal Nutrition* 91(5–6), 263–268.

Vervuert, I., Voigt, K., Hollands, T., Cuddeford, D. and Coenen, M. (2008) Effects of processing barley on its digestion by horses. *Veterinary Record* 162(21), 684–688.

Vervuert, I., Voigt, K., Hollands, T., Cuddeford, D. and Coenen, M. (2009a) The effect of mixing and changing the order of feeding oats and chopped alfalfa to horses on: glycaemic and insulinaemic responses, and breath hydrogen and methane production. *Journal of Animal Physiology and Animal Nutrition* 93(5), 631–638.

Vervuert, I., Voigt, K., Hollands, T., Cuddeford, D. and Coenen, M. (2009b) Effect of feeding increasing quantities of starch on glycaemic and insulinaemic responses in healthy horses. *The Veterinary Journal* 182(1), 67–72.

Whitaker, T.B. (2006) Sampling foods for mycotoxins. *Food Additives and Contaminants* 23(1), 50–61.

9 Which Fibre? Choosing a Forage and Understanding a Forage Analysis

Teresa Hollands

School of Veterinary Medicine, University of Surrey

Learning Objectives

LO1 Be able to read and understand a forage analysis.
LO2 Relate the role of fibre/forages in relation to the anatomy and physiology of the horse's digestive system.
LO3 Explain the relationship between forage feeding management and eating behaviour.
LO4 Maintain dry matter intake of horses eating forages that are high in water – haylage and grass.
LO5 Explain how to manage forage feeding to replicate the horse's normal feeding behaviour and minimise the development of nutritionally related diseases.

On completion of this chapter, you will be able to use forage analysis to choose a forage that is most appropriate for the horse relative to its workload and fat score and advise clients on the best feeding management to maintain gut health.

Introduction

It has been stated elsewhere in this book that forage and, more importantly, fibre are of fundamental importance to the horse's health and should be the foundation of the diet. Chapter 4 discussed the different types of forages available to your clients. This chapter explains the practical aspects of feeding forage and assumes an understanding of the pros and cons of the different forages your client might have on their yard.

Interpreting Forage Analysis

A forage analysis is only as good as the sampling technique (see Chapter 4: 'Sampling hay or haylage for analysis'); clearly a handful of forage taken from one bale will not be representative of the stack nor indeed the field. For many single-horse owners who might not buy their hay/haylage in bulk, a forage analysis is just academic; instead consult that year's typical analysis from the farming press.

Most horse feed companies will offer a complementary forage analysis for vets and large yards; and for owners who do buy in their annual supply of hay from one supplier, the cost is not expensive unless you want a mineral analysis.

There are two methods of forage analysis commonly used: (i) wet chemistry/proximate analysis, which is the most accurate and involves the dissolution of various nutrients with chemicals and thus is used less frequently; and (ii) near-infrared (NIR), which produces different wavelengths/curves depending on the concentration of the nutrient.

NIR requires calibrating on a regular basis with wet chemistry and is only as accurate as the last calibration – check that the laboratory you are using takes part in ring testing and calibrates their equipment regularly. Many agricultural labs do not have calibrations suitable for horse forages/pasture, because they analyse mostly cattle forages – the giveaway is that they declare energy as metabolisable energy (ME). Germany has started to develop ME values

DOI: 10.1079/9781789245134.0009

for horses (Coenen *et al.*, 2011) so this may change in the future.

Be wary of any company that does not provide an interpretation of the results together with their lab's means and ranges – just as you would expect from any 'diagnostic' test.

Haylage analysis

All reputable companies should provide your client's results together with a typical range and results on both a dry-matter and as-fed basis (Fig. 9.1).

When checking a forage report, make sure that the descriptors relate to the type of forage the client sent to the lab and that the interpretation matches the analysis and is not too generic (Fig. 9.2). If the results are provided as dry matter (DM), then so should the interpretation.

Please remember that any wet forage (haylage and grass) should be sampled, sealed and sent immediately (preferably having booked your lab slot first) at the beginning of the week to minimise any postal delay; loss of water will impact on the results. The results from haylage and grass samples sent to the USA will be of limited value, due to the changes in dry matter content.

Hay analysis

There will be no pH or lactic acid on a hay analysis report; interpret the nutrient values – the means and ranges will differ (Fig. 9.3) because the grass is harvested later than grass harvested for haylage. It is useful to have UK ranges for forages, as they do differ from grass crops in the USA. Most UK hays are low in water-soluble carbohydrates (but this will vary according to year, time of cutting and grass varieties).

You can learn a lot about the quality of hay (but not its nutrient content) by looking at it and smelling it – teach your clients to be observant (Table 9.1, p. 179).

Interpreting the analytes

All forages are low in minerals (reflective of where they are grown), whereas vitamin content reflects the speed and efficiency of the drying process. Haylage retains more vitamins compared with hay, but the micronutrients will only be as good as the original grass crop. Most grazing in the UK does not provide recommended intakes of minerals (Jones *et al* 2005a,b). Unless there is a specific pathology related to mineral deficiency or excess (see Chapter 6: Tables 6.2, 6.3, 6.4 and 6.5), recommend a good vitamin and mineral supplement or appropriate hard feed – all of which are formulated to balance the nutrient deficiencies in UK forages, rather than paying for a mineral analysis of their forages. Table 9.2, p. 180, provides a quick summary of the analytes.

The Role of Fibre and Forage

Feeding behaviour

Horses are unique as herbivores because they mechanically process their food completely before swallowing – unlike ruminants that regurgitate and rabbits that practise caecotrophy. Their grazing behaviour also differs, as they move continuously to trickle-graze throughout the day.

Horses have a psychological need to chew. Horses naturally chew for 16–18 h out of 24 h; ideally this is met by a minimum dry matter intake of a low-quality forage equivalent to 2.5% of their bodyweight to meet their appetite without provision of excess calories; when prevented from doing so they are at higher risk of developing stereotypies and obesity. Horses only produce saliva when they are physically chewing; saliva buffers the upper stomach from the acidic lower stomach. Wild horses spend 62% more time moving, 20% less time eating and 30% more time resting compared with the same herd in captivity (Boyd and Bandi, 2002).

Forages should not be meal fed but managed to stimulate the natural trickle-grazing behaviour when horses travel to seek out grazing, rarely eating large meals of forage (or concentrates) in one graze but taking a few bites of grass before walking a few steps to a new area to graze (Duncan, 1980). Fibre (plant cell walls) is essential for hind gut health. Clearly domestication changes the natural eating behaviour of horses. Feed-seeking behaviour decreases to walking 5–15 steps/min during paddock grazing (Matsui *et al.*, 1990).

As workload increases, horses are taken off grazing and kept in stables, further reducing their feed-seeking to less than 5 steps/min during feeding (Matsui *et al.*, 1990). Forage intake is generally reduced, sometimes by 50%, despite a recommendation of maintaining forage intake at 2% BW (Coenen *et al.*, 2011), and replaced by concentrates, reducing their feeding time because they spend less time chewing concentrates compared with forages on a dry matter basis, (Bochnia *et al.*, 2019). Horses complete a full lateral chewing pattern, take longer to chew and chew more slowly when fed forage compared with when they chew

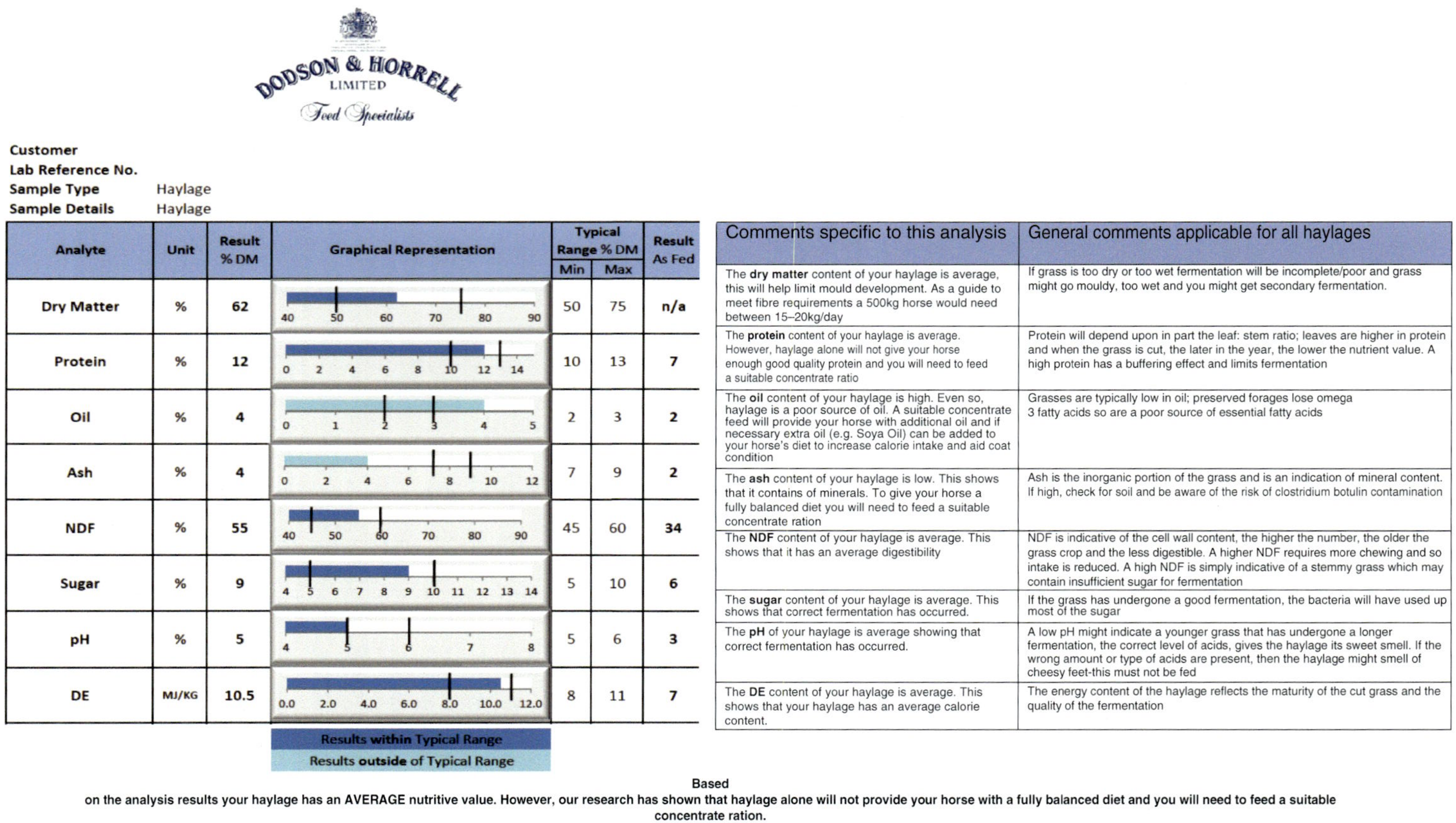

DODSON & HORRELL LIMITED Feed Specialists

Customer
Lab Reference No.
Sample Type Haylage
Sample Details Haylage

Analyte	Unit	Result % DM	Graphical Representation	Typical Range % DM Min	Typical Range % DM Max	Result As Fed
Dry Matter	%	62	40 50 60 70 80 90	50	75	n/a
Protein	%	12	0 2 4 6 8 10 12 14	10	13	7
Oil	%	4	0 1 2 3 4 5	2	3	2
Ash	%	4	0 2 4 6 8 10 12	7	9	2
NDF	%	55	40 50 60 70 80 90	45	60	34
Sugar	%	9	4 5 6 7 8 9 10 11 12 13 14	5	10	6
pH	%	5	4 5 6 7 8	5	6	3
DE	MJ/KG	10.5	0.0 2.0 4.0 6.0 8.0 10.0 12.0	8	11	7

Results within Typical Range
Results outside of Typical Range

Comments specific to this analysis	General comments applicable for all haylages
The **dry matter** content of your haylage is average, this will help limit mould development. As a guide to meet fibre requirements a 500kg horse would need between 15–20kg/day	If grass is too dry or too wet fermentation will be incomplete/poor and grass might go mouldy, too wet and you might get secondary fermentation.
The **protein** content of your haylage is average. However, haylage alone will not give your horse enough good quality protein and you will need to feed a suitable concentrate ratio	Protein will depend upon in part the leaf: stem ratio; leaves are higher in protein and when the grass is cut, the later in the year, the lower the nutrient value. A high protein has a buffering effect and limits fermentation
The **oil** content of your haylage is high. Even so, haylage is a poor source of oil. A suitable concentrate feed will provide your horse with additional oil and if necessary extra oil (e.g. Soya Oil) can be added to your horse's diet to increase calorie intake and aid coat condition	Grasses are typically low in oil; preserved forages lose omega 3 fatty acids so are a poor source of essential fatty acids
The **ash** content of your haylage is low. This shows that it contains of minerals. To give your horse a fully balanced diet you will need to feed a suitable concentrate ration	Ash is the inorganic portion of the grass and is an indication of mineral content. If high, check for soil and be aware of the risk of clostridium botulin contamination
The **NDF** content of your haylage is average. This shows that it has an average digestibility	NDF is indicative of the cell wall content, the higher the number, the older the grass crop and the less digestible. A higher NDF requires more chewing and so intake is reduced. A high NDF is simply indicative of a stemmy grass which may contain insufficient sugar for fermentation
The **sugar** content of your haylage is average. This shows that correct fermentation has occurred.	If the grass has undergone a good fermentation, the bacteria will have used up most of the sugar
The **pH** of your haylage is average showing that correct fermentation has occurred.	A low pH might indicate a younger grass that has undergone a longer fermentation, the correct level of acids, gives the haylage its sweet smell. If the wrong amount or type of acids are present, then the haylage might smell of cheesy feet-this must not be fed
The **DE** content of your haylage is average. This shows that your haylage has an average calorie content.	The energy content of the haylage reflects the maturity of the cut grass and the quality of the fermentation

Based on the analysis results your haylage has an AVERAGE nutritive value. However, our research has shown that haylage alone will not provide your horse with a fully balanced diet and you will need to feed a suitable concentrate ration.

Fig. 9.1 An example of a useful haylage analysis report and interpretation. Used with permission of Dodson and Horrell Limited.

Information provided in haylage report	Clarification of interpretation
Digestible Energy - This is a measure of the energy available in your forage. In the UK this is measured in MJ/kg. A digestible energy content of around 8MJ/kg is average in the UK. Lower than this level and you will have to feed more forage to maintain weight, higher than this level and you will need to feed less	The amount of **calories** a horse needs from and workload. It is always best to advise forage as the main calorie supply. If the horse is putting on weight, do not reduce DMI rather change to a lower calorie forage.
Crude Protein - This is a measure of the total protein in the sample including true protein and non-protein nitrogen. A protein level of around 8% is adequate; however, protein levels in the UK are usually much lower than this. Where your report shows a poor protein level, below 8%, you should check the amount of forage fed is covering the protein requirements of your horse. The report does not inform about the individual amino acids that make up the protein in your hay. We have included a nitrogen/sulphur ratio which is an indication of protein quality; however, this will only be calculated if you have also carried out a full mineral analysis of the forage as well as a nutritional analysis. When the ratio of nitrogen/sulphur is above 10 then this indicates poor protein quality, so supplementation with methionine and other essential amino acids is recommended along with feeding other high protein sources such as copra, linseed or alfalfa. Many forages in the UK report above this 10:1 figure so many horses need supplementing with extra individual amino acid.	No preserved forage in the UK provides adequate **protein** quality which is why you will recommend a balancer. This haylage looks to be high in protein but it is a very wet sample so clients would need to consider DMI
Lysine - This is an estimated level and in the UK the average is usually lower than needed for maintenance of horses even on adlib forage. An average 500 kg horse needs around 25 lysine for maintenance, if working this level will need to be higher. For this reason, we recommend 10 grams of supplementation per day for an adult horse. Performance horses will need at least 20 grams extra, pregnant, lactating mares and young horses 30 grams extra	If fed a feed or Balancer suitable for the workload, the diet will be balanced in **lysine**
Acid Detergent Fibre and Neutral Detergent Fibre – These figures measure fibres (there are 5 types). The higher the ADF and NDF values are, the more lignin the hay contains and the more of this type of hay your horse will have to eat to maintain their weight. The ideal ADF value is less than 35% and the ideal NDF value is less than 45%. However, most hays have values that are 10% higher than these ideal levels. Levels 10% or more than the ideal level is not a problem but to compensate your horse will need to consume more of this type of hay.	Although the explanatory notes refer to hay, this is a haylage analysis. A horse that is a good doer will be better fed hay with a high **NDF** rather than haylage as they will get less calories, a performance horse needs a higher nutritive value forage with a lower NDF
Water-Soluble Carbohydrates (WSC) - This is a measure of the simple sugar and fructan levels in the forage. It has been thought in the past that fructan can contribute to laminitis; however, the amount of fructan contained in forage has not been shown to be a problem so it is now thought the levels of simple sugar and starch are the values to be aware of when trying to control laminitis in horses. **Ethanol-Soluble Carbohydrates (ESC)** - This is a subset of WSC with-out the fructan fraction and includes primarily monosaccharides and disaccharides. These simple sugars are digested in the foregut and raise insulin levels. Too much can lead to laminitis because of elevated blood insulin. The ESC measure gives you a much better idea of the simple sugar level. This combined with the starch level is the figure that you should be interested in when controlling laminitis in horse. Dr Kellon and the ECIR Crushing's Group have found the ideal level for managing Laminitic horses is an ESC and Starch combination of below 10%. Rinsing hay will reduce the sugar but you need to rinse in a specific way that is like washing detergent out of clothes	It would be unusual to find high levels of **sugars** in haylage as they are used up by the bacteria that ferment the grass. NEVER advise soaking haylage as secondary fermentation might take place. Horses still need to consume adequate dry matter even when fat but should be fed low calorie forages
Starch – This compound is normally digested in the foregut into individual glucose (blood sugar) molecules; therefore, it has a strong elevating effect on blood insulin levels. You cannot lower starch levels by soaking or rinsing hay or haylage. It is therefore wise to feed hay or haylage which is low in starch. As stated above it is wise to feed hay to IR/Laminitic horses which has a combined ESC and Starch amount of less than 10%. Some horses will do better on an even lower percentage so experimenting with rinsing hay below the 10% level is also sometimes necessary	Grasses do not store **starch,** only in their seed heads – if there is starch, it might be indicative of some clover or other legume

Sample Details
.ab Reference:
Sample Type: Haylage
Sample Received:
Order Number:

Dietary Nutritional Report (values are based on 100% dry matter basis)

Dry Matter (as sampled)	Analysis	Units
Dry Matter	48.3	%
Digestible Energy	**Mcal/kg**	**MJ/kg**
Digestible Energy	2.33	9.76
Nutritional Analysis	**%**	**g/kg**
Crude Protein	21.6	216.0
Estimated Lysine	1.0	9.5
Acid Detergent Fibre (ADF)	38.0	380.0
Neutral Detergent Fibre (NDF)	44.6	446.0
Water Soluble carbohydrates (WSC)	4.7	47.0
Ethanol Soluble Carbohydrates (ESC)	3.0	30.0
Starch	1.3	13.0
Non-Fibre Carbohydrates (NFC)	20.8	208.0
Nitrate Analysis	**Units**	
%Nitrate (below)	Not Tested	%
PPM Nitrate-Nitrogen (below)	Not Tested	ppm
Nitrogen / Sulphur Ratio		
Nitrogen / Sulphur Ratio		

Digestible Energy This is a measure of the energy available in your forage. In the UK this is measured in MJ/kg. A digestible energy content of around 8MJ/kg is average in the UK. Lower than this level and you will have to feed more forage to maintain weight, higher than this level and you will need to feed less.

Fig. 9.2 An example of a haylage forage report whose interpretation is not compatible with the analysis. (Left-hand column explains the discrepancies.). Used with Permission.

DODSON & HORRELL
LIMITED
Feed Specialists

Forage Analysis Report

Customer nds **Lab Reference No.** 1

Sample Details Hay **Sample Type** Hay

Based on the analysis results your hay has an AVERAGE nutritive value. However, our research has shown that hay alone will not provide your horse with a fully balanced diet and you will need to feed a suitable concentrate ration.

Analyte	Result % DM	Guide	Average Range % DM	Comments	Result As Fed
Dry Matter %	84	Low	85 – 90	The dry matter content of your hay is low and it contains a high amount of water. High water content may increase the risk of mould development; mouldy hay should not be fed. As a guide to meet total fibre requirements a 500kg horse would need between: 9 – 15 kg/day or 20 – 33 lbs/day	n/a
Protein %	8	Average	6 – 9	The protein content of your hay is average. However, hay alone will not give your horse enough good quality protein and you will need to feed a suitable concentrate ration.	7
Oil %	2	Average	2 – 3	The oil content of your hay is average. However, hay is a poor source of oil. A suitable concentrate feed will provide your horse with additional oil and if necessary extra oil (e.g. Soya Oil) can be added to your horse's diet to increase calorie intake and aid coat condition.	2
Ash %	6	Average	6 – 10	The ash content of your hay is average. This shows that it contains average levels of minerals. However, hay alone will not provide you horse with a fully balanced diet and you will still need to feed a suitable concentrate ration or vitamin and mineral supplement.	5
NDF %	70	High	50 – 65	The NDF content of your hay is high. This shows that it contains more mature indigestible fibre. This means it has a lower nutritional value but indigestible fibre is a normal part of your horse's diet.	59
DE MJ/kg	8.0	Average	8 – 10	The DE content of your hay is average. This shows that your hay has an average calorie content.	6.7
Sugars %	8	Average	8 – 10	The sugar content of your hay is average. The sugar level will vary depending on the time of day, weather conditions and the stage of plant growth during harvest.	7

This analysis was undertaken using NIR. It represents the sample received and should only be used as a guide to overall quality. Water (moisture) is contained in forages and the water content can vary, grass typically has a high water content whereas hay has a lower water content. Nutrient analyses expressed as dry matter (DM) represent the percentages of nutrients present excluding water content. Nutrient analyses expressed as as fed include this water component and is what your horse consumes as fresh forage.

Authorised By:

11/04/2013

DODSON & HORRELL LIMITED

Fig. 9.3 A useful hay analysis which provides ranges, results on a dry-matter and as-fed basis.

pellets (Bonin *et al.*, 2007) and are thus less likely to develop dental irregularities.

Despite these changes in husbandry, you can still advise managing fibre feeding, maintaining ration dry matter intake (DMI) at 2.5% BW, maintaining a healthy digestive system and normal feeding behaviour.

Chewing behaviour

A meta-analysis (Auer *et al.*, 2021) of the time budgets of 144 horses established that the horses (25% free-ranging; 17% in semi-reserve and 58% domesticated) spent between 10% and 66% of 24 h

Table 9.1 Hay characteristics that can be visually appraised to judge suitability for feeding to horses.

Sensory evaluation	Description/comment
Visual Stage of maturity	Look for the presence of seed heads (grass forages) or flowers or seed pods (legumes), indicating more mature forages
Leaf-to-stem ratio	Are the stems or leaves more obvious; good-quality legume forages will have a high proportion of leaves, and stems will be less obvious and fine
Colour	Colour is not a good indicator of nutrient content, but bright green colour suggests minimal oxidation; yellow hay indicates oxidation and bleaching from sun, and hay will have lower vitamins A and E content
Foreign objects	Look for presence and the amount of inanimate objects (twine, wire, cans, etc.), weeds, mould, or poisonous plants
Touch	Feel stiffness or coarseness of leaves and stems; see if alfalfa stems wrap around your finger without breaking; good-quality hay will feel soft and have fine, pliable stems
Smell	Good quality hay will have a fresh mowed grass odour; no musty or mouldy odours

either eating or foraging; with free-ranging spending the most time eating and foraging.

When eating, horses chew about once per second and only swallow food when it has been mechanically processed to less than 4 mm (mean 1.6 mm) in length (Mueller *et al*., 1998).

Horses produce 1 mm saliva at every chew; the number of chews varies depending on the forage or feedstuffs that the client is feeding the horse (Table 9.3, p. 181).

It is important that the dry matter of a horse is maintained at 2.5% BW, with a minimum of 50% forage (1.25% BW) on a dry weight basis for performance horses to ensure adequate saliva production.

Chewing and fibre content of forages

The amount of time a horse spends chewing its forage depends on the ratio of cell wall to cell content. The amount of cell wall (NDF) (Fig. 9.4) in the forage will determine how long the horse needs to chew; mature plants contain more cell wall (higher NDF) and need more chewing compared with younger forages.

In ruminant nutrition, forage intake rate is advised not just on bodyweight but also a minimum and maximum intake of NDF. High-yielding dairy cows must have their intake of high-NDF forage restricted (it takes them too long to eat), otherwise they cannot eat enough calories. We do not tend to ration NDF intake of horses, as even a racehorse needs 62% less digestible energy (DE)/day compared with a dairy cow producing 50 l of milk; but you will intuitively be recommending forages with different NDF depending upon the workload of the horse.

Chewing fibre is of psychological and physiological importance to the horse, so do take advantage of the time needed to chew high-NDF forage, especially for the fatter horse.

Horses take 2½ times (98 min/kg NDF) longer to eat 1 kg of barley straw (78% NDF/kg DM) compared with 1 kg meadow hay (52% NDF/kg DM; 56 min/kg NDF) (Brokner *et al*., 2008). Horses took longer to eat late-season haylage (August cut: 36 min/kg DM) compared with that cut earlier (June cut: 29 min/kg) (Muller, 2012) – a reflection of the NDF content.

Stomach health

Leaving horses without forage for more than 6 h (Luthersson *et al*., 2009) or reducing forage below 1.25% BW (DM) (see Chapter 12: 'Equine gastric ulcer syndrome (EGUS)') is associated with an increased risk of the horse developing gastric ulcers.

Horses on poor grazing as part of a weight management regime might be at increased risk of ulceration unless other low-nutritive-value forage is provided to ensure saliva production. Ensure that clients substitute a lack of grass with alternative low-calorie forages. Horses that had gastric ulcers when left out on winter grazing had an improvement in gastric ulcer scores when brought in and fed hay for 14 days (1.5% BW) and grain (0.5% BW) (Woodward *et al*., 2014).

Hind gut health

Remind clients that if they do not feed enough fibre, as well as affecting hind gut health, it can impact on their horse's behaviour. Replacing forage (8 kg) with concentrates (6 kg) changes the VFA profile of the hind gut (if the starch is not fed in small meals < 1 g starch/kg BW/meal) with an increase in caecal propionate. High levels of propionate are correlated

Table 9.2 A summary of the analytes of a forage analysis

Analyte	Hay	Haylage
Moisture	Be concerned if over 15% – more likely to go mouldy If more than 25% moisture, get it out of the barn quickly and de-stack: it is a fire risk	Be concerned if under 50% as likely to be more acidic or if over 70% incomplete fermentation
Dry matter	Some people talk about dry hay being brittle; if drier than 90%, unlikely in the UK All alfalfa chaffs are dried to 90% DM	If drier than 75%, then unlikely to be enough moisture for fermentation High DM 'haylage' might go mouldy rapidly when exposed to oxygen
Crude protein	60–90 g/kg DM Protein of UK hays is of low quality – will be balanced if on hard feed	100–130 g/kg DM More digestible compared with hay, because the grass was cut earlier in its growth stage
NDF (not so digestible fibre)	Horses need some NDF; can ferment up to 65% NDF The higher the NDF, the longer it takes to chew and the less the horse eats If very high, will reduce the amount of cell wall that can be fermented in the hind gut	Usually lower than hay – simply a reflection that the grass is not so mature and so the horse can extract more calories
Digestible energy	7–10 MJ/kg DM A horse on ad lib hay can consume enough hay to meet calorie requirements for light work	8–11 MJ/kg DM If fed to meet DM requirements, then higher in calories and thus good for performance horses
Water-soluble carbohydrates (WSC)	Any sugar that dissolves in water – mono- and disaccharides and fructans	
Non-structural carbohydrates (NSC)	WSC plus starch – very few UK hays contain starch unless the grass has gone to seed (seeds store starch) Horses with insulin resistance (IR) should be fed hays/haylages with less than 10% NSC (limited evidence base); horses with polysaccharide storage myopathies (PSSM) should be fed hays with < 17% NSC (Borgia *et al.*, 2011) but all overweight horses (aka IR) should be fed soaked hay, which reduces calories. Haylage cannot be soaked	
Ethanol-soluble carbohydrates (ESC)	WSC without the fructans (fructans are not soluble in ethanol) – fructans are fermented by bacterial enzymes in the stomach and small intestine of the horse to volatile fatty acids – occasionally reaching the large intestine	

with an increase in the amount of time spent chewing wood, 2% versus 11%, respectively (Willard *et al.*, 1977) and an increase in cribbing and plasma endorphins (Gilham *et al.*, 1994).

The Relationship Between Forage Feeding Management and Eating Behaviour

Stereotypies

A large body of evidence shows that restricting fibre, whether for performance horses or to try to achieve weight loss, has a negative effect on the behaviour of the horse.

The development of behavioural pathologies such as stereotypies are common in horses fed a low-fibre, high-energy diet (Arena *et al.*, 2021). Horses unable to express their normal eating behaviour will find other means to express this behaviour.

Clients will typically keep overweight horses in a stable to restrict the amount of grass they can eat – which is rather strange because periods of 'bed rest' are not normally associated with a successful fat-loss regime; it would be much better to maintain an increased activity but limit the quantity and quality of grass.

Grass intake will vary according to the time of year (see Chapter 11, Fig. 11.1) but dry matter intake can be as high as 5% BW (Smith *et al.*, 2007). Given a choice between short grass (< 4.5 cm) and longer grass (15 cm), horses will spend more time consuming the longer grass in preference to the short grass (see Chapter 4: 'Growth stage') (Naujeck *et al.*, 2005).

Table 9.3 A comparison between the mean number of chews a horse eats and the feed provided

Feed	Chews/second	Chews/kg DM	Chews/g NDF	NDF (%DM)
[a]Alfalfa hay	1.23	1880	4.240	44.5
[a]Timothy hay	1.04	2540	4.270	59.4
[a]Mixed hay	1.13	3160	5.160	61.3
[a]Fresh grass (provided cut)	1.2	4610	7.970	57.8 (picked to match NDF of timothy hay)
[b]Muesli (horses vs ponies)	1.4 vs 1.43	1106 vs 1163		
[b]Oats (horses vs ponies)	1.28 vs 1.4	1215 vs 1163		
[b]High-fibre pellets (horses vs ponies)	1.43 vs 1.45	899 vs 1154		
[c]Hay pellets (horses vs ponies)	1.06 vs 1.35 10,036.8 chews/day			
[c]Hay	0.92–1.1 43, 476.5 chews/day			
[d]Donkeys legume/grass hay	0.88 120 min to eat 1 kg DM	6200	9.5	
[d]Donkeys grass hay	0.9 121 min to eat 1 kg DM	6500	9.9	

[a]Janis *et al*., (2010); [b]Bochnia *et al*. (2017); [c]Elia *et al*., (2010); [d]Mueller *et al*., (1998)

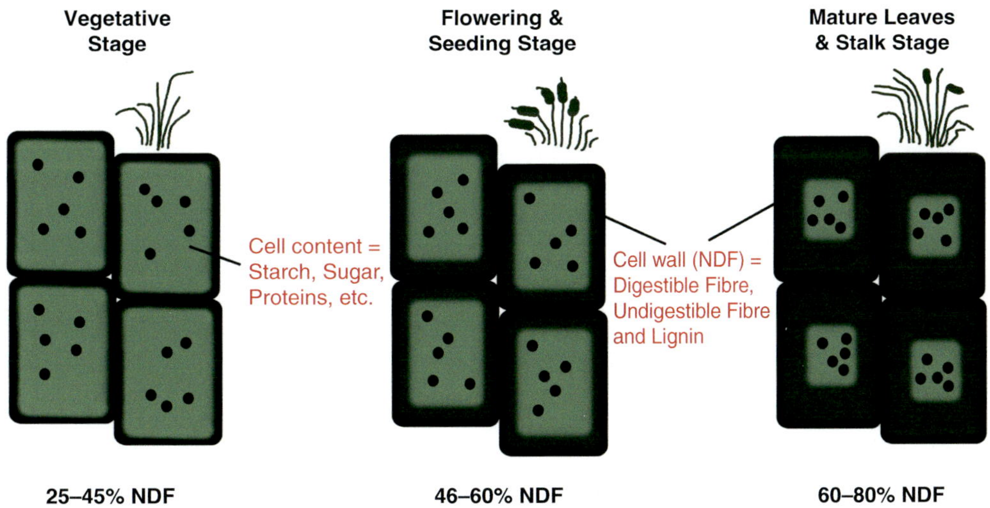

Fig. 9.4 The amount of neutral detergent fibre (cell walls) in forages at differing maturities. (Redrawn from various sources.)

Top tip

Poor nutritive value pasture (high NDF) takes feral horses longer to eat, which results in an 8% BW loss in the winter (Scheibe and Streich, 2003).

Please point out to clients that this level of fat loss is natural and should happen in leisure horses that are not ridden much in the winter.

Advising grazing to support normal feeding behaviour

Your aim should always be to maximise time in paddocks but provide clients with tips and tricks to restrict grass intake when necessary. Timing of turnout will depend upon the horse and whether you want to minimise the sugar content of the grass or replicate the natural eating bouts of wild horses, which in the northern hemisphere are highest between 0600–0800 h and 1800–2200 h (Boyd and Bandi, 2002) when temperatures are coolest.

A horse kept in a 1 acre field is likely to 'travel' about 4 km/day compared with feral horses that travel 17 km/day (Hampson *et al.*, 2010). The value of grazing is clear in terms of activity when compared with dressage horses moving between 1 km and 2.4 km in a hard 30–40 min training session (Hampson, 2010) or a racehorse that moves 2–3 km in each training session lasting up to 1 h maximum (Perkins *et al.*, 2005)

Using muzzles

If you recommend that a pony wears a muzzle, they will eat less grass (Fig. 9.5). Wearing a muzzle for 3 h reduces grass intake by 30% (Glunk *et al.*, 2013; Glunk, 2014). Muzzled ponies ate less grass (0.5 kg DM grass DMI 0.13% BW) in the autumn, compared with unmuzzled ponies (3.3 kg DM grass; DMI 0.8% BW) (Longland *et al.*, 2016). Wearing a muzzle in the summer reduces intake by 77%; in the spring by 78% and by 83% in the autumn (compared to unmuzzled ponies (Longland *et al.*, 2012). These ponies were subsequently stabled with hay – not ideal as they are likely to lose fitness compared with horses being exercised or kept at pasture (Graham-Thiers and Bowen, 2013). It would be better to advise longer periods of muzzling and turnout.

Muzzling for 10 h will reduce weight even if the pony tries to compensate for the rest of the 24 h. Horses that are pastured for 24/7 but muzzled for 10 h (0800–1800 h) during the summer (meadow grass sward height 8–10cm) had a daily mean weight loss of 0.04% BW compared with a daily 0.3% BW gain for those not muzzled over 7 days (Longland *et al.*, 2016). Reassuringly, restricting grazing for 12 h followed by 12 h grazing has no effect on hind gut pH or fluid balance (Siciliano and Schmitt, 2012)

Time-limiting grazing to reduce calories

If ponies have less time grazing, they cannot eat as much grass. Ponies grazing for 3 h over 6 weeks during the summer ate between 1.4 kg and 2.6 kg DM grass (dry matter intake of 0.49–0.91% BW), well below the recommended DMI. When subsequently stabled and provided with free access to haylage, they all ate enough dry matter haylage (1.6–2.2% BW) (Ince *et al.*, 2011) to mostly meet their recommended minimum of 2% BW (Coenen *et al.*, 2011).

If ponies have a limited time grazing, their hourly consumption rate is quicker than those left to graze for 24/7 (Glunk *et al.*, 2013) but they still eat fewer calories (Table 9.4), even accounting for the ad lib hay eaten when not grazing. If you choose to advise straw rather than hay, then the calorie reduction will be even greater.

Strip grazing

If you recommend strip grazing, then the ponies will eat less grass compared with free access. Ponies grazing grass in 10 m × 75 m paddocks (potential DMI of 1.5% BW/day) for 28 days ate less grass when strip grazed with either (i) a lead fence (1.8% DMI) or (ii) a lead fence and a fence restricting access to the back (1.6% DMI compared with horses not on strip grazing, 2.3% DMI) (Longland *et al.*, 2021). All ponies not in work are likely to gain weight on spring and summer grazing. Weight gain/body fat score will reflect their grass intake. Horses allowed unrestricted grass gained 4.28% BW (no restriction) compared with those restricted with

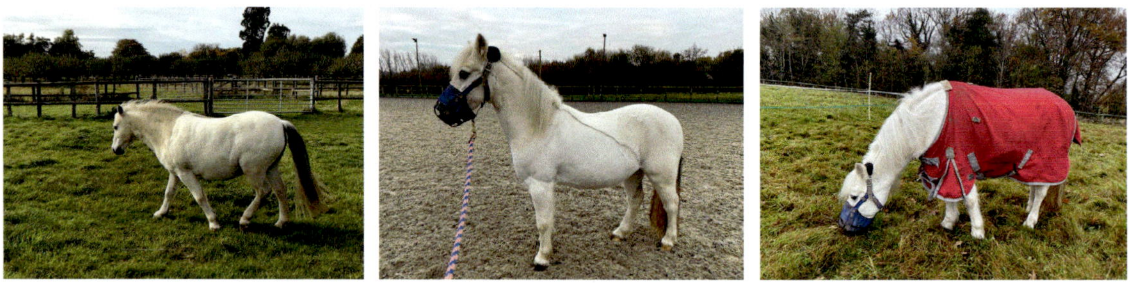

Fig. 9.5 The use of muzzles will result in weight loss if used correctly. Weight loss can be achieved even when using a rug, which should be lightweight only and used to keep the pony dry for riding. If not being ridden, then rugging is not necessary even if the pony is partially clipped. (Photo: Creative Marketing.)

just a lead fence (+1.82% BW) and with a lead and back fence (+ 1.5% BW) (Longland *et al.*, 2021). Remember to advise winter weight/fat loss.

Longland *et al.* (2021) measured the growth of the grass that was not grazed by ponies by fencing off an area. The grass not grazed increased from 15 cm to more mature stemmy grass of 30–50cm by weeks 3 and 4 but digestibility decreased from 58% (NDF 50%) to 44% (NDF 68%).

Track systems

There is very limited evidence as to the effect of track grazing systems on grass intake in horses. A conference proceeding suggested that horses on a track system versus a paddock grazed more in groups and ate from haynets more frequently but also moved more. There was no measurement of DMI or bodyweight changes.

Removing grass by mowing

Dry matter intake can be restricted by either 'over-grazing' with more horses or by removing the grass by mowing in tandem with any of the above options or as a stand-alone option.

Cutting the grass reduces the calorie content (sugar). Young growing grass has higher cell contents and is generally analysed with higher sugars compared with more mature grass. But actively growing grass uses up the sugars in growth and only stores excess sugars (as fructans, not starch) when able to photosynthesise but not grow (e.g. frost or drought) (see Chapter 4: 'Growth stage').

If your clients need further convincing that there is enough grass for their horses, they can do the supermarket bag test and poo pick (see Chapter 11: 'Measuring grass in the field'). Visually, it is helpful for clients to compare the growth and quantity of grass in their paddocks with grass growing just outside the fence (Fig. 9.6). The horses have been eating the equivalent of the grass growing outside the fence – the paddock is only 'bare' because the horses have eaten the grass as fast as it is growing.

Relationship Between Timing of Grazing and Feed Value

Clients generally turn horses out to graze at times to suit their management and working lives rather than consideration in terms of nutritional values. If they have a fat horse or one that is insulin resistant, then it would be good if the client could turn out on low-sugar grass.

It might help them to understand your advice if you discuss photosynthesis: grass needs moisture and sunlight to make sugars and warmth to grow. Plants usually use the sugar to grow but if growth is slowed, grass will store the extra glucose as fructans

Table 9.4 The effect of restricting horses' grazing times on the amount of grass and hay eaten and the total calories consumed compared with daily digestible energy requirements. (Modified from Glunk *et al.*, 2013.)

Turnout time	Hourly intake rate (g DM/kg BW/h)	Dry matter intake (% BW)	% of recommended daily digestible energy (DE) requirements from grazing	Total DE intake (pasture and ad lib hay combined) as % of requirements
3 h	1.96	0.6	40	66
6 h	1.52	0.9	66	85
9 h	1.12	1	67	67
24 h	0.57	1.3	94	94

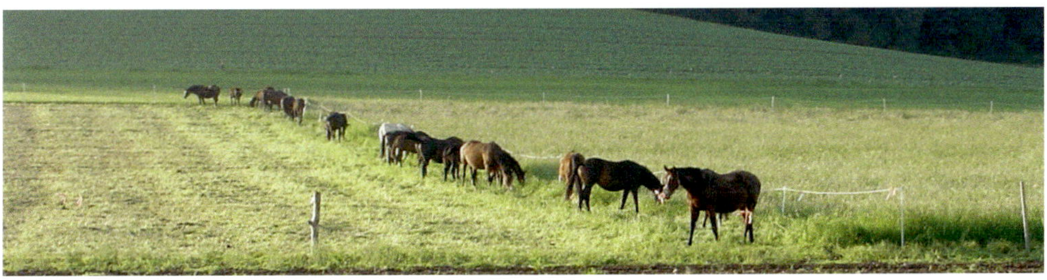

Fig. 9.6 Horses consume grass as fast as it can grow. Use grass outside the field as an indicator of intake.

in the stems/stubble. Ryegrass contains higher levels of fructans compared with meadow grasses (see Chapter 4). Remember that the amounts of sugars (WSC) will depend upon grass species and weather.

Changes in glucose over 24 h

During the spring, the concentration of glucose falls through the night as the grass is no longer photosynthesising and is lowest at 0400 h and 0800 h in cool-season grasses (Williams *et al.*, 2019). Farmers usually cut grass in the early afternoon to ensure the highest sugar levels for ensiling.

To minimise calorie intake from grass when it is actively growing, advise night turnout when sugars are lower and horses eat less (Husted *et al.*, 2009).

Seasonal changes

All grasses tend to have lower levels of WSC in the autumn (October to April).

Grass contains less fructans in the spring compared with the end of summer, because spring grass is using the storage carbohydrates (fructans) during fast growth (Benot *et al.*, 2019).

Although sugars are lowest in early morning, June grass contains more sugars in the early morning (0400 h and 0800 h) compared with October, when sugars are highest at 1600 h. High insulin response in horses is correlated with high grass sugar (Pratt-Phillips *et al.*, 2013; Williams *et al.*, 2019) and timing of grazing should take this into account.

You are more likely to advise restricting grass intake in the summer compared with the winter.

Maintaining Normal Eating Behaviour and Dry Matter Intake When Grass Cannot Be Restricted

Advising straw as a low-calorie forage for overweight horses

> **Top tip**
>
> Advise oat or barley straw as bedding or as a partial or complete hay/grass replacer to keep fat horses chewing whilst reducing calories.

Horses bedded on straw rather than shavings spend 7% of their time eating their bedding and 17% more time sleeping compared with horses bedded on shavings, which spend more time engaged in other behaviours that were not defined but could have included stereotypies (Greening *et al.*, 2013).

Horses bedded on shavings eat their hay and bucket feed faster compared with horses bedded on straw and they are subsequently left without food for longer (Baumgartner *et al.*, 2020).

You might have read that straw should not be fed to horses because it increases the risk of equine gastric ulcer syndrome (EGUS). This is because it was found that horses stabled on straw bedding and fed very restricted forage rations (less than 0.25% BW as DM hay or haylage) and horses fed just straw (quantities and straw variety were not provided) were shown to be at increased risk of ulceration (Luthersson *et al.*, 2009), no doubt because their feeding was very infrequent. It is possible that EGUS might be associated with feeding straw, but it is more likely, as supported throughout the literature, that the small quantities chewed did not produce enough saliva to buffer the acid from the lower stomach.

Remember that infrequent feeding increases the risk of ulceration (Murray and Eichorn, 1996); horses fasted for 24 h have lower median intragastric pH (1.6) compared with horses that are able to eat hay ad lib (pH 3.1) (Murray and Schusser, 1993).

It is helpful sometimes to consider evidence from other species. In cows, 'long periods of low abomasal pH are believed to increase the risk of injury to the abomasal mucosa and abomasal ulceration in ruminants' (Hund and Wittek, 2018). The protective advantage of chewing is recognised in pigs, where 'the presence of straw, continuously provided in small amounts, may represent an important protective factor against the onset of oesophago-gastric ulcers' (Rutherford *et al.*, 2018). The explanation may be related to the protective action of continuous chewing and ingestion of small amounts of fibres (Di Martino *et al.*, 2013; Herskin *et al.*, 2016).

There has been some discussion that the physical 'toughness' of the straw might scratch the stomach lining; this was one of the hypotheses suggested to support the finding that alfalfa chaff when fed with oats increased ulceration in foals; 'mechanical damage due to the chopped edges in this alfalfa chaff' (Pfaff *et al.* 2015). This is potentially an issue in horses that have compromised dentition, but most horses are perfectly capable of chewing fibrous materials to between 1.6 mm and 4 mm before swallowing, even lignified straw.

Evidence supports advising straw to provide low-calorie fibre

Many welfare organisations feed straw as their sole forage to horses requiring weight reduction. Ponies (23 ponies; 13 UK native cross, 13 Welsh and Welsh cross and 10 cobs) fed straw as 50% of forage intake with hay lost 20% of bodyweight (with no reports of ulceration) compared with a gain of 20% in ponies fed 100% hay (Dosi *et al.*, 2020), Older horses with dentition issues should not be fed straw, as the higher cell wall content means they cannot mechanically process the straw.

There were no reports of EGUS in donkeys fed ad lib barley straw whilst being restricted to 8, 12 and 23 h of grazing in the winter and summer; even when they ate more straw in the winter to maintain their DMI and consumed significantly less grass when grazing time was limited, no reports of ulceration were recorded (Wood *et al.*, 2012). More recently some of the group that had originally advised that feeding straw was linked to increased risks of ulceration updated their advice based on their published work showing no relationship between gastric ulceration and feeding straw (50:50 with hay) to ponies as part of weight loss management (Jansson *et al.*, 2021) – a great illustration of open-minded scientists and reassuring for those who have advised feeding straw since the 1990s.

Advising soaking hay to provide low-calorie forage

No doubt you have advised soaking hay for horses, as it has become common place since Webster *et al.* (1987) identified hay as being the main source of airborne dust in stables and Clarke (1987) demonstrated that soaking hay reduced inspirable dust.

Soaking times as part of weight management were increased when it became clear that soaking reduced the nutrient content of hay (Warr and Petch, 1992), resulting in lower fat scores (Stephenson *et al.*, 2011). Soaking hay reduces calories; horses fed 1.25% BW dry matter hay (subsequently soaked) for 6 weeks lost 0.98–2% BW/week (Argo *et al.*, 2015).

If soaking hay does not achieve fat loss, then you would normally advise replacing some of the soaked hay with straw.

Soaking and nutrient reduction

Calories

Most hays fed to horses in the UK contain less than 10% WSC (Fig. 9.7). However, if you are advising a client with an overweight horse, it is always advisable to recommend soaking hay.

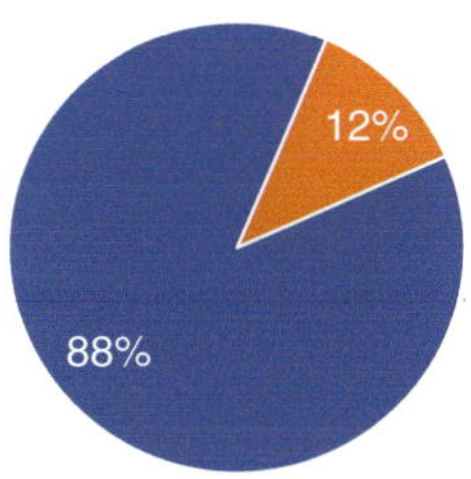

% of hays with less than 10% water soluble carbohydrates analysed between July 08 & July 09, n=250

Year	Average sugar content (WSC) % DM	N
2010	9.2	303
2011	8.8	480
2012	7.7	487
2013	7.3	500

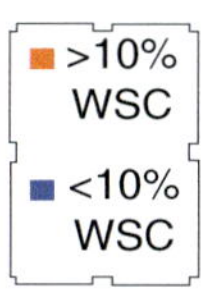

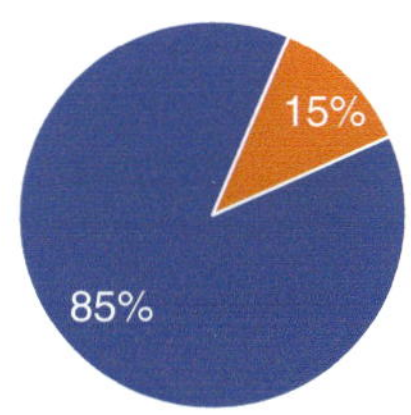

% of hays with less than 10% water soluble carbohydrates analysed between July 16 & July 17, n=550

Fig. 9.7 Typical water-soluble carbohydrate content of UK hays as analysed by NIR.

Soaking hay leaches out water-soluble carbohydrates (WSCs), reducing calorie content (Table 9.5); the calorie content post-soak will be affected by the original sugar content of the hay.

As a result of lower sugars, the insulinaemic and glycaemic responses of ponies fed soaked hay is lower than ponies fed the same weight (0.25% BW) soaked (WSC 10.6% DM) compared with unsoaked hay (WSC 13.8% DM) from the same batch or haylage (WSC 16.5% DM) (Carslake *et al.*, 2018).

It is unusual for haylage to be high in WSC, as the sugars should be used by the bacteria to ferment the grass; haylage more typically contains 49 g WSC/kg DM (4.5%) compared with hay containing 93 g WSC/kg DM (9.3%) made from the same batch of grass (Muller, 2009).

Often your client's compliance for soaking hay reduces in the winter but some facts and figures might help them persevere (Table 9.6): it *is* worth soaking.

Top tip

Soaking hay is an effective method of reducing the calorie content of hay, but it also reduces other nutrients.

Protein loss

Protein loss from soaked hay is not consistent (Warr and Petch, 1992; Moore-Colyer, 1996; Longland *et al.*, 2011b); some studies have shown that soaking decreases small intestine protein digestibility (Bochnia *et al.*, 2021) others that it increases apparent protein digestibility (Argo *et al.*, 2015), maybe as a consequence of differences in fibre content and soaking times.

Minerals

Soaking hay for 12 h decreases minerals by 58% (Moore-Colyer, 1996). Potassium is reduced by

Table 9.5 The reduction in water-soluble carbohydrates (sugars and fructans) (% DM) in hay relative to different soaking times and pre-soak analysis.

Time of soak and conditions	Forage	Pre-soak nutrient (% dry matter)	Nutrient loss after soaking (% dry matter)	Reference
16 h 8°C water, 1 kg hay in 12 litres of water	Ryegrass or timothy hays	13.3–23% WSC Mean 17% WSC Fructans 10% Sucrose 1.6% Glucose 2.2% Fructose 3.9%	12.5% WSC Fructans 8.2% Sucrose 0.9% Glucose 1% Fructose 2.3%	Longland *et al.* (2011b)
60 min 30 min hot	Hay		31% 29%	Watts and Chatterton (2004)
12 h 250 g in 5 litres of water	Hay	7.3–10.2% WSC	4.6–7.1% WSC WSC in water that was used for soak 2–4%	Warr and Petch (1992)
24 h in water (5–7°C) using 17 l water/kg hay	Timothy 50%; red clover 10%; meadow fescue hay 40%	Glucose 3.9% Fructose 2.9% Sucrose 1.2% Fructans 1.2% 9.3% WSC	Glucose 1.2% Fructose 2.1% Sucrose 0.1% Fructans 0.4% 3.8% WSC	Müller *et al.* (2016)
12 h 750 g in 10 l of water at 22°C and 20°C	1st cut meadow hay– ryegrass, meadow fescue, timothy, smooth stalked meadow grass and cocksfoot mix	2.5–12.5% WSC Fructans 4%	Fructans 3.4% 1.7–8.8% WSC	Bochnia *et al.* (2021)
14 h	Hay	13.8% WSC	10.6%WSC	Carslake *et al.* (2018)

Table 9.6 The effect of time of hay soak on sugar loss and calorie reduction[a] for a 500 kg horse (adapted from Longland *et al.*, 2014) assuming a daily digestible energy intake of 65 MJ and fed 10 kg hay[b] providing 1.92 kg sugar

Time soaking (h)	Sugar lost (%)	Sugar weight (g)	Calorie reduction (kcal)	MJ reduction	Reduction in daily calorie intake (%)	Sugar equivalent (tablespoons)
1	26	499	1871	8	12	39
3	34	653	2449	10	16	52
16	42	806	3022	12.8	20	63

[a]1 g sugar = 3.75 kcal (16 kJ)
[b]Hay analysed as 192 g sugar in 1 kg hay providing 40% of the calorie content of the dry hay and 31 MJ DE (7404 human kcal)

1.44% after a 30 min soak (Blackman and Moore-Colyer, 1998); 3% calcium, 4% magnesium and 3% sodium were leached from an overnight soaking of hay into water (Owens *et al.*, 2019).

Dry matter

Soaking hay reduces dry matter (Martinson *et al.*, 2012; Argo *et al.*, 2015) with similar dry matter losses to that recorded after rainfall before baling (Scarborough *et al.*, 2005), because of WSC and other nutrients loss into the liquor. When the amount of dry matter from soaking is calculated on a dry matter basis (Scarborough *et al.*, 2005), rather than estimated from a fresh weight (Argo *et al.*, 2015), 5–8% dry matter was leached when the hay was rained on at 76 mm/h; a similar loss might be expected from soaking.

Top tips

- Advise clients to buy a luggage- or fish-scale/sling.
- Clients should weigh their hay out *before* they soak it, and feed as close as possible to 2.5% BW/day.
- On a 5 kg haynet the dry matter loss from soaking is 0.25 kg DM or 0.2 kg fresh weight, which practically speaking is negligible when stuffing haynets.
- A slice of small bale hay is about 2 kg.
- You must advise a balancer to provide protein and vitamins and minerals. No forage provides a balanced diet in terms of micronutrients or protein – advise feeding a high-quality balancer at 100 g/100 kg BW compensating for the low buffering of straw and the leaching of nutrients from soaked hay.

Soaking or steaming for dust suppression

You should advise soaking hay for performance horses but for a much shorter duration to reduce respirable dust – soaking for 30 min reduces dust by 90% (Moore-Colyer, 1996) and is as effective at reducing dust as a 16 h soak (Clements and Pirie, 2007) but less nutrients are lost compared with a longer soak (Warr and Petch, 1992; Moore-Colyer, 1996).

Alternatively, steaming hay for 50 min results in similar dust suppression but with none (Blackman and Moore-Colyer, 1998) or less nutrient loss (–WSC 4%) compared with soaking (–35% WSC) (Moore-Colyer *et al.*, 2014); this is preferable for the performance horse needing forage with a high nutrient content. Others have measured a 13% reduction of WSC and a 27% decrease in protein after a 90 min steam (Earing *et al.*, 2013), which may be a reflection of the longer steam or the original hay crop.

Is soaking safe?

The 'dust' and leaf shatter that are being soaked or steamed from the hay (a large percentage of which can be dislodged from the hay by vigorous shaking, (Gregory *et al.*, 1963); remind clients to wear a mask. Our vegetables are covered with a mixture of moulds and yeasts (< 100 to 4.0×10^4 cfu/g) (Tournas, 2005) and total bacterial populations of 10^6 cfu/g (Qadri *et al.*, 2015). Many of the bacteria only multiply when moisture is available (soaking), resulting in a high biological value of the liquor (Warr and Petch, 1992).

There has been some concern raised in the literature that soaking hay might increase bacterial numbers and be a health risk, based on hay soaked for 10 min increasing bacterial numbers compared with steaming for 40 min (Moore-Colyer and Fillery, 2012). These results were not comparable, because of the differences in treatment times. Further work has provided mixed results (Table 9.7).

> **Top tip**
>
> Researchers generally conclude that growth of bacteria might increase after a 10 min soak, but longer soaking appears to have less effect or kills the bacteria (Moore-Colyer *et al*., 2020) and reduces mould counts in hay (Müller *et al*., 2015).

Be reassured that enterobacteria found in forages are not pathogenic (Müller *et al.*, 2015) but if you are advising a client whose horse has persistent diarrhoea, then it would be worth checking the bacterial load of the forage.

The presence of bacteria and mould on forages has been established and measured (Scudamore and Livesey, 1998) and upper limits are established for cereal crops destined for human consumption. What is missing is the correlation between soaking forages and any gastric disturbances and disease in the horse. There is no correlation between the WSC of hay and bacterial numbers after soaking and little difference in bacteria species with different grass hays (Moore-Colyer *et al.*, 2020).

Until further work indicates otherwise, do continue to recommend soaking hay for all horses and carefully read any new evidence.

The major factor influencing extent of fungal activity in baled hay is its water activity, not moisture content (Wittenberg *et al.*, 1996). Clearly the water cannot be reused and this might not be environmentally sustainable on large yards; thus haylage would be a better fibre source for performance horses.

Maintaining fibre intake for performance horses

Advising less than 50% forage dry matter intake for performance horses compromises their gut health and increases the risk of gastric ulceration, colic and development of stereotypies. On the other hand, recommending more than 60% forage DMI compared with 50% forage DM (when fed isocalorifically with concentrates) to horses working hard and fast may compromise their performance; because it increases their insensible bodyweight, their maximum heart rate and duration for heart rate to recover, with a trend in higher rectal temperatures, after a set exercise test (Ellis *et al.*, 2002) – 'a compromise needs to be made between the potential detrimental effects of high forage intake on performance and the potential detrimental effects of low forage intake on equine welfare' (Ellis *et al.*, 2002).

The insensible weight gain is likely due to the fact that horses will drink more when fed high dietary fibre (orchard grass hay versus alfalfa or timothy hay) or a high soluble fibre (sugar beet) but have lower faecal dry matter (Warren *et al.*, 1999), increasing bodyweight by 10% – corresponding to the litres of water drunk (Greco-Otto and Léguillette, 2019).

If you advise too much fibre (45% of digestible energy) and too little concentrates (non-structural carbohydrates reduced to 18%) then muscle glycogen after intense exercise is not replenished (Mesquita *et al.*, 2014), which is why clients reduce forage and increase concentrates for performance horses.

It is important to consider alternatives to simply reducing forage to ensure that performance (and leisure) horses can exhibit natural foraging behaviour and trickle feeding.

Replicating Natural Eating Time Budgets

Advising haynets, bags and grids

Slowing forage intake is one method of increasing eating and chewing time. Horses fed a total of 1% BW as hay in two feedings in a net ate slower (0.88 kg/h), taking 62% longer compared with the hay fed on the floor (1.42 kg/h); the overall daily intake was the same (Glunk *et al.*, 2015).

Stabled horses fed hay at 2% BW split into two meals in a net (square holes 3.8 cm × 3.8 cm) reduced their hay intake by 20% compared with feeding hay on the ground; if both were fed ad lib, then there were no differences in eating (Aristizabal *et al.*, 2013).

The time it takes a horse to eat 6 kg of forage can be further increased by 2 h when putting hay into double-layered haynets at multiple points in the stable (Ellis *et al.*, 2015).

To reduce stereotypies, think about advising haynets (45 mm holes) instead of feeding hay in a manger (both fed at 52% of diet), which reduced coprophagy and weaving from 110 min/24 h to 80 min/24 h and increased the time it took the horses to eat by 87% (Correa *et al.*, 2020).

Table 9.7 The effect of steaming or soaking hay on bacteria, yeast and mould numbers

Treatment	Dust: respirable particles/litre air/kg hay (as fed)	Mould (lowest detection log1.7 cfu/g)	Bacterial counts	References
Dry	1180	53,703 cfu/g	234,422	Moore-Colyer *et al.*
10 min soak in water	2.8	Not measured		(2016)
Steamed commercial steamer	4.0	12	5	
Steamed homemade steamer	63	549, 540	5012	
Steamed kettle	142	No reduction		
Dry		1047	51,286	Moore-Colyer *et al.*
Steamed 40 min		2	741	(2014)
Soaked 16°C 9 h		380	186,209	
Steamed 40 min and then soaked for 9 h		288	10,233	
Soaked for 9 h and then steamed for 40 min		1.8	309	
Dry	1.3	1,174,897	21,877,616	Moore-Colyer and
Soaked 10 min and drained for 10 min	0	316,227	37,153,522	Fillery (2012)
Steamed 40 min	1.5	1,072	83,176	
Mean of 2 meadow and 1 perennial ryegrass hay			4 phyla represented 96% of all bacteria Log10 cfu/g	Moore-Colyer *et al.* (2020)
Dry			7.45	
1.5 h soak			7.42	
9 h soak			7.74	
16 h soak			7.51	
	Yeast		(i) Enterobacteria (ii) Lactic acid bacteria (iii) Clostridial spores (log cfu/g)	
Dry hay (DM 85%)	3.6	4.7	4.9, 2.7, 1.9	Müller *et al.* (2015)
Hay 24 h soak	4.7	3.6	5.1, 5.2, 1.7	
Unsoaked haylage (DM 61.5%)	2.4	1.7	1.7, 4.5, 1.9	
[a]Haylage 24 h soak	3.5	1.7	4.8, 7.1, 1.8	
Unsoaked silage (DM 40.6%)	3.7	1.8	1.1, 6.6, 2.0	
[a]Silage 24 h soak	5.8	1.7	2.7, 8.1, 1.9	

[a]Do not recommend soaking fermented forages as it will change their fermentation and no studies on safety have been reported.
cfu, colony-forming unit

Slow feeders (Fig. 9.8) have the further advantage of allowing greater lateral movement of the jaw and result in less frustrated behaviour (Rochais *et al.*, 2018) as well as slowing intake with hay left in the morning and reduced consumption of the straw bed.

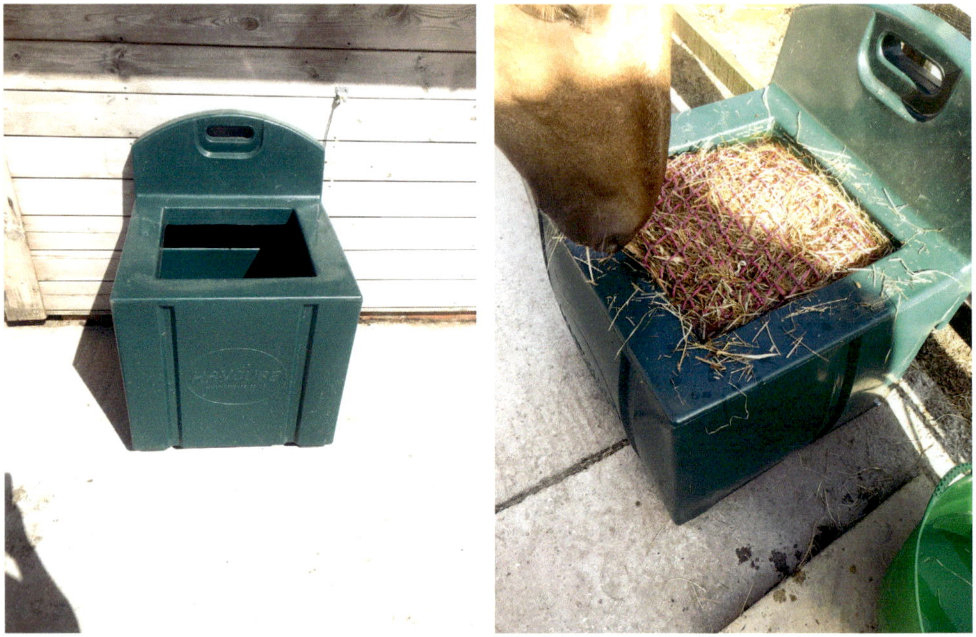

Fig. 9.8 Hay grids to slow intake in horses.

Adding chaff to bucket feed (grains, cereals, concentrates)

A horse takes longer to chew fibre compared with pellets and this is one of the reasons that clients add chaff to their horse's bucket food. Increasing the chaff fibre length from 2.5 cm to 4 cm and increasing inclusion from 10% to 30% increased the number of chews compared with the horse's normal feed (Table 9.8) (Ellis *et al.*, 2005).

Adding more than 15–50% (by weight) of wheat straw chaff at 1.9 cm and 4 cm in length to a meal of oats fed at 3 g/kg BW slowed the intake rates (Campbell *et al.*, 2020) but no measure was made on the digestion of the oats.

Top tip

Chaff should only be used in the bucket alongside low-starch leisure feeds.

Always advise feeding chaff first if clients are feeding higher-starch meals to performance horses (Miraglia *et al.*, 1992; Brüssow *et al.*, 2005; Vervuert *et al.*, 2009; Philippeau *et al.*, 2009; Jensen *et al.*, 2012; Sadet-Bourgeteau *et al.*, 2017).

Feeding forage before concentrates

Feeding forage before concentrates does not reduce performance (Pagan and Harris, 1999) but some form of glycogen replenishment is necessary.

Top tip

- You should advise feeding hay or chaff before concentrates to slow the intake time of the hard feed, increasing small-intestine digestion of starch (Brüssow *et al.*, 2005).
- You can still advise adding chaff to small meals of concentrates (< 1 g starch/kg BW) as this does not overwhelm the holding capacity of the stomach. A smaller bolus is produced with slower rate of passage through the small intestine ensuring maximal starch digestion

Horses fed alfalfa chaff separately from and before oats (2 g starch/kg BW) ate their oats more slowly (15.9 min/kg) compared with horses fed oats alone (11 min), oats mixed with alfalfa (11 min) or oats fed before alfalfa (14 min), possibly because they were less hungry (Brüssow *et al.*, 2005) (see Chapter 5: Fig. 5.3).

Table 9.8 The number of chews and quantities consumed by horses offered feed without chaff and various inclusion rates of chaff (adapted from Ellis *et al.*, 2005)

Feed	Chews/kg (as fed)	Time taken to consume 1 kg (min)	Amount eaten in 1 min (g)
Pellets alone	446 ± 113.8	6.5 ± 1	161 ± 32.1
10% chaff straw 2.5 cm	735 ± 120	10.4 ± 1.9	99 ± 19.4
10% chaff straw 4 cm	735 ± 149.8	10.9 ± 1.5	94 ± 15.7
20% chaff straw 2.5 cm	918 ± 205.4	13.7 ± 3.7	75 ± 13.1
20% chaff straw 4 cm	896 ± 189.8	13.7 ± 2.4	77 ± 15.6
30% chaff straw 2.5 cm	1103 ± 269.2	15.9 ± 3.35	64 ± 15.2
30% chaff straw 4 cm	1074 ± 261.8	15.8 ± 3.05	66 ± 15.4

Horses can eat a meal very quickly to start with and then slow down the longer the duration of the meal (Campbell *et al.*, 2020); thus a small meal of forage (chaff or hay) first might mitigate this and slow the consumption of starch-based feeds.

Feeding just under 1 kg hay 30 min before concentrates improves starch digestion measured by hourly postprandial blood samples of d-lactate and interleukin-b related to intestinal digestion (1–4 h of small intestine digestion and 6–8 h hind gut fermentation), confirming that 'feeding a small amount of hay before feeding a meal of moderate starch and sugar content reduced the negative effects of rapid starch and sugar fermentation in the equine digestive tract, evidenced by reduced postprandial d-lactate and IL-1b concentrations' (Suagee-Bedore *et al.*, 2020).

Top tip

Reassure clients that the slower the horse eats and the more chews they take, the healthier the digestive tract is. If their horse does not eat up straight away it is preferable, as long as they have finished the food before the next meal.

Providing forages in 'dry' paddocks

Many clients are aware that keeping a horse in a stable for long periods of time is a welfare issue and will turn them out into sand paddocks or yards. It is important that they still provide forages during this time. Groups of 50 mares were turned out for 6 h/day in bare paddocks without or with haynets (50× 5 kg haynets set 3 m apart). Mares without hay did not lie down; social interactions tended to be aggressive and they spent twice as much time walking the paddock and standing idle compared with mares with hay, who spent three times as long eating (Benhajali *et al.*, 2009).

Allowing horses to exhibit foraging behaviour

Horses provided with different forages in different positions in their stables exhibit more natural feeding behaviours compared with those fed from a single haynet.

Horses reduce the time they stand doing nothing, eat less of their straw bed and spend more time foraging when fed multiple forages such as hay, haylage and leafy twigs provided in different haynets, as well as root vegetables and some high-fibre cubes (1.5 kg) or short-chop chaffs, compared with a single haynet (Goodwin *et al.*, 2002; Thorne *et al.*, 2005). Similarly, 75% of pastured horses browse and forage feedstuffs other than grass (Van den Berg *et al.*, 2015).

Maintaining Dry Matter Intake for Horses Eating Forages High in Water (e.g. Haylage and Grass)

All horses should eat 2.5% of their bodyweight as dry matter, irrespective of the water content of the forage.

Water content does not influence how much a horse eats; but horses that are not eating enough fibre/dry matter may have an acidic hind gut and diarrhoea, are often more challenging to ride and of course will be at risk of stereotypies (Walters *et al.*, 2002), gastric ulcers (Murray and Eichorn, 1996) and colic (Pinchbeck *et al.*, 2008).

Clients still associate these clinical signs with feeding concentrates and so struggle sometimes with the advice to double the 'fresh weight' of haylage that they are feeding.

> **Top tip**
>
> Haylage contains 30–50% water. In other words, for every kilogram of haylage a horse eats, it is only consuming between 500 g and 700 g of fibre (dry matter). If the water content is not taken into account, then the horse's fibre intake is compromised.

If you provide an example of the numbers (Table 9.9), this helps your client to understand the principle. The client has weighed out what they think is 2% of the pony's bodyweight of various forages but this is fresh weight. In reality the hay is being fed at 1.75% BW as dry matter and the small-bale haylage at 0.95% BW (DM), which is not ideal.

You should recommend a dry matter intake (DMI) of 2.5% BW as dry matter (DM) for *every* horse. The ratio of the feeds to forage will vary according to the workload.

Help your owners work out the impact of water content of their haylage and grass on their horse's fibre intake; encourage them to weigh out the forage at least once a month to check that they have been feeding enough (Box 9.1).

Sometimes it is helpful to do this calculation for grass, showing them how much fresh grass their

Table 9.9 The amount of fibre (DM) and energy provided by owner feeding 4 kg of typical UK preserved forages to a 200 kg pony

Intake/day	Typical hay	High-fibre haylage	Large-bale haylage	Small-bale haylage
[a]Digestible energy (MJ)	33.9	22	28	19
[b]Dry matter (fibre) (kg)	3.5	2.76	3.1	1.9
% bodyweight (DMI)	1.75	1.38	1.55	0.95

[a]Mean MJ/DE/kg DM: hay 9.5; small-bale haylage 10; large-bale haylage 9; high-fibre haylage 8
[b]Mean dry matter: hay 88%; high-fibre haylage 69%; large-bale haylage 77.8%; small-bale haylage 48%.

Box 9.1 How to work out how much forage your client should weigh out and feed

Think about describing dry matter as fibre. Whilst not scientifically precise, it will help your client's understanding.

1. How much does the horse weigh? BW kg	500kg	
2. How much should their horse be eating	2.5% BW DM kg/day	500 X 0.25 = 12.5kg **(assuming adlib forage)**
3. What forage are they feeding their horse- what is the dry matter of the forage?	i. Hay = 85% DM (15% water) ii. Haylage = 70% DM (30% water) iii. Haylage = 55% DM (45% water)	i. horse is eating 850g fibre for every kg hay it eats (0.85kg fibre) ii. horse is eating 700g fibre for every kg weighed out (0.7kg fibre) iii. horse is eating 550g fibre for every kg weighed out (0.55kg fibre)
4. How much (fresh weight) should they weigh out?	Divide the total dry matter that the horse should eat by dry matter (kg) of the forage) **X 100**	i. Hay o 12.5/0.85 = 14.7 kg Need to weigh out 14.7 kg hay ii. Haylage (big bale): o 12.5/0.7 = 17.8 kg Need to weigh out 17.8 kg big bale haylage iii. Haylage (small bale): o 12.5/0.55 = 22.7 kg Need to weigh out 22.7 kg small bale haylage

horse eats in a day versus how much water it has 'drunk' (Box 9.2).

The grass belly they notice on their horse when they bring it in at night is due to massive water intake (50 litres in the example in Box 9.2); the wet bedding the next morning bears witness to how much water their horse has 'drunk'.

Grass intake and hours grazing

Ration programmes (see Chapter 10) calculate how much grass a horse might eat based on their DMI, accounting for what else is eaten, the time of year, quantity of grazing available and hours grazing. Horses grazing 24/7 will eat for 16–18 h, potentially eating 2.5–5% BW DM (0.13–0.3% BW DMI/h) (Table 9.10).

If clients are worried that there is not enough grass, get them to do the supermarket bag test (see Chapter 11: 'Measuring grass in the field').

Advising forage based on calorie content

Remember to check whether the forage calories (digestible energy (DE)) is stated on a dry matter or as-fed basis. Spring grass has the highest calorie content and straw the lowest (Table 9.11) but clearly intake will depend on quantities fed.

Summary

1. Pasture grazing whenever possible
   - Control quantity of grass, if necessary, by aggressive management by cutting or overstocking.
   - Meadow grass rather than perennial ryegrass.
   - If pasture not managed, then strip grazing with front and back fences.
   - Muzzle for up to 12 h.
   - Turn out late evening to 0800 h in spring/summer.
2. High forage dry matter intake – 2.2–2.4% BW leisure horses; minimum of 1.25% performance horses but preferably 1.5%
   - Replicate foraging behaviour by providing multiple forages and haynets.
   - Feed forage before concentrates.
   - Slow forage intake and advise feeding at floor level, using small grids.
   - Small meals of < 1 g starch/kg BW for performance horses after a small meal of forage.
   - Advise techniques to slow intake.
3. Low-nutritive-value forages for leisure horses
   - Timothy hay (help clients spot the seed heads).
   - Soak hay for 12 h to reduce WSC.
   - Oat or barley straw.
4. High-nutritive forages for performance horses
   - Take haylage water content into account to maintain DMI.
   - Soak hay for 30 min to reduce dust and retain nutrition.
   - Advise ryegrass hays.
5. Feed balancers if on predominantly forage diets.
6. Forages and importantly the fibre they contain are fundamental to the horse's health. Always maximise the forage intake of all horses.
   - All horses should be allowed to eat a minimum of 2.5% BW as dry matter, but calorie intake needs to be appropriate to the type of horse and its workload.

Box 9.2 Grass dry matter and water consumption by a 500 kg horse out 24/7

How much does the horse weigh (BW kg)?	500 kg	
How long is the horse grazing?	24/7, grazing spring grass	
What is the dry matter of the grass?	20% DM	Horse is eating 200 g fibre (DM) for each kg of fresh grass
How much dry matter should the horse be eating?	2.5% BW as dry matter	12.5 kg DM
How much fresh grass is the horse eating to meet its DM?	(Total amount of dry matter grass eaten in a day (kg) divided by kg DM in 1 kg intake of fresh grass) × 100	(12.5/0.2) = 62.5 kg fresh weight grass, providing 12.5 kg fibre (DM) and 50 kg (litres) water

Table 9.10 Effect of hours grazing and season on the horse's consumption of grass dry matter (and spring versus winter fresh weight)

	Grass kg of dry matter (DM) (kg fresh weight of spring grass (20% DM,) – winter grass (45% DM))			
	16 h grazing		18 h grazing	
DMI of grass (% BW)	2.5%	5%	2.5%	5%
250 kg	6 kg DM (30–13 kg fresh weight)	12 (60–23)	6.75 (33–150)	22.5 (112–50)
400 kg	9.6 (48–21)	19 (96–42)	11 (55–24)	22 (110–48)
500 kg	12 (60–26)	24 (120–46)	13.5 (66–30)	45 (224–100)

Table 9.11 The average calorie content (MJ digestible energy) of forages fed to horses in the UK, in descending order of calorie content on a DM basis

Forage source	Per kg (DM)	Per kg as fed (fresh weight)
Spring grass	12	1.8
Summer grass	10	2
Ryegrass haylage	11	7
High-fibre haylage	10	6
Meadow hay (late-cut–early-cut)	7–10	5.8–8.4
Autumn/winter grass	6	1.5
Soaked hay	5	4
Straw (barley/oat)	4.5	4

Table 9.12 The difference in fibre/forage management for leisure versus performance horses

	Overweight	Leisure	Performance / underweight
Pasture			
Timing	Late evening to before 0800 h in spring/summer	Can be 24/7, determined by body fat score	Daytime – continue to turn out as the horse comes off pasture and starts to get fit
Muzzle	For up to 12 h	Might be needed if fat score increases	Not normally needed
Strip grazing	Front and back fences needed	Not normally needed	Not needed
Grass length	Short (2–4 cm)	4–6 cm	Longer (4–10 cm)
Grass quantity	Limited Cut or over-graze	As dictated by fat scores	As dictated by fat scores
Pasture management	Limited fertilising; 'poo' pick	Limited fertilising; 'poo' pick	Fertilising increases grass nutrition content
Grass species	Meadow grasses – timothy, bent, creeping fescue, cocksfoot	Meadow grasses – timothy, bent, creeping fescue, cocksfoot	Perennial ryegrass, clover, meadow grasses
Conserved forages			
Type	Soaked meadow hay Barley or oat straw (only if horse has good dentition)	Meadow hay (soaked if gaining fat) High-fibre haylage	Haylage fed correctly Perennial ryegrass or alfalfa hay

Continued

Table 9.12 Continued.

	Overweight	Leisure	Performance / underweight
Quantity	2.4% BW as DMI if sole source of fibre	Minimum 2% BW as DMI	Minimum DMI of 1.25% – consider maximum 1.5% DMI for high-performance horses
Process	Soak for 12–16 h	Soak hay for minimum of 30 min	Soak hay for 30 min Steam hay for 50 min
Management	Small-holed haynets or gridded containers Several feedings/day Four small nets or containers rather than one single 'meal'.	Small holed haynets or gridded containers Several feedings/ day Four small nets or containers rather than one single 'meal'	Small holed haynets or gridded containers Several feedings/ day Four small nets or containers rather than one single 'meal' Feed in lorry and up to 1 h before competing
'Hard' feed (balance nutrient deficiencies of forage)			
Type	Balancer – check vitamin E (see Chapter 11: Table 11.3)	Product from leisure or light work range	Product from performance/ competition /hard work range – must not feed leisure feeds
Quantity	100 g/100 kg BW	Normally 300–600 kg/100 kg BW	Normally 800 g–1.2 kg/100 kg BW
Management	Mix with a small quantity of low-nutritive-value chaff (less than 100 g/100 kg BW) Divide into two meals/day Use techniques to slow intake	Feed after forage Small meals – divide daily intake into a minimum of two meals/day Use techniques to slow intake	Feed after forage at less than 1 g starch/kg BW/meal – normally need ration divided into four meals/day Use techniques to slow intake

- Forage/fibre should never be at less than 50% by dry matter for even the hardest working horse.
- Remember that reducing DMI as a weight loss tool does not always reduce calorie intake but always has welfare consequences for the horse and reduces client compliance.

7. Hard feeds are only fed to balance the deficiencies in forage and should only be advised once the type, quantity and management of the forage has been established.
8. Whilst all horses must have forage in their diet, your clients need to manage the fibre intake so it is appropriate for their horse (Table 9.12).

All clients should be repeatedly reminded that, regardless of the type of work their horse is doing, fibre is first and foremost the fundamental foundation of any diet. Fortunately, there are many ways of feeding fibre to horses, even providing twigs to encourage some browsing; 75% of horses have been recorded by their owners as browsing trees and twigs (van den Berg *et al.*, 2015).

Finally, do make sure owners can recognise poisonous plants.[i]

Note

[i] https://www.msd-animal-health-hub.co.uk/Healthy-Horses/Health/PoisonousPlants

Bibliography

Arena, I., Marliani, G., Sabioni, S., Gabai, G., Bucci, D. *et al.* (2021) Assessment of horses' welfare: behavioral, hormonal, and husbandry aspects. *Journal of Veterinary Behavior* 41, 82–90.

Argo, C.M., Dugdale, A.H.A. and McGowan, C.M. (2015) Considerations for the use of restricted, soaked grass hay diets to promote weight loss in the management of equine metabolic syndrome and obesity. *The Veterinary Journal* 206, 170–177.

Aristizabal, F., Nieto, J., Yamout, S. and Snyder, J. (2013) The effect of a hay grid feeder on feed consumption and measurement of the gastric pH using an intragastric electrode device in horses: a preliminary report. *Equine Veterinary Journal* 46, 484–487.

Auer, U., Kelemen, Z., Engl, V. and Jenner, F. (2021) Activity time budgets – a potential tool to monitor equine welfare? *Animals* 11(3), 850.

Baumgartner, M., Boisson, T., Erhard, M.H. and Zeitler-Feicht, M.H. (2020) Common feeding practices pose a risk to the welfare of horses when kept on non-edible bedding. *Animals: An Open Access Journal from MDPI* 10(3), 411. doi: 10.3390/ani10030411.

Benhajali, H., Richard-Yris, M.A., Ezzaouia, M., Charfi, F. and Hausberger, M. (2009) Foraging opportunity: a crucial criterion for horse welfare? *Animal: An International Journal of Animal Bioscience* 3(9), 1308–1312.

Benot, M.L., Morvan-Bertrand, A., Mony, C., Huet, J., Sulmon, C. *et al.* (2019) Grazing intensity modulates carbohydrate storage pattern in five grass species from temperate grasslands. *Acta Oecologica* 95, 108–115.

Blackman, M. and Moore-Colyer, M. (1998) Hay for horses: the effects of three different wetting treatments on dust and nutrient content. *Animal Science* 66(3), 745–750.

Bochnia, M., Boesel, M., Bahrenthien, L., Wensch-Dorendorf, M. and Zeyner, A. (2017) Feed intake patterns of sport ponies and warmblood horses following iso-energetic intake of pelleted fibre-rich mixed feed, muesli feed and semicrushed oat grains. *Journal of Animal Physiology and Animal Nutrition* 101(Suppl. 1), 37–42.

Bochnia, M., Goetz, F., Wensch-Dorendorf, M., Koelln, M. and Zeyner, A. (2019) Chewing patterns in horses during the intake of variable quantities of two pelleted compound feeds differing in their physical characteristics only. *Research in Veterinary Science* 125, 189–194.

Bochnia, M., Pietsch, C., Wensch-Dorendorf, M., Greef, A. and Zeyner, A. (2021) Effect of hay soaking duration on metabolizable energy, total and prececal digestible crude protein and amino acids, non-starch carbohydrates, macronutrients and trace elements. *Journal of Equine Veterinary Science* 101, 103452.

Bonin, S.J., Clayton, H.M., Lanovaz, J.L. and Johnston, T. (2007) Comparison of mandibular motion in horses chewing hay and pellets. *Equine Veterinary Journal* 39(3), 258–262.

Borgia, L., Valberg, S., McCue, M., Watts, K. and Pagan, J. (2011) Glycaemic and insulinaemic responses to feeding hay with different non-structural carbohydrate content in control and polysaccharide storage myopathy-affected horses. *Journal of Animal Physiology and Animal Nutrition* 95(6), 798–807.

Boyd, L. and Bandi, N. (2002) Reintroduction of takhi, *Equus ferus przewalskii*, to Hustai National Park, Mongolia: time budget and synchrony of activity pre- and post-release. *Applied Animal Behaviour Science* 78, 87–102.

Brøkner, C., Nørgaard, P. and Hansen, H.H. (2008) Effect of feed type and essential oil product on equine chewing activity. *Journal of Animal Physiology and Animal Nutrition* 92(6), 621–630.

Brüssow, N., Voigt, K., Vervuert, I., Hollands, T., Cuddeford, D. *et al.* (2005) The effect of the order of feeding oats and chopped alfalfa to horses on the rate of intake and chewing activity. *Pferdeheilkunde* 21, 37–38.

Campbell, T.E., Doughty, H., Harris, P.A., de Laat, M.A. and Sillence, M.N. (2020) Factors affecting the rate and measurement of feed intake for a cereal-based meal in horses. *Journal of Equine Veterinary Science* 84, 1–7.

Carslake, H.B., Argo, C.M., Pinchbeck, G.L., Dugdale, A. and McGowan, C.M. (2018) Insulinaemic and glycaemic responses to three forages in ponies. *Veterinary Journal (London, England: 1997)* 235, 83–89.

Clarke, A.F. (1987) Stable environment in relation to the control of respiratory disease. In: Hickman, J. (ed.) *Horse Management*, 2nd edn. Academic Press, London, pp. 125–170.

Clements, J.M. and Pirie, R.S. (2007) Respirable dust concentrations in equine stables. Part 2: the benefits of soaking hay and optimising the environment in a neighbouring stable. *Research in Veterinary Science* 83, 263–268.

Coenen, M., Kienzle, E., Vervuert, I. and Zeyner, A. (2011) Recent German developments in the formulation of energy and nutrient requirements in horses and the resulting feeding recommendations. *Journal of Equine Veterinary Science* 31, 219–229.

Correa, G.C., Rodrigues e Silva, C.F., Dias, L.A., Silva Rocha, S. Jr, Thomes, F.R., do Lago, L.A., Carvalho, A.M. and Faleiros, R.F. (2020) Welfare benefits after the implementation of slow-feeder hay bags for stabled horses. *Journal of Veterinary Behavior* 38, 61–66.

Curtis, G., Barfoot, C., Dugdale, A., Harris, P. and Argo, C. (2011) Voluntary ingestion of wood shavings by obese horses under dietary restriction. *British Journal of Nutrition* 106(S1), S178–S182.

Di Martino, G., Capello, K., Scollo, A. *et al.* (2013) Continuous straw provision reduces prevalence of oesophago-gastric ulcer in pigs slaughtered at 170 kg (heavy pigs). *Research in Veterinary Science* 95(3), 1271–1273. doi: 10.1016/j.rvsc.2013.08.012.

Dosi, M., Kirton, R., Hallsworth, S., Keen, J.A. and Morgan, R.A. (2020) Inducing weight loss in native ponies: is straw a viable alternative to hay? *The Veterinary Record* 187(8), e60.

Duncan, P. (1980) Time-budgets of Camargue horses II. Time-budgets of adult horses and weaned sub-adults. *Behaviour* 72, 26–49.
Earing, J.E., Hathaway, M.R., Sheaffer, C.C., Hetchler, B.P., Jacobson, L.D. *et al.* (2013) Effect of hay steaming on forage nutritive values and dry matter intake by horses. *Journal of Animal Science* 91(12), 5813–5820.
Elia, J.B., Erb, H.N. and Houpt, K.A. (2010) Motivation for hay: effects of a pelleted diet on behavior and physiology of horses. *Physiology & Behavior* 101(5), 623–627.
Ellis, J.M., Hollands, T. and Allen, D. (2002) Effect of forage intake on bodyweight and performance. *Equine Veterinary Journal* 34(6), 66–70.
Ellis, A.D., Thomas, S., Arkell, K. and Harris, P. (2005) Adding chopped straw to concentrate feed: The effect of inclusion rate and particle length on intake behaviour of horses. *Pferdeheilkunde*, 21.
Ellis, A.D., Redgate, S.E., Zinchenko, S., Owen, H., Barfoot, C. *et al.* (2015) The effect of presenting forage in multi-layered haynets and at multiple sites on nighttime budgets of stabled horses. *Applied Animal Behaviour Science* 171, 108–116.
Gillham, S.B., Dodman, N.H., Shuster, L., Kream, R. and Rand, W. (1994) The effect of diet on cribbing behavior and plasma β-endorphin in horses. *Applied Animal Behaviour Science* 41(3–4), 147–153.
Glunk, E.C. (2014) *Methods of restricting forage intake in horses*. Retrieved from the University of Minnesota Digital Conservancy. Available at: https://hdl.handle.net/11299/163753.
Glunk, E.C., Pratt-Phillips, S.E. and Siciliano, P.D. (2013) Effect of restricted pasture access on pasture dry matter intake rate, dietary energy intake, and fecal pH in horses. *Journal of Equine Veterinary Science* 33, 421–426.
Glunk, E.C., Hathaway, M.R., Grev, A.M., Lamprecht, E.D., Maher, M.C. *et al.* (2015) The effect of a limit-fed diet and slow-feed hay nets on morphometric measurements and postprandial metabolite and hormone patterns in adult horses. *Journal of Animal Science* 93(8), 4144–4152.
Goodwin, D., Davidson, H.P. and Harris, P. (2002) Foraging enrichment for stabled horses: effects on behaviour and selection. *Equine Veterinary Journal* 34(7), 686–691. doi: 10.2746/04251640277625045.
Graham-Thiers, P.M. and Bowen, L.K. (2013) Improved ability to maintain fitness in horses during large pasture turnout. *Journal of Equine Veterinary Science* 33, 581–585.
Greco-Otto, P. and Léguillette, R. (2019) Assessment of body fluids and blood parameters associated with rapid weight change in heavy horses. *The Canadian Veterinary Journal [La revue veterinaire canadienne]* 60(7), 721–724.
Greening, L., Shenton, V., Wilcockson, K. and Swanson, J. (2013) Investigating duration of nocturnal ingestive and sleep behaviours of horses bedded on straw versus shavings. *Journal of Veterinary Behavior* 8, 82–86.
Greening, L., Williams, J. and Mitson, K. (2017) A preliminary investigation comparing the frequency of grazing and movement behaviour between a track paddock system and a conventional paddock system. *In: 13th International Conference of the International Society of Equitation Science*, Charles Sturt University, Wagga Wagga, Australia.
Gregory, P.H., Lacey, M.E., Fenstenstein, G.W. and Skinner, F.A. (1963) Liberation of spores from mouldy hay. *Transactions of the British Mycological Society* 46, 73–80.
Hampson, B. (2010) Training working horses. In: Hodgson, D., McKeever, K. and McGowan, C. (eds) *The Athletic Horse: Principles and Practice of Equine Sports Medicine*. Elsevier Science, Sydney, Australia, pp. 347–353.
Hampson, B.A., de Laat, M.A., Mills, P.C. and Pollitt, C.C. (2010) Distances travelled by feral horses in 'outback' Australia. *Equine Veterinary Journal* (Suppl. 38), 582–586.
Herskin, M.S., Jensen, H.E., Jespersen, A., Forkman, B., Jensen, M.B. *et al.* (2016) Impact of the amount of straw provided to pigs kept in intensive production conditions on the occurrence and severity of gastric ulceration at slaughter. *Research in Veterinary Science* 104, 200–206. doi: 10.1016/j.rvsc.2015.12.017.
Houpt, K.A. (2012) A preliminary answer to the question of whether cribbing causes salivary secretion. *Journal of Veterinary Behaviour* 7(5), 322–324.
Hund, A. and Wittek, T. (2018) Abomasal and third compartment ulcers in ruminants and South American Camelids. *The Veterinary Clinics of North America. Food Animal Practice* 34(1), 35–54. doi: 10.1016/j.cvfa.2017.10.003.
Husted, L., Sanchez, L.C., Baptiste, K.E. and Olsen, S.N. (2009) Effect of a feed/fast protocol on pH in the proximal equine stomach. *Equine Veterinary Journal* 41, 658–662.
Ince, J.C., Longland, A., Moore-Colyer, M., Newbold, C.J. and Harris, P.A. (2011) Changes in proportions of dry matter intakes by ponies with access to pasture and haylage for 3 and 20 hours per day respectively, for six weeks. *Journal of Equine Veterinary Science* 31, 283.
Janis, C.M., Constable, E.C., Houpt, K.A., Streich, W.J. and Clauss, M. (2010) Comparative ingestive mastication in domestic horses and cattle: a pilot investigation. *Journal of Animal Physiology and Animal Nutrition* 94(6), e402–e409.
Jansson, A., Harris, P., Davey, S.L., Luthersson, N., Ragnarsson, S. *et al.* (2021) Straw as an alternative to grass forage in horses – effects on post-prandial metabolic profile, energy intake, behaviour and gas-

tric ulceration. *Animals: An Open Access Journal from MDPI* 11(8), 2197. doi: 10.3390/ani11082197.
Jensen, R.B., Austbø, D. and Tauson, A.H. (2012) Feeding forage before or after oats affects caecum pH profiles of the horse. In: Saastamoinen, M., Fradinho, M., Santos, A. and Miraglia, N. (eds) *Forages and Grazing in Horse Nutrition*. Wageningen Academic Publishers, Wageningen, The Netherlands, pp. 327–330.
Jones, L., Lax, J. and Hollands, T. (2005a) The mineral content of spring and summer pasture grazed by young growing Thoroughbred in the UK. *Pferdeheilkunde* 21(Suppl.), 21–23.
Jones, L., Lax, J. and Hollands, T. (2005b) Analysis of the mineral content of spring summer grazing used for thoroughbred breeding stock in the UK. *44th BEVA Annual Congress*, Harrogate, UK.
Kim, H.J., Lee, D.S. and Paik, H.D. (2004) Characterization of *Bacillus cereus* isolates from raw soybean sprouts. *Journal of Food Protection* 67(5), 1031–1035.
Longland, A.C., Barfoot, C. and Harris, P.A. (2011a) The effect of wearing a grazing muzzle vs not wearing a grazing muzzle on pasture dry matter intake by ponies. *Journal of Equine Veterinary Science* 2011, 31, 282–283.
Longland, A.C., Barefoot, C. and Harris P.A. (2011b) Effects of soaking on the water-soluble carbohydrate and crude protein content of hay. *Veterinary Record* 168, 618.
Longland A.C., Barfoot C. and Harris P.A. (2012) The effect of wearing a grazing muzzle vs. not wearing a grazing muzzle on intakes of spring, summer and autumn pastures by ponies. In: Saastamoinen, M., Fradinho, M.J., Santos, A.S. and Miraglia, N. (eds) *Forages and Grazing in Horse Nutrition. EAAP* vol. 132. Wageningen Academic Publishers, Wageningen, Netherlands, pp. 186–186.
Longland, A.C., Barfoot, C. and Harris, P.A. (2014) Effect of period, water temperature and agitation on loss of water-soluble carbohydrates and protein from grass hay: implications for equine feeding management. *The Veterinary Record* 174(3), 68.
Longland, A.C., Barfoot, C. and Harris, P.A. (2016) Efficacy of wearing grazing muzzles for 10 hours per day on controlling bodyweight in pastured ponies. *Journal of Equine Veterinary Science* 45, 22–27.
Longland, A.C., Barfoot, C. and Harris, P.A. (2021) Strip-grazing: reduces pony dry matter intakes and changes in bodyweight and morphometrics. *Equine Veterinary Journal* 54(1), 159–166.
Luthersson, N., Hou Nielsen, K., Harris, P. and Parkin, T.D.N. (2009) Risk factors associated with equine gastric ulceration syndrome in 201 horses in Denmark. *Equine Veterinary Journal* 41, 625–630.
Martinson, K.L., Hathaway, M., Jung, H. and Sheaffer, C. (2012) The effect of soaking on protein and mineral loss in orchardgrass and alfalfa hay. *Journal of Equine Veterinary Science* 32, 776–782.
Matsui, K., Shiose, E. and Okubo, T. (1990) Automatic determination of grazing and feeding behavior of horse in paddock and stall. *Japanese Journal of Zootechnical Science* 61(7), 648–654.
Mesquita, V., Pagan, J., Valberg, S., Waldridge, B. and Whitehouse, C. (2014) Effect of non-structural carbohydrate, fat and fiber intake on glycogen repletion following intense exercise. *Equine Veterinary Journal* 46, 33–33.
Miraglia, N., Poncet, C. and Rosset, W.M. (1992) Effect of feeding level, physiological state and breed on the rate of passage of particulate matter through the gastrointestinal tract of the horse. *Annales de zootechnie* 41(1), 69–69.
Moore-Colyer, M.J.S. (1996) Effects of soaking hay fodder for horses on dust and mineral content. *Animal Science* 63, 337–342.
Moore-Colyer, M.J.S. and Fillery, B.G. (2012) The effect of three different treatments on the respirable particle content, total viable count and mould concentrations in hay for horses. In: Saastamoinen, M., Fradinho, M.J., Santos, A.S. and Miraglia, N. (eds) *Forages and Grazing in Horse Nutrition*. Wageningen Academic Publishers, Wageningen, The Netherlands, pp. 101–106.
Moore-Colyer, M.J.S., Lumbis, K., Longland, A. and Harris, P. (2014) The effect of five different wetting treatments on the nutrient content and microbial concentration in hay for horses. *PLoS ONE* 9(11), e114079.
Moore-Colyer, M.S., Taylor, J.L.E. and James, R. (2016) The effect of steaming and soaking on the respirable particle, bacteria, mould, and nutrient content in hay for horses. *Journal of Equine Veterinary Science* 39, 62–68.
Moore-Colyer, M., Longland, A., Harris, P., Zeef, L. and Crosthwaite, S. (2020) Mapping the bacterial ecology on the phyllosphere of dry and post soaked grass hay for horses. *PLoS ONE* 15(1), e0227151.
Mueller, P.J., Protos, P., Houpt, K.A. and Van Soest, P.J (1998) Chewing behaviour in the domestic donkey (*Equus asinus*) fed fibrous forage. *Applied Animal Behaviour Science* 60(2–3), 241–251.
Muller, C.E. (2009) Long-stemmed vs. cut haylage in bales–effects on fermentation, aerobic storage stability, equine eating behaviour and characteristics of equine faeces. *Animal Feed Science and Technology* 152, 307–321.
Müller, C. (2012) Equine digestion of diets based on haylage harvested at different plant maturities. *Animal Feed Science and Technology* 177, 65–74. doi: 10.1016/j.anifeedsci.2012.06.002.
Müller, C. and Udén, P. (2007) Preference of horses for grass conserved as hay, haylage or silage. *Animal Feed Science and Technology* 132, 66–78.
Müller, C.E., Nostell, K. and Bröjer, J. (2015) Microbial counts in forages for horses – effect of storage time

and of water soaking before feeding. *Journal of Equine Veterinary Science* 35, 622–627.

Müller, C.E., Nostell, K. and Bröjer, J. (2016) Methods for reduction of water soluble carbohydrate content in grass forages for horses. *Livestock Science* 186, 46–52.

Murray, M.J. and Eichorn, E.S. (1996) Effects of intermittent feed deprivation, intermittent feed deprivation with ranitidine administration, and stall confinement with ad libitum access to hay on gastric ulceration in horses. *American Journal of Veterinary Research* 57(11), 1599–1603.

Murray, M.J. and Schusser, G.F. (1993) Measurement of 24-h gastric pH using an indwelling pH electrode in horses unfed, fed, and treated with ranitidine. *Equine Veterinary Journal* 25, 417–421.

Naujeck, A., Hill, J. and Gibb, M.J. (2005) Influence of sward height on diet selection by horses. *Applied Animal Behaviour Science* 90, 49–63.

Owens, T.G., Barnes, M., Gargano, V.M., Julien, L., Mansilla, W.D. *et al.* (2019) Nutrient content changes from steaming or soaking timothy-alfalfa hay: effects on feed preferences and acute glycemic response in Standardbred racehorses. *Journal of Animal Science* 97(10), 4199–4207.

Pagan, J.D. and Harris, P.A. (1999) The effects of timing and amount of forage and grain on exercise response in thoroughbred horses. *Equine Veterinary Journal* (30), 451–457.

Perkins, N.R., Reid, S.W.J. and Morris, R.S. (2005) Profiling the New Zealand Thoroughbred racing industry. 1: Training, racing and general health patterns. *New Zealand Veterinary Journal* 53, 59–68.

Pfaff, M., Venner, M. and Vervuert, I. (2015) *Effects of different forage-based diets on gastric mucosa in weanling*. In: *Proceedings of the Equine Workshop on Equine Nutrition*, pp. 8–9.

Philippeau, C., Faubladier, C., Goachet, A.G. and Julliand, V. (2009) Is there an impact of feeding concentrate before or after forage on colonic pH and redox potential in horses? In: *Equine NUtrition and TRAining COnference (ENUTRACO)*, 26–29 September 2009, Madrid, Spain.

Pinchbeck, G.L., French, N.P., Proudman, C.J. and Archer, D.C. (2008) Risk factors for epiploic foramen entrapment colic in a UK horse population: a prospective case-control study. *Equine Veterinary Journal* 40(4), 405–410.

Pratt-Phillips, S.E., Wycoff, C., Sykes, C., Kutzner-Mulligan, J. and Siciliano, P.D. (2013) Glucose and insulin concentrations in restricted pasture-fed horses. *Journal of Equine Veterinary Science* 33, 351.

Qadri, O.S., Yousuf, B. and Srivastava, A.K. (2015) Fresh-cut fruits and vegetables: critical factors influencing microbiology and novel approaches to prevent microbial risks – A review. *Cogent Food & Agriculture* 1(1), Article 1121606.

Rochais, C., Henry, S. and Hausberger, M. (2018) 'Haybags' and 'Slow feeders': testing their impact on horse behaviour and welfare. *Applied Animal Behaviour Science* 198, 52–59.

Rutherford, K.M.D., Thompson, C.S., Thomson, J.R., Lawrence, A.B., Nielsen, E.O. *et al.* (2018) A study of associations between gastric ulcers and the behaviour of finisher pigs. *Livestock Science* 212, 45–51. doi: 10.1016/j.livsci.2018.03.013.

Sadet-Bourgeteau, S., Philippeau, C. and Julliand, V. (2017) Effect of concentrate feeding sequence on equine hindgut fermentation parameters. *Animal* 11(7), 1146–1152.

Scarbrough, D.A., Coblentz, W.K., Humphry, J.B., Coffey, K.P., Daniel, T.C. *et al.* (2005) Evaluation of dry matter loss, nutritive value, and in situ dry matter disappearance for Wilting Orchardgrass and Bermudagrass forages damaged by simulated rainfall. *Agronomy Journal* 97, 604–614.

Scheibe, K.M. and Streich, W.J. (2003) Annual rhythm of body weight in Przewalski horses (*Equus ferus przewalskii*). *Biological Rhythm Research* 34(4), 383–395.

Scudamore, K.A. and Livesey, C.T. (1998) Occurrence and significance of mycotoxins in forage crops and silage: a review. *Journal of the Science of Food and Agriculture* 77, 1–17.

Siciliano, P.D. and Schmitt, S. (2012) Effect of restricted grazing on hindgut pH and fluid balance. *Journal of Equine Veterinary Science* 32, 558–561.

Smith, D., Mayes, R., Hollands, T., Cuddeford, D., Yule, H. *et al.* (2007) Validating the alkane pair technique to estimate dry matter intake in equids. *The Journal of Agricultural Science* 145(3), 273–281.

Stephenson, H.M., Green, M.J. and Freeman, S.L. (2011) Prevalence of obesity in a population of horses in the UK. *The Veterinary Record* 168(5), 131.

Suagee-Bedore, J.K., Linden, D.R., Bennett-Wimbush, K. and Splan, R.K. (2020) Feeding grass hay before concentrate mitigates the effect of grain-based concentrates on postprandial plasma interleukin-1β. *Journal of Equine Veterinary Science* 86, 102899. doi: 10.1016/j.jevs.2019.102899.

Thorne, J., Goodwin, D., Kennedy, M., Davidson, H. and Harris, P. (2005) Foraging enrichment for individually housed horses: practicality and effects on behaviour. *Applied Animal Behaviour Science* 94, 149–164.

Tournas, V.H. (2005) Moulds and yeasts in fresh and minimally processed vegetables, and sprouts. *International Journal of Food Microbiology* 99(1), 71–77.

Van den Berg, M., Brow, W.Y., Le, C. and Hinch, G.N. (2015) Browse-related behaviors of pastured horses in Australia: a survey. *Journal of Veterinary Behavior* 10(1), 48–53.

Van Weyenberg, S., Sales, J. and Janssens, G. (2006) Passage rate of digesta through the equine gastrointestinal tract: a review. *Livestock Science* 99(1), 3–12.

Vervuert, I., Voigt, K., Hollands, T., Cuddeford, D. and Coenen, M. (2009) The effect of mixing and changing the order of feeding oats and chopped alfalfa to horses on: glycaemic and insulinaemic responses, and breath hydrogen and methane production. *Journal of Animal Physiology and Animal Nutrition* 93(5), 631–638.

Walters, A.J., Nicol, C.J. and French, N.P. (2002) Factors influencing the development of stereotypic and redirected behaviours in young horses: findings of a four-year prospective epidemiological study. *Equine Veterinary Journal* 34, 572–579.

Warr, E.M. and Petch, J.L. (1992) Effects of soaking hay on its nutritional quality. *Equine Veterinary Education* 5(3), 169–171.

Warren, L.K., Lawrence, L.M., Brewster-Barnes, T. and Powell, D.M. (1999) The effect of dietary fibre on hydration status after dehydration with frusemide. *Equine Veterinary Journal* (Suppl. 30), 508–513.

Watts, K.A. and Chatterton, J. (2004) A review of factors affecting carbohydrate levels in forage. *Journal of Equine Veterinary Science* 24, 84–86.

Webster, A.J., Clarke, A.F., Madelin, T.M. and Wathes, C.M. (1987) Air hygiene in stables. 1: effects of stable design, ventilation and management on the concentration of respirable dust. *Equine Veterinary Journal* 19(5), 448–453.

Willard, J.G., Willard, J.C., Wolfram, S.A. and Baker, J.P. (1977) Effect of diet on cecal pH and feeding behavior of horses. *Journal of Animal Science* 45(1), 87–93.

Williams, C.A., Kenny, L.B. and Burk, A.O. (2019) Effects of grazing system, season, and forage carbohydrates on glucose and insulin dynamics of the grazing horse. *Journal of Animal Science* 97(6), 2541–2554. doi: 10.1093/jas/skz103.

Wittenberg, K.M. Undi, M. and Bossuyt, C. (1996) Establishing a feed value for moulded hay. *Animal Feed Science and Technology* 60(3–4), 301–310.

Wood, S.J., Smith, D.G., Morriss, C.J. and Cuddeford, D. (2012) The effect of pasture restriction on dry matter intake of foraging donkeys in the United Kingdom. In: Saastamoinen, M., Fradinho, M.J., Santos, A.S. and Miraglia, N. (eds) *Forages and Grazing in Horse Nutrition*, Vol. 132. Wageningen Academic Publishers, Wageningen, The Netherlands.

Woodward, M.C., Huff, N.K., Garza, F. Jr, Keowen, M.L., Kearney, M.T. *et al.* (2014) Effect of pectin, lecithin, and antacid feed supplements (Egusin) on gastric ulcer scores, gastric fluid pH and blood gas values in horses. *BMC Veterinary Research* 10 (Suppl. 1), 54–62.

10 Intake versus Requirements: Using Computer Programs

Lizzie Drury

Saracen Horse Feeds, Aylesford

Learning Objectives

LO1 Describe the common software programs available for checking a horse's ration.
LO2 Decipher the outputs from a ration software program.
LO3 Use and explain common feeding errors and questions using outputs from a ration program.
LO4 Explain the limitations of software programs

At the end of this chapter, you will be able to use and interpret common software, whilst being aware of its limitations, as part of a nutritional assessment.

Introduction

Putting a diet together is part of everyday husbandry for clients but many are unaware of how to check if the diet is meeting the specific requirements of their horse.

They are very capable of doing a simple check to see if their horse is eating enough food but, to be accurate, you need to know the quantity of nutrients the horse needs to meet maintenance and workload, the health goals and the nutrient content of the feeds available. You need to be able to check if the horse can eat the ration and if the ration is affordable and practical and check intake against requirements.

In production species, checking the ration is an essential part of the regular herd health checks and farmers are very familiar with the numerous ration packages used by nutritionists in conjunction with farm vets (Table 10.1). Production farm animal feed rations are very precise and accurate, based on extensive, exhaustive research, and are vital for the economics of the farm and the welfare of the animals. Most rations are specific to the individual farm, balancing their own regularly analysed forages. Commercial pet food manufacturers make it quite challenging to do basic checks for dogs and cats.

You need to consider the three horse factors (weight, fat score and workload: see Chapters 2 and 3) and the three diet factors (quantities of forages: Chapter 4; concentrates: Chapter 5; and supplements: Chapter 6) before you can check the ration.

Ration Evaluation

To evaluate the ration, you need clients to weigh the amount of concentrate feed and forage they are feeding, as well as any that is not eaten (Kronfeld, 1978; Pagan *et al.*, 1996).

Nutritionists can visit the stables and speak to the grooms, owner or rider to determine the volumes of hay, concentrates and other supplements that are being fed and, where there are 'leftovers', weigh any amounts that have not been consumed. Hopefully, in time, this will become part of your health check visits, with clients happy to pay for your advice.

 Evidence-based Equine Nutrition: A Practical Approach for Professionals (T. Hollands and L. Drury)
DOI: 10.1079/9781789245134.0010

The calculations of diets and rations by hand is a simple task to carry out but can be inaccurate and time consuming. Usually you will only work out energy, protein, calcium and phosphorus, and dry matter intakes.

Software programs

Programs specifically designed for the horse are simple to use and save you a lot of time and calculations. They are updated with new research, allowing you to enter specific individual feeds and forages that your client is using. You can update nutrient values as the available forage choice changes through different purchased batches or suppliers.

These programs are useful to illustrate the common feeding mistakes and this chapter provides you with some templates.

Accurate rationing is essential for all performance-horse clients. Use software to accurately evaluate the complete ration of their horse, optimising the opportunity to maximise performance, recovery and overall health of that individual or group of horses, and ensure their feeding is cost effective with no 'under' or 'over' supplementation (Fig. 10.1).

Table 10.1 Various ration packages available across the species

Farm animals	Horses
https://www.feedexpert.com/	https://feedxl.com
https://agmodelsystems.com/	https://pchorse.se/index.php/en/
https://www.nutrientmanagement.org/assets/12028 Manual calculations	https://ker.com/tools/microsteed/
https://www.sheepandgoat.com/rationsoftware	**Small animals**
https://www.canr.msu.edu/spartandairy/	https://secure.balanceit.com/ez/?rotator=NewEz#
https://www.dietcheck.co.uk/	https://www.pfma.org.uk/_assets/docs/fact-sheet/PFMA-fact-sheet-calories.pdf
https://www.agrovision.com/uk/products/agri-business/optifeed	Manual calculations
https://www.forfarmers.co.uk/dairy/dairy/dairy-nutrition/dairy-nutrition-products/optifeed.aspx	
https://www.fao.org/ag/againfo/home/en/news_archive/2017_FAO_Ration_Formulation_Tool.html	
https://www.feedipedia.org/node/23164	

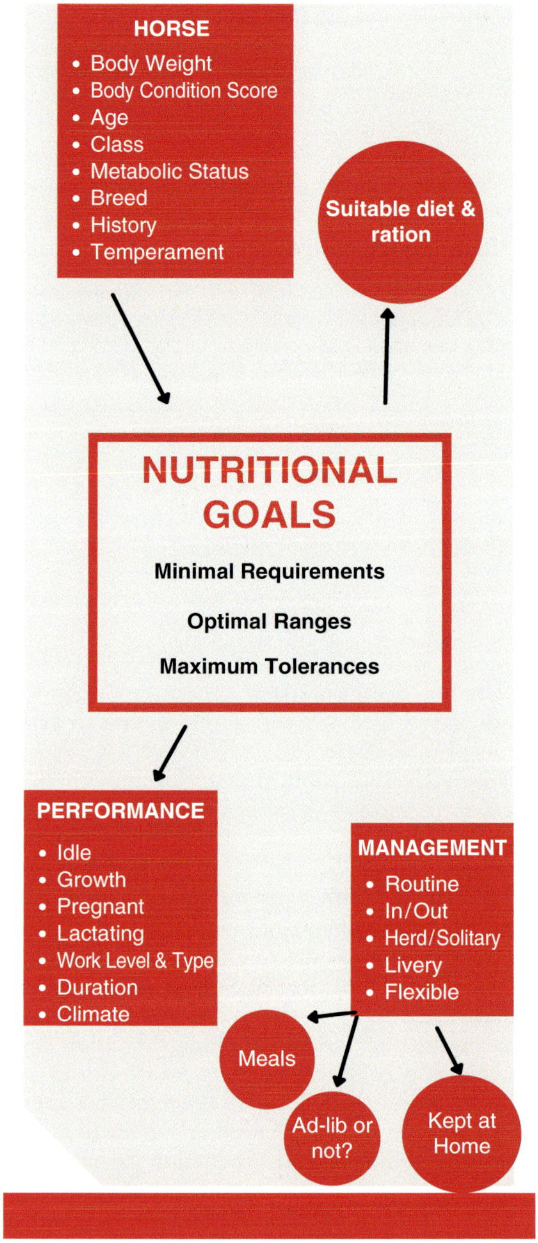

Fig. 10.1 The protocol for a nutritional assessment using a computer software program.

Care still needs to be taken over the interpretation of the data output, because the system is based solely upon the information that *your* client has provided *you*.

The programs (Table 10.1) use large databases of feeds and feed ingredients, forages and supplements from around the world to provide ration analysis that can be graphically represented to show the breakdown and contribution of each feed ingredient. The intake of these is then checked against recommendations of the National Research Council (NRC), Institut National de la Recherche Agronomique (INRA), Gesellschaft fur Ernährungsphysiologie (GfE) (Coenen *et al*., 2011) or Kentucky Equine Research (KER). These might differ, as some use the minimum requirement for most nutrients, others increase values to 1.25–3x those of NRC (2007) based on their own research rather than the body of evidence provided by NRC.

How to Use the Software

Input data: horse details

Every nutritional evaluation should follow the same series of steps (see Chapters 2 and 3) (Fig. 10.2).

Determining metabolic rate

The software allows you to modify requirements based on metabolic rate, enabling you to adjust energy or calorie requirements without altering the intake of other micronutrients. The higher the metabolic rate, the more calories will be required by the horse to maintain its body fat score (BFS); and the lower the metabolic rate, the fewer calories will be required (Table 10.2). You can change the metabolic rate of the horse within the software program to alter the calorie requirement to reflect the BFS of the horse, so that it eats the correct amount of calories. This change might need to be done in stages and do check that this is achievable by noting if the dry matter intake (DMI) is being met and not exceeded.

Exercise level

Most clients will typically overestimate the amount and intensity of the work that their horses are doing, and this results in an excess of calories being fed and increased weight gain. A discussion about the type of work and the speed and longevity of the exercise can then be used to refer to basic guides (Table 10.3) (see also Chapter 3: Table 3.3).

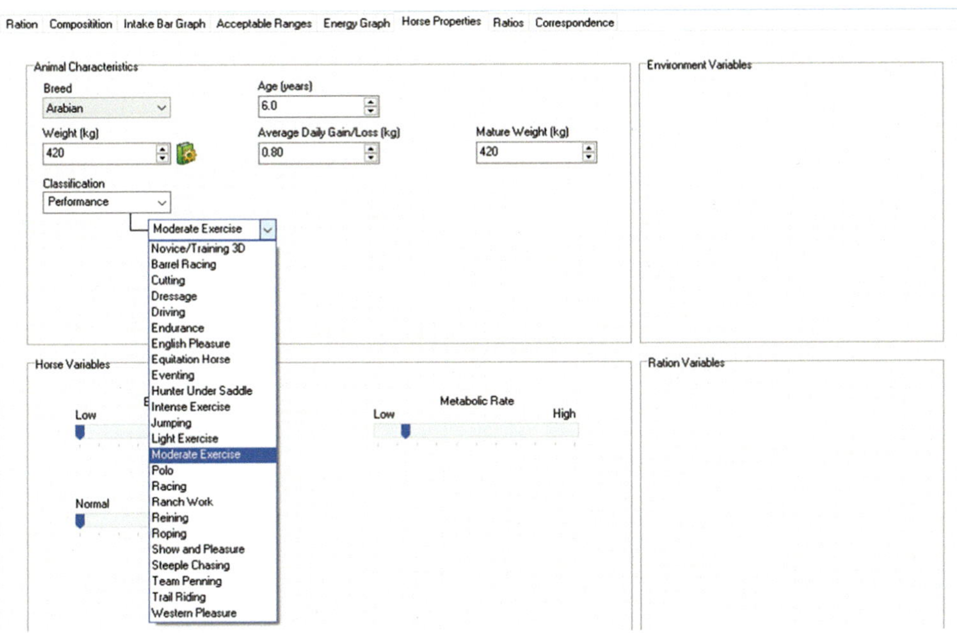

Fig. 10.2 Horse details.

Input data: diet details

You need to input the information about the feed, forage and supplements that are being fed. A database of feeds including comprehensive nutrient analysis is often provided and updated by the software developer, although there is the facility for the nutritionist to add their own feed or forage analysis if it is available.

There may also be the ability to enter feed and supplement costs so that more commercial feeding programmes can be developed.

Enter the kilograms or grams of each feed in the ration (Fig. 10.3), not scoops or cups. Check if you are entering dry matter or as-fed intakes.

Interpreting the data output

The comparison of a ration against the requirements can be viewed in tabular or graphical form.

Table 10.2 Metabolic rate relative to body fat scores (KER) (source: NRC, 2007)

Body fat score	Metabolic rate
Has difficulty losing weight and puts on weight easily	Low
Maintains a consistent body weight	Medium
Is difficult to put weight on	Medium to high
Will not put weight on	High

Table 10.3 Exercise levels by hour and type

Type of exercise	Time/day Days/week	Exercise level
Casual riding	30–45 min 4–5 days	Low
Light work	45–60 min Up to 6 days	Low to medium
Competitive flat work, schooling and dressage and affiliated show jumping/eventing or dressage	45–60 min 5 days Plus competition	Medium
Competitive low-level endurance, FEI-level sport	1 h–1 h 30 min 6 days Plus competition	Medium to high
Intense work, elite-level sport, all disciplines, endurance 100 km+	1 h + 6 days Plus competition	High

These representations allow your client to easily appreciate the benefits or the disadvantages of a particular ration.

You can save reports as pdfs, upload to practice software or share between other members of the team, such as nutritionists, groom, owner and rider, making discussion, record keeping and progress of the horse more accurate.

Contribution of each feed to requirements

The analysis of the feeds can be checked to allow you to compare feeds against one another to show which are proportionately higher in the nutrients that you are interested in. You can then adjust accordingly and this can help your client to appreciate why you are recommending a feed or removing a feed or supplement from an existing diet. The program adds up the nutrients based on the relative intakes to calculate the mean composition of 1 kg of the overall diet (intakes as percentage of protein, total MJ of energy and all vitamins and trace minerals).

These tables rely on the full and accurate input of the analysis of the individual ingredients, and this full information may not always be available or provided willingly by feed manufacturers or supplement providers (Fig. 10.4).

The ration: intake versus requirements

You can check if the ration is meeting NRC or modified KER recommended requirements and the nutrient contribution from the quantity of each individual feed given to the horse (Fig. 10.5).

Contribution of each feed to nutrient intakes

To make it clear which feed ingredient is contributing to the overall diet, each bar is divided up to show the specific ingredients in different colours and how they contribute to the nutrients supplied by the total diet.

The bar graph works as a visual tool of the diet and enables your client to view the effects when feed ingredients, supplements, chaffs and forages are added to or subtracted from the ration (Fig. 10.6).

Energy

Check the digestible energy first, which is equally important for horses in hard work and for horses that are prone to becoming overweight, metabolically challenged and at greater risk of obesity and laminitis.

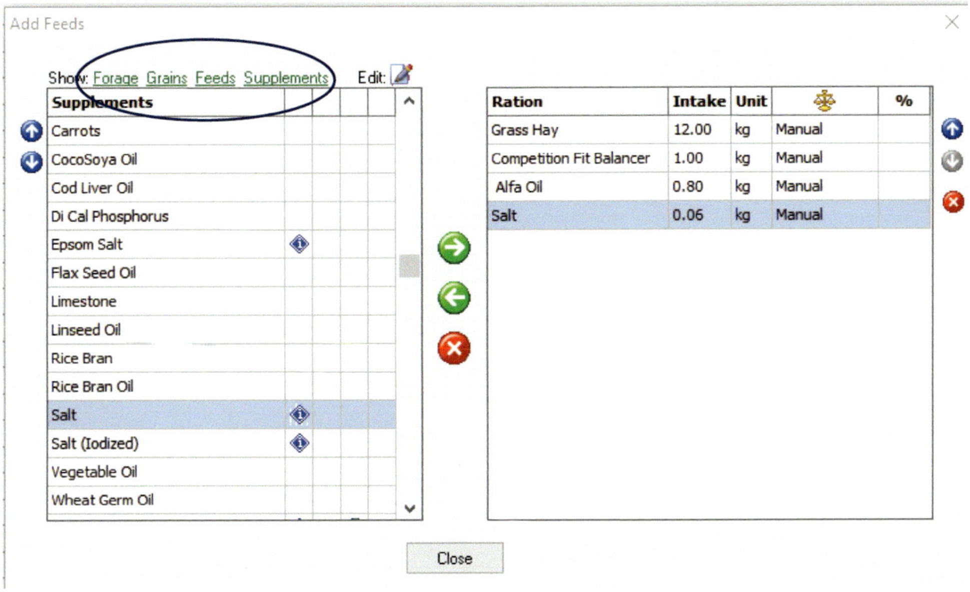

Fig. 10.3 How to select feeds and enter quantity using Microsteed.

Ration | Compositition | Intake Bar Graph | Acceptable Ranges | Energy Graph | Horse Properties | Ratios | Correspondence

	Unit	Salt	Lucerne Chop	Enduro Performance	Grass Hay	Total
DRY MATTER	%	98.000	90.000	89.600	90.000	89.94
DE	Mj/kg	0.000	9.63	12.89	7.45	8.66
PROTEIN	%	0.000	18.000	11.000	9.300	10.19
LYSINE	%	0.000	0.700	1.510	0.200	0.51
CALCIUM	%	0.000	1.230	1.230	0.350	0.59
PHOSPHORUS	%	0.000	0.300	0.490	0.200	0.27
MAGNESIUM	%	0.000	0.280	0.140	0.180	0.18
MAGNESIUM	%	0.000	0.280	0.140	0.180	0.18
SALT	%	0.000	0.000	0.840	0.000	0.17
SODIUM	%	40.000	0.010	0.240	0.010	0.16
CHLORIDE	%	60.000	0.100	0.400	0.100	0.31
POTASSIUM	%	0.000	1.500	1.140	1.280	1.26
COPPER	mg/kg	0.000	9.000	38.000	9.000	14.85
ZINC	mg/kg	0.000	20.000	110.000	25.000	41.85
MANGANESE	mg/kg	0.000	57.000	62.000	52.000	54.23
IRON	mg/kg	0.000	200.000	40.000	53.000	59.78
VITAMIN E	IU/kg	0.000	60.000	485.000	40.000	131.43

Fig. 10.4 Ration output. The columns provide the analysis (composition) of each feed, which can be checked against bags or labels.

Remember that the actual requirements can differ from the calculated recommendation, so it is important to take a clinical judgement and to encourage your client to use the horse's body fat/condition score as the key indicator of the daily energy requirement (see Chapter 3: 'Body fat scoring').

The interpretation of the printout must be compared with and considered against the horse that you are assessing and the information that has been provided by your client.

If the horse is eating less than required energy/calories but is fat, then clearly the energy intake for that horse exceeds its requirements, regardless of what the printout is telling you; adjust the metabolic rate before you share with the client!

Protein

Protein levels need to be monitored carefully. Lysine, an essential amino acid, is often deficient. Nutritionists will use lysine as an indicator of protein quality.

Vitamins and minerals

The output for trace minerals and vitamins may show excesses around 200% or 300%; this is often unavoidable when working with horses where forage source and other aspects of the diet cannot be changed. Though excesses may be wasteful, toxicity occurs at much higher levels than those recommended and would be highlighted if close to those levels.

The output is very useful for illustrating the effects of multiple additions of different supplements, many of which contain the same minerals or vitamins.

As a clinician and nutritionist, you will not recommend a diet if there are mineral imbalances that could jeopardise the health of the horse and eliminating some supplements from the diet will help towards cost savings for your client.

Some short-term mineral deficiencies at around 90% are unlikely to cause health issues but should be rectified over the long term.

Acceptable ranges of all nutrients

Recommended intakes are based on evidence (NRC, 2007) to meet optimal levels of nutrients rather than just minimal recommended levels.

The recommended amounts should be at or close to 100% but there will be situations where the actual amount may be over or under 100% of

Ration | Composition | Intake Bar Graph | Acceptable Ranges | Energy Graph | Horse Properties | Ratios | Correspondence

	Unit	Salt	Lucerne Chop	Enduro Performance	Grass Hay	Recommended KER beta	Totals
Intake	kg/day	0.030	0.800	2.500	9.000		12.330
DRY MATTER	kg/day	0.029	0.720	2.240	8.100	8.750	11.089
DE	Mj/day	0.000	7.7	32.2	67.0	85.8	107.0
PROTEIN	g/day	0.000	144.0	275.0	837.0	766.7	1256.0
LYSINE	g/day	0.000	5.6	37.8	18.0	26.8	61.4
CALCIUM	g/day	0.000	9.8	30.8	31.5	33.0	72.1
PHOSPHORUS	g/day	0.000	2.4	12.3	18.0	22.0	32.6
Ca:P ratio	g/g	0.000	4.1	2.5	1.8	1.5	2.2
MAGNESIUM	g/day	0.000	2.2	3.5	16.2	12.5	21.9
SALT	g/day	0.000	0.000	21.0	0.000	0.000	21.0
SODIUM	g/day	12.0	.1	6.0	.9	26.3	19.0
CHLORIDE	g/day	18.0	.8	10.0	9.0	39.4	37.8
POTASSIUM	g/day	0.000	12.0	28.5	115.2	61.3	155.7
COPPER	mg/day	0.000	7.2	95.0	81.0	131.3	183.2
ZINC	mg/day	0.000	16.0	275.0	225.0	393.8	516.0
MANGANESE	mg/day	0.000	45.6	155.0	468.0	393.8	668.6
IRON	mg/day	0.000	160.0	100.0	477.0	0.000	737.0
VITAMIN E	IU/day	0.000	48	1213	360	700	1621

Fig. 10.5 An example of a ration output illustrating intake (kg) versus requirements (g/mg/day), based on KER modified from NRC (2007).

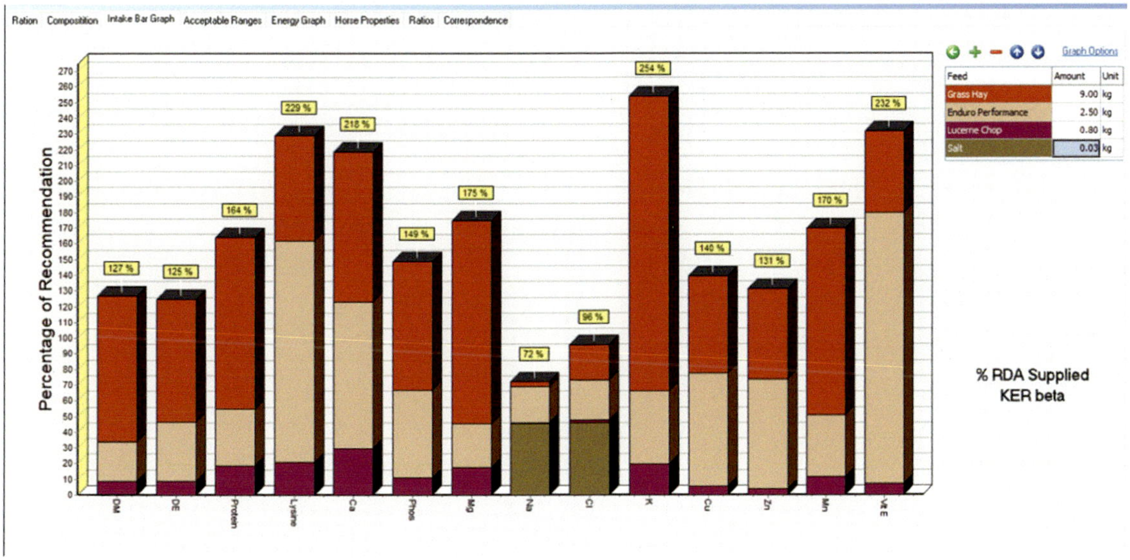

Fig. 10.6 The contribution of each feed to requirements (%).

Top tip

Help your client to understand the overall contribution of individual feeds by breaking each bar down to the percentage of each nutrient as actual intakes. For example, in Fig. 10.6, hay provides 62.6% of the total ration and hard feed 29.9% of the total ration.

recommendations for each nutrient, with the bars showing whether that nutrient is short or in excess.

Acceptable ranges help to indicate whether excesses or deficiencies are acceptable (green), whether they represent an actual excess or deficiency (red) and whether that excess or deficiency (yellow) falls within the unacceptable range (colours as shown in, for example, Figs 10.8–10.11, below). Most diets will generally fall within required parameters (Fig. 10.7).

Using the Software to Highlight Common Feeding Errors and Questions

You will know the more common errors that you encounter in practice and it might be useful to develop some templates and help leaflets to go alongside those typical for your specific practice.

The following questions encompass the myths that are commonly queried in nutritional helplines.

How to advise a diet for a retired horse out 24/7 maintaining good body condition (Fig. 10.8)

Q. Do they need to feed anything extra?

Factors to consider

It rather depends upon the time of year (see Chapter 11: Fig 11.1).

- Energy/calorie intake is above requirements (at 140% of requirement).
- The horse maintains good body condition, is not carrying excess body fat and is not gaining weight.
    - A visual assessment of the horse, to include a fat score, should help confirm if this is in fact the case.

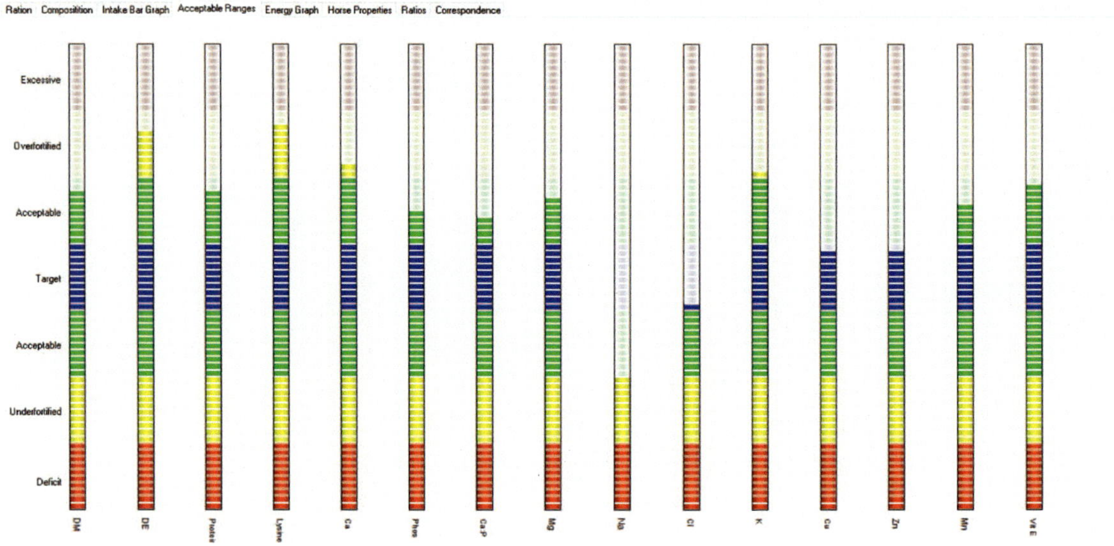

Fig. 10.7 Nutrient intakes plotted to show deficits and safe upper limits. DE, calcium, lysine and potassium are oversupplied but not excessive; sodium is deficient.

- If the horse starts to gain excess weight, consider restricting calorie intake, such as using a grazing muzzle or strip grazing.
- Crude protein and lysine levels are within optimum recommendations.
  - Autumn and winter pastures maybe of poorer quality.
  - Average protein and lysine intakes can be below optimal ranges.
  - Protein and lysine intakes should be addressed in horses that are older, resting or recuperating.
- Mineral levels in grass are affected by several factors:
  - grass species and growth stage;
  - the mineral content of the soil; and
  - the interactions of other minerals.
  - Mineral levels will vary through the year.
  - Seasonal fluctuations in mineral content generally mean that, as the growing season slows, levels of some minerals will decrease.
  - In most practical situations it is not feasible to analyse the pasture for mineral content.
  - Use average analysis.
  - Key minerals, such as zinc and manganese, are below recommendations, although within optimum ranges.
  - No grazing will never provide optimum intakes of minerals.
- Recommend a feed balancer.

All horses in light work will eat excess calories from spring and summer grass.

- Support clients in accepting this as long as they exercise their horse at least 5/7 days for a minimum of 30 min at a heart rate of 80 bpm.
- Ensure that the horse loses fat in the winter, even if they go down to 2/5 on some areas, replicating natural winter weight loss (assuming only in little to light work).

How to recommend a diet for a horse eating ad lib conserved forage (Fig. 10.9)

Q. My horse is resting, and I am feeding him ad lib average quality meadow hay. I have weighed this and his daily intake averages 2.5% of his current body weight. Do I need to feed him anything else or will this be enough? He weighs 500 kg and eats 10–12 kg daily.

Factors to consider

- Energy/calorie intake meets optimal requirements.

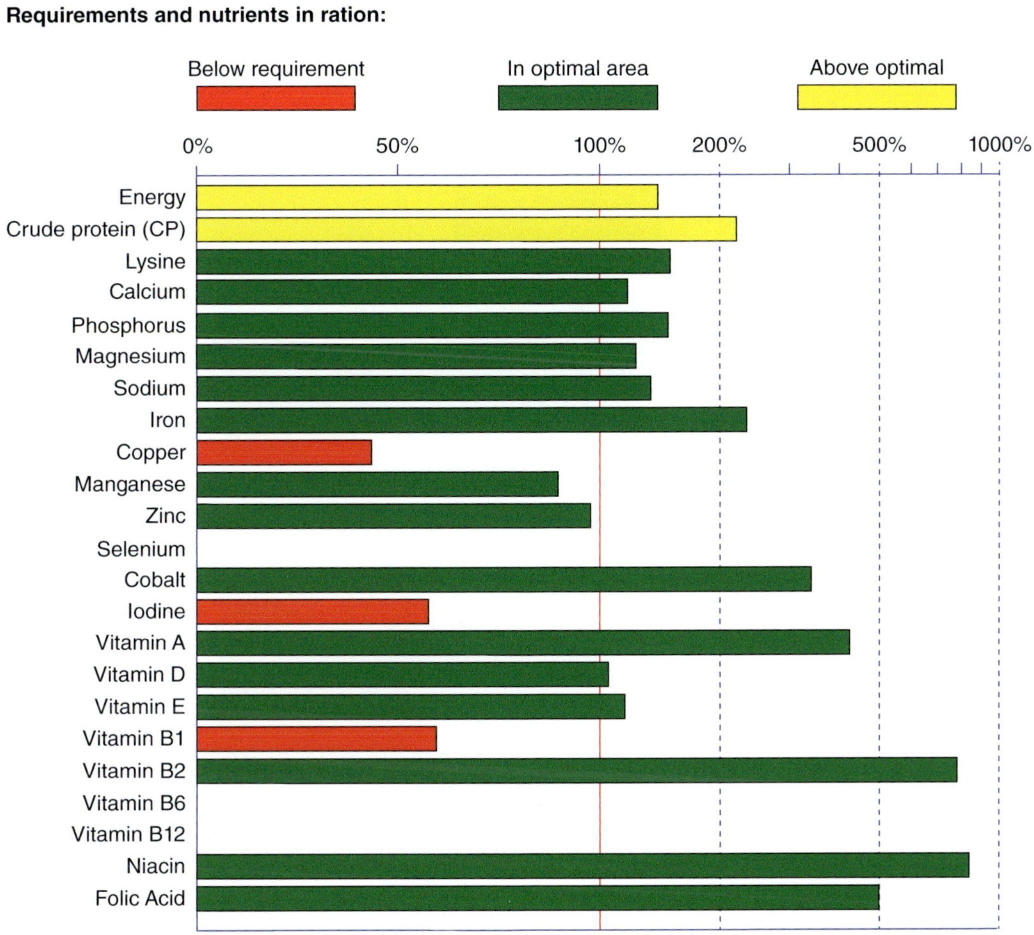

Fig. 10.8 Intake vs requirements of a 500 kg retired horse out 24/7 on summer pasture assuming a 2.5% BW (dry matter intake). (Ration courtesy of Briony Witherow.)

- Most horses in light work/maintenance will get adequate/excess calories from hay.
- Protein intake: adequate
  - An average hay = 8–9% crude protein, sufficient for horses that are at maintenance, but quality is poor and this horse is deficient in lysine.
- Trace minerals and vitamin E are below the recommended requirements.
  - Need balancing
- Advise a low-calorie balancer (100 g/100 kg BW)
  - For an estimated bodyweight of 500 kg: 500 g

Most horses fed ad lib hay will be overfed calories but undernourished with protein, vitamins and minerals. The clinical signs you are likely to encounter will include:

- dull coat;
- poor hoof quality;
- poor muscle development; and
- decreased immune responses.

Diet advice for horses being fed less than recommended amounts of feed (Fig. 10.10)

Q. I can only feed a handful of horse and pony nuts because my horse gets too fat.

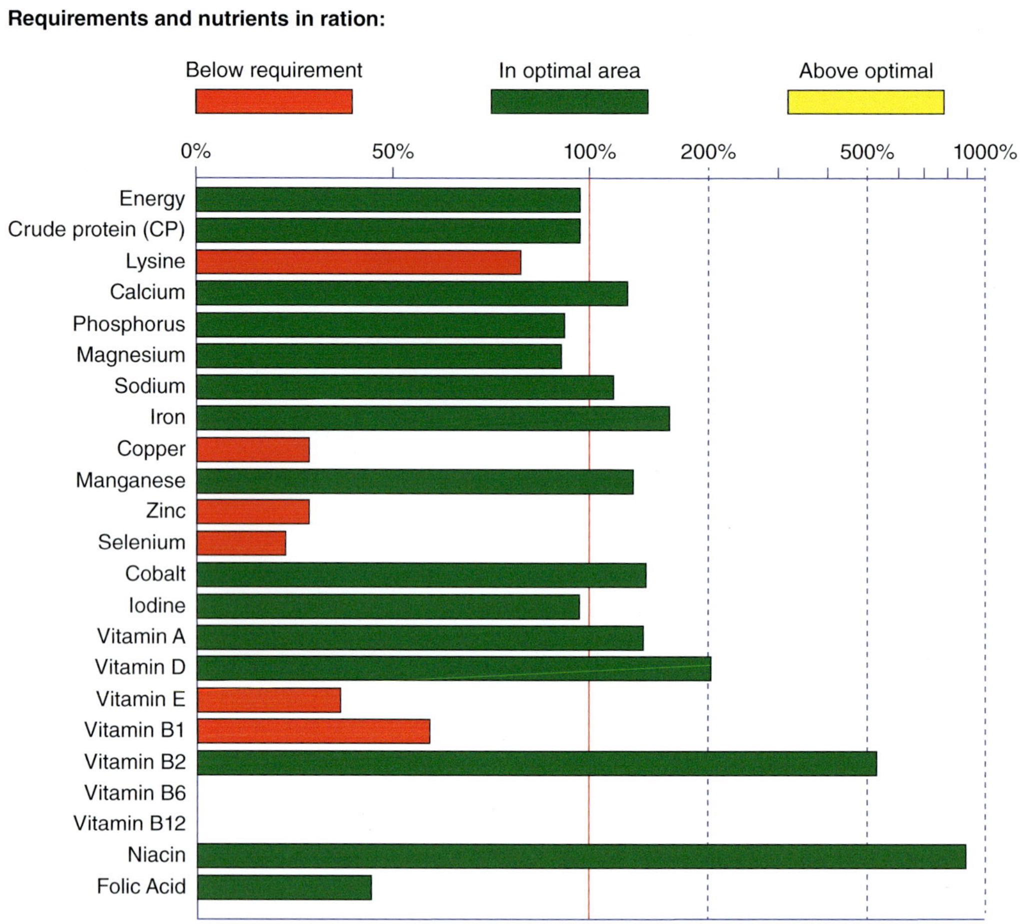

Fig. 10.9 The nutrient provision of a 500 kg horse at rest, eating ad lib conserved forage. Average meadow hay DMI 2.5% BW.

Factors to consider

This is a very common feeding scenario. Clients feed optimal intakes of forage but feel that they 'need' to be feeding a concentrate feed.

- This is usually an emotional decision rather than one that is based on actual ration knowledge and nutrient contributions.
- It may also be because this client has other horses that are being fed and therefore the horse is given a 'token' feed to reduce stress levels.
- Feed manufacturers formulate feeds to ensure that, when they are fed at the minimum recommended feeding rate, the ration is balanced when fed alongside the recommended intakes of forage. This minimum feeding rate is usually 400–600 g/100 kg BW (minimum of 2–3 kg per day for a 500 kg horse).
- In this situation, if the horse was fed 2 kg of the cooling nuts per day, this would exceed the energy recommendation and increase the risk of obesity. However, a handful of cubes is not providing enough vitamins and minerals and so this deficit needs to be addressed.
- A feed balancer fed at 100 g/100 kg BW will provide a balanced ration.
  - Recommend splitting into two meals.
  - Add 250 g alfalfa chaff to improve lysine.
  - Find a container that holds *exactly* the right quantity.

Requirements and nutrients in ration:

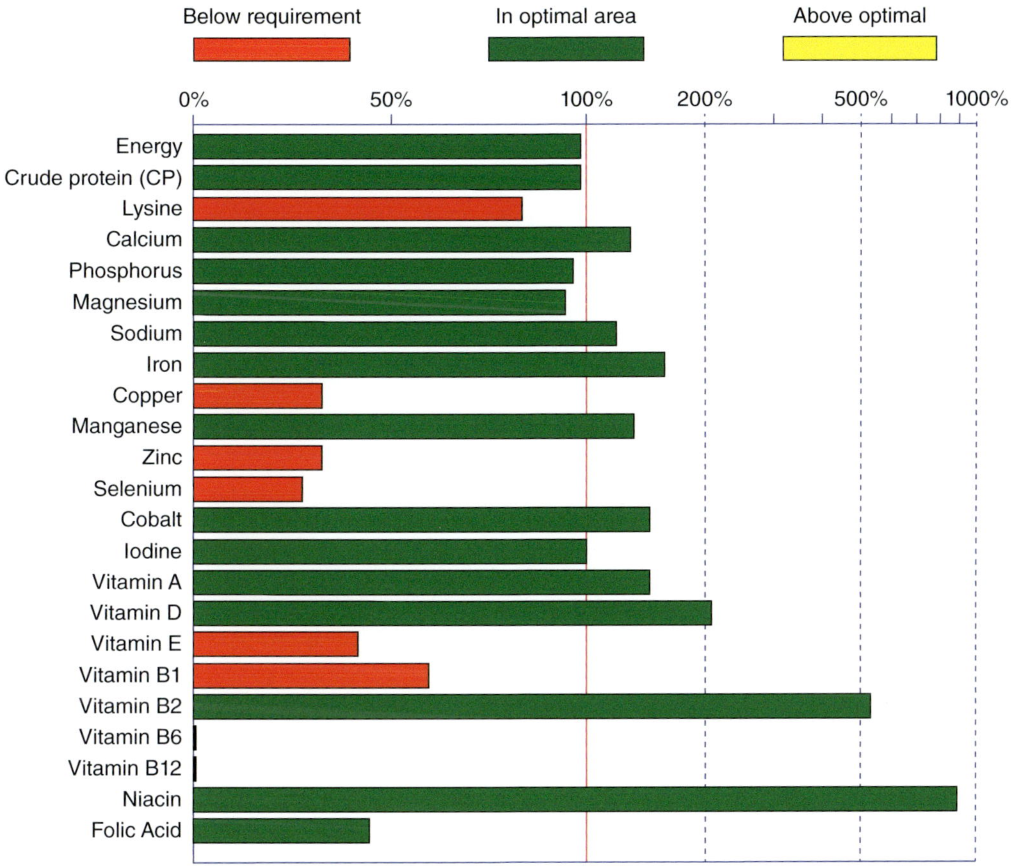

Fig. 10.10 Nutrient provision of an average meadow hay (2.5% BW DM) and a handful (100 g) of High Fibre Nuts for a 500 kg horse at rest. (Ration courtesy of Briony Witherow.)

Diet for a horse prone to laminitis (Fig. 10.11)

Q. My horse is a good doer and prone to laminitis, so I am feeding him a scoop of feed that is suitable for laminitics.

Factors to consider

- Energy and protein requirement are being met.
- Deficient in key trace minerals and some vitamins.
  - The daily intake of 600 g/day is below the manufacturer's recommended 400–600 g/100 kg BW/day.
  - Not providing a balanced ration.
  - Clients often underestimate the actual weight of chaff that they are feeding, as they are voluminous products.
  - Accurate weighing of chaffs is essential.
- Increasing the intake of Safe and Sound will increase the calorie intake, resulting in body-weight gain and body fat score, and laminitis.
- Your client is insistent that they would like to continue using Safe and Sound.
- You will need to recommend a calorie reduction in the forage allowance.
  - Carry out a forage analysis to see if the hay being fed has a lower calorie content than the forage source used in the programme database.
  - Advising your client to soak the current hay reduces the calorie content, provided that it is practically possible (see Chapter 9: Tables 9.5–9.7).
  - If soaking the hay is not possible, then advise forage with a lower calorie content.

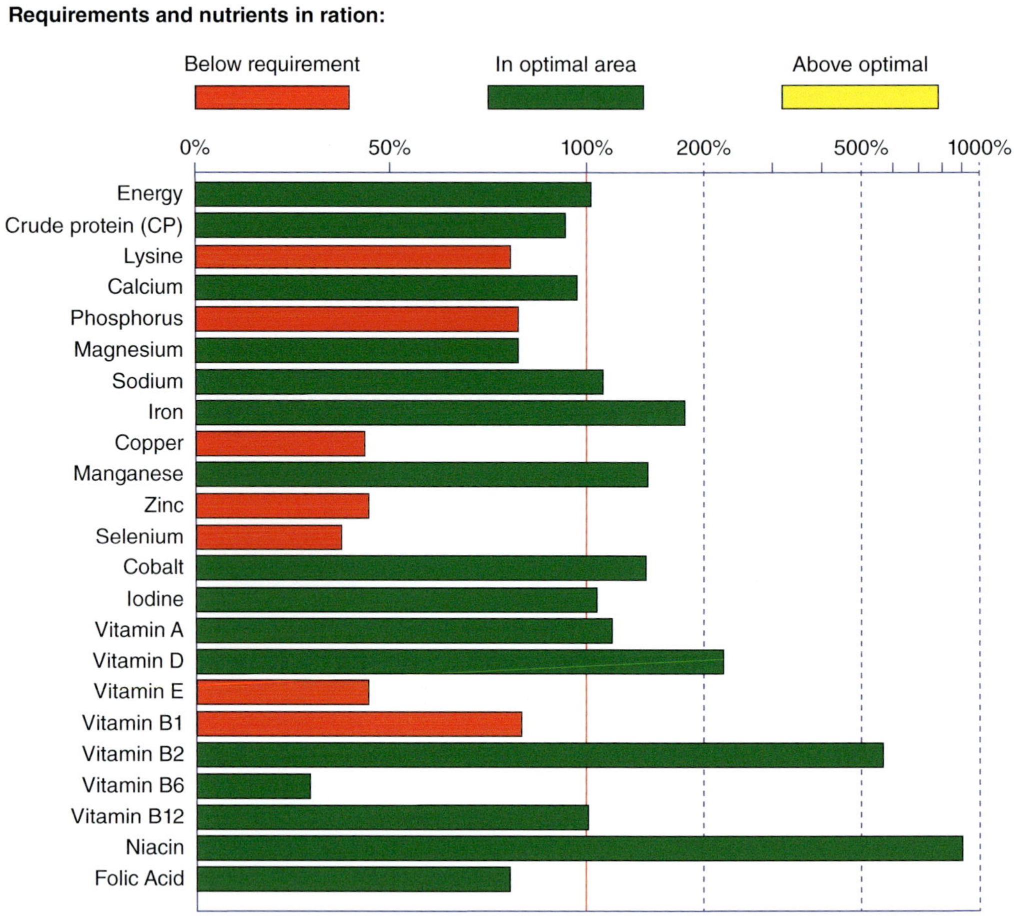

Fig. 10.11 Nutrient provision of average meadow hay (2.0% BW DM) and a Stubbs scoop (600 g) of Safe and Sound for a 500 kg horse prone to laminitis. (Ration courtesy of Briony Witherow.)

- Straw, fed at 50% of the daily allowance, extends feeding time and promotes a metabolic profile more suitable for overweight horses (Jansson *et al.*, 2021).

Advising a diet for a competition horse fed a leisure feed (Fig. 10.12)

Q. I have a competition horse who maintains his weight well but is naturally very excitable and gets 'too hot' on normal competition feeds. I feed him a low-energy Cooling Mix. He weighs 500 kg and has a BCS of 5 on a scale of 1–9. He has a good appetite, and his energy levels are good, although I struggle with his coat condition and my farrier says he has poor hoof quality. He is fed the manufacturer's minimum recommended daily feeding level.

Factors to consider

- The horse is in good body condition but has naturally high energy levels, and tends to react to fast-release energy ingredients that exaggerate the natural behaviour.
  - The low-energy/calorie feed is formulated for horses that are resting or in light work and is deficient in many nutrient levels.
- Usually an excitable horse needs more calories compared with a 'lazier' or less exuberant horse but they are maintaining good body condition on a lower than recommended intake of calories.
  - Adjust the metabolic rate to reflect this before discussing with the client.

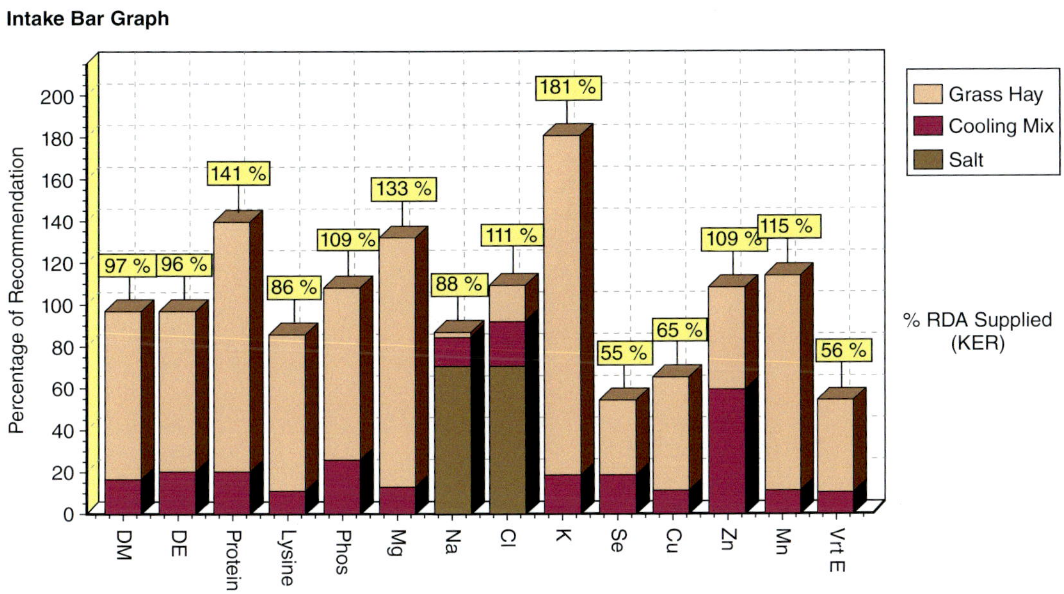

Fig. 10.12 The nutrient provision for a 500kg competition horse in medium work, with a body fat score of 5 and an excitable temperament, being fed 2kg of a low energy cooling feed and average grass hay (2% BW DM).

  - Ask client to monitor, especially if this is at the start of the competition season, and to record bodyweight and fat score fortnightly.
- The diet is not meeting protein, lysine, minerals and vitamins.
  - You need to advise your client that a ration adjustment is required to meet the requirements to support performance.
  - Lysine deficiency might result in clinical signs, such as failure to build muscle bulk properly.
  - Poor hoof and coat condition are also early indicators that the diet is lacking or unbalanced.
- The diet is deficient in sodium and chloride.
  - This will be further exacerbated as work increases and through sweat.
- Advise a gradual diet transition from the current leisure cooling feed to a performance feed that provides slow-release energy from fibre and oil; for example, Saracen Re-Leve or Dodson and Horrell StayPower, Spillers Slow Release energy competition feeds.

How to advise a client with a showjumper who wants to feed a high-protein diet (Fig. 10.13)

Q: My horse is competing and requires a high-protein diet, so I am feeding a stud diet base which is high in protein. My horse is 600 kg, 10 years old and showjumping.

Factors to consider

There are still many misconceptions that high protein levels are required to support high performance. Stud feeds are a common choice of feed for this class of horse.

- The diet exceeds the requirements for energy and protein and is overfortified for lysine.
  - Horses in hard work do have an increased requirement for protein but the increase is not as large as many people would believe.
  - Excess protein intake will compromise performance.
  - Protein quality is important, not the % protein content of the concentrate feed.
- Lower crude protein diets can be fed provided that they are high in quality protein sources and include limiting amino acids, such as lysine, methionine and threonine (Graham-Thiers *et al.*, 2001).
- Competition feeds from reputable horse feed manufacturers will typically contain 12–13% crude protein levels and 0.4–0.6% lysine.

How to recommend a diet for a horse that is anaemic (Fig. 10.14)

Q. I have been told that because my horse is lethargic with poor work recovery rate it needs an iron supplementation.

Ration Composition

Nutrient	D&H Alfa Oil	STAMM 30	STUD MIX	Grass Hay	Requirement	Total
Intake (kg/day)	0.800	1.000	4.000	12.000		17.800
DRY MATTER (kg/day)	0.720	0.900	3.540	10.800	13.500	15.960
DE (MJ/day)	7.7	11.7	49.5	89.4	134.3	158.4
PROTEIN (g/day)	144.0	300.0	580.0	1116.0	907.0	2140.0
LYSINE (g/day)	5.6	17.1	35.6	24.0	31.7	82.3
METHIONINE (g/day)			12.0			12.0
CALCIUM (g/day)	9.8	46.7	47.6	42.0	43.2	146.1
PHOSPHORUS (g/day)	2.4	21.4	20.8	24.0	28.8	68.6
MAGNESIUM (g/day)	2.2	8.6	7.2	21.6	18.0	39.6
SALT (g/day)			34.0			34.0
SODIUM (g/day)	.1	5.2	9.2	1.2	40.5	15.7
CHLORIDE (g/day)	.8	7.8	15.2	12.0	60.8	35.8
POTASSIUM (g/day)	12.0	14.0	32.8	153.6	94.5	212.4
SELENIUM (mg/day)	0.08	2.50	2.00	1.20	3.38	5.78
COPPER (mg/day)	7.2	200.0	152.0	108.0	202.5	467.2
ZINC (mg/day)	16.0	545.0	440.0	300.0	607.5	1301.0
MANGANESE (mg/day)	45.6	308.0	248.0	624.0	607.5	1225.6
IRON (mg/day)	160.0		160.0	636.0		956.0
VITAMIN E (IU/day)	48	605	1140	480	1080	2273

Fig. 10.13 The nutrient provision for a 600kg, 10 year old showjumper in medium work, fed 1kg of a stud balancer and 4kg of a stud mix and average grass hay (2% BW DM).

Factors to consider

Iron (Fe)-deficiency anaemia is extremely rare in horses. Hay, pasture and other feed provide dietary excess.

- UK soils and forages are generally high in iron (> 100 mg Fe/kg DM).
- Commercially formulated feeds can contain from 40 mg up to 700 mg of iron.
- Some of this iron is likely to be poorly absorbed or bound to the pectin constituents in some fibre products.
- High Fe intakes may compromise the absorption of other minerals in the diet.

The main causes of anaemia in horses are blood loss, blood-cell destruction and reduced red blood cell production.

- Some infections, including equine infectious anaemia, babesiosis and trypanosomiasis, lead to the destruction of red blood cells.
- Internal parasites, in particular large strongyles (also known as blood worms or red worms), can damage tissue to the extent that blood loss leads to anaemia.
- Daily requirement is 0.8 mg/kg BW for horses and 500 mg for growing foals, pregnant and lactating mares (NRC, 2007).

Following client feedback of horses feeling lethargic or experiencing lower energy levels, particularly as a competitive season progresses, many are advised to supplement with iron to improve performance

- Supplementation is commonly carried out without any formal analysis of the diet to determine if additional iron is required.
- In typical scenarios where optimum forage is being fed, iron intake exceeds requirements.
- Event horses supplemented with iron had plasma total iron concentrations up to 2–3 times higher than the typical normal range (Mills *et al.*, 1996).
- The average horse does not need an iron supplement, assuming they are being fed optimum quantities of forage and that the recommended amount of a commercial feed is being fed (Fig. 10.7), which often provides over 300% of iron requirements.

Requirements and nutrients in ration:

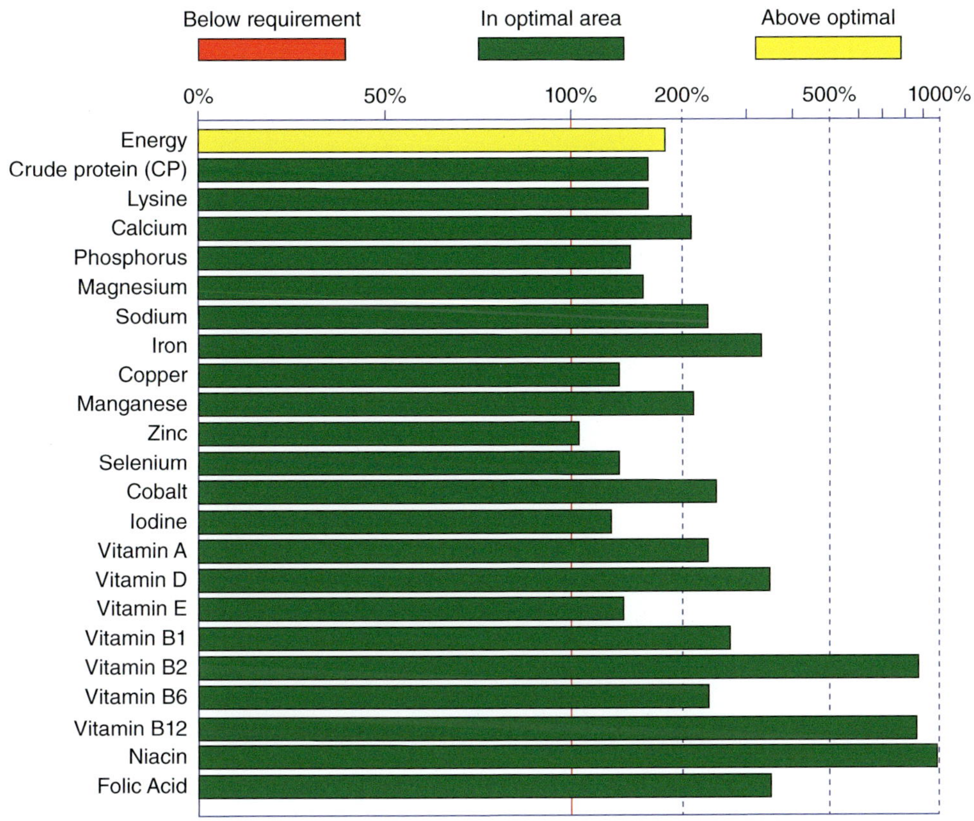

Fig. 10.14 The nutrient provision for a 500kg horse in medium work, being fed 3kg of a slow energy release competition feed and average grass hay (2% BW DM).

Top tip

Over-supplementation of iron rather than a low dietary level is more likely to be a problem in performance horses.
You should advise against the use of iron supplementation until you have carried out further investigations.
Investigate and focus on other reasons for a lack or loss of energy and performance.
Rule out any possible clinical issues, such as dehydration, gastric ulcers, upper airway disease or lameness.
Discuss type of feed being fed.
Explore the opportunity to advise a feed that provides fast-releasing energy (see Chapter 5).

How to advise supplements for an endurance horse (Fig. 10.15)

Q. My horses are competing in endurance rides and the training and work is long and intense. My feed and forage is not enough at this level and I need to feed a variety of supplements to maintain the work and performance level

Factors to consider

Feeding multiple supplements is often done to find that 'magic bullet' for that dramatic change in performance level. The belief comes from marketing and advertising and the basic instinct of wanting to do the best for the horse.

Rations such as this example are expensive and wasteful and in the long term are more likely to create a dietary imbalance.

- This horse is being fed the recommended level of forage, which is balanced with a fully fortified feed that is being fed at a suitable intake.
- Energy and protein requirements are balanced and assessment of the horse has shown that this is maintaining body condition and weight.
- Minerals: client is correct in adding additional salt and electrolyte to the diet but can be advised that the other supplements are in excess to requirements.
  - Using the coloured bar chart, you can show your client what each individual supplement is contributing to the diet and how removing them from the diet will still leave nutrients within recommended levels.

How to check a 'normal' horse's diet (Fig. 10.16)

Q. My horse has a normal temperament and is in light daily work of hacking and arena schooling 2–3 times per week and may compete occasionally at weekends. Horse maintains good body condition and is a 5 on a 9 scale. Sports horse bred and 9 years old and weighs approximately 500 kg on a weightape. He has access to ad lib hay, and intake has been monitored to average 11 kg per day.

Factors to consider

- This horse is being fed the correct choice of a fortified feed, fed at the correct daily intake, alongside the optimum level of forage (2.5% of BW DM), and meets recommended requirements.
- This ration would need no alteration, based on the information provided by the client.
  - You would amend the calorie requirement by changing the metabolic rate before sharing with client.
  - You might advise a teaspoon of salt/day.

How to recommend a diet that contains straights or individual feed ingredients (Fig. 10.17)

Q. I have a hunting horse and I prefer to feed straights mixed with bran, it's what I have always done. I can then see what I feed him. I add a cup of oil to each feed. Horse is hunted twice per week and will usually do a full day. Horse has always maintained good body condition and is kept in the stable through the hunting season. He is 500 kg and 12 years old.

Factors to consider

Feeding straights is often seen as a cheaper option than feeding compound feeds, but it is more challenging to ensure that the horse gets all the correct nutrients.

- Oats, barley, maize, bran and wheat are all straights. They are a non-complete feed when fed with forage and they are unbalanced in protein, vitamins and minerals.
- The horse needs to be eating optimum levels of a good-quality forage. Ensure that:
  - the forage has been analysed to confirm its actual nutrient contribution;
  - you have checked with your client that the horse is eating its daily allocation; and
  - this forage is providing sufficient protein and lysine.
- However, you do need to remember that many forages are commonly low in essential minerals such as calcium, vitamins and the essential amino acid lysine.
  - Insufficient lysine will mean the horse cannot process protein correctly and will result in loss of condition, poor hoof growth and poor coat condition.
- Feeding cereals without supplementation will unbalance the calcium:phosphorus ratio, which can cause bone problems.
- Advantages of feeding straights:
  - Appear cheaper
  - Palatable
  - Offer the client more control
- Disadvantages of feeding straights:
  - Quality can vary
  - Difficult to ensure a balanced diet
  - Imbalances can lead to laminitis, colic and tying-up
- Advise a specific oat balancer. There are specifically formulated oat balancers:
  - minimum rate of 1–2.0 kg per day (e.g. Saracen Horse Feeds Kentucky Balancer)
- Advise varying the amount of oats according to workload and BFS.
- Oat balancers are more appropriate compared with broad-spectrum vitamin and mineral supplements that do not provide enough quality protein or the correct balance of calcium and phosphorus.

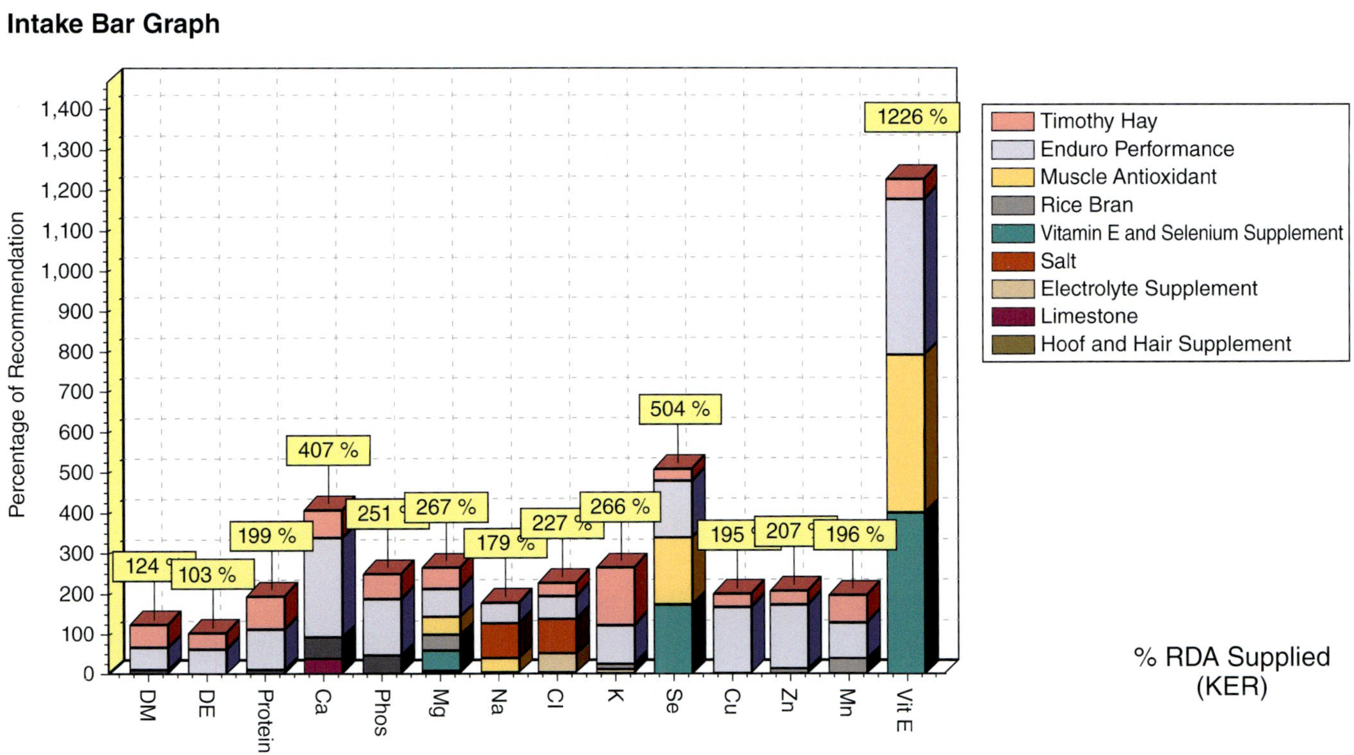

Fig. 10.15 The nutrient provision for a 420kg endurance horse competing in 100km endurance rides, being fed 6kg of a specialist endurance feed, additional supplements to maintain performance and Timothy hay (1.5% BW DM).

Intake Bar Graph

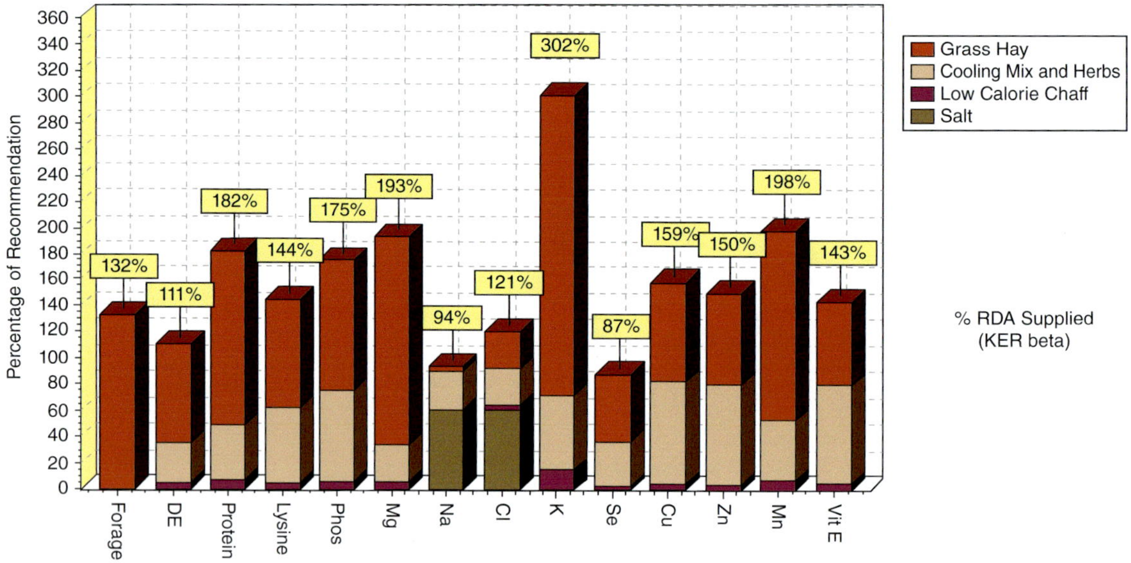

Fig. 10.16 The nutrient provision for a 500kg leisure horse in light work being fed 2kg of a leisure feed and average grass hay on an ad-lib basis actually consuming 11kg per day when monitored.

How to advise a client feeding small-bale haylage to meet DM intake (Fig. 10.18)

Q: My horse is starting to eat his droppings. I have been told to increase his fibre intake, so I have increased his haylage to about 2.5% of his bodyweight. He is around 400 kg, so I have weighed out 10 kg and he is still eating his droppings. I have bought small-bale haylage, as the yard only provides hay.

Factors to consider

It is more common for people to underfeed haylage than overfeed, due to the perception that it has higher energy content or because they have replaced hay on a weight-for-weight basis. This pony is eating 2.5% fresh weight of his body weight as 'forage', which is meeting 100% of his calorie requirement. What the client has not done is take into account the water content of the haylage (60% DM).

- Reduced dry matter intake leads to increased risk of gastrointestinal diseases
  - Equine gastric ulcer disease
  - Colic
  - Loose droppings
  - Development of behavioural vices such as wood chewing or eating droppings.

Your client has been correctly advised that she needs to increase her pony's fibre intake to 2.5% of BW.

- You need to check the nutritional analysis of the haylage that she has bought in or arrange for a forage analysis to check the dry matter value and the calorie/energy content.
- Eating droppings is an indication that dry matter intake is not being met and so the pony is exhibiting behaviour to try to 'increase' his fibre and roughage intake.
- If you have access to the dry matter content of the haylage being fed (60%) you can carry out a simple calculation to check the dry matter requirement:
  - 400 x 2.5% BW = 10 kg DM
  - 1 kg haylage contains only 600 g of 'fibre' (60% DM)
  - 10/0.6 = 16 kg fresh weight haylage
- You should recommend:
  - feeding additional haylage up to an extra 6 kg *if* the pony is in regular exercise and not at risk of becoming overweight; or
  - adding in an additional fibre product such as a high-fibre and low-calorie chaff product as an 'extra haynet' or extending with straw (if the horse does cough).

Intake Bar Graph

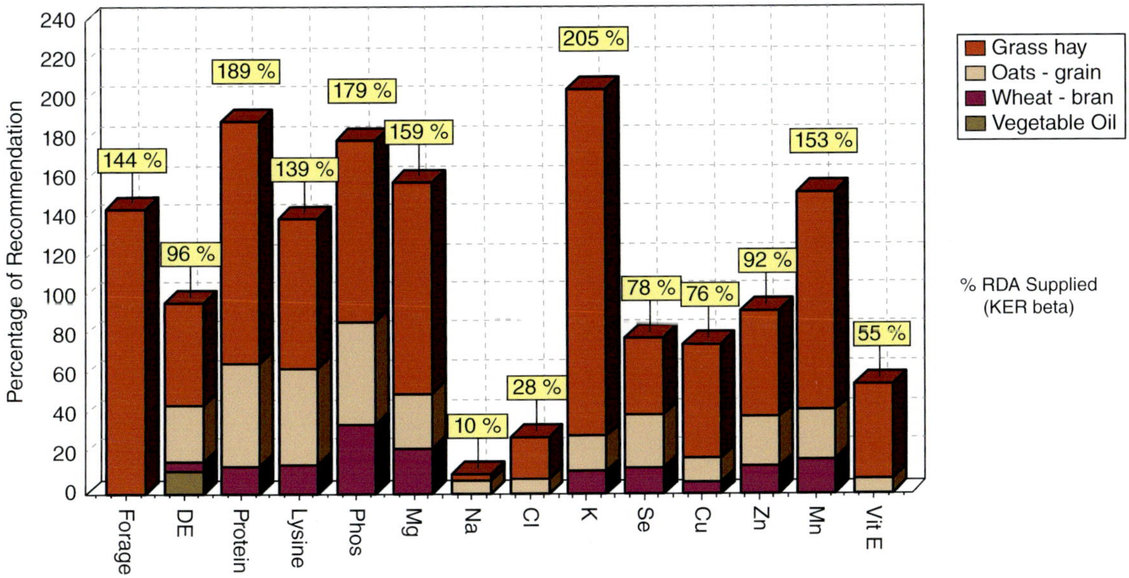

Acceptable Ranges

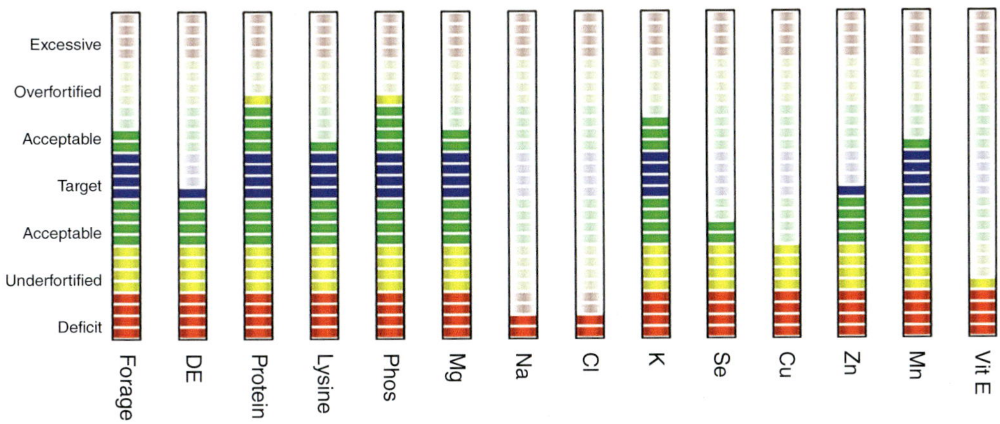

Fig. 10.17 The nutrient provision for a 500kg, 12 year old hunting horse in hard work being fed 4kg oats, 0.8kg of wheat bran and 3 cups of oil, and average grass hay (2% BW DM).

Advantages and Disadvantages of Software Programs

It is important that the basis of carrying out a ration evaluation and the derivation of the calculations is understood, so that you can provide a knowledgeable understanding of the computer software print-out and understand its limitations.

Pros

- Offers a method of simplifying the ration evaluation process.
- Provides a practical and visual tool for your client and students to understand the impact of feeding plans and rations.
- Illustrates the effect of the addition of various supplements or feeds etc.

Intake Bar Graph

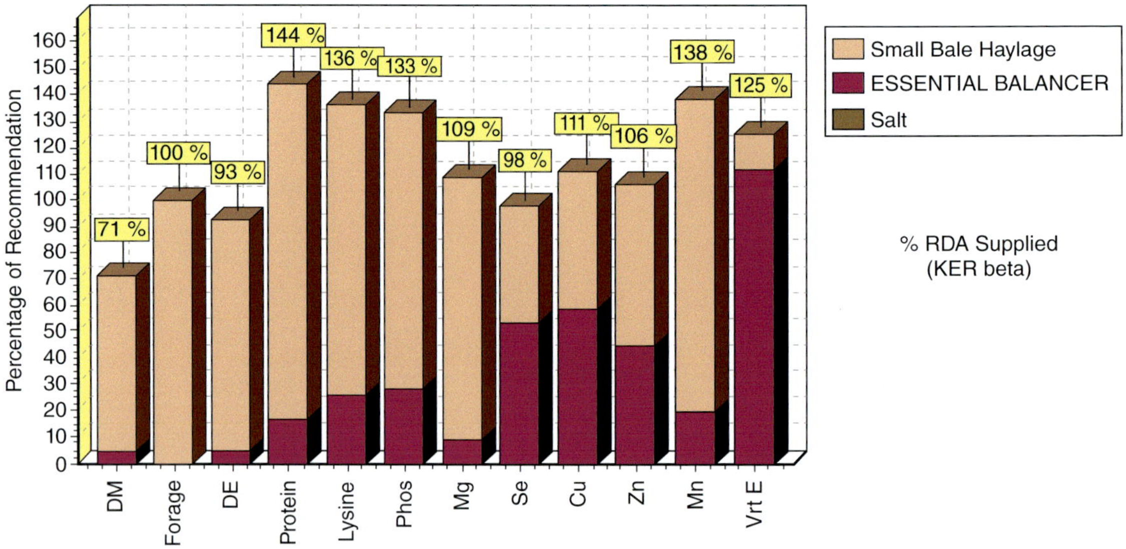

Fig. 10.18 The nutrient provision for a 400kg pony in light work eating 400grams of a feed balancer and average haylage (2.5% BW DM).

- Large databases of nutrient analysis of feeds, forages and supplements.
- Regular data updates, for average forages.
- Most programs allow for adjustments to be made for metabolic rate, enabling the user to adjust the energy intake accordingly.
- Enables accurate interpretation 'adding value' to a health check.

Cons

- No accounting for imprecise input data; or variability in the energy and nutrient requirements of individual horses.
- Mean values for nutritional requirements and analytical compositions of ingredients.
- Failure of the client to appreciate the limitations of the output.
- Lack of understanding as to how some of the calculations have been derived.
- Ration analysis can be inaccurate if databases contain old information and are not kept regularly updated.
- Keeping up to date with the huge array of available compound feeds and supplements can be time consuming. Not all the information is always easily obtained, or companies may be unwilling to disclose.
- The accuracy and the reliability of the output data from the ration evaluation software remains very reliant on the input data, the correct assessment of the horse and the variables for that individual.
- Emphasis can be erroneously placed on the requirements in terms of absolute values, especially for the micronutrient requirement, where the reality is often that an optimum range for intake may exist (Kronfeld, 2001).
- Check if the program provides information on the energy provision of water-soluble carbohydrate, starch fibre and oil.

The quality of the ingredients and diet cannot be determined simply by using a software evaluation program, so a visual assessment of forage and feeds and a clinical history should always play a key part of a ration evaluation (see Chapters 4, 8 and 9).

Summary

With any type of ration evaluation, it is important that your client knows how much they are feeding in weight rather than volume; the only way to do this is to weigh each feed ingredient that is used daily, using a set of weigh scales.

Miscalculations of bodyweight can have a dramatic effect on requirements. Energy requirements can vary by as much as 10% above or below the calculated daily requirement on the programme, due to metabolism or climate.

Software programs are based on a set of numbers and recognised parameters and therefore must be used as a guide only. Ration evaluation software can most certainly be used successfully to assess the suitability of an existing diet and can be used to make a new ration in a similar manner.

It is likely that clients will become more familiar with the use of digital tools and your practice software will hopefully develop to include the 5th vital sign. Remote consultations and telemedicine are on the increase and software programs can help provide the required dietary advice to the owners, both remotely and face-to-face offering a 'visual assessment' of the ration.

Bibliography

Coenen, M., Kienzle, E., Vervuert, I. and Zeyner A. (2011) Recent German developments in the formulation of energy and nutrient requirements in horses and the resulting feeding recommendations. *Journal of Equine Veterinary Science* 31, 219–229. doi: 10.1016/j.jevs.2011.03.204.

Graham-Thiers, P.M., Kronfeld, D.S., Kline, K.A. and Sklan, D.J. (2001) Dietary protein restriction and fat supplementation diminish the acidogenic effect of exercise during repeated sprints in horses. *The Journal of Nutrition* 131(7), 1959–1964.

Harris, P., Ellis, A., Fradinho, M., Jansson, A., Julliand, V. *et al*. (2017) Review: feeding conserved forage to horses: recent advances and recommendations. *Animal* 11(6), 958–967. doi: 10.1017/S1751731116002469.

Jansson, A., Harris, P., Davey, S.L., Luthersson, N., Ragnarsson, S. *et al*. (2021) Straw as an alternative to grass forage in horses—effects on post-prandial metabolic profile, energy intake, behaviour and gastric ulceration. *Animals* 11(8), 2197. doi: 10.3390/ani11082197.

Kronfeld, D.S. (1978) Feeding on horse breeding farms. *American Association of Equine Practitioners* 24, 461–464.

Kronfeld, D.S. (2001) A practical method for ration evaluation and diet formulation: an introduction to sensitivity analysis. In: Pagan, J.D. and Geor, R.J. (eds) *Advances in Equine Nutrition II*. Kentucky Equine Research, Versailles, Kentucky, pp. 13–28.

Mills, P.C., Smith, N.C., Casas, I., Harris, P., Harris, R.C. *et al*. (1996) Effects of exercise intensity and environmental stress on indices of oxidative stress and iron homeostasis during exercise in the horse. *European Journal of Applied Physiology and Occupational Physiology* 74(1), 60–66.

NRC (National Research Council) (2007) *Nutrient Requirements of Horses: Sixth Revised Edition*. The National Academies Press, Washington, DC. doi: 10.17226/11653.

Pagan, J.D., Jackson, S. and Duren, S. (1996) Computing horse nutrition: how to properly conduct an equine ration evaluation using Microsteed™ equine ration evaluation software. *World Equine Veterinary Review Archives* 1(2), 10B1–10B7.

11 Feeding the Leisure Horse

TERESA HOLLANDS

School of Veterinary Medicine, University of Surrey

Learning Objectives

LO1 Explain the advantages and disadvantages of different feedstuffs.
LO2 Describe feeding management techniques to meet the horse's physiological and anatomical adaptations.
LO3 Justify your choice of feeds, ration and feeding management.
LO4 Compare and contrast diet plans for a range of leisure horses.

At the end of this chapter, you will be able to choose the correct ration for the leisure horse to maintain healthy longevity and minimise the risk of diet-related diseases.

Overview

Over 80% of horses in the UK are kept for leisure (the client is not benefiting financially from keeping the horse) and are exercised for around 6 h/week (Hotchkiss *et al.*, 2007; Boden *et al.*, 2013). Whilst leisure riding has been shown to increase energy expenditure for the rider (Devienne and Guezennec, 2000) – a 45 min stage 2 lesson was recorded as needing the same metabolic energy demand as moderate exercise (Beale *et al.*, 2015) – it is well recognised that most clients overestimate the workload of their horses (Honoré and Uhlinger, 1994; Hale *et al.*, 2016). This perception of workload means that clients feel that they should feed concentrates to meet their horse's 'work': 87% of horse owners reported feeding concentrates, which were mostly premixed commercial feeds, 'using scoops, cans, cups or by eye' (68%), despite 54% being leisure riders (most leisure horses do not need hard feed) (Murray *et al.*, 2015). Whilst clients tend to overfeed their horse for energy – 44% excess (Honoré and Uhlinger, 1994) – supplementary feeding of concentrates is only a moderate risk factor for overweight/obesity compared with the consumption of grass (Giles *et al.*, 2015).

Feeding increased amounts of concentrates was recorded as a protective factor against obesity (Salonen *et al.*, 2009). This is because horses fed larger quantities of concentrates tend to be in harder work with less access to grass. Grass can provide 2–4× the energy requirements of a horse in light work (Smith *et al.*, 2007) and is the main source of calories/energy for many leisure horses, resulting in more than 50% of the equine population (41% of ponies and 26% of horses) being overweight or obese (Salonen *et al.*, 2009; Robin *et al.*, 2015).

This grass needs replacing with a lower-energy forage such as soaked hay, but most clients are unaware of how much hay their horses eat; only 34% of clients provided accurate records of hay intake (Honoré and Uhlinger, 1994). Cutting down the amount (dry matter intake) the leisure horse eats is detrimental to its health and increases the risk of gastric ulcers (Murray and Schusser, 1993; Videla and Andrews, 2009; Pedersen *et al.*, 2015), colic (Scantlebury *et al.*, 2015) and stereotypy behaviours (McGreevy *et al.*, 1995; Waters *et al.*, 2002), resulting in an imbalanced diet. It is also a challenging concept for the owner, as clients consider feeding an act of caring (Furtado *et al.*, 2020).

DOI: 10.1079/9781789245134.0011

This chapter is as much about minimising the dietary risks to prevent horses becoming fat or obese as it is about feeding the 'normal' horse. You may also find it helpful to refer to Chapter 15 ('The chronically inflamed (obese) horse: understanding adipose biology') so that you can expand on your advice and explain the reasons behind the need to maintain fitness, not fatness. In the case of leisure horses, 75% are cared for by their owner, with between 37% and 68% kept on private premises (Hotchkiss *et al.*, 2007). You are one of their main sources of nutritional information (Gemmill *et al.*, 2014, 2016), so make sure that your advice is evidence based and follow the steps needed to take a dietary history (see Chapters 2 and 3).

The Contribution of Pasture to the Diet

Most leisure (also known as overweight) horses have access to grazing all year round. Mean annual turnout is 8 h. In the winter 73% of horses are turned out during the day; 80% in the spring and summer, with 50% turned out 24/7 in the summer (Hotchkiss *et al.*, 2007; Ireland *et al.*, 2011).

Depending on the quality and quantity of the grass, horses grazing for 24 h can eat up to 5% of their bodyweight as dry matter, consuming 2–4× the calorie requirements for a leisure horse in light work (Smith *et al.*, 2007). Limiting horses to grazing short grass for 3 h will always reduce the calories the horse consumes – together with a combination of strip grazing, muzzles, and active grass management through cutting or overstocking. Providing alternative low-calorie forages (see Chapter 9) when the horse does not have access to pasture will provide the horse with adequate fibre and ensure that it can exhibit its natural foraging behaviour.

You need to account for the numerous variables that affect the amount of grass the horse can eat as part of your dietary history taking.

Grass quantity

Industry-accepted recommendations state that an individual horse needs 1–1.5 acres of pasture (BHS, 2019), with the caveat that adjustments might be needed according to grass availability, quality, workload and fat score of the horse. Clearly there is a seasonal aspect too (Fig. 11.1).

Do make sure that you do not make academic judgements based just on season: global warming has affected seasonal availability and grass growth. Remind clients that if the temperature is above 6°C and there is enough sunlight and water, then grass will grow; conversely, in a very wet spring or hot summer, grass will not grow.

Restricting pasture

Stabling horses

Reducing access to high-calorie grass will reduce the calorie intake of the horse, but the alternative to pasture is normally an increased time in a stable, which is the equivalent of the client staying in bed to lose weight.

In natural grazing environments, horses have access to low-quality forages, mainly grass, and travel 16 km/day seeking food, with some travelling as far as 55 km (Hampson *et al.*, 2010a); whereas paddocked horses travelled 7.5 km/day and horses kept in a 6 m^2 yard only moved 1 km/day (Hampson *et al.*, 2010b). Leisure horses that are kept stabled for 13–16 h/24 h are harder to handle, as are those bedded on shavings rather than straw. The longer the horse is stabled, the more aggressive it is to people and, like the performance horse, increased time in a stable is correlated with an increase in oral stereotypies (Hockenhull and Creighton., 2014).

Disadvantages of pasture restriction: fibre restriction, gastric ulcers, stereotypies and colic

A reduction in forage increases the risk of gastric ulcers (Murray and Schusser, 1993; Luthersson *et al.*, 2009; Videla and Andrews, 2009), because the fibre mat is diminished and the horse chews less (Meyer *et al.*, 1985). Whilst commonly associated with performance horses, 22% of feral horses sampled from an abattoir had squamous ulceration and 30% had glandular ulceration (Ward *et al.*, 2015), as did 54–68% of leisure horses (Hepburn, 2014).

Less chewing means that less saliva is produced. Saliva buffers the top part of the horse's stomach from the acid splashback from the lower stomach; specifically, during exercise (Lorenzo-Figueras and Merritt, 2002).

Horses that cannot satisfy their need to chew find other ways to satisfy that need, such as wood chewing or crib biting, (McGreevy *et al.*, 1995; Waters *et al.*, 2002).

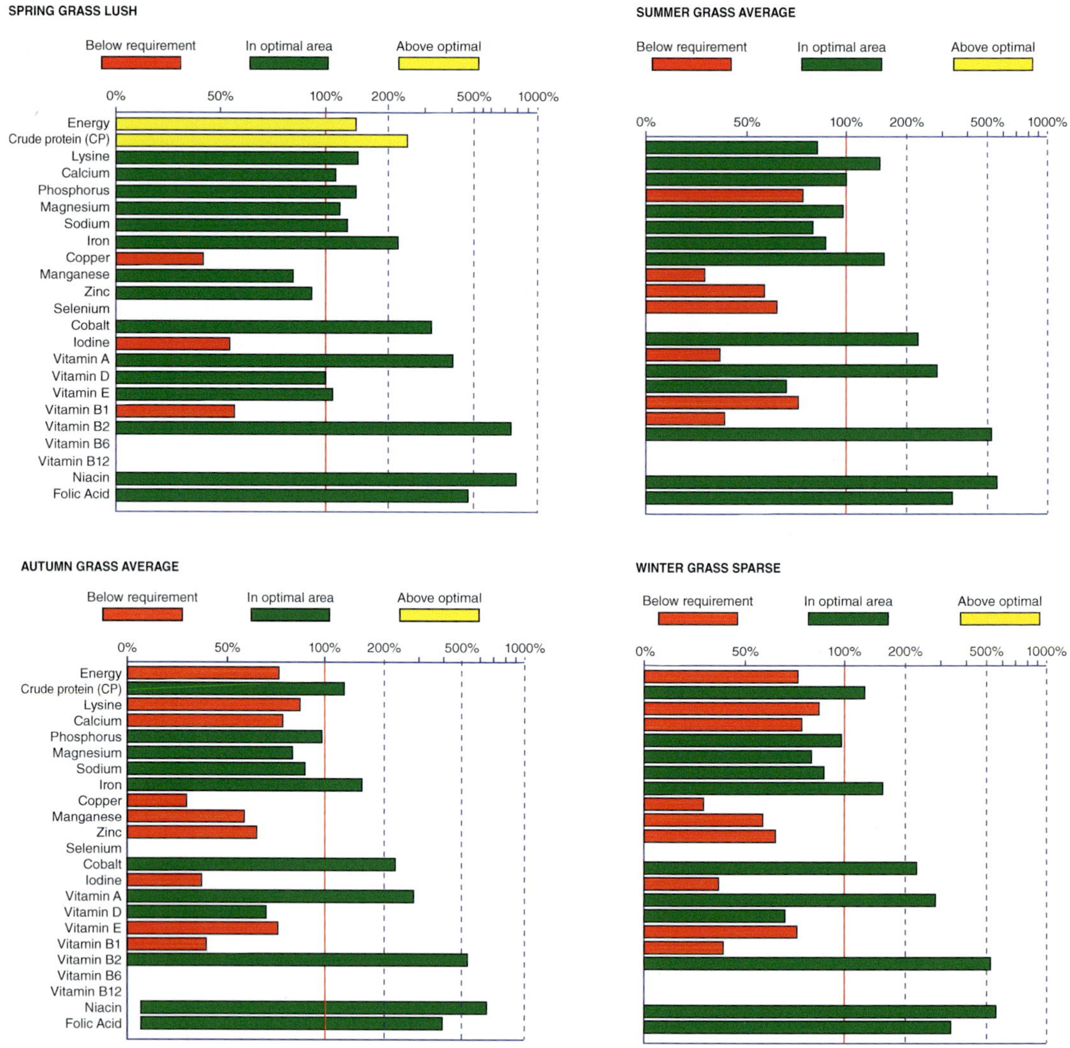

Fig. 11.1 The impact of the season on nutrient intake expressed as % of requirements of a 500 kg horse in light work, grazing 24/7. Red = deficiency; green = adequate/optimum or, if in excess, no toxicity or health issues; yellow = excess and needs addressing. (From PC-Horse, Norway, available at https://pchorse.se/index/php/en/)

- Crib biting increases the risk of colic (Scantlebury *et al.*, 2015).
  - Low-fibre diets increase the risk of acidic hind guts (Jouany *et al.*, 2009) as well as certain colics, due to the disruption of the microflora (Willing *et al.*, 2009).
  - Reducing food intake increases the risk of insulin resistance (see Chapter 15: 'Fibre restriction, insulin resistance and cortisol levels').

Advantages of pasture restriction

Restrictive (night-time) versus ad lib (24/7) grazing reduces calorie intake but has no effect on hind gut pH or fluid balance (Siciliano and Schmidt, 2012).

Restricting grass DMI from 2% to 1.25–1.5% BW for 8 months from September to May reduced the calorie intake of client-owned horses by 80–85%, resulting in a mean BW loss of 5.98% and decrease in BFS of 1.4/9 (Gill *et al.*, 2016).

There were differences in how much weight the clients' horses lost, depending on the management of the horses. Horses pastured with muzzles lost 4.8% BW and 1 fat score; horses that were kept on a mix of sand paddocks and pasture lost 7.2% BW and 1.14 fat score; and horses that had no access to pasture lost 9.8% BW and 2.3 BFS. Horses that continued to have their normal access to grass gained 12% BW and +0.7 BFS (Gill *et al.*, 2016). The differences between partial and no pasture access were not significant.

Even though clients often struggle with the concept of keeping their horses stabled, there is some evidence suggesting that compliance is greatest when pasture is removed completely, simply because it is easier to manage. Owners struggle with partial pasture restrictions, citing not being able to keep muzzle on, the livery yard being uncooperative, or not having alternative options (Gill *et al.*, 2016).

Top tip

Evidence shows that when the livery yard comes on board, facilitates sand paddocks/dry lots and provides and supports muzzle use, then client compliance results in the greatest weight and BFS loss (Giles *et al.*, 2015).

Your role

On most yards, there will be a mix of overweight and normal horses, and it is possible for clients to manage both these groups on the same pasture – by utilising muzzles and strip grazing for the good doers whilst allowing the other horses free access.

Encourage client compliance to prevent their horse from maintaining dysfunctional adipose tissue by ensuring that the horse keeps moving, interacts with a 'herd', continues to eat but at the same time reduce calories (see Chapter 9: 'The relationship between forage feeding management and eating behaviour').

Feeding Management of the Leisure Horse

The client needs to ensure that the horse is eating enough dry matter whilst controlling calories; they need to balance the ration, especially with respect to minerals and protein, and accept the fact that you are not wanting them to diet their horse but rather to ensure that they are managed correctly for life.

Provide them with three target areas:

1. Count calories.
2. Maintain dry matter intake (bulk/forage).
3. Balance micronutrients.

Count calories

Horses should be fed a minimum of 2.5% of their bodyweight to maintain their health and welfare. Please do not tell the client to reduce food intake, as this might not decrease calories sufficiently (Table 11.1) but it will be detrimental to the horse's health and welfare.

Even 1.5% DM high-fibre haylage or good-quality meadow hay exceeds the calorie requirement of a horse at maintenance, as does the same DM intake of winter pasture (17 h), summer grazing (8 h) and night-time grazing of spring grass; so fat and weight loss would be unsuccessful.

Most clients forget that fibre/forages provide their leisure horse with excess calories and spend more time considering the hard feed rather than quantifying forage intakes.

Perhaps a better way of gaining client understanding would be to use a human example. A 60 kg human restricting their food intake to 1.5% of their bodyweight will consume 900 g DM food (Table 11.2) but calorie intake will differ.

Maintain dry matter intake (DMI)

It is possible for a horse in light work to eat 2.5% of its bodyweight as forage and consume fewer calories compared with requirements (Table 11.1).

Choosing a low-calorie forage

Advise feeding low-calorie forages to meet calorie requirements and maintain DMI (see Chapter 9, Table 9.11: 'The average calorie content of forages fed to horses in the UK, in descending order of calorie content on a DM basis'). Advising the right type of forage depends upon several factors (see Chapter 9), including:

- soaking (Chapter 9: 'Advising soaking hay to provide low-calorie forage');
  - using multiple haynets and small-hole haynets (Chapter 9: 'Advising haynets, bags and grids'); and

Table 11.1 A comparison of calorie intake from different forages fed at 2.5% BW as dry matter to a 500 kg horse in light work as a % of requirements[a]

Forage	2.5% DMI (kg)	Fresh weight (kg)	Total calorie intake (MJ/DE)	Calorie as % of requirements	Energy/calories intakes
Spring grass	12.5	62.5	150	164–192	Excess calories – weight gain
Summer grass	12.5	41.6	125	137–160	
Ryegrass haylage[b]	12.5	25	112–144	123–185	
Ryegrass hay	12.5	14.7	120	131–154	
High-fibre haylage[b]	12.5	19	87.5–125	96–160	Check estimated digestible energy of forage or get analysed
Meadow hay (late-cut–early-cut)	12.5	14.7	87.5–112	96–144	
Autumn/winter grass	12.5	25	75	82–96	Calories controlled, dry matter intake maintained; should lose weight
Soaked hay	12.5	14.7[c]	62.5	69–80	
Straw (barley/oat)	12.5	14.7	56	62–72	

[a]500 kg horse in light work needs 78–91 MJ DE/day
[b]All values approximate or taken from manufacturers' websites
[c]Weighed out before soaking for 12 h

Table 11.2 Calorie content of 900 g DM of different human foods

Food	Calories (kcal) in 900 g fresh weight of food	Dry weight (g) equivalent to 900 g fresh weight	Calories (kcal) in 900 g DM	[a]Fresh portion size equivalent of 900 g DM
Carrot cake (Costa) (20% water)	3774 (6 × 150 g slices)	720	4717.5	7.5 × 150 g slices
Dried dates (20% water)	2871 (6 large handfuls)	720	3587	7.5 large handfuls
Medium potatoes (80% water)	693 (10 potatoes)	180	3465	50 potatoes
Fresh spinach (91% water)	207 (7.2 × 125 g bags)	81	2300	82 × 125 g bags

[a]Kcals are converted from fresh weight to 900 g DM equivalent and the comparable fresh portion size, which is disproportionate, so just use the first column to illustrate your point.

- muzzling (Chapter 9: 'Using muzzles') to allow grazing rather than keeping a horse in bed (stable).

Be aware that it is better for horses to have access to a mix of forages rather than one source. Rapid changes from ad lib grass to ad lib hay and vice versa changes the microbiome of the hind gut of ponies, which might be a higher risk for gut disturbances, although this is not common and most ponies do not suffer any digestive disturbances (Garber *et al.*, 2020).

Controlling and monitoring grass intake

Remind clients that their horses do not obtain calories from 'fresh air' (Fig. 11.2); grass can provide excess calories. Advise them to check if their horse has excess grass.

If a 250 kg pony eats 4% of their BW as DM, then they will be eating 10 kg DM grass or 50 kg fresh weight, which provides 40 litres of water, 1 kg of sugar, 1 kg of fibre, 1.2 kg of protein, 300 ml of oil and 90–120 MJ DE.

Measuring grass in the field

A 'bare paddock' (Fig. 11.3) can easily support most leisure horses. Clients can check how much grass there is in the field by doing the supermarket bag and poo pick test.

The supermarket bag test

- Ask clients to follow several Ws across all the areas that the horse grazes; at each point of the W cut the grass with a pair of scissors.

1 scoop holds 0.5kg of fresh grass (15%DM) or 0.075kg DM grass	
Per day	**Per hour**
10kgDM 66kg fresh weight 133 scoops of grass	0.625kg 4.1kg 8 scoops

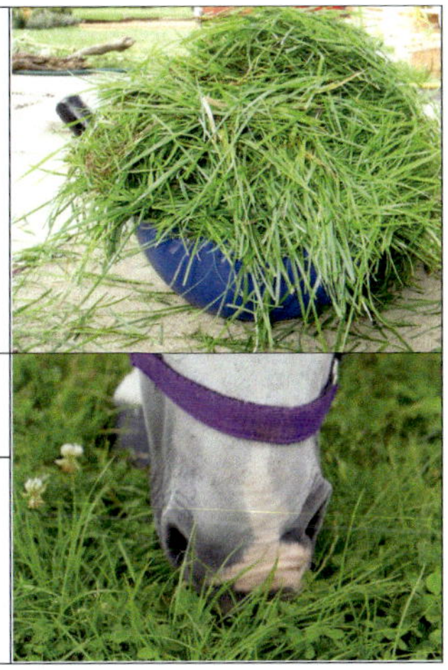

Fig. 11.2 A comparison between grass intake and the scoop equivalent of a 400 kg pony eating 16/24 h and consuming 2.5% BW as dry matter

- Put the cut grass into a supermarket plastic bag (the old single-use ones).
- If they take less than 30 min to fill the bag, there is excess grass.
- If they take over an hour to 2 hrs means there is appropriate grass availability for a horse that is a good doer.

The poo pick

(which they should be doing anyway)

- If clients need further reassurance that there is enough grass on a 'bare' paddock (Fig. 11.3), remind them that horses cannot produce faecal output if they are not consuming food.
  - The owner needs to collect all the droppings in a 24 h window and weigh them.
  - If the horse is producing less than 1% of its bodyweight in faeces, then it is not eating enough dry matter.
  - If producing closer to 3%, then it is eating excess dry matter.
  - Compare quantity of grass in the field to an ungrazed area. This is the amount of grass their horse has eaten (see Chapter 9: Fig. 9.6).

Feeding hay

Soaking hay

More clients feed hay (69%) than feed haylage (44%) (see Chapters 4 and 9); 26% of clients soak hay but not correctly – either not submerging it or only soaking for 30 min (Hotchkiss *et al.*, 2007). Soaking for 30 min is fine for supressing dust, but if fat cover needs reducing then you need to advise that the hay needs soaking for 12 h + (see Chapter 9: Tables 9.5 and 9.6). Steps to advise are as follows.

- Weigh out the daily quantity, stay upwind of hay (wear a mask) and shake aggressively.
  - Divide into equal quantities depending on the number of times/day clients will be providing the hay.
  - Split each feeding into four haynets.
  - Completely submerge the haynets in cold or warm water, using dustbins or baths or water troughs.
  - Soak for between 30 min and 16 h (depending on calorie reduction required).
  - Hang nets to drip to remove excess water for around 30 min out of direct sunlight (hay needs to be wet when fed).
  - Remove hay from nets and place in containers with hay grids.

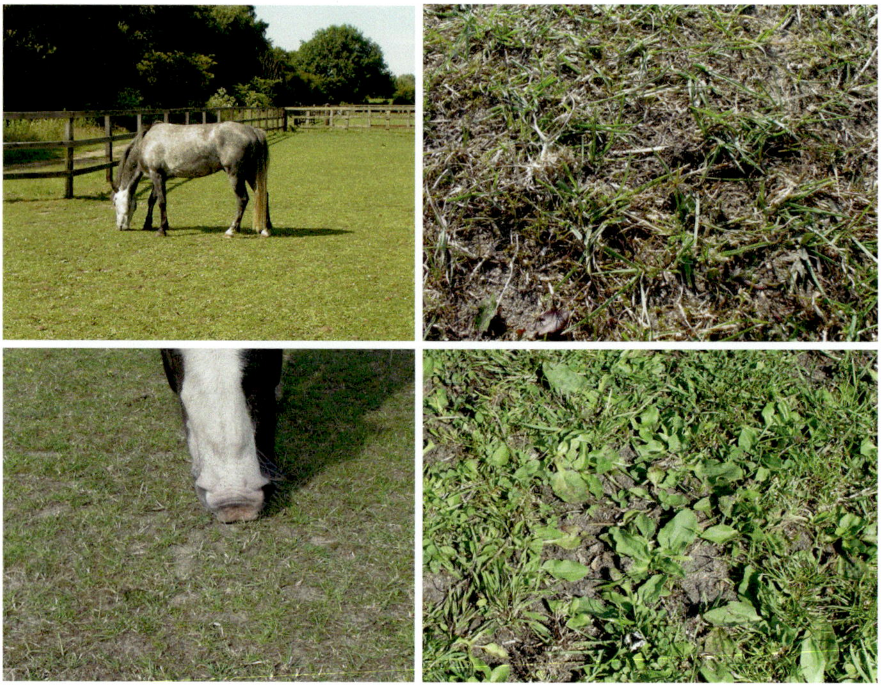

Fig. 11.3 A bare paddock can be deceptive.

Feeding hay at floor level to mimic natural eating position

- Haynets slow intake but increase the risk of cranial and caudal hooks developing, because the lower jaw cannot make a full lateral movement.
- Haygrids allow the horse to eat with its head at ground level and slow intake (see Chapter 9: Fig. 9.8). Various options are available for your clients.[i]

Advising straw

If horses are not losing weight on soaked hay, then recommend replacing some or all the hay with oat or barley straw. Check dentition first and advise the client to keep an eye on fibre faecal length, which should be mostly less than 4 mm (see Chapter 9: 'Advising straw as a low-calorie forage for overweight horses').

Whilst maintaining a high dry matter (bulk, forage fibre) intake is necessary for the horse's gut and behavioural health, it will not provide adequate micronutrients or protein; it is vital that the diet is balanced.

Top tips

- Not wheat straw, because it is high in silica as well as lignin, so stops bacteria fermenting the cell walls and increases risk of impaction.
  - Get the client to check that their horse is chewing well by monitoring fibre lengths in the droppings.
  - Ensure that the horse is drinking enough.
  - Introduce slowly.
  - Can be used as a partial or total hay replacer.
  - Balance minerals and protein by advising a balancer.

Balancing Micronutrients

Many horses are overfed but undernourished; in other words, they are eating enough/too many calories, but not enough protein, vitamins and minerals.

There is a strong correlation between low micronutrient intakes and obesity (Astrup and Bugel, 2010; Via, 2012). Biotin is needed for insulin receptor transcription improving pancreatic function (Via, 2012); other B vitamins are cofactors in glucose metabolism. B vitamin production (Hintz *et al.*, 1978) and vitamin E intake (Beeckman *et al.*, 2010; Cappai *et al.*, 2020) will be lower in horses that are fed restricted forage.

Horses exposed to reduced hours of sunlight might be deficient in vitamin D (Azarpeykan *et al.*, 2016).

There appears to be some association with low calcium and raised levels of certain hormones in obese people (Via, 2012). For horses, well-managed spring and summer grazing is low in certain minerals, including calcium (Jones *et al.*, 2005); hay is low in vitamins and soaking hay (vital for reducing calorie intake and maintaining dry matter intake) for more than 30 min leaches out valuable minerals as well as calories (Moore-Colyer, 1996).

It is therefore important that you check that the owner is balancing their horse's diet.

Balancing a ration

Recommend a balancer formulated to be fed at 100 g/100 kg BW – these provide negligible calories but are vitamin and mineral rich and should have a good protein source included. Feeding a small quantity of a low-energy feed at less than recommended on the back of the bag will simply add more calories but inadequate vitamins and minerals.

Which Balancer?

Check ingredients and analysis (not the marketing info on the front of the bag), specifically levels of vitamins and minerals. Vitamin E is a great guide as it is expensive to include. Check for products where the company has invested in a good-quality micronutrient package. Lysine content is also important – a good indicator of protein quality (Table 11.3).

Trickle feeding concentrates to replicate more closely the feeding behaviour of a horse eating forage

Assuming that the leisure horse needs to be fed a balancer or other hard feed, then anything that slows consumption is better for gut health – large boulders in buckets, muzzles or specially designed feeders (Fig. 11.4) that horses have to learn to operate to obtain food. The slower the horse eats, the less guilty the client feels about the 'small meal'.

Table 11.3. A comparison of UK equine feed balancers (intake 100 g/100 kg BW unless otherwise stated)

Balancer manufacturer/brand	[a]Vitamin E declaration (iu/kg)	[d]Daily intake vitamin E IU/day (iu/kg BW)[b]	Lysine (g/kg)	Protein (%)	[d]Calories/day (MJ DE)
Simple Systems – MetaSlim	No added vitamins	0	n/a	19–25	7
Spillers Lean and Lite	2000	1000 (2)	30	18	4.25
Forageplus Laminae-Plus (25–30 g/100 kg BW)	20100[c]	3000 (6)	66	17.3	0.9
TopSpec AntiLam (125 g for 12 hh pony mean wt 250 kg (50 g/100 kg BW)	2500	625 (1.25)	n/a	12	4.5
Blue Chip Lami Lite	270 mg/kg	135 (0.27)	n/a	15	n/a
Baileys Low Cal	800	400 (0.8)	n/a	16	n/a
Dodson and Horrell Go Lite	2300	1150 (2.3)	6.8	12.5	4.25
Saracen Essential Balancer	2000	1000 (2)	14	26	6.1

[a]Info from manufacturer's website December 2021
[b]NRC requirements for vitamin E = 1–2 iu/kg BW
[c]Product information states 3000 iu vitamin E in 150 g; so in 1 kg = 6.7 × 3000 iu vitamin E = 20100 iu vitamin E/kg.
[d]500kg horse

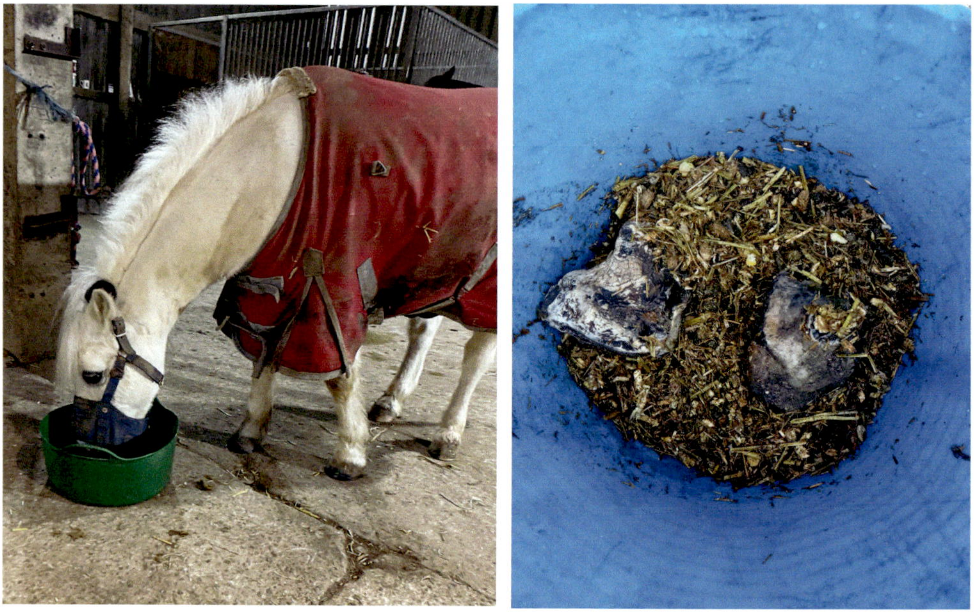

Fig. 11.4 There are various options for slowing down concentrate intake.

Advising the Correct Diet

Following the steps outlined in Chapters 2 and 3, and described in more detail in Chapters 9 (choosing a forage) and 10 (intake versus requirements), means that you will do the following.

1. Take horse details:
   - Bodyweight
   - Fat score
   - Workload
     - Time in field, exercise and competitions
   - Age
2. Take diet details and check ration and feeding management:
   - Forage (sample)
     - Grass availability and any restrictions
     - Conserved forages – quantities and frequency of feeding
     - Current hard feed, if any.

If clients wish to change products, discuss the information from Chapters 7 and 8 and check their choice of brand/manufacturer. Then simply choose the most appropriate product from that brand's light/leisure range.

Make sure that clients are not using feed to achieve the impossible and confusing the properties of feed.

How to advise the correct compound feed

Often owners feed 'bucket' food to provide their laid-back horse with more energy. The challenge is that scientific terms are used colloquially, leading to confusion. Do clarify the confusion around these terms. Most leisure horses do not need feeding to provide more energy (see Chapter 5: Table 5.12).

Energy

Normally the word 'energy' in relation to ourselves (or the horse) describes a feeling of weariness and we often turn to food to give us a buzz, even if we have consumed our daily calorie requirements.

Calorie

The word calorie, on the other hand, is used to describe how fattening a food is and provides us with an idea of how much food we can eat to meet our daily calorie requirements.

You may need to explain to clients that when food is broken down and metabolised to provide cells with energy for life, we measure this energy in different units, including calories for ourselves and megajoules for our horses. Calories are simply a unit of energy.

Horses that have a fat score of more than 3/5 anywhere on their body do not need additional calories (energy) – quite the contrary.

Neither of the horses in Fig. 11.5 needs more calories (energy).

Remind clients to always maintain the dry matter appetite by changing products to provide variable calorie intakes but meet vitamin and mineral requirements (Table 11.4).

Case Examples

- For any diet, it is first necessary to use a weight tape to establish the horse's bodyweight (see Chapter 3: 'Weight tapes').
- Calculate 2.5% BW – this is their **dry matter intake.**
- Forage-to-concentrate ratio (by bodyweight) for the leisure horse varies according to workload but would usually be between:
  - 2.4% BW fibre/forage to 0.1% BW hard feed (95% forage, 5% concentrates);
  - 2% BW fibre/forage to 0.5% BW hard feed (80% forage, 20% concentrates).

How to check the diet of a Riding Club horse

During a routine visit for flu jabs, a client has asked you to check that their horse's diet is OK. You are limited for time as you have quite a large backlog but clearly wish to provide suitable support. You have already taken a brief history as part of the health check visit. You therefore ask the client to take you to the feed and hay store to show you what they are currently feeding. The client shows you the feed and the scoops they use, you take a photo of the scoops and the bags. You then ask them to fill a plastic bag from several bales (see Chapter 4: 'Taking a forage sample').

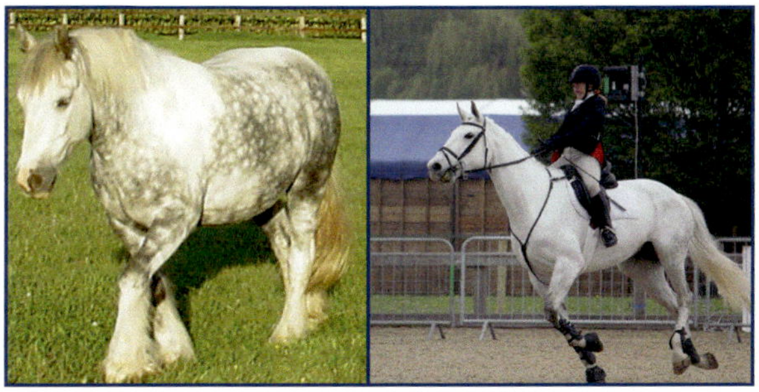

'My horse needs more energy, he needs some 'pep'; what can i feed him?'

'He needs a bit more energy, to get him moving more quickly off my leg; what can I feed him?'

Fig. 11.5 Misunderstanding of energy.

Table 11.4 The difference in calories intakes from a selection of leisure horse feeds formulated to be fed at different intakes but all providing vitamin/mineral and protein requirements when fed with forage

Product	MJ/kg	Feed rate/ 100 kg BW	Scoops	Daily calorie intake (MJ)	Main source of calories
Balancer	11.5	100 g	0.5	5.75	Minimal
Leisure Mix	10	300 g	1.5	15	High-fibre cereals and by-products
Healthy Hooves	8.5	500 g	5	21	Chopped fibre
High Fibre Nuts	9.5	300 g	1.25	14.25	Slow fibre

Table 11.5 Diet check for a Riding Club horse

Horse signalment	Horse 16 hh TB × WB, 3.5, 3, 3.5; 550 kg
Horse workload	• Out at night; in during day in summer and vice versa winter. • Hacked out three times/week with friends – active walk, trotting and some canter. • Weekly lesson for 1 h, horse gets into sweat. • Schooled twice a week, jumping, dressage and sometimes travel to Jump Cross. • Riding Club competitions monthly.

Current diet	• 1 Stubbs scoop Pasture mix (1.6 kg – 17.2 MJ DE)
	• 1 Stubbs scoop All Round Competition Mix (1.4 kg – 17.5 MJ DE)
	• Spilt into two feeds
	  ○ plus scoop alfalfa chaff (0.5 kg × 2 – 10 MJ DE) in each meal.
	• 9 h grazing on sparse paddock with four other horses
	  ○ 4–5 kg DM intake – 13–16 kg fresh wt, 19.5–32 MJ DE)
	• 3 slices of hay at night (6 kg – 42 MJ DE)

Advice	No changes needed
	80% forage:20% concentrates (2% BW forage: 0.5% BW concs)
	• Mean DMI = 13.75 kg,
	• DE intake = 118.7 MJ DE
	  ○ Recommended intake = 99 (light) to 107 (medium) MJ/DE/day
	  ○ If you can access a heart rate monitor to measure workload, would provide a better guestimate.
	• The fact that the horse is eating more than the mean requirements is reflected in the 3.5 fat scores, but every horse is an individual and there is no need to adjust ration unless the horse gets fatter.

	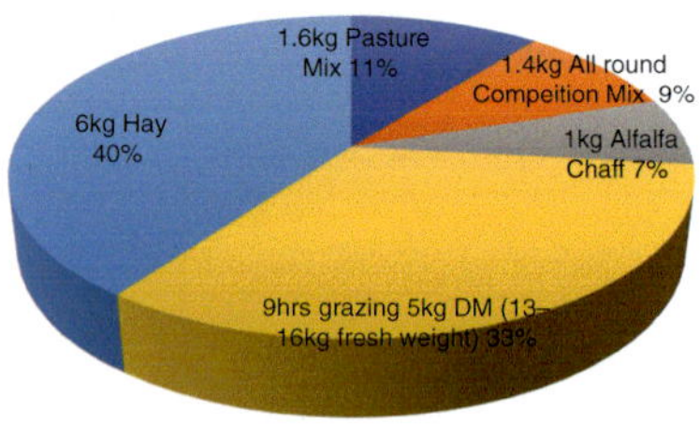

Ongoing husbandry	• The horse has no problems, is carrying a little too much fat on the neck and bottom, but you know it loses that in the winter.
	• It is competing well.
	  ○ The client has no issues with the horse.
	• Its DMI is being met and, based on its fat score, it is not eating excess calories.
	• You have cautioned the client to monitor the neck and bottom fortnightly,
	  ○ by fat scoring and taking photos
	  ○ and to soak the hay if the score goes up
	• The hard feed ration is meeting nutrient requirements.
	  ○ The client is feeding a mix of feeds and brands but each is being fed at 50% of recommended intake, so mixed together, the horse is getting their daily requirements.
	• The hay analysis comes back within typical ranges (see Chapter 9).
	• You ask the feed company to run the ration through their ration checker and it comes back balanced.
	• You suggest the client monitors grass availability and poo picks and consider a muzzle if the quantity of grass increases.

You explain to the client that you intend to contact the manufacturer of the feed to get the hay analysed and, in the meantime, you need them to weigh out the exact weight of the hay, the time spent grazing and the weight of each feed they are using. On your way out, you stop and take a photo of the grazing. Having received the information, you filled in a dietary history (Table 11.5).

How to advise using straw as a hay replacer

Your client has explained that the yard cuts its own hay and it got rained on before it was baled. The first three bales they opened were mouldy in the middle and their pony has started to cough. They've already thrown away some bales and the yard charges them for every bale they open. Table 11.6 is a diet check for using straw as a low-calorie forage.

How to advise using dusty hay as a sole forage source

Your client tells you that 'I am stuck with dusty hay. I'm on a livery yard where the owner produces the hay, it's included in my bill. There is no room to store my own and if there was it would probably be borrowed by other people. I don't know how long to soak for and I do not have time to soak hay before I turn her out in the morning as I have to get to work after sorting the kids.'

Table 11.7 is a diet check for using dusty hay.

How to advise a diet for a horse in good condition

I do local shows and usually get placed in the first 3, although most judges tell me that my horse is in good condition, some say my horse needs more condition on his bum and neck, so I need to change her diet to increase her condition.

Table 11.8 is a diet check for a horse in good condition.

Summary: Which Feed for the Leisure Horse?

There may seem to be a plethora of feeds, as there are browbands or rugs, but the inappropriate choice of feeds will have health consequences.

- Note the type and quantity of forage being fed (including grass) (see Chapters 4 and 9).
  - Ensure that it is at least 2% BW as dry matter.
  - Make sure they are managing the diet correctly to replicate normal eating behaviour.
- Teach how to fat score (see Chapter 3).
  - If the horse is fat score 3.5 or above on neck, middle or bottom or they are feeding less than recommended intakes, then advise a balancer.
- Encourage clients to focus on feeds formulated for light work or leisure.
  - Advise recommended intakes if the horse is 'normal' (see Chapter 7: Table 7.4).
  - Ignore any tempting marketing.
  - Check they are not just feeding a double handful of something before choosing a feed.
  - Feeding ½ scoop of 'conditioning' anything will not muscle up a horse in light work.
  - Encourage an increase in exercise.
- Check if they prefer mixes or pellets (see Chapter 7).
- Check the brand or feed you advise is reputable (see Chapter 8).
  - Work out their total daily dry matter intake (2.5% BW) and take the recommended intake of feed from the total. The difference will be the forage (grass and conserved forages).

It is important to acknowledge that most leisure horse owners relate a well-rounded horse with being well. 'While monitoring the horse to ensure it did not become too thin was considered an integral part of responsible ownership, monitoring for overweight was not usually considered by owners, unless the owner had been previously made aware of excess weight on their horse' (Furtado *et al.*, 2020). Maintaining or achieving weight loss in the clinical situation is as achievable, but the key is the degree of client compliance (Gill *et al.*, 2016).

Nutritional support for the leisure horse is one of preventative medicine. You must be prepared to use all the tools in your armoury to help clients choose the appropriate diet to maintain the correct fat cover on their horses.

Table 11.6 Diet check for using straw as a low-calorie forage

Horse signalment	Pony, 12.2; fat score neck 4, middle 4, bottom 5 Estimated weight of pony 300 kg; dry matter appetite 7.5 kg
Horse workload	• Out during the day for 5 h, in at night • Very good doer, prone to laminitis in the spring • Ridden at weekends and school holidays
Current diet	• Fed a low-energy coarse mix for light work, ½ scoop am and pm and double handful molassed chaff
Advice	96% forage to 4% hard feed (2.4% BW forage to 0.1% BW concentrates) i. Oat straw • Mouldy hay should never be fed to horses, not even when soaked, so it has been replaced with oat straw: o to provide bulk; o to satisfy appetite; o low calories; o less dusty than hay; o keeps pony occupied; o can be fed in haynet or slow feeder; and o available in big or small bales but must be kept under cover and dry ii. Grazing • The grass is sparse and of low feed value, so time out could be increased. Winter dry matter intake will be lower: keep an eye on droppings – straw might need feeding in the field. • In the summer consider advising a muzzle for up to 12 h and maybe strip graze with back and front fences for the rest of the time. Alternatively turn pony out in a sand paddock or similar with oat straw as forage. iii. Hard Feed • A leisure mix fed at less than recommended intake will not meet vitamin/mineral or protein requirements, so it is just empty calories • Recommend a balancer (100 g/100 kg BW) iv. Alfalfa/straw chaff • Fed extensively to laminitics, low calories but improves protein intake and slows intake of the balancer. • If the pony loses too much fat, then recommend changing to alfalfa chaff
	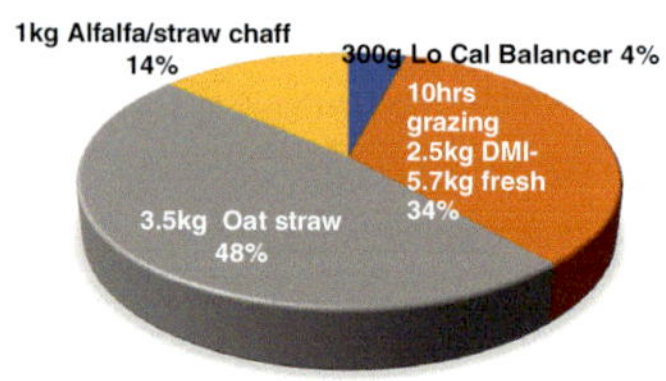
Ongoing husbandry	Special considerations for a straw- based diet: • Introduce straw slowly – takes 10–14 days. • Ensure good dentition – teeth need checking regularly as the pony needs to be able to chew the 'tougher' fibre. Get owners to keep any eye on fibre length in droppings. • In cold weather ensure that water intake stays high. o Dampen straw before feeding but throw away any left over after 12 h. o Feed bucket food dampened (maybe some unmolassed sugar beet shreds in the winter). o Add daily 1 carrot and 1 apple (tell the client to slice them appropriately). o Ensure water troughs and buckets stay ice free and topped up. • It is highly probable that the pony will increase in fat score during the spring and summer to above 3.5, 3.5, 3.5 despite being ridden. It is important that the fat score reduces in the winter and when it falls to 2.5, 2.5. 2.5 please reassure the client of the health benefits.

Table 11.7 Diet check for using dusty hay

<table>
<tr><td>Horse signalment</td><td>15.2 450 kg TB ×; fat score, 3, 3.5, 3</td></tr>
<tr><td>Horse workload</td><td>• Out day, in night.
• Working owner.
• Schooled for 30 min in floodlit arena after work.
• Ridden out at weekends.</td></tr>
<tr><td>Current diet</td><td>Fed 2 kg low energy coarse mix, 0.25 kg dry weight sugar beet, 1 kg straw/alfalfa chaff.</td></tr>
<tr><td>Advice</td><td>450 kg horse dry matter appetite 11.25 kg – the adjusted ration below provides adequate DMI and is balanced for protein, vitamins and minerals.
86% forage to 14% concentrates (2.15% BW forage to 0.35% concentrates).</td></tr>
<tr><td colspan="2">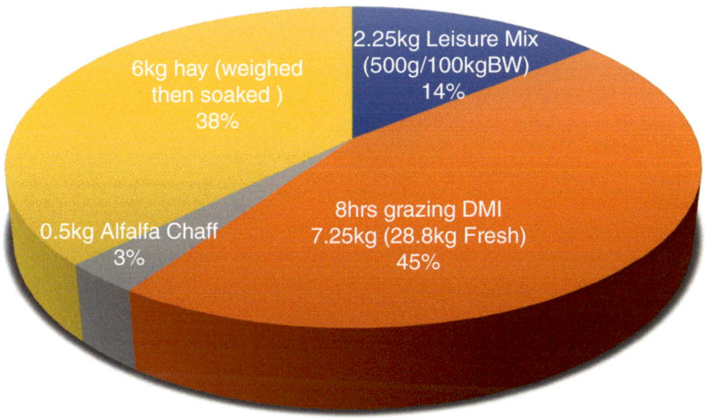

i. Hay soaking
• Soak the hay for the 30 min that client is schooling.
○ Split open the slices and completely submerge in water.
○ Drip for 5 min and then feed the hay split into four containers with grids at each corner of the stable.
• Provide 30 min before giving hard feed.
ii. Alfalfa chaff
• If not time to feed hay 30 min before the feed, then advise feeding 125 g alfalfa before feeding the mix.
○ Alfalfa is recommended because hay is low in quality protein.
▪ Soaking hay leaches some protein.
○ The amount of chaff would be increased in the winter, when the horse is more reliant on hay and has less access to grass.
○ Alfalfa is also a good source of calcium, which is also low in most forages.
iii. Hard feed
• Should be split into two feeds of 1.25 kg (1¼ scoops) with 125 g alfalfa chaff.
○ Feed after the small meal of alfalfa chaff
▪ before turnout and after riding.
○ The amount of hard feed will depend upon the recommended intake by the manufacturer.
• Make sure the client knows how much their scoop holds; if feeding nuts then the volume will be less.</td></tr>
<tr><td>Ongoing husbandry</td><td>Special considerations:
• Ideally no one would feed dusty hay to horses.
• It is accepted that due to the growing (drying) conditions in the UK, 90% of hay is not of sufficient hygienic quality to be fed to horses.
• All horses (not just competition horses) deserve ‘dust-free’ hay, so all hay for all horses should be soaked.
• If the horse starts to put on weight, then recommend replacing the mix with a suitable balancer and a longer soak for the hay</td></tr>
</table>

Table 11.8 Diet check for a horse in 'good' condition

Horse signalment	14.2 hh Fat score 4, 3.5, 4 Bodyweight 450 kg
Horse workload	• Out for 4 h a day (estimated DMI 2.8 kg; fresh wt 9.4 kg; 14 MJ; 13% DE intake). • Schooled 3× a week for 30 min – 1 h in sand school. • 1 day off in field (rugged). • Hacked once a week. • Exhibits most weekends at local and affiliated qualifiers.
Current diet	• Fed scoop conditioning mix (2 kg, 26 MJ; 33% of DE intake). • Scoop Alfalfa Oil (1 kg; 10 MJ). • 50 g PharmaPlast Ultimate Topline, am and pm. • Two haynets: one when comes in; one at night (2 slices/meal = 8 kg; 56MJ; 52% DE intake).

Advice	• Calorie requirements 56 × 1.1 = 61 MJ; currently eating 106 MJ.
	  ○ Horse is fat.
	  ○ Needs to lose fat and gain muscle.
	  ○ No need to feed a condition/show mix as the horse is only in light work.
	  ○ Needs to lose around 11.25 kg (2.5% BW) to reduce fat score by 0.5 (see Chapter 15: 'Control calorie intake').
	• Reduce calories to requirements and maintain DMI.
	i. Soaked hay
	  • Reduces calories but maintains DMI.
	    ○ Soak for 12 h minimum.
	    ○ Split into several meals using several hay grids or small-holed haynets to encourage foraging.
	    ○ Encourage client to analyse hay. If high calorie, might need to replace some with oat straw.
	ii. Hard feed
	  • Advise a show balancer to maintain client compliance.
	    ○ Divide into two meals and mix with Hi Fi Lite.
	    ○ Ensure client has container that holds exactly the correct weight.
	iii. Grazing increases energy expenditure
	  • Adjust time according to grass quality and availability.
	    ○ Consider advising muzzles or strip grazing with back and front fences.

	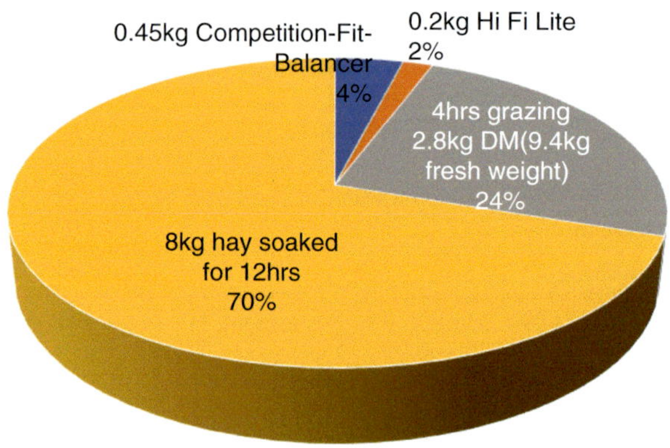

Continued

Table 11.8. Continued.

Ongoing husbandry	Special considerations:
	• The condition (outline) of the horse should be improved by appropriate exercise to build muscle on the hindquarters and neck.
	  ○ The workload needs increasing.
	  ○ Work with their trainer to establish a fitness regime.
	• Remind client that the topline is in fact fatline.
	  ○ Teach them how to do a cresty neck score (see Chapter 3: Fig. 3.11).
	• Contact farrier, explain your advice and get them on board as support.
	• A leisure balancer would meet this horse's nutrient requirements but would decrease client compliance.
	• As workload and calorie expenditure increases, the client should not change the ration until the fat score is reduced.
	  ○ Consider changing Hi Fi Lite for Alfalfa Chaff if better quality protein is required.
	• Important to emphasise that exercise reduces risk of hyperinsulinaemia (Pagan *et al.*, 2009) in fat horses.
	  ○ If she reduces the exercise her horse will be at risk of insulin resistance.

Note

[i] https://www.eazigrazer.co.uk/eazigrazer/hay-soaker?v=79cba1185463; https://www.slowfeeding.org; https://www.haybar.co.uk/

Bibliography

Astrup, A. and Bügel, S. (2010) Micronutrient deficiency in the aetiology of obesity. *International Journal of Obesity* 34, 947–948.

Azarpeykan, S., Dittmer, K.E., Gee, E.K., Marshall, J.C., Wallace, J. *et al.* (2016) Influence of blanketing and season on vitamin D and parathyroid hormone, calcium, phosphorus, and magnesium concentrations in horses in New Zealand. *Domestic Animal Endocrinology* 56, 75–84.

Beale, L., Maxwell, N.S., Gibson, O.R., Twomey, R., Taylor, B. *et al.* (2015) Oxygen cost of recreational horse-riding in females. *Journal of Physical Activity and Health* 12(6), 808–813. doi: 10.1123/jpah.2012-0428.

Beeckman, A., Vicca, J., Van Ranst, G., Janssens, G.P. and Fievez, V. (2010) Monitoring of vitamin E status of dry, early and mid-late lactating organic dairy cows fed conserved roughages during the indoor period and factors influencing forage vitamin E levels. *Journal of Animal Physiology and Animal Nutrition* 94(6), 736–746.

BHS (2019) *Advice on Pasture Management*. British Horse Society, Kenilworth, UK. Available at: https://www.nationalponysociety.com/wp-content/uploads/2019/02/Pasture-Managment-BHS.pdf (accessed 10 January 2023)

Boden, L.A., Parkin, T.D., Yates, J., Mellor, D. and Koa, R.R. (2013) An online survey of horse-owners in Great Britain. *BMC Veterinary Research* 9, 188. doi: 10.1186/1746-6148-9-188.

Cappai, M.G., Flavia Pudda, F., Wolf, P., Accioni, F., Boatto, G. *et al.* (2020) Variation of hematochemical profile and vitamin E status in feral Giara horses from free grazing in the wild to hay feeding during captivity. *Journal of Equine Veterinary Science* 94, 103220.

de Laat, M.A., Hampson, B.A., Sillence, M.N. and Pollitt, C.C. (2016) Sustained, low-intensity exercise achieved by a dynamic feeding system decreases body fat in ponies. *Journal of Veterinary Internal Medicine* 30(5), 1732–1738.

Devienne, M.F. and Guezennec, C.Y. (2000) Energy expenditure of horse riding. *European Journal of Applied Physiology* 82(5–6), 499–503. doi: 10.1007/s004210000207.

Furtado, T., Perkins, E., Pinchbeck, G., McGowan, C., Watkins, F. *et al.* (2020) Exploring horse owners' understanding of obese body condition and weight management in UK leisure horses. *Equine Veterinary Journal* 1–11. doi: 10.1111/evj.13360.

Garber, A., Hastie, P., McGuinness, D., Malarange, P. and Murray, J.A. (2020) Abrupt dietary changes between grass and hay alter faecal microbiota of ponies. *PLoS ONE* 15(8), e0237869.

Gemmill, R., Agar, C., Freeman, S. and Hollands, T. (2014) Factors affecting owners' choice of nutritional supplements in dressage and eventing horses. *Veterinary Record Open* 46, 31–32.

Gemmill, R., Agar, C., Freeman, S.L. and Hollands, T. (2016) Factors affecting owners' choice of nutritional supplements for use in dressage and eventing horses. *Veterinary Record Open* 3, e000155.

Giles, S.L., Nicol, C.J., Rands, S.A. and Harris, P. (2015) Assessing the seasonal prevalence and risk factors for nuchal crest adiposity in domestic horses and ponies using the Cresty Neck Score. *BMC Veterinary Research* 11, 13. doi: 10.1186/s12917-015-0327-7.

Gill, J.C., Pratt-Phillips, S.E., Mansmann, R. and Siciliano, P.D. (2016) Weight loss management in client-owned horses. *Journal of Equine Veterinary Science* 39, 80–89.

Hale, C., Hemmings, A. and Randle, H. (2016) Accuracy of horse workload perception by owners when compared to published workload parameters. *Journal of Veterinary Behavior: Clinical Applications and Research* 15, 94–94. doi: 10.1016/j.jveb.2016.08.065.

Hampson, B.A., de Laat, M.A., Mills, P.C. and Pollitt, C.C. (2010a) Distances travelled by feral horses in 'outback' Australia. *Equine Veterinary Journal* 38, 582–586. doi: 10.1111/j.2042-3306.2010.00203.x.

Hampson, B.A., Morton, J.M., Mills, P.C., Trotter, M.G., Lamb, D.W. *et al.* (2010b) Monitoring distances travelled by horses using GPS tracking collars. *Australian Veterinary Journal* 88(5), 176–181. doi: 10.1111/j.1751-0813.2010.00564.x.

Hepburn, R.J. (2014) Endoscopic examination of the squamous and glandular gastric mucosa in sport and leisure horses: 684 horses (2005–2011). In: *Proceedings of the 11th International Equine Colic Research Symposium*. p. 5.

Hintz, H.F., Schryver, H.F. and Stevens, C.E. (1978) Digestion and absorption in the hindgut of nonruminant herbivores. *Journal of Animal Science* 46(6), 1803–1807. doi: 10.2527/jas1978.4661803x.

Hockenhull, J. and Creighton, E. (2014) Management practices associated with owner-reported stable-related and handling behaviour problems in UK leisure horses. *Applied Animal Behaviour Science* 155, 49–55.

Honoré, E.K. and Uhlinger, C.A. (1994) Equine feeding practices in central North Carolina: a preliminary survey. *Journal of Equine Veterinary Science* 14(8), 424–429. doi: 10.1016/S0737-0806(06)82009-5.

Hotchkiss, J.W., Reid, S.W. and Christley, R.M. (2007) A survey of horse owners in Great Britain regarding horses in their care. Part 1: Horse demographic characteristics and management. *Equine Veterinary Journal* 39(4), 294–300.

Ireland, J.L., Clegg, P.D., McGowan, C.M., McKane, S.A. and Pinchbeck, G.L. (2011) A cross-sectional study of geriatric horses in the United Kingdom. Part 1: demographics and management practices. *Equine Veterinary Journal* 43(1), 30–36. doi: 10.1111/j.2042-3306.2010.00145.x.

Jones, L., Lax, J. and Hollands, T. (2005a) Analysis of the mineral content of spring summer grazing used for thoroughbred breeding stock in the UK. In: Proceedings of 44th BEVA Congress, Harrogate.

Jouany, J.P., Medina, B., Bertin, G. and Julliand, V. (2009) Effect of live yeast culture supplementation on hindgut microbial communities and their polysaccharidase and glycoside hydrolase activities in horses fed a high-fiber or high-starch diet. *Journal of Animal Science* 87(9), 2844–2852. doi: 10.2527/jas.2008-1602.

Lorenzo-Figueras, M. and Merritt, A. (2002) Effects of exercise on gastric volume and pH in the proximal portion of the stomach of horses. *American Journal of Veterinary Medicine* 63(11), 1481–1487. doi: 10.2460/ajvr.20022.63.1481.

Luthersson, N., Nielsen, K.H., Harris, P. and Parkin, T.D. (2009) Risk factors associated with equine gastric ulceration syndrome (EGUS) in 201 horses in Denmark. *Equine Veterinary Journal* 41(7), 625–630. doi: 10.2746/042516409x441929.

McGreevy, P.D., Cripps, P.J., French, N.P., Green, L.E. and Nicol, C.J. (1995) Management factors associated with stereotypic and redirected behaviour in the thoroughbred horse. *Equine Veterinary Journal* 27(2), 86–91. doi: 10.1111/j.2042-3306.1995.tb03041.x

Meyer, H., Coenen, M. and Gurer, C. (1985) Investigations on saliva production and chewing effects in horses fed various feeds. *Proceedings of the Equine Nutrition and Physiology Society* 9, 38–42.

Moore-Colyer, M.J. (1996) Effects of soaking hay fodder for horses on dust and mineral content. *Animal Science* 63, 337–342.

Murray, M.J. and Schusser, G.F. (1993) Measurement of 24-h gastric pH using an indwelling pH electrode in horses unfed, fed, and treated with ranitidine. *Equine Veterinary Journal* 25, 417–421.

Murray, J.A.M.D., Bloxham, C., Kulifay, J., Stevenson, A. and Roberts, J. (2015) Equine nutrition: a survey of perceptions and practices of horse owners undertaking a massive open online course in equine nutrition. *Journal of Equine Veterinary Science* 35, 510–517. doi: 10.1016/j.jevs.2015.02.005.

Pagan, J., Martin, O., Crowley, N. and Hooks, K.L. (2009) Relationship between body condition and metabolic parameters in sport horses, pony hunters and polo ponies. *Journal of Equine Veterinary Science* 29(5), 418–420.

Pedersen, S., Windeyer, C., Read, E., French, D., Cribb, A. *et al.* (2015) Prevalence of and risk factors for gastric ulceration in showjumping Warmsbloods. *Journal of Veterinary Internal Medicine* 29, 1239–1240.

Robin, C., Ireland, J., Wylie, C., Collins, S., Verheyen, K. *et al.* (2015) Prevalence of and risk factors for equine obesity in Great Britain based on owner-reported body condition scores. *Equine Veterinary Journal* 47(2), 196–201. doi: 10.1111/evj.12275.

Salonen, L.K., Hollands, T., Piercy, R.J. and Verheyen, K.L.P. (2009) Epidemiology of equine obesity in south-east England: preliminary findings. In: *Proceedings of the 48th British Equine Veterinary Association Congress*, ICC, Birmingham, 9–12 September 2009, p. 247.

Scantlebury, C.E., Archer, D.C., Proudman, C.J. and Pinchbeck, G.L. (2015) Risk factors for recurrent colic in UK general equine practice. *Equine Veterinary Journal* 47, 202–206. doi: 10.1111/evj.12276.

Siciliano, P.D. and Schmitt, S. (2012) Effect of restricted grazing on hindgut pH and fluid balance. *Journal of Equine Veterinary Science* 32, 558–561.

Smith, D., Mayes, R., Hollands, T., Cuddeford, D., Yule, H. *et al*. (2007) Validating the alkane pair technique to estimate dry matter intake in equids. *The Journal of Agricultural Science* 145(3), 273–281. doi: 10.1017/S0021859607006788.

Via, M. (2012) The malnutrition of obesity: micronutrient deficiencies that promote diabetes. *ISRN Endocrinology* 2012, 103472.

Videla, R. and Andrews, F.M. (2009) New perspectives in equine gastric ulcer syndrome. *Veterinary Clinics: Equine Practice* 25(2), 283–301.

Ward, S., Sykes, B.W., Brown, H., Bishop, A. and Penaluna, L.A. (2015) A comparison of the prevalence of gastric ulceration in feral and domesticated horses in the UK. *Equine Veterinary Education* 27, 655–657.

Waters, A.J., Nicol, C.J. and French, N.P. (2002) Factors influencing the development of stereotypic and redirected behaviours in young horses: findings of a four-year prospective epidemiological study. *Equine Veterinary Journal* 34, 572–579.

Willing, B., Vörös, A., Roos, S., Jones, C., Jansson, A. and Lindberg, J.E. (2009) Changes in faecal bacteria associated with concentrate and forage-only diets fed to horses in training. *Equine Veterinary Journal* 41, 908–914. doi: 10.2746/042516409X447806.

12 Feeding the Performance Horse

Teresa Hollands and Lizzie Drury

School of Veterinary Medicine, University of Surrey;
Saracen Horse Feeds, Aylesford

Learning Objectives

LO1 Critically evaluate the changes in feeding management and diet needed to support the performance horse.
LO2 Describe how to maximise glycogen replacement without compromising performance.
LO3 Choose an appropriate feed to balance fibre intake according to performance type/temperament.
LO4 Manage feeding during travelling.
LO5 Explain how to feed to minimise the risk of nutritionally related diseases of the performance horse:
- Equine gastric ulcer syndrome (EGUS)
- Colic
- Recurrent exertional rhabdomyolysis (RER) and polysaccharide storage myopathy (PSSM).

LO6 Describe how to feed different performance horses.

At the end of this chapter, you will be able to summarise the way that the diet and ration need to be adapted to maximise performance and minimise the risk of nutritionally related diseases

Introduction and Overview

Whether you are advising a client with a yard of racehorses or competition horses or a client with a single child's pony, the horse needs to forage, to exhibit normal herd behaviour and to eat a balanced diet to keep the digestive tract healthy. But clearly the requirements are different (output) and thus the input (diet) is different. Feeding performance and leisure horses is as different as it is for human athletes versus the general population (Fig. 12.1). Problems occur when clients try to extrapolate the feeding of leisure horses to performance horses or vice versa.

Many of your performance horse clients will already be competing at a high level and thus you might be a little reticent as to how you might be able to help. Don't be. All top human athletes now rely on nutritionists for dietary advice; our results in the last few Olympics are evidence of that support.

It is also worth reflecting that, despite that level of knowledge, we still see unfit and inappropriately fed horses competing at top levels (Fig. 12.2).

The aim of your input and advice is to minimise the impact of performance on gut health and behaviour by:

- ensuring appropriate forage intake;
- managing forage intake to mimic natural feeding behaviour;
- safe starch feeding;
- choosing appropriate energy ingredients;
- maintaining dry matter intake of 2.5% bodyweight;
- advising electrolyte supplementation;
- advising supplements only when required; and
- making sure that feeds are suitable for performance horses competing under rules/NOPS.

Performance feeds are formulated to support work, although clearly diet alone does not predict

  Evidence-based Equine Nutrition: A Practical Approach for Professionals (T. Hollands and L. Drury)
DOI: 10.1079/9781789245134.0012

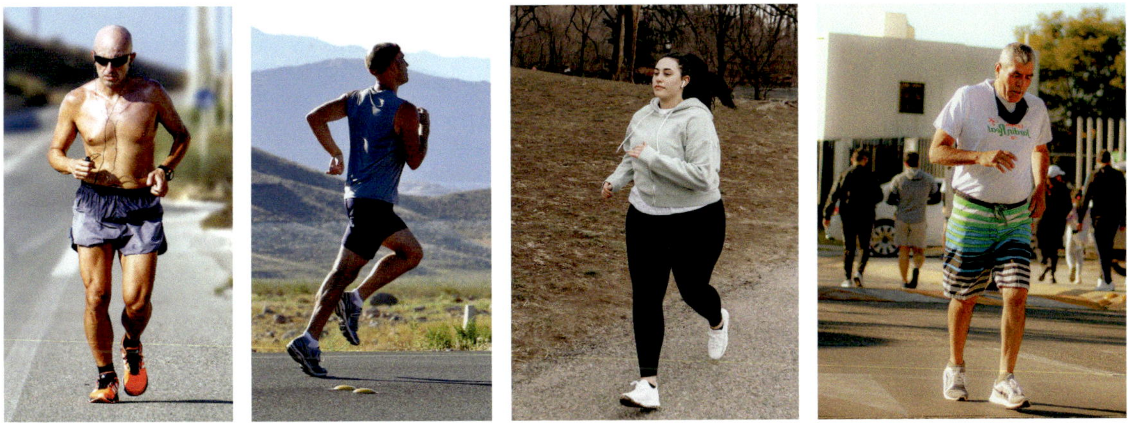

Fig. 12.1 A comparison between the physique and fitness of human athletes and the general population

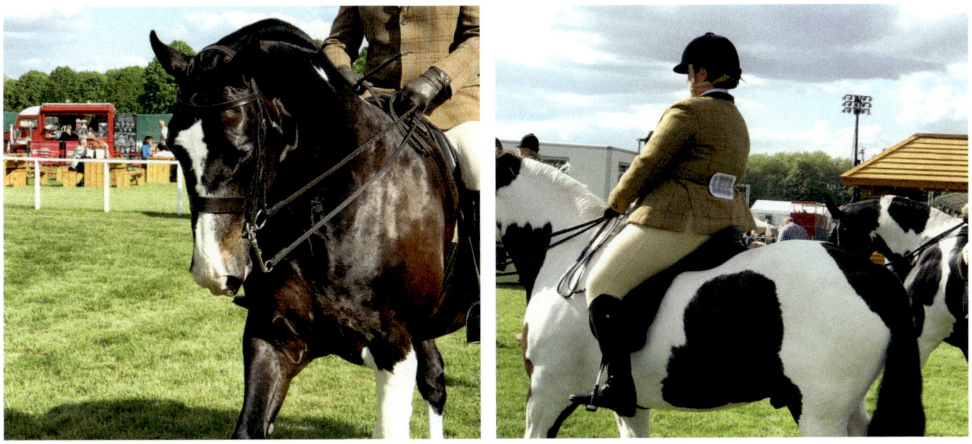

Fig. 12.2 Horses competing in championship classes at Royal Windsor.

success. Performance is limited by fatigue induced by physical activity due to several factors, which in humans are listed as muscle mass and metabolic characteristics, cardiovascular capacity and genetics, which in turn depend upon suitability of the exercise training, diet, altitude and ambient temperature (Maughan, 2005).

Remember those lessons in biochemistry? The muscle obtains fuel to work by breaking down food energy stored as fat or glycogen to ATP, either quickly via glycolysis (anaerobic) or more slowly via the TCA cycle (aerobic). This biochemistry is shared by horses and humans, although there are some differences in terms of muscle glycogen storage capacity and speed of replenishment. This biochemistry can help you use comparative evidence when the evidence might be lacking for the horse and thus advise an appropriate ration that might slow time to fatigue.

Working across the disciplines from Excel Talent Squad level through to World Class, key issues of interest, confusion or concern in the nutrition of the sports horse are consistent regardless of the disciplines and similar at grassroots as well as elite levels.

In some cases, the way clients feed their horses has not changed for many years, which is why it is important to consider sports nutrition in other athletes so that we can debate whether human nutritional management might be applicable for the athletic horse (showjumper = human hurdler; eventer = human triathlon; dressage = human gymnast). The three areas of performance nutrition of greatest importance are:

- energy/calories (the equine concept of heating versus non-heating) – how these are delivered and replenished will vary between disciplines;
- protein (requirements for muscle development and recovery); and
- micronutrients (immune support and electrolyte restoration).

When horses and humans exercise at a similar percentage of maximal oxygen consumption (VO_2 max), the horse's metabolic rate and absolute energy requirements are 2–3× higher compared with the human's (Geor *et al.*, 2000), emphasising the importance of dietary support.

Aspects of Diet Associated with Fatigue

Dietary energy

Several metabolic parameters affected by diet can quicken or slow the fatigue that limits performance. These include low blood glucose, depletion of muscle glycogen, loss of muscle ATP, metabolic acidosis and lactate and ammonia accumulation (Malone *et al.*, 2021). Carbohydrate and fat are the main energy sources for the horse and whilst depletion of carbohydrate is associated with fatigue, the horse rarely depletes its fat reserve.

As anyone who runs in marathons knows, eating or drinking carbohydrates during exercise improves their endurance. Several explanations have been explored and these include: stimulation of CHO receptors in the mouth, which reduces the perception of tiredness; maintenance of blood glucose; and sparing of glycogen (Malone *et al.*, 2021).

Consequences of eating a large meal of carbohydrates

What many might not appreciate is that ingesting large quantities of some CHO (fructose) has similar adverse effects on the human gastrointestinal tract (GIT) as it does in horses, including gut pain, flatulence, diarrhoea and, unlike in horses, vomiting (de Oliveira *et al.*, 2014). Thus, in both species, the key is to manage the ration to minimise the risk to gut health.

Maintaining blood glucose: starch versus simple sugars to reduce fatigue

Whilst horses have limited salivary amylase and a decreased capacity to digest starch compared with the pig, they are very efficient at digesting small starch meals in the small intestine, thus removing or reducing risks to hind gut health.

In addition, horses have an amazing enzymic capacity to absorb simple sugars from their small intestine (Dyer *et al.*, 2002). Glucose absorption via Na-dependent membrane vesicles is highest in the duodenum, followed by the jejunum, and lowest in the ileum (Dyer *et al.*, 2002). The glucose co-transporter (SGLT1) in the equine small intestine (SI) has a 90–92% similarity to other species at the amino acid level and similar levels of sucrase, whose activity is highest in the duodenum, with some expression of lactase enzymes compared with other non-ruminant species. Levels of maltase are 18–76 times higher compared with humans and 71 times higher compared with sheep throughout the small intestine (Dyer *et al.*, 2002). Horses are very clearly adapted to digesting simple sugars in their diet – hardly surprising as grass is their natural diet.

Introducing concentrates into a horse's ration

Feed management advice is rooted in anecdotal experiences, and it is challenging for the clinician to try to facilitate change to better evidence-based management. One of the more common questions is how quickly diet should be changed: most clients take 7–10 days to allow the hind gut to adapt to the changes. It is just as important to allow time for the small intestine enzymes to adapt; clearly if absorption of carbohydrates (CHOs) in the SI is maximised, then the risk of unabsorbed CHO reaching the hind gut is reduced.

The small intestine enzyme activity of horses eating grass has been compared with that of those eating hay (< 1 g starch /kg BW/day); 60% hay to 40% oats (3.3 g starch/kg BW/day) and 40% hay to 60% oats (6 g starch/kg BW/day). The absorptive activity adapts to higher starch intakes, for whilst glucose uptake in the duodenum was similar, horses fed starch had 1.9× higher glucose uptake in the jejenum and 3.7× higher in the ileum (Dyer *et al.*, 2009).

Adaptation to starch diets

Clearly the horse can adapt to high-starch diets, increasing its ability to absorb glucose by doubling the number of SGLT1 molecules in the jejunum and

Table 12.1 The adaptation of the horse's small intestine enzymes[a] in response to increasing dietary starch[b]. (Modified from Dyer *et al.*, 2009.)

Time	Duodenum *SGLT1 mRNA units*	Ileum *SGLT1 mRNA units*
Grass fed/hay fed	1.28	0.49
After 1 week of concentrate feeding (3.3 kg starch/kg BW/day)	1.28	1.15
After 1 month of feeding concentrate	2.31	1.23
After 1 month of increased starch intake (6 g starch/kg BW/day)	2.31*(2× original level)*	1.91*(3.8× original level)*

[a]SGLT1. [b]SGLT1 is upregulated by mono- and disaccharides, not starch; but clearly starch hydrolysis must have increased to provide the glucose, showing that amylase can be upregulated with time

quintupling in the ileum compared with those on hay or grass (Dyer *et al.*, 2009). This adaptation continues over time (Table 12.1) and despite a 500 kg horse eating 3.3 kg of starch/day from 6.2 kg of oats and maize, split into three meals of 2 kg which provided 2.2 g starch/kg BW/meal, no horse suffered intestinal pain or any digestive disease that can be associated with feeding this level of starch (Dyer *et al.*, 2009), although glycaemic and insulinaemic responses were not measured. At the same time, the horse must also upregulate the production of pancreatic amylase in response to high-starch diets (double compared with hay) (Kienzle *et al.*, 1994), to provide the mono- and disaccharides for subsequent enzymic breakdown and absorption.

Be careful if you are advising clients with overweight show or dressage horses. Work in pigs (Pierzynowski *et al.*, 2017) and people (Muneyuki *et al.*, 2012) has shown that insulin resistance delays or even prevents the upregulation of amylase activity; and appears to be age dependent.

People who eat high-starch diets have higher expressions of amylase; whereas those who are obese have lower amylase activities (Bonnefond *et al.*, 2017). Whilst at first read this might seem counterintuitive (less amylase, less glucose uptake), it is suggested that the undigested starch has an impact on the fermentation by-products in the human lower gut, increasing energy availability (Mejía-Benítez *et al.*, 2015). Others suggest that the higher amylase prevents glucose absorption into the blood and the glucose is used by the intestinal cells, thus reducing insulin secretion (Pierzynowski *et al.*, 2017). Plasma amylase acts on the beta-cells of the pancreatic islets and reduces the glucose-stimulated insulin response: the same amount of glucose requires less insulin in healthy pigs; glucagon release seems to be unaffected (Pierzynowska *et al.*, 2020).

Top tip

Regardless of the biochemical mechanism, evidence shows that 7–10 days is not long enough to increase starch feeds to recommended quantities.

- Ensure that the horse is adapted to lower starch intakes during fittening over at least 2 weeks.
- Add a further 6 weeks to increase starch.
- Continue to recommend small starch meals (< 1 g starch/kg BW/meal)

This should ensure:

- maximal digestion of carbohydrates within normal physiological parameters;
- minimal risk of undigested starch reaching the hind gut; and
- maximal muscle glycogen replacement.

Diet can support the muscle to adapt to and recover from exercise by sparing glucose, increasing fat oxidation, reducing free-radical accumulation and replenishing glycogen.

Muscle glycogen depletion

Blood glucose, free fatty acids (from fat or liver) and muscle triglycerides are the main sources of energy in low-intensity work. Horses rely on muscle glycogen to sustain their workload (muscle contraction) after the first few minutes of work. Glycogen depletion can result in a 60% decrease in anaerobic capacity during subsequent exercise, which is relevant for those horses doing fast work or competing over several days (Table 12.2) but less likely for those doing prolonged

Table 12.2 Disciplines in which performance might be reduced due to energy depletion

FAT DEPLETION UNLIKLEY	GLYCOGEN DEPLETION LIKELY
ENDURANCE 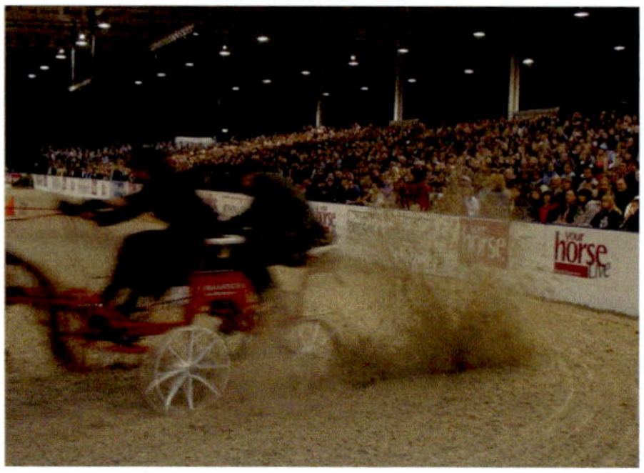	CROSS COUNTRY 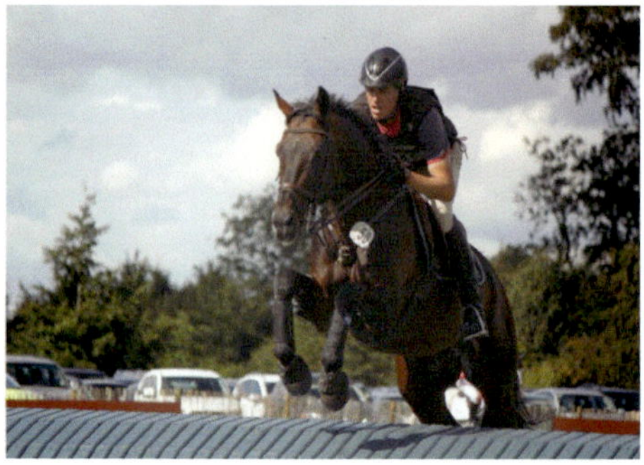
WALK/TROT 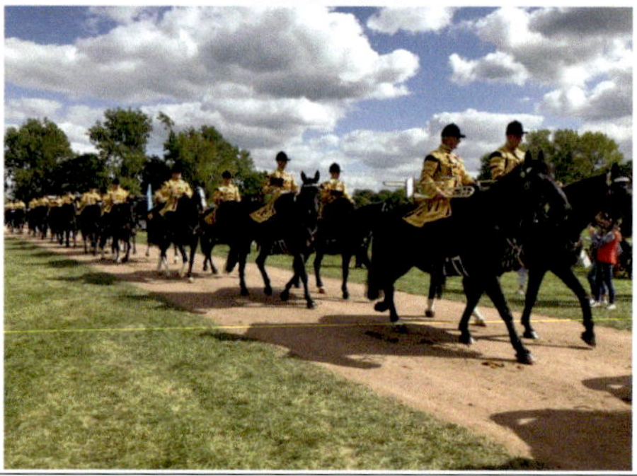	JUMP OFF 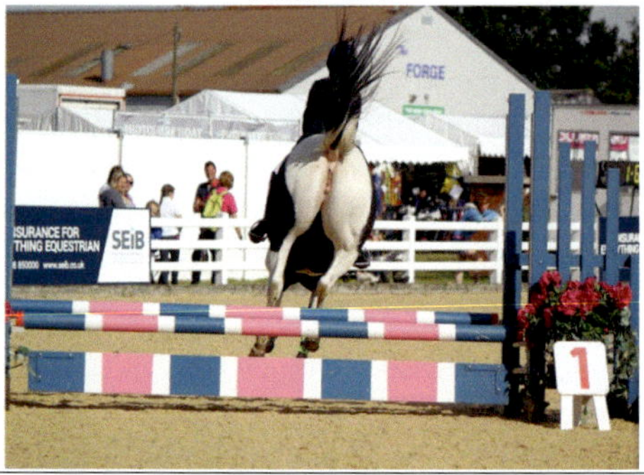
TRANSPORT 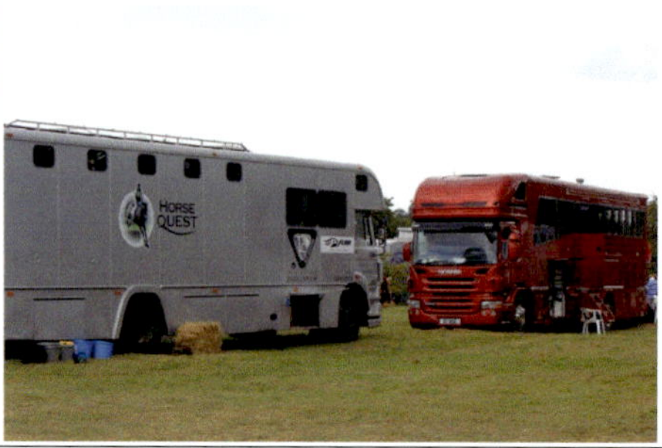	SOME DRESSAGE MOVES 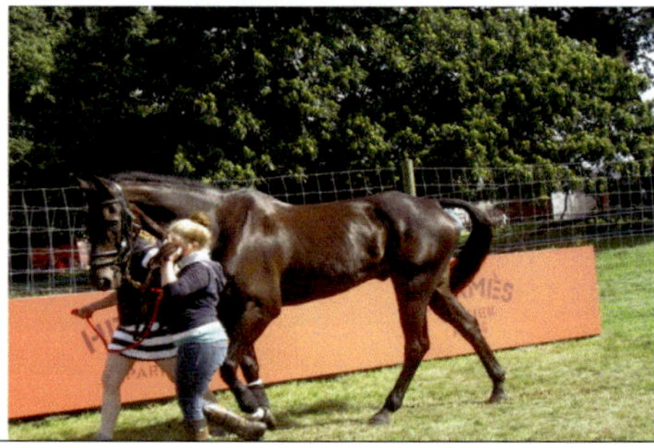

low- to moderate-intensity exercise (Lacombe and Hinchcliffe, 2003).

Glycogen depletion is also dependent on the duration of exercise (Table 12.3) and muscle type (Table 12.4). Pre-exercise, type I fibres have lower glycogen content compared with type IIA or IIB (Hodgson *et al.*, 1985). Fitness regimes will impact on muscle fibre development and muscle mass (TBs have over 55% muscle mass (Gunn, 1987)).

Carbohydrate-derived muscle fuels are the dominant factor in both power production and fatigue resistance, and this has proven true in practical application, from high-speed racehorses to 100-mile endurance horses (Ivers, 2002). To minimise fatigue, muscle glycogen repletion is tailored for the human athlete according to the type of work they are doing and carbohydrates eaten at specific times relative to exercise to replenish muscle glycogen.

The horse can lose up to 50% of its muscle ATP (how the energy is released from glycogen) after galloping and the losses are greater than in humans. Timing of carbohydrate feeding relative to the type, duration and intensity of exercise has been extensively studied in humans, providing an international

Table 12.3 Quantification of the effect of exercise on muscle glycogen in horses

Horses	Speed	Rate of use	Depletion	Recovery	Reference
Racehorses	1–3 min: 70 km/h for 400–1000 m and 1600–3100 m	149 mmol/kg muscle DW/min[a]	↓ 20–40%[b]		[a]Nimmo and Snow, 1983; [b]Hodgson *et al*., 1984
Racehorses	1000 m gallops, 70 s, heart rate > 200 bpm 1600 m, 113–122 s, heart rate > 200 bpm		19–25% of resting content		Snow and Harris, 1991
Endurance	9 h, 15–20 km/h	[c]Glycogen used < 1 mmol/kg muscle DW/ min	[d]Endurance rides of over 100 km, total muscle glycogen ↓ by 67%		[c]Essén-Gustavsson *et al*., 1991; [d]Hodgson *et al*., 1983
Endurance	Seven endurance-trained horses competing in 'Roslagsritten'		Post-race muscle glycogen content 262 mmol/kg DW	8 days after completion 634 mmol/kg DW	Jensen-Waern *et al*., 1999

position paper on nutrient timing for different sports (Kerksick *et al*., 2017; Mata *et al*., 2019).

A human athlete eating 78–90 g CHO/h during exercise spares liver glycogen which in turn regulates the adaptation of the glycolytic signalling pathways in response to exercise (Mata *et al*., 2019). The daily CHO intake for a person who is not exercising is 130 g/day to maintain liver glycogen at 80 g and blood glucose levels at 4–5.5 mmol/litre. Human athletes consume 8–12 g CHO/kg BW, (Murray and Rosenbloom, 2018), the consumption varying depending upon the exercise programme (Mata *et al*., 2019).

This level of detail is not available for the equine athlete, but despite strong evidence that horses have:

- higher glycogen stores (490–625 mmol/kg DW (Geor *et al*., 2006)) compared with people (300–400 mmol/kg DW (Harris *et al*., 1974));
- greater relative capacity (/kg BW) for energy production via aerobic and anaerobic metabolism; and
- depletion of glycogen stores after exercise (Tables 12.3 and 12.4) and slower glycogen replenishment.

There are still ways that you can advise timing of feeding to maximise glycogen replenishment (Lacombe *et al*., 2004).

It makes sense to point out to clients that replenishment needs maximising to compensate for the slower glycogen replenishment in equine athletes compared with their human counterparts.

Feeding to Replenish Glycogen Muscle Stores

In humans, carbohydrates eaten either before or during intermittent high-intensity exercise improve performance (Welsh *et al*., 2002). This increase in carbohydrate intake suppresses fat metabolism and increases carbohydrate metabolism almost immediately but it takes time (days) for the metabolism to adapt to eating a high-fat diet (Jeukendrup, 2003). Feeding starch to replenish muscle glycogen cannot be considered in isolation; you must consider fat and protein intakes too, as well as the implications for insulin metabolism.

Feeding fat

Fat is often fed because it spares glycogen but, unless the horse is adapted to the fat diet, feeding fat slows muscle glycogen replenishment. There is some evidence to show that even after adaptation there is no advantage to feeding fat in terms of glycogen replenishment (Hyppa *et al*., 1997) when horses are exercised in a treadmill (Table 12.5). Reducing starch/glucose intake by 55% by partially replacing oats (fed at 0.99 g starch/kg BW/meal) with sugar beet (fibre) (0.44 g sugar/kg BW/meal) (Palmgren Karlsson *et al*., 2002) increases muscle glycogen stores (before and after exercise) of working horses.

Carbohydrate intake of human athletes is manipulated according to exercise type in a very similar

Table 12.4 Glycogen depletion in muscle fibre types of horses undertaking various workloads

Horses	Exercise level	Resting	Type I	Type IIA	Type IIB	Post-exercise levels	Utilisation rate	Reference
			% glycogen content					
Eleven standardbreds (SB) – muscle biopsies 15 min after race	Warm-up submaximal levels 2140 race; mean speed 12.5 m/s. Recorded glycogen depletion in muscle fibres after exercise					Type I 5% low levels 95% medium levels Type IIA 1% high 98.5% medium 0.5% low Type IIB 40% high 60% medium		Valberg, 1989
Three SB horses – muscle biopsies mid-exercise	Three trotting sessions on treadmill i. 10 m/s (short distance) ii. 8 m/sec (middle distance) iii. 6 m/s (long distance)		After exercise: i. depletion of type I only ii. marked depletion iii. complete depletion	After exercise: ii. some depletion (35–73%) iii. over 50% depleted	After exercise: iii. only low and medium levels left	After exercise tolerance test Mean 325–418 mmol/litre		
Seventeen SBs	Standardised submaximal exercise tolerance test (6, 7, 8 and 9 m/sec)		15% medium 85% high	100% high	100% high	Type I: 10% high, 90% medium Type IIA: 30% high, 70% medium Type IIB: 60% high, 40% medium Mean 286–610 mmol/kg		
Six TBs	Competing in day 2 (roads and tracks, steeplechase and cross-country) of 3-day event	546.7 mmol glucose/kg muscle DM	Pre-exercise: 25% medium, 75% low glycogen Post-exercise: 80% low, 10% no glycogen, 10% medium	Pre-: 30% high, 70% medium Post-: 2% high, 48% medium, 50% low	Pre-: 5% very high, 75% medium, 20% low Post-: 0% very high, 4% high, 55% medium, 41% low	248.7 mmol glucose/kg DM muscle	4.08 mmol glucose/kg DM muscle/min.	Hodgson *et al.*, 1985

Table 12.5 The effect of feeding on glycogen replenishment in exercising horses

Horses	Exercise	Diet	Effect on glucose/ glycogen	Authors' conclusions	Reference
Twelve Finn horses	Exercise test 5 min 1.7 m/s; 11 min 4 m/s; 4 min 7 m/s ×3 – treadmill at 3° incline SET 15 min 1.7 m/s, 4 × 2 min at 4, 6, 7 and 8 m/s treadmill	***Added fat*** *Control ration provided 176 g fat (2.4% DM/day) *Experimental diet supplement with 400 g rapeseed oil (7.5% fat DM/ day) to give total intake 358 g fat (5% DM)	Lower plasma glucose, insulin, triglycerides and glycerol in fat-fed. Lower muscle glycogen when fed fat without time to adapt	'... giving fat supplementation during recovery to fat-adapted horses did not enhance post exercise repletion of muscle glycogen when compared to the basal diet or the CHO-supplemented diet. Furthermore, when horses were not adapted to fat, repletion of muscle glycogen was slowed down.'	Hyppa *et al.* (1997)
Four Standardbred geldings	Three phases: *Phases 1, 2: 3.5 min submaximal exercise, 2 h stabled *Phase 3: 26 min walk (1.8 m/s for 17 min), trot (6–10 m/s for 9.25 min)	***Starch replaced by fermentable fibre*** 3X/day: hay 14.8ghay/kg BW and 7.1 g oat diet/kg BW or 7.6 g/kg BW MSBP diet: (54.7% oats, 38.9% molassed sugar beet pulp (MSBP) and 6.4% dried brewers grains (DBG).	No differences in plasma glucose/ insulin at rest, or during exercise. Post-exercise: MSBP diet glycogen decreased from 597 to 484 mmol/kg DW Oat diet muscle glycogen decreased from 546 to 394 mmmol/kg DM	'... the glycogen saving effect of the MSBP diet produces more short-chain fatty acids (SCFA; i.e. acetate, propionate and butyrate) in the hindgut and increase in SCFA absorption in the portal blood.' 'A major part of the absorbed acetate would pass the liver without being metabolised and available for extra-hepatic tissue utilisation via the tricarboxylic metabolic pathway.' OR: '... glycogen saving effect of the MSBP diet could be the increase in sugar intake (increase of about 350 g sugar/day) and an increased utilisation of blood-borne glucose'	Palmgren Karlsson *et al.*, 2002

way to practical horse diets. A high availability of CHO before and after high-intensity exercise is essential to minimise depletion of glycogen levels triggering exercise-induced adaptations to resistance training, whereas endurance-exercise-induced adaptations (mitochondrial biogenesis and enhanced lipolysis) respond to low CHO availability (Mata *et al.*, 2019).

This makes sense because once VO_2 max is over 65% then fat oxidation declines and carbohydrate oxidation takes over; high levels of one energy source improves the ability to oxidise that nutrient supply. In people, high-CHO diets increase muscle glycogen concentration whereas high-fat diets decrease muscle glycogen at the same time as increasing intramuscular triglycerides (Purdom *et al.*, 2018).

TBs exercised at supramaximal exercise to exhaustion (115% VO_2 max) had higher levels of three plasma unsaturated fatty acids and six phospholipids but decreased signal intensity of four saturated fatty acids and five triacylglycerols (Nolazco Sassot *et al.*, 2019). Whilst there was no information on diet or time to exhaustion, the fact that the horses were in race training would suggest that they would be on high-CHO diets. The authors suggested that the changes reflected exercise-induced lipolysis and muscle metabolism of saturated fats and queried whether the fats were being used for cell membrane repairs; they noted that further work would be needed in terms of diet manipulation and exercise intensity to increase an understanding of the impact of fat metabolism in horses exercising anaerobically.

Feeding starch

There is a difference in muscle glycogen replenishment when horses are fed isocalorific diets containing high starch (HS) versus low starch (LS) post-exercise (Table 12.6). The HS diet resulted in a higher glycaemic response, meaning that there was more glucose available to convert to glycogen, and the increased insulin means that more glycogen synthase is activated compared with the LS diet (Lacombe *et al.*, 2004). The effect on the glycogen replenishment needs to be considered in conjunction with gut health (g starch/kg BW/meal).

Timing of starch feeds relative to exercise

Please remember to advise feeding a high-starch diet as small starch meals. In this example HS should be fed in five meals and the MS in four meals to reduce the starch intake/meal to 1.5 g starch/kg BW/meal. Equally important is to consider timing of feeding so that it can support maximum rate of glycogen synthesis, which is immediately after (Fig. 12.3) to 3 h after exercise; decreasing by 60% at 12 h with a further 50% decrease at 24 h and 73% decrease at 72 h (Lacombe *et al.*, 2004).

> **Top tip**
>
> Consider advising a small meal of alfalfa chaff followed by a high-starch diet fed in several small starch rations/meals within 1–6 h of completing exercise.

Starch intake and insulin sensitivity

There is a concern in the literature regarding the impact of high-starch diets on insulin sensitivity in the horse. It is important to make sure that the papers you are reading are relevant for the performance horse. Clearly starch fed to a fat leisure horse that is only in light work is a risk to their health and **it cannot be reiterated enough that there is no justification for the feeding of starch to the leisure horse** – please do not extrapolate results from the leisure to competition horse and vice versa.

Athletes adapted to high-starch diets have higher levels of GLUT 4 and enzymes associated with muscle glycogen storage; those training on a low-CHO diet adapt to using fat but can suffer from fatigue and a lack of concentration, impairing their ability to use CHO during competition (Kanter, 2018). Exercise attenuates the body's insulin response and of course if you are advising small starch meals (albeit a high-starch diet) then the insulinaemic response stays within normal physiological parameters.

Starch-fed horses have a higher insulin sensitivity (decrease in insulin resistance) compared with fat-fed, when measured over a training and fattening period (Stewart-Hunt *et al.*, 2010), although this depends on the duration of training (Pratt *et al.*, 2006) and the size of the meal (Table 12.7).

> **Top tip**
>
> - The feeding of a high-starch diet to an unexercised horse is an oxymoron and inexcusable.
> - Diet effects investigated in the leisure horse should not be extrapolated to a performance horse.
> - Racehorses are fed more starch/meal compared with other horses. There is limited, if any, evidence of insulin resistance in this group of horses.

Table 12.6 The effect of different starch intakes on muscle glycogen fed to horses (mean BW 473 kg) on isocalorific diets. (Modified from Lacombe *et al*., 2004.)

Diet description	Daily intake (kg)	Starch in feed (% and g/kg)	Starch (kg/day)	g starch/kg BW/day g starch/kg BW/meal	Water intake (l)	Muscle glycogen 24 h post-exercise as % of pre-exercise	Muscle glycogen 72 h post-exercise (mmol/kg DW)	Muscle glycogen synthesis rate
High starch (HS): 21% forage to 79% concentrates	6.5	50.9% 509 g/kg	3.3	6.97 g 2.32 g	43	64.4	133	1.5
Medium starch (MS): 66% forage to 33% concentrates (control)	7.8	26.4% 264 g/kg	2.07	4.37 g 1.45 g	67	54.2	106	1.1
Low starch (LS): hay only	9.7	4.3% 43 g/kg	0.417	0.88 g 0.29 g	88	52.9	102	0.9

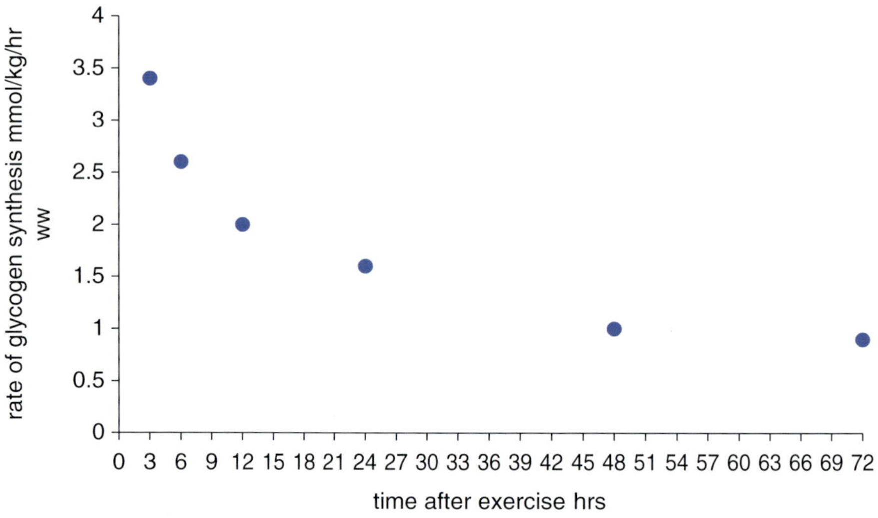

Fig. 12.3 Rate of muscle glycogen replacement in response to diet (mean of HS, MS and LS) after strenuous exercise. (Made with data from Lacombe *et al.*, 2004.)

Protein Intake

Whilst most of your clients will know that protein is needed for muscle development and maintenance, they are unlikely to have considered the physiology of muscle synthesis in relation to feeding and indeed in some disciplines tend to forget that muscle develops because of work rather than simply feeding a conditioning or topline feed.

Human athletes tailor their protein intake according to exercise type but the NRC recommends different protein intakes according to energy expenditure rather than work type, although it is possible to equate output to work type (Fig. 12.4).

In horses, exercise (as well as insulin and amino acids) triggers muscle protein synthesis as long as amino acids (AA) are not limited (1.26 g/kg BW/day; lysine 54 mg/kg BW) (Urschel *et al.*, 2011). Although total tract digestion of forage protein is high, only 20–30% of protein from forage is absorbed prior to fermentation in the hind gut. Forage does not provide enough protein for the performance horse; and there is no correlation between caecal amino acids and blood amino acids (NRC, 2007).

In human athletes it has been established that certain amino acid supplements (whey protein) increase serum levels of essential and branched-chain amino acids (BCAAs) with a decrease in myoglobin and creatine kinase levels compared with controls (Lam *et al.*, 2019). Supplementing resistance-training athletes with BCAAs whilst on a low-calorie diet increases lean body mass and skeletal performance, with the added benefit of losing fat mass (Dudgeon *et al.*, 2016). Human researchers have also modelled protein turnover and suggest that there might be an increased demand for tyrosine, threonine and valine during intensive exercise and that deficiencies would limit anabolic metabolism (Dunstan *et al.*, 2019). It is likely that a similar biochemical response exists for the horse and the timing of feeding relative to exercise might affect the availability of AA during and after exercise.

When fed after glycogen-depleting exercise in horses, leucine (a BCAA) given as bolus (0.1 g/kg BW) twice a day with glucose increased the BCAAs leucine, isoleucine, valine, tyrosine and phenylalanine as well as glucose and stimulated insulin response to increase post-exercise muscle glycogen synthesis, compared with a bolus of water or glucose alone (Nostell *et al.*, 2012). Remember that insulin also increases cellular uptake of amino acids and reduces protein breakdown in the muscle.

Timing of protein intake relative to exercise

Horses fed 1 h after exercise had lower creatine kinase (less muscle damage, improved recovery) and

Table 12.7 The effect of exercise duration and starch intake on the insulin sensitivity of working horses

Horses	Maximum starch intake kg/day g/kg BW/meal	Maximum fat intake kg/day g/kg BW/meal	Training duration and level	Insulin sensitivity	Authors' comments	Ref.
Fourteen mature Standardbred horses (mean BW 424 kg)	Mean WSC 530 g/kg conc. mean conc. intake = 4.3–4.4 kg feed 2.27–2.3 kg starch/day 2.7 g starch/kg BW/meal	Mean fat = 142 g/kg conc. Mean conc. intake = 4.4–4.5kg 0.6–0.61 kg/day 0.75 g fat/kg BW/meal	6 weeks no exercise (D) 7 weeks exercise 5 days/week, *3 days treadmill *weeks 1and 2,* 12 min of trotting at 35% of pretraining VO_2 peak 4 min at 50% VO_2 peak. *weeks 3 and 4*, plus 2 min canter approx. 75% of VO_2 max *weeks 5–7*, all trotting 14 min at 50% VO_2 peak 3 min canter at 75% *2 days 15–20 min of trotting (4 m/s) on automated exercise machine (Equine Exerciser)	Unexercised horses on starch diet decreased insulin sensitivity compared with fat fed and with no feeding Exercised horses regardless of diet had no change in insulin sensitivity compared with no feed	Physical conditioning modified the effects of dietary energy source on insulin-mediated glucose disposal. 7-week period of physical conditioning reverses the effect of the high NSC concentrate fed to non-exercised horses and increases insulin sensitivity	Pratt *et al.*, 2006
Fourteen mature Standardbreds (mean BW 424 kg)	Mean dietary NSC (starch and sugar) 6.9 g/kg BW/day Total starch intake 2.9 kg/day Fed in two meals 3.45 g NSC/kg BW/meal	Mean dietary NSC 1.8 g/kg BW/day Total starch intake 0.763 kg /day Fed in two meals 0.9 g NSC/kg BW/meal Fat 142 g/kg feed Mean conc. intake = 4.4–4.5 kg 0.6–0.61 kg/day 0.75 g fat/kg BW/meal	Phase 1 (3 weeks), Phase 2 (6 weeks), Phase 3 (7 weeks) 4 m/s for 15–20 min 2 ×/week treadmill (3° incline) 3 ×/week. Treadmill training same as Pratt *et al.*, 2006	Insulin sensitivity increased on high starch diet after exercise	Muscle glycogen (mmol/kg DM) higher on the starch diet (687.6) compared with fat diet (548) at end of exercise in phase 3 together with an approx. 58% increase in GLUT4 Exercise increases insulin sensitivity	Stewart-Hunt *et al.*, 2010
Twelve Arabian geldings, 456 kg BW	447 g NSC/kg concentrate 894 g NSC/day 0.9 g NSC/kg BW/day	131 g NSC/kg concentrate 262 g NSC/day 0.6 g NSC/kg BW/day	1 h, 3×/week;treadmill work minimum once/week or work in an automatic walker (walk, trot); ridden (light trail riding) or lunged (walk, trot, canter) when the treadmill and walker were not available	No significant differences in insulin sensitivity between diets – exercise increased insulin sensitivity for both diets	'Insulin sensitivity (SI) was not different between SS adapted horses and FF adapted horses in the trained state'	Treiber *et al.*, 2006

WSC water soluble carbohydrate; NSC Non structural carbohydrates; FF fat and fibre; SS starch and sugar

Human	Horse
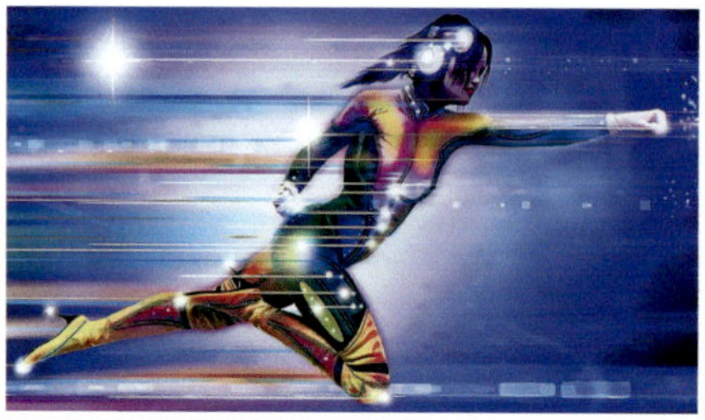	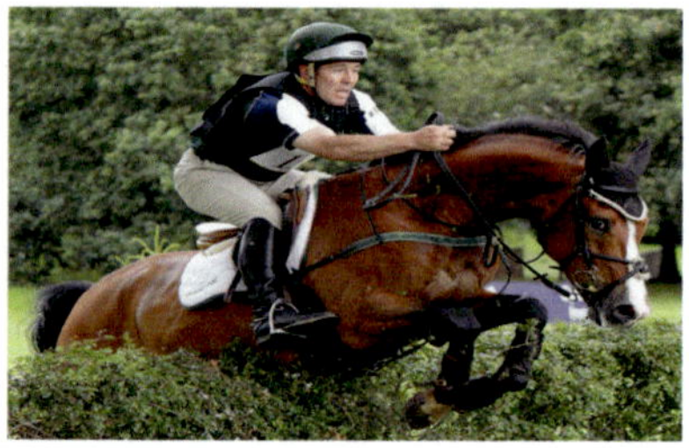
Maintenance/light work 0.8	Maintenance/light work 1.08–1.44
Resistance /strength trained 1.6–1.7	Medium work (Showjumpers/Dressage) 1.24–1.61
Endurance 1.2–1.4	Hard work (Eventers/endurance) 1.34–1.7

Fig. 12.4 'Disciplinising' diets. Protein requirements (g protein/kg BW/day) of human and equine athletes. Human image by alan918, https://pixabay.com/illustrations/superhero-girl-speed-runner-534120/

increased AA (except for leucine and isoleucine) compared with feeding 2 h before exercise, or exercised after an overnight fast. Muscle recovery resulted in rapid decrease of some plasma AA concentrations and increase in others, suggesting that feeding post-exercise may facilitate better muscle protein balance (synthesis versus breakdown) in the recovery period following exercise. Timing of feeding protein in relation to exercise can help improve muscle recovery and muscle protein synthesis/degradation balance (Graham-Thiers and Bowen, 2021) (Table 12.8).

In men there is a significant drop in leucine after aerobic exercise, but the evidence is not clear whether increasing dietary leucine reduces the net rate of protein degradation (Mero, 1999), mainly because the effect of leucine cannot be separated from that of the other BCAAs fed. In unfit men, a mix of AA including leucine (1.44 g) and lysine (0.6 g/day) reduced creatinine kinase (Matsui *et al.*, 2019); in fit basketball players a mix of AA including lysine eaten 3×/day reduced inflammatory cytokines (IL6) and muscle soreness (0.0065–0.012 g lysine, 0.014–0.026 leucine/kg BW) (An *et al.*, 2020).

Clearly more work is needed to determine horses' requirements of g AA/kg BW in relation to exercise and timing of feed, but it makes sense to advise clients to feed shortly after exercise to maximise AA absorption for muscle recovery.

Top tip

- Plasma AA highest 3–6 h after feeding (Russell *et al.*, 1986)
  - This coincides with increased muscle protein synthesis.
- Check that the feed contains the appropriate amount of lysine.
  - Crude protein (CP), which is declared on the label, is not a good indicator of protein quality or digestibility.
- The general assumption for horses in work is that as their energy intake increases, so does their protein intake.
  - but if you have advised adding fat to the diet, rather than a formulated feed, then this will not be the case.

You can check the protein requirements for exercise (Table 12.9) versus intake (Table 12.10) using one of several software packages (see Chapter 10: 'Intake versus requirements').

You will find that many horses eat much higher levels of protein compared with Table 12.9 with no detrimental effects except for a lower dietary cation–anion balance (DCAB) (higher is better) and this is supported by the literature.

Table 12.8 The effect of feeding protein in relation to exercise on muscle metabolism in horses

Horses	Mean daily intake amino acids(g)	Exercise	Timing relative to exercise	Results	Reference
Eight lightweight horses BW 585 kg	Arginine 21 Histidine 9 Isoleucine 13 Leucine 24 (0.04 g/kg BW) Lysine 20 Methionine 6 Phenylalanine 15 Threonine 12 Valine 18	5 min walk (1.5 m/s), 5 min trot (3.5 m/s), 3 min canter (5 m/s), 2 min hard gallop (7 m/s), 10 min walk (1.5 m/s)	2 h before 1 h after Fasted	2 h before: had lower NH_4, glucose and AA Fed 1 h after exercise: higher AA, creatinine; lower isoleucine, leucine, creatine kinase, lactate	Graham-Thiers and Bowen, 2021

Table 12.9 The horse's protein requirements relative to exercise levels. (Made using data from NRC, 2007.)

Exercise level	Crude protein (CP) requirements g C/kg BW/day[a]			Lysine requirements
Maintenance (M)	BW × 1.26 (min BW × 1.08; elevated BW × 1.44)			
Working horses	M + (BW × MG + ((BW × SL × 7.8 g[b]/kg)/0.5[a])/0.79[a])			
	Crude protein (CP) requirements for muscle gain (MG) in addition to maintenance requirements (g CP/kg BW/day)	Sweat loss (SL) % pre-exercise BW loss	Additional protein requirements from sweat loss (SL) (g CP/kg BW/day)	4.3% CP
Light	0.089	0.25	0.019	
Moderate	0.177	0.5	0.039	
Heavy	0.266	1	0.078	
Very heavy	0.354	2	0.16	

[a]NRC (2007) assumes that the horse only has a 50% efficiency of CP use and that CP has a digestibility of 79%
[b]No information provided on this integer

If you want to maximise the horse's chance of building muscle, consider that after exercise in humans there is an increase in protein synthesis which overrules the degradation rate and this increase stays high for 48 h after exercise, even in the fasted state and in older adults (Esmarck *et al.*, 2001). There is an additive effect of building lean body mass stimulated by protein intake and hyperaminoacidaemia post-exercise (Mazzulla *et al.*, 2020).

Interestingly the best increases in muscle hypertrophy in humans are greatest during the early stages of training (Mazzulla *et al.*, 2020).

Top tip

- Horses in early training are often fed a leisure mix
  - which compared to a competition mix is lower in quality protein
- Whilst exercise is still light,
  - the horse does not need the additional calories from a competition mix,
- Consider advising:
  - Performance Balancer
  - alfalfa chaff
  - maybe an amino acid supplement
  - high quality forage.

Table 12.10 Crude protein, lysine and amino acid content of common competition horse feeds

Feed	Crude protein (g/kg feed)	Lysine (g/kg feed)	Other amino acids	Intake rate (g/100 kg BW)
Saracen Competition Fit Mix	13.5	6.0	Methionine 2.0 Threonine 4.0	400 g–1 kg
Saracen Race 13	13.0	6.0	Methionine 2.0 Threonine 5.0	500 g–1 kg
Saracen Enduro Performance	11.2	6.0	Methionine 2.0 Threonine 4.0	400 g–1 kg
Saracen Re-Leve Cubes	13.0	6.3	Methionine 1.8 Threonine 4.0	400 g–1 kg

Feeding and Transport

One of the main concerns of clients is how the inevitable increase in transport duration and overnight stays associated with higher levels of competitions affects feeding. Travelling disrupts the normal feeding routine of the horse as well as potentially at the final venue. Even a 2 h journey changes faecal biota and increases the neutrophil-to-lymphocyte ratio (Faubladier *et al.*, 2013).

Two hours after arriving from a 1 h journey (50 km) the cortisol levels of horses are higher than when they left; they eat their concentrates more quickly than at home, but hay takes longer. When travelled for longer (4 h), the same horses were thirstier on arrival (Tateo *et al.*, 2012).

Do remind clients that travel requires energy, and it is important that the horse does not arrive at the competition with depleted muscle glycogen stores. Horses ate less food travelling (hay or feed) on the lorry as opposed to during rest periods, probably because they were spending their time trying to maintain balance (Waran *et al.*, 1996), which is associated with severity of gastric ulceration (Padalino and Radal, 2020; Padalino *et al.*, 2020). Long journeys will likely result in weight loss from dehydration and fat loss. Thoroughbred horses transported for 4000 km over 4 days lost weight, had compromised immune systems in terms of increased neutrophil numbers and oxidative stress as well as increased heart rates compared with controls (Padalino *et al.*, 2017); those travelling for 6 h but offered food lost 2.5% BW (Waran, 1993).

Top tips

- Encourage clients to ensure adequate rest periods at times that reflect normal routine for feeding and watering, minimising the risk of nutritionally related diseases.
- Smaller, wetter meals are often advisable.
- Some horses need leading out in hand to settle them enough to eat and allow them to urinate.
- Encourage clients to consider changing to feeding haylage before travelling, to reduce dust on the lorry.
- Flavour water and accustom horses to drinking from buckets before leaving home (Fig. 12.5).

Minimising the Risk of Nutritionally Related Disease Associated with Feeding Management of Performance Horses

For any athlete, competing at a high level means a change in routine and also exercise supported by specific diets, which without doubt differs from normal; but this does not mean that the health and welfare of that athlete (human or horse) should be compromised. Many of the nutritionally related diseases associated with performance horses can be mitigated simply by ensuring that clients relate feeding management to the anatomy and physiology of the gut, reducing the risk of gastric ulceration, colic and repetitive exertional rhabdomyolysis (RER). It is fair, though, that the implication of diet in the disease is complicated by the many management changes associated with performance and thus generally accepted that most of these diseases are multifactorial in cause.

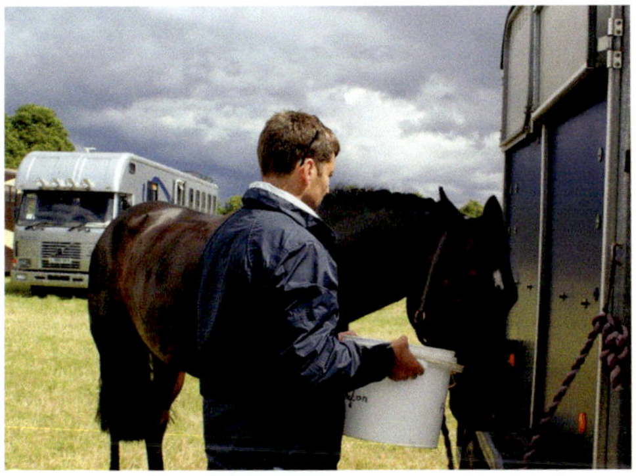

Fig. 12.5 Flavour water and accustom horses to drinking from buckets before leaving home, to support drinking at competitions.

Equine Gastric Ulcer Syndrome (EGUS)

Although you will be aware of the anatomy of the horse's stomach, do not assume that your clients have that knowledge. When describing the stomach, it might aid understanding if you simply describe the stomach as upper (alkaline) and lower (acid), which are visibly different and segregated (Fig. 12.6).

As you know, all parts of the stomach can be at risk of ulceration and whilst dietary management is a risk factor for ulcers in the upper stomach (equine squamous gastric disease) (ESGD) there is currently little evidence that it is part of the aetiology of ulceration in the lower stomach (equine glandular gastric disease) (EGGD).

Stress appears to be a trigger factor for ulcers in the lower stomach (Banse and Andrews, 2019), and incidence increases in line with exercise intensity in warmblood show jumpers, whereas those fed sugar beet pulp (SBP) were at lower risk (Pedersen *et al.*, 2018); it is not clear (but it is likely) that the horses in lighter work would have been fed SBP. A 10-day course of Bute appeared to be a risk factor for ulceration, reducing the mucosal protection of the lower stomach (Whitfield-Cargile *et al.*, 2021), whereas NSAID seemed to reduce the risk of upper stomach ulceration in polo ponies, although numbers were low (Banse *et al.*, 2018). The fact that more experienced polo ponies had less ESGD compared with inexperienced ponies might be added evidence of stress being a risk factor.

It is important clinically not just to record and name the type of gastric ulceration (Sykes *et al.*, 2016) but also to make it clear to the client that the causes and management of ulcers in the upper and lower stomach are different, to ensure understanding and compliance – especially if they are swapping notes with other owners. The two types of ulceration should be considered as different diseases (Sykes, and Jokisalo, 2015; Sykes *et al.*, 2019): diet is clearly implicated in ESGD but may not be in EGGD.

Equine squamous gastric syndrome (ESGD)

Consider how you wish to describe the anatomy of the upper part of the stomach. It is not dissimilar to the rumen of the cow, insofar as it is a site of fermentation facilitated by the alkaline conditions, and both fibre and concentrate fermentation produce volatile fatty acids. The integrity of the upper stomach relies heavily on the buffering capacity of the saliva to protect it from any acid splash 'up' from the lower stomach and to neutralise the volatile fatty acids. Saliva is only produced when a horse chews and thus depends on feed type (see Chapter 9, Table 9.3); most performance horses eat less forage and saliva production might be compromised unless their diet is managed appropriately.

Fibre intake and stomach health

Horses whose forage intake is reduced produce less saliva and are at an increased risk of developing ESGD (Murray and Schusser, 1993; Murray and Eichorn, 1996) and oral stereotypies (Waters *et al.*, 2002). Horses provided with ad lib hay eat 63% of their intake between 0900 h and 2100 h, meaning that some horses eat less than 0.3 kg in a 4 h period at night, with a resultant drop in proximal pH to 4 (Husted *et al.*, 2009). Maybe it could be argued that some degree of ulceration is normal; 25% of feral horses have ESGD and 30% EGGD (Ward *et al.*, 2015), which is not surprising when they have limited access to food through the winter and that even a few hours fasting reduces the pH of the upper stomach, particularly during the day (Husted *et al.*, 2009); more than 6 h without hay increases the risk of ESGD (Luthersson *et al.*, 2009).

Cribbing and saliva production

Horses that crib due to a reduction in forage intake produce 15–30 times less saliva compared with when they chew food (Houpt, 2012), so they may well be more susceptible to ulceration. Ulcers appear not to stimulate crib biting in horses with gastric ulceration; but they might be the cause of ESGD in some horses, simply due to the reduction in saliva production. Please be aware that only 5–10% of horses with gastric ulcers crib (Albright *et al.*, 2009).

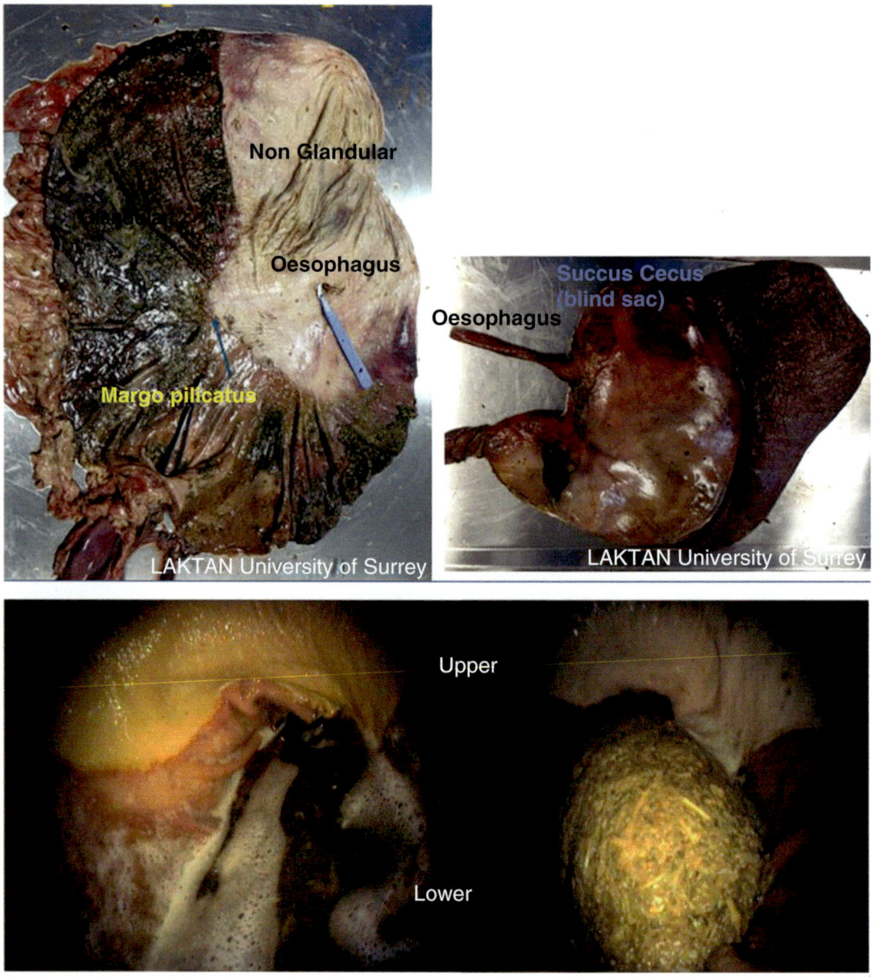

Fig. 12.6. Simplifying the anatomy of the equine stomach.

Forage 'meal' size

Large starch concentrate meals stay in the stomach for longer compared with small starch and small high-fibre concentrate meals (Metayer *et al.*, 2004). This is worth noting, because gastrin, which stimulates HCl, is produced in proportion to stomach distension (Merritt, 1999). Feeding a high-fibre diet to 8-month-old foals increased gastrin for a longer period, due to an increased distension and decreased gastric emptying of the lower stomach compared with feeding a high-starch diet, although the increase in acidity appeared to be in part buffered by increased saliva production (Wilson *et al.*, 2007).

It has been known for a long time that hay increases the acidity (decreases pH) of the ventral stomach compared with concentrates, due to the increase in stomach distension. In people, increased acid secretion and stomach distension seem to prolong gastric emptying slightly (Camilleri, 2019). Similarly delays in equine gastric emptying prolonged contact of the ingested meal with gastrin receptors, resulting in sustained high levels of serum gastrin (Smyth *et al.*, 1989). Mechanical distension was responsible for the gastrin release similar to colicky horses with stomach distension (Sandin *et al.*, 1998) (Fig. 12.6) (Table 12.11).

Large 'meals' of forages also stay in the stomach longer, lowering pH, and may result in longer exposure to splashback; others argue that the fibre mat actually stops the splashback. Retained food within the upper stomach (whether concentrates or forages) will continue to be fermented by bacteria until the pH drops sufficiently to kill them. These bacteria produce volatile fatty acids (VFAs), includ-

Table 12.11 The effect of hay versus concentrate feeding on the pH of the ventral equine stomach

pH ventral stomach	Diet and ration	Reference
1.9	Adlib hay	
	Adlib hay	Berschneider *et al.* (1999)
4.88	2 meals concentrates	
2.69	Adlib hay at 2.4g /100kgBW	Damke *et al.* (2015)
3.35	1.5 g hay/100 kg BW 1 kg conc/100 kg BW	
Plasma gastrin (pg/ml)		
100–120 Peaked at 30min after feeding Stayed > 100 for 12.5 hrs	8–9 kg hay	
100 Peaked at immediately after feed Returned to fasting levels 4hrs after feeding	0.6kg hay/100kgBW 0.2kg concs/100kgBW	Sandin *et al.* (1998)
65–85 (Peaked at 2.5hrs after feeding with gradual return to fasting levels after 6hrs	0.2kg concs /100kgBW	
67–77	Overnight fasting	

ing acetate, which lower the pH to < 4, damaging the upper stomach (Andrews *et al.*, 2006). Starch overload from large meals of starch can change the ratio of VFA (increase in propionate and lactate and decrease in acetate), decreasing pH conditions and causing mucosal damage (Willard *et al.*, 1977).

Advising small meals of forage fed multiple times a day

The volume of 250 g of hay before ingestion is 4.35 litres, compared with 250 g grain, which is 0.45 litres. When saliva is added the volume of grain remains unchanged, but the hay becomes denser, decreasing the volume to 3 litres (Lorenzo-Figueras *et al.*, 2002).

The way your clients manage feeding haylage (or hay) is important.

A group of horses fed on an 'as-fed' basis of 12–13 kg haylage (DM 54%) or 2–3 kg haylage retained the forage differently: 66% of the former group still had visible ingesta 12 h after fasting during gastroscopy (40% of horses retained ingesta occupying 25% gastric volume; 20% retained 50% gastric volume and 40% retained 75% gastric volume) compared with those fed the smaller quantity of haylage (Boswinkel *et al.*, 2007).

The horses fed the large 'meal' of haylage had worse (more and higher scores) ESGD compared with the horses fed the smaller 'meal', probably due to continued stomach distension promoting gastrin or continued fermentation of the fibre producing VFAs.

Thus, a balance is needed between providing enough fibre for chewing and minimising stomach distension and stimulation of gastrin.

Top tips

Managing forage feeding is of foremost importance to reduce the risk of ESGD.

- Ad lib fibre, in small haynets, frequently.
- Good-quality hay in small meals:
- increases chewing and saliva production; and
  - decreases gastrin produced compared with large haynets or lower-quality forage.
  - Adjust haylage quantities:
- water content versus adequate fibre intake
  - adequate fibre intake is required for chewing and subsequent saliva production.
- Adding alfalfa chaff (protein and minerals) to small meals or feeding before a meal will aid buffering and chewing.
- Ensure horse has access to grazing 2–3 h/day.
- Feed forages before concentrates (see Chapter 9: 'Feeding forage before concentrates').

Starch intake and stomach health

As you know, you need to recommend ≤ 1 g starch/kg BW to ensure safe starch solutions and, rather conveniently, Luthersson *et al.* (2009) found that feeding > 1 g starch/kg BW significantly increased the risk of ESGD, which gives two reasons to be very firm with your clients.

Exercise and feeding

Racehorses have a higher incidence of ESGD (85–95%) (Bell *et al.*, 2007) compared with sports horses (65–75%) (Hepburn, 2014; Murray *et al.*, 1996) and leisure horses (45%) (Luthersson *et al.*, 2009), in part because of the effect of exercise on stomach physiology.

Even at walk, the pressure in the stomach and the abdomen increases; this increase is linear with an increase in speed. The increase in pressure compresses the stomach, pushing the acid from the lower stomach into the upper stomach and decreasing pH to 4. The harder and longer the exercise, the more the upper stomach is exposed to acid (Lorenzo-Figueras and Merritt, 2002b). This can be mitigated in part by making sure the client does not exercise the horse after an overnight fast. The upper stomach of horses exercised 18 h after feeding (riding before breakfast) had lower pHs (measured by surgically placed pH meters) at all speeds as well as 1 h and 6 h after exercise (Table 12.12) (Merritt *et al.*, 2003). Simple management changes can minimise the risk of EGUS (Table 12.13).

Minimising the risk of EGUS will also reduce the risk of some colics; 81% of horses with colic also had signs of EGUS, with EGUS determined to be the primary cause of colic in 51% of the horses (Murray, 1992). It might be that ESGD reflects an alteration in GI motility or that medically treated horses are fasted for longer, increasing the risk of ESGD (Dukti *et al.*, 2006; Rabuffo *et al.*, 2009).

Top tips for feeding before exercise

- Forage 2 h before exercise
  - 200–300 g/100 kg BW
  - 1 kg hay produces 4500 ml of saliva
  - 225 meq of buffering
- Small meal 2 h before exercise
  - 50–100 g/100 kg BW
  - 0.5 kg concentrate produces 600 ml of saliva
  - 30 meq buffering

Table 12.12 The effect of feeding before exercise on pH of the upper stomach of the horse compared with riding before breakfast

Time /exercise	Fed 2 h before exercise (pH)	Fed the night before and exercised before breakfast (pH)
Before exercise	5.3	5.23
Walk	3.95	3.15
Trot	2.52	1.07
Canter/gallop	2.39	0.92
1 h after exercise	3.6	3.4
6 h after exercise	5.46	4.58

Colic

Diet or ration is perceived as being the main risk factor for colic, with some suggesting that a high level of concentrates is the main risk (Cohen *et al.*, 1999; Hudson *et al.*, 2001; Tinker *et al.*, 1997). As with most things diet related, the risk is multifactorial and depends upon feeding management, such as a sudden change to the diet, lack of forage, excessive intake of indigestible forage (e.g. eating straw bedding), large meal size, feeding unprocessed cereals with a low pre-caecal digestibility and reduced water intake. Often the challenge with the evidence base is that diet information is collected after the event and details are missing, leaving more questions than answers (Table 12.14).

Pulling together all the information from Table 12.14 and combining with what you know about the time it takes the digestive enzymes to adapt to changes in diet: sudden changes, poor feeding management and a dry diet are the main dietary risk factors.

Top tip

Management solutions to reduce risk of colic

- Recommend daily turnout
- Pastured horses – exhibit natural feeding behaviour.
- will eat more continuous and higher volume of intake of forage.
- grass is a forage with a higher water content,
- in addition, pastured horses spend a more time moving and eating. (4.7–7.2 km/day) compared to stabled (1.1km/day).
- 12hr turnout at pasture decreases colic risk by 50%.
- Stabled horses spend 15% of time eating compared to 50% when out grazing.
- Stabling reduces large intestine motility.
- Make any changes to diet slowly because gut needs time to adapt to forage and concentrates.
- Advise feeding starch at <1g/kgBW/meal (Chapter 5) i.e. small meals.
- Keep hydrated.

Table 12.13 How to provide dietary advice for a horse with EGUS

<table>
<tr><td>Horse signalment</td><td>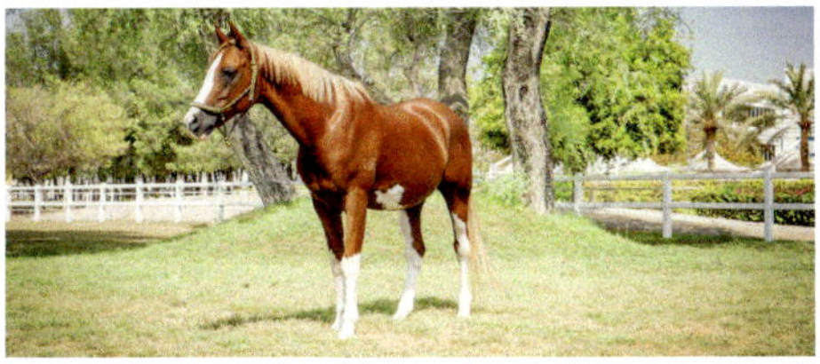</td><td>14 y
420 kg
BCS/BFS 4.5/9 dropped to 4/9</td></tr>
<tr><td>Workload</td><td colspan="2">• All-round sports horse,
  ◦ dressage and show jumping.
• Worked up to 5×/week,
  ◦ flat work training and jumping
• 1.5–2 h/day,
  ◦ walk, mostly trot and some canter
• Competes 2×/month.
• 2–3 h in sand pen
• ½ h on the walker
• Stabled 19 h</td></tr>
<tr><td>Horse history</td><td colspan="2">• History of EGUS, relating to previous endurance career
  ◦ struggles to hold body condition
• Limited appetite; easily over-faced
  ◦ often leaves hay, but will clear concentrate feed</td></tr>
<tr><td>Diet</td><td colspan="2">• 5.5 kg hay (client describes as ad lib)
• 1.5 kg of a low-calorie feed, split into three feeds fed at recommended intake
• 0.6 kg of alfalfa chaff split into three feeds/day
• 60 g of salt</td></tr>
<tr><td></td><td colspan="2">
<table>
<tr><th>Ration kg/day</th><th>Salt 0.06</th><th>Lucerne chop 0.6</th><th>Shape Up 1.5</th><th>Hay 5.5</th><th>Requirement</th><th>Intake</th></tr>
<tr><td>Nutrient[a]</td><td></td><td></td><td></td><td></td><td></td><td></td></tr>
<tr><td>Dry matter</td><td>0.059</td><td>0.54</td><td>1.343</td><td>4.95</td><td>10.5</td><td>6.892</td></tr>
<tr><td>Digestible energy (DE MJ/day)</td><td></td><td>5.8</td><td>13.8</td><td>41</td><td>90.8</td><td>60.6</td></tr>
<tr><td>Protein g/day</td><td></td><td>108</td><td>150</td><td>511.5</td><td>654.5</td><td>769.5</td></tr>
<tr><td>Lysine g/day</td><td></td><td>4.2</td><td>25.4</td><td>16.5</td><td>22.9</td><td>46</td></tr>
</table>
[a]Full vitamin and mineral intake vs requirements would be provided – current diet meets requirements</td></tr>
<tr><td>Advice</td><td colspan="2">Eating 6.8 kg DM
• Should be 10.5 kg (2.5% BW).
• Only eating 64% of DMI, not enough fibre or calories.
Increase fibre intake to increase chewing and subsequent saliva production
• In addition to the hay, recommend a 'hay replacer' which horse might 'enjoy' and eat better because it is provided in a bucket
  ◦ Either one the client puts together
  ◦ Or a low-calorie, fortified chaff-based product, e.g. Fast Fibre, Pure Grass, Fibre Plus Nuggets (soaked), Happy Hoof
  ◦ Split into four 'meals' of 1 kg each
    ▪ increases calories by 40 MJ/day
Increase turnout to 5 h a day
• Make sure there is enough grass; if not, provide alternative fibre
• Hay replacer might need reducing if grazing good</td></tr>
</table>

Continued

Table 12.13 Continued.

	Concentrates
	• The current diet is meeting the daily requirements for vitamins and minerals
	• Was on a low-calorie pellet
	• Change to a competition feed as work increases
	  ◦ Might want to consider a performance balancer fed with alfalfa chaff
	  ◦ Or high-fibre, high-oil feed

Ongoing husbandry	• Keep meal sizes small.
	  ◦ Increase meal frequency from 3 to 4/day
	  ◦ Ensure < 1 g starch/kg BW/meal
	• Advise feeding fibre in a cafeteria style of feeding to encourage browsing behaviour
	  ◦ Provide small haynets around stable
	• Do not overload the stomach
	  ◦ Feed hay/chaff before concentrates
	  ◦ Feed hay 2 h before exercise
	• Feed alfalfa chaff to maintain protein intake (helps buffer the stomach)
	• Weigh out feed and hay monthly to check quantities
	  ◦ Use appropriate containers to measure out

The horse's gut is well suited to 'drinking' its diet, with large chambers to hold digesta which reduce to tight bends, not expecting high dry matter mass but rather feed containing 70–90% water. Williams *et al.*, (2011, 2015) took a multifactorial approach investigating stabling management, not isolating diet or exercise, to measure the impact on the physiology of the gut (Fig. 12.7).

Top tip

Useful resources for your clients:
https://www.bhs.org.uk/our-work/welfare/our-campaigns/react
Links to the different colic titles:
https://www.bhs.org.uk/our-work/welfare/our-campaigns/react/further-colic-information
Vet REACT Colic Champions:
https://www.bhs.org.uk/our-work/welfare/our-campaigns/react/vet-react-colic-champions
For yourself:
https://www.beva.org.uk/Guidance-and-Resources/Practice-Managers/colic-resources

Equine Exertional Rhabdomyolysis

Not all colic signs are gastrointestinal. Some horses suffering exertional rhabdomyolysis may present with non-GI signs of colic (Hewetson, 2006). There are two intrinsic muscle diseases common in certain groups of performance horses: polysaccharide storage myopathy (PSSM) and recurrent exertional rhabdomyolysis (RER). The dietary support for both differs from sporadic exertional rhabdomyolysis caused extrinsically due to over- or inappropriate exercise (see Chapter 13: Tables 13.4 and 13.5).

Tying up, or 'Monday morning disease', as it has been commonly called for decades, was thought to be caused by feeding high-carbohydrate diets following a day of rest. These are not considered risk factors for human athletes; in fact, athletes replenish carbohydrates (CHOs) and rarely spend the day in bed after heavy exercise. Despite some differences in muscle physiology, there are more similarities from a biochemical perspective between horse and human muscle; thus the role of CHOs in the nutritional pathophysiology of myopathies needs further thought, because despite similar clinical presentations, the role of diet in the aetiology of muscle damage is varied (Fig. 12.8).

A simple explanation of the underlying biochemistry of each disease will help your clients to understand your dietary advice and appreciate why it might vary from their friend's.

Polysaccharide storage myopathy (PSSM)

Of horses diagnosed with muscle problems, 21% (McGowan *et al.*, 2009) to 40% (McCue *et al.*, 2008c) have PSSM. These horses tend to be breeds recognised as good doers (Table 12.15) with calm temperaments, and episodes of muscle damage common in the initial stages of getting fit, normally light aerobic exercise (Firshman *et al.*, 2005).

Table 12.14 Diet and diet-related management factors that are associated with an increased risk of equine colic

Documented risk factor	Reference	Reasoning	Debate/information missing
Sugar beet in large colon torsion	Suthers *et al*. (2013).	Whilst authors conclude SB might be risk factor, it should be remembered that SB is fed through the winter, and change of season is an increased risk for colic Horses with simple colonic disruption and distension colic have been reported to have an increase in Streptococci and Lactobaccilli and a decrease in the proportion of Fibrobacter spp. Sugar beet is a fermentable fibre, does not contain starch and is an excellent source of fermentable fibre which supports Fibrobacter, which increases butyrate production. Additionally SB is a much-needed succulent through the winter when the horse is on a predominantly dry diet of conserved forages	Authors noted: 'Horses that had received medication, other than a routine anthelmintic, in the previous 7 days were at increased risk of LCV.' Was SB used to disguise these drugs in the feed?
Increased hours in stable	Suthers *et al*. (2013).	'An increase in hours of stabling in the previous 14 days'	Sudden change in management and associated dietary changes, gut stasis, decreased water intake Gut stasis High DM diet/hay Increased exercise and competition all associated with increase in time stabled. Exercise alters gastrointestinal function by reducing the digestibility of dry matter in feed, and reducing mean retention time (Williams *et al*., 2011)
	Hillyer *et al*. (2002)	Increasing number of hours spent in a stable, 24 h greatest risk	
	Escalona *et al*. (2014)	Increased duration of stabling in the autumn months (September–November)	Higher dry matter forages (or not enough), gut stasis
	Williams *et al*. (2011)	'Motility assessed by ultrasound was significantly lower in stabled horses compared to pasture-kept horses. Intestinal motility contractions/min for caecum (pastured = 2.0, stabled = 1.4), sternal flexure (pastured = 1.7, stabled = 1.5), left ventral colon (pastured = 1.0, stabled = 0.7).'	Large intestinal motility is reduced in stabled horses compared with those kept at grass '… possible mechanism for the increased risk of large intestinal impactions in stabled horses.'

Continued

Table 12.14 Continued.

Documented risk factor	Reference	Reasoning	Debate/information missing
	Williams *et al.* (2015)	Drinking water intake was significantly increased (mean ± s.d. pasture 2.4 ± 1.8 vs stabled 6.4 ± 0.6 l/100 kg BW/day), Total faecal output was significantly decreased (pasture 4.62 ± 1.69 vs. stabled 1.81 ± 0.5 kg/100 kg BW/day) and faecal dry matter content was significantly increased (pasture 18.7 ± 2.28 vs. stabled 27.2 ± 1.93% DM/day) on all days post-stabling compared with measurements taken at pasture	'… significant changes in large intestinal motility patterns and parameters relating to gastrointestinal water balance during a transition from pasture to stabled management, particularly during the first 5 days.'
Change in forage	Suthers *et al.* (2013)	'An alteration in the amount of forage fed in the last 7 days'	Sudden change in management and associated dietary changes, gut stasis, decreased water intake. Likely to be confounded by increase in time stabled and seasonality
Change in pasture (decrease)	Suthers *et al.* (2013)	'Change in pasture in the previous 28 days'	Likely to be seasonal autumn/spring; large intestinal motility is reduced in stabled horses compared with those kept at grass
Crib-biting/wind-sucking/ weaving		Crib-biting/windsucking (odds ratio 10.1) Weaving behaviour (OR 3.9) had an increased risk of recurrence of colic	
	Scantlebury *et al.* (2011, 2015)	'Horses that displayed crib-biting/windsucking behaviour were 12 times more likely to have a history of recurrent colic compared to horses that did not display these behaviours'	Uneven wear of teeth Less saliva Reduced fibre intake Ineffective processing of fibre
	Suthers *et al.* (2013)	Horse being noted to quid in the previous 90 days increased the likelihood of LCV. Crib-biting/windsucking behaviour twice as likely to have a history of colic than those that did not exhibit the behaviour	
	Hillyer *et al.* (2002)	Wood chewing increases risk of simple colonic obstruction and distension colic	Decreased intake of forage
Change in pasture (increased time grazing)	Scantlebury *et al.* (2015)	Reduced the risk of recurrence	'A horse with 12 h/day (i.e. a total of 84 h/week) access to pasture had almost half the risk compared to a horse that is always stabled'

Turnout h/day	**Recurrence colic risk Odds ratio**
3	0.93
6	0.66
24	0.18

Type of forage hay vs haylage or grass	Suthers *et al.* (2013)	Horses fed hay, rather than haylage or grass, had an increased risk of LCV	'Increased dry matter content of hay, compared to haylage or grass might predispose horses fed hay to impactions'
	Escalona *et al.* (2014)	Horses that were fed haylage = twice the increased risk of colic	Intake needs documenting as it could be simply inappropriate dry matter intake (DMI) as owners don't take water content into account
	Cohen *et al.* (1999)	Hay of poorer quality and low digestibility predisposes horses to colic	Rate of passage of high digestible fibre and low digestible fibre (mix of straw and alfalfa) were compared with donkeys, ponies and TBs Fibre content marked effect on nutrient digestibility; water intake increased as straw % increased (be aware of winter and cold weather effects) Transit time for low-quality fibre significantly longer compared with high-quality fibre
Probiotics	Scantlebury *et al.* (2015)	Increased risk of recurrent colic	Cuddeford *et al.*, (1995) '... possible that administering probiotics is a marker for certain types of horse that already have an inherent risk of colic, e.g. older horses, those with dental problems'
Seasonality	Archer *et al.* (2006)	More common in the spring and autumn months '... all colic and all medically or surgically treated colic groups with small peaks evident around the months of March/April and October/November" Epiploic Foramen Entrapment (EFE) 'the main peak occurred in the months of November, December and January with a secondary, less pronounced peak in the months of April, May and June' '... large colon impaction colic group an increasing number of cases identified in the autumn and winter months (peak December/ January) decreasing over the spring months with the lowest incidence over the months of July and August'	UK sudden changes in diet and management – mostly associated with leisure and low-level competition horses 'Equine Grass Sickness (EGS) exhibited significant 12- and 6-month cyclical components, cases peaking in the month of May with a secondary less pronounced peak in the month of October. 'Risk factors for EGS that have been identified in epidemiological studies previously include increased risk associated with change of field in the previous 2 weeks non-feeding of hay or haylage and change of feed type or quantity 14 days prior to disease. 'The seasonal pattern of EGS identified in the present study coincides with months of the year that may be associated with change in grazing practices and feed types in the UK.' '... seasonality of EFE may reflect changes in stabling, turnout, exercise and feeding practices common to these times of the year' Reflects forage type and probably decreased water intake and reduced exercise = increased stasis, standing in stable for longer

Continued

Table 12.14 Continued.

Documented risk factor	Reference	Reasoning	Debate/information missing
	Hillyer *et al*. (2001)	',,, seasonal pattern of colic in the race-horse population under investigation in their study may have been associated with stage of training or level of activity."	Or feeding
Exercise	Hillyer *et al*. (2002)	Recent change in a regular exercise programme	Likely to be different to leisure/competition horses; adjust advice according to use and management of horse
Feeding concentrates	Hillyer *et al*. (2002)	Feeding more than 4 lb concentrates/day odds ratio 2.7	No report on meal size, what type of concentrates and starch concentrate, or order of feeding and whether chaff was added
	Hillyer *et al*. (2002)	If a change of concentrates had happened in the last week, odds ratio increased to 12	Info more useful if compared to the actual consumption and quantities
	Traub-Dargatz *et al*. (2002)	No association with feeding of concentrates	Explain the risks of a high-starch meal Explain that a horse can easily eat a high-starch diet as long as it is provided in low-starch meals Explain the effect of large meals on glycaemic index Explain that the cooked starch fed in small meals is primarily digested in the small intestine Need to check the starch content with the manufacturer, needs to be fed at less than 1-g starch/kg BW/meal If hay is fed first, this slows the speed of eating and the rate of passage through the SI, improving enzymic digestion Can also consider feeding the chaff separately as long as the horse is not a greedy eater Changes in feed must be done slowly to allow microbiome to adapt
	Tinker *et al*. (1997)	High levels of concentrate (> 2.5 kg/day dry matter, OR=4.8; > 5 kg/day dry matter, OR=6.3) relative to feeding no concentrate	Confounding management factors. If fed large meals of starch, overwhelms SI enzymic digestion and starch utilised by lactobacilli in hind gut with decrease in pH and increase in acidity.
		Changes in concentrate feeding during the year (1 per year, OR=3.6)	Change in fermentation parameters, endotoxaemia and inflammation and pain.
Dental care		Reduced mastication of feed may lead to the ingestion of longer dietary fibres passing to distal portions of the gastrointestinal tract, increasing the risk of impaction	May be a similar mechanism to horses that windsuck etc, which leads to inappropriate wear on teeth and reduced masticatory efficiently.

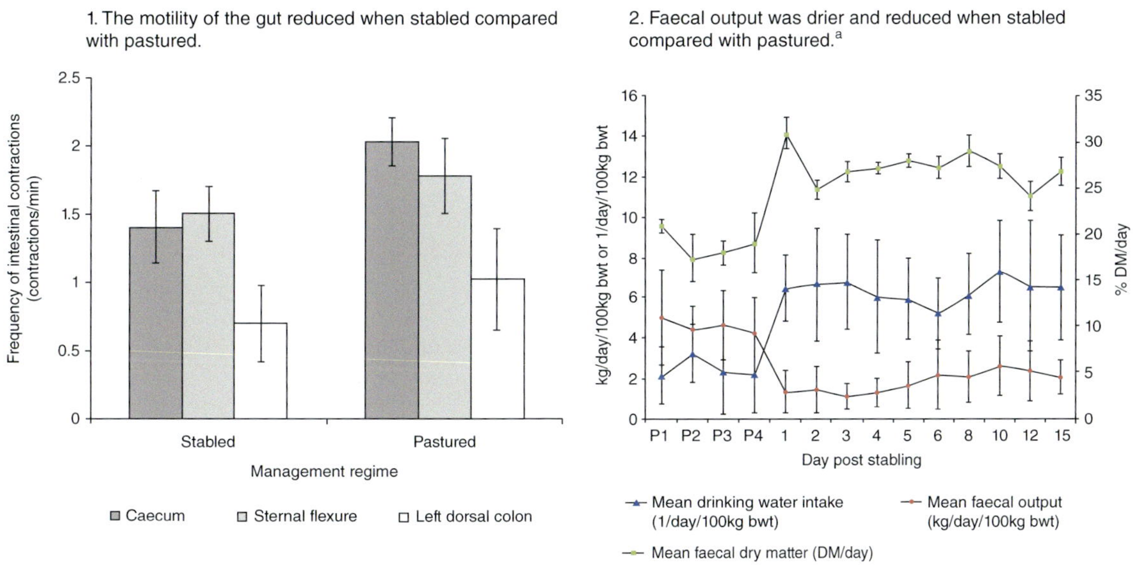

Fig. 12.7 The effect of changing from pasture to stabling on various gut parameters associated with colic. (Modified from Williams *et al.*, 2011, 2015.)

[a]There are a number of factors that may predispose a horse to colic under stabled conditions, including differences in: feed type; feeding patterns and intervals; and exercise levels

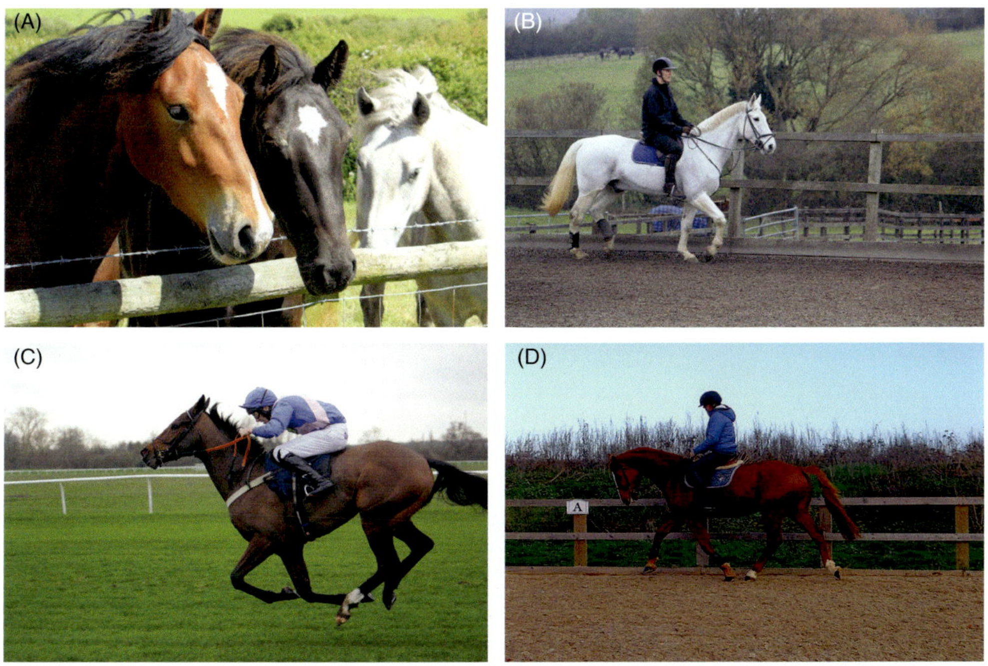

Fig. 12.8 Diet, exercise, fitness and breeds differed despite common clinical signs of muscle damage. Diet very varied, from no carbohydrates to large intakes. (A) Leisure horse hacked out twice a week. (B) Heavy Hunter on day off. (C) Fit racing filly. (D) Warmblood initial fittening programme.

Table 12.15 Prevalence of PSSM in horse breeds

Type of horse	USA (McCue *et al.*, 2008c) (*n* = 831, 17 breeds)	UK (McGowan *et al.*, 2009) (*n* = 150)	
Quarter-horses	72%	¼ Xs 67%	Cobs 34.5%
Draught/heavy breeds	87%	38%	
Warmbloods	18%		
Light breeds	24%	17% (TB Xs 13%)	
Ponies		0%	

Type 1 PSSM is a dominantly inherited defect in the gene encoding glycogen synthase (GYS1) which maintains a persistent activity, so horses accumulate 1.5–4× higher levels of CHO complexes in 1–40% of skeletal muscle fibre. The normal flux of energy metabolism in the muscle is disturbed during exercise because of this glycogen storage disease (McCue *et al.*, 2008c). Horses can be diagnosed via DNA testing of hair roots or blood (McCue *et al.*, 2008a).

Dietary advice

From a dietary perspective, your clients need to understand that their horse has the following.

- Normal glycogen metabolism:
- Increased glycogen use in anaerobic exercise.
- Abnormal regulation of glycogen synthesis rather than defect in use.
- Enhanced insulin sensitivity and glucose uptake at light exercise, leading to:
- higher glucose-6-phosphate concentration; and
- increased number of glycogen granules (Firshman *et al.*, 2005).

The aim of the diet is to:

- reduce glucose load;
- decrease glucose uptake into cells; and
- decrease insulin sensitivity.

'A low-starch diet reduces glycogen accumulation in muscle which combined with a daily exercise regime, has been fairly successful in ameliorating the signs of rhabdomyolysis associated with PSSM' (Steph Valberg, personal communication). 'a low-starch diet reduces glycogen accumulation in muscle which combined with a daily exercise regime, has been fairly successful in ameliorating the signs of rhabdomyolysis associated with PSSM'.

Concentrates

- **Increase fat to provide above 10% calorie intake**

There is still limited information on appropriate quantities (12–25% of DE) – fat is energy dense, so you need to reduce the calorie content of the forage to compensate.

Feeding fat to ponies increases insulin resistance, resulting in 25% higher plasma insulin (Schmidt *et al.*, 2001); it lowers hepatic fatty acid (FA) synthesis, increases FA oxidation in aerobic muscle and decreases masseter, gluteus and semitendinosus muscle glycogen concentration by 65% (Geelen *et al.*, 2001), providing evidence as to its efficacy for PSSM. It is challenging to put together a ration for light work with a high % of DE from fat whilst still meeting dry matter intakes (Table 12.16).

- **Reduce water-soluble carbohydrates (WSC) as calorie source**

PSSM horses fed < 15% of daily DE as starch appeared to have lower CK but no differences in insulin sensitivity or glycogen concentration, although post-prandial insulin and glucose were lower, compared with PSSM on higher-starch diets (Ribeiro *et al.*, 2004)

- **Advise forages with less than 11% water-soluble CHO**

PSSM horses fed hay with 17% WSC versus hay with 4% or 9% elicited a higher peak insulin (Borgia *et al.*, 2011). Most hays in the UK are < 10% WSC (see Chapter 9) but advise clients to have their forage analysed. Using lower-calorie forages means that you can ensure that DMI is maintained even with high fat intake.

- **Daily turnout when not being exercised**

It is important that these horses have daily exercise and turnout to enhance glycogen use and reduce accumulation (Valberg *et al.*, 1999) but please utilise all the tips for controlling grass WSC intake (see Chapter 9) or it will be counterproductive (grass WSC content g/kg DM: autumn 80, winter 36, spring 107, summer 102) (Table 12.17).

PSSM – type 2

Typically for type 2 PSSM, or myofibrillar myopathy, currently there is no genetic test[i] because the genetic variants are not consistent. Muscle biopsy

Table 12.16 Effect of different percentages of digestible energy (DE) from fat on the reduction in dry matter intake from 12.5kg DM for 500kg exercising horses[c].

Workload	Digestible energy requirements MJ/day	% DE from oil			Amount of hay[a] (kg/day) if feeding just hay and oil			Amount of hay[a] if feeding concentrates[b]		
		10% (A)	15% (B)	20% (C)	A	B	C	A	B	C
Maintenance	62.5–70		**DE provided by oil (MJ)**							
Light (L)	75–84	7.5–8.4	11.25–12.6	15–16.8	11.5	10.9	10.4	8.8	8.25	7.7
			Oil fed (ml)							
		234–262	351–394	468–524						
			DE provided by oil (MJ)							
Medium (M)	87.5–98	8.75–9.8	13.1–14.7	17.5–19.6	11.25	10.6	10	7.8	7.2	6.6
			Oil fed (9ml)							
		273–306	409–459	546–612						

[a]Calculated for lowest DE intake in each category; assuming Hay DE of 7 MJ/kgDM
[b]Light work: fed Balancer 12 MJ/kg (0.5 kg intake) = 6MJ/DE Medium work: fed low starch competition mix 11.8 MJ/kg (2 kg intake) = 23.6MJ/DE
[c]Hay without oil fed at 2.5% BW (12.5kg); Hay fed with concs but no oil Light work = 9.8kg. Medium work without oil = 9.1kg

to aid glycogen clumping (not necessarily high levels), which is found in the fibre cytoplasm and under the cell membrane, is needed for diagnosis. Some similarity of clinical signs with PSSM1 (Box 12.1) and similar dietary advice will help alleviate but not eliminate the drop in performance, with the caveat that this group need higher protein intakes (Williams *et al.*, 2018).

Recurrent exertional rhabdomyolysis (RER)

RER is associated with changes in genetic pathways that regulate myoplasmic Ca^{2+} mitochondrion and protein degradation. Because there is a decreased capacity to remove Ca^{2+} from the myoplasm, these horses have 8× higher levels of Ca^{2+} compared with normal horses, which, together with enhanced storage of Ca^{2+} in the sarcoplasmic reticulum, enhances muscle force and energy metabolism within a physiological range of myoplasmic Ca^{2+} (Aldrich *et al.*, 2021). The clinical signs you see are because of persistent muscle contracture, and loss of mitochondrial and myofibre integrity (Aldrich *et al.*, 2021).

Box 12.1 Clinical signs of PSSM**2**

- Lazy – drop in energy level and unwillingness to perform after 5–10 min of exercise.
- Gait abnormality:
- painful firm back and hindquarter muscles;
- reluctance to collect and engage the hindquarters;
- poor rounding over fences.
- Slow onset of atrophy, especially when out of work.
- Warmbloods 8–11 years of age:
- median CK 323 AST 331 u/l.

The susceptibility appears to be heritable in about 10% of all Thoroughbred racehorses (Fritz *et al.*, 2012) and risk factors include changes in training (MacLeay *et al.*, 1999), being a filly (McGowan *et al.*, 2002) or maybe chronic stress in a race training environment (measured by cortisol) which affects younger mares more than older mares in race training (Nogueira and Barnabe, 1997).

Although it has been noted that horses fed more than 5 kg of starch-based feed are more susceptible to RER, there is mixed evidence that diet influences RER. All racing TBs are fed more than 5 kg of hard feed, yet only 10% suffer from RER, thus the link is not clear cut.

Some researchers argue that high starch increases the nervousness of fillies and thus might exacerbate the stress trigger (Table 12.18) but more work with blinded observers and objective behavioural ethograms are needed to fully elucidate the physiological links.

Whilst in practice high-fat diets have been successful in reducing RER in fillies, in the long term the performance of the horse seems to suffer and many trainers return to a higher-starch diet but

Table 12.17 How to advise a diet for a horse with PSSM type 1

Horse signalment	6 y, 16 hh Draft × Appaloosa 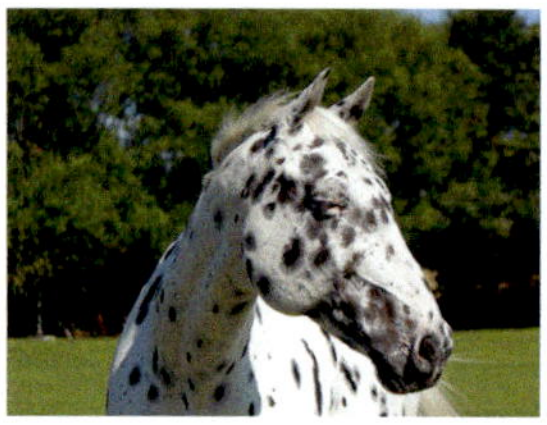	Horse is a good doer Weight tape indicates 650 kg BFS 4, 3, 3.5
Horse history	• Little stiff when first ridden and has a reluctance to come on the bit when schooling. • Gets rather sweaty. • Light work, getting fit for Riding Club dressage competitions. • Trying to build topline but weak neck. • Often reluctant to canter; does not like being shod. • Thought was just a late developer. • Lazy, particularly for the first 30 min when just walking and trotting. • Tenses up when tighten the girth after 5 min exercise.	
Differentials	• Solid muscles over hind quarters, do not 'ripple' when 'thumped'. • Positive for PSSM1 with N/PSSM1 genotype. • Pre exercise CK > 1600, post-exercise > 4000.	
Current diet	5 h grazing 1 large net of haylage ½ scoop conditioning mix ½ scoop competition mix	
Advice	1. Decrease water-soluble carbohydrates (WSC) and starch to reduce muscle glycogen stores. 2. Increase gentle exercise as soon as possible. Increase intensity to allow for oil feeding. Rest is counterproductive. 3. Increase fibre intake. 4. Add oil and vitamin E to diet to increase insulin resistance. 5. Balance vitamins and minerals. • Increase turnout (if possible, 24/7) on low-quality pasture: ◦ with another active horse to encourage moving; ◦ muzzle to decrease grass/WSC intake. ▪ Winter grazing 6–8 kg DMI; DE intake 30–40 MJ. ◦ Summer grazing 16 kg DMI. ▪ 128 MJ DE if not muzzled. ▪ Check droppings to ensure eating enough DM. • Feed hay when shortage of grass. ◦ Weigh out 9 kg (1.5% BW) and soak for 8 h to decrease WSC. ◦ Split into three and distribute around stable (see Chapter 9). ▪ DE intake 45 MJ • Limited rugging to increase fat loss (horses use 80% of feed energy to keep warm; rug them and the calories go on their back as fat). ◦ Will need rugging in winter. ◦ Will need warming up and down carefully so muscles do not get cold. • Exercise daily. ◦ Needed to increase DE requirements to 97 MJ (DE_m × 1.2), otherwise very difficult to shift fat. ◦ Minimum 45 min–1 h with trot and canter after warmed up. • Alfalfa chaff (0.25 kg) twice a day: ▪ 5 MJ/DE. • Performance vitamin and mineral supplement (275 g) 0 MJ/DE.	

Continued

Table 12.17 Continued.

	• Vegetable oil: ◦ Start with 50 ml, making sure the horse starts to lose fat before increasing slowly ◦ Feed to provide 10% DE intake (DE_m = 81 MJ ▪ Work out for M, no need to add extra for work as eating excess calories. ▪ 10% of 81 = 8 MJ. ▪ 1litre/kg oil = 32 MJ. • 250 ml oil. ▪ Can increase as workload increases and when horse loses fat – aim for BFS 3, 3, 3. • Vitamin E supplement: ◦ 100 iu vitamin E/100 ml of additional oil. ◦ Check label (see Chapter 7: 'Interpreting a feed label')
Electrolytes	• Depending on sweat loss: ◦ Weight tape can pick up kg loss after exercise (see Chapter 13). ◦ Only advise if vitamin/mineral supplement not adequate.

manage the horse better to minimise stress[ii] and avoid having rest days.

Adjusting the advice to the individual horse takes time and trust but is necessary because most research provides us with information for the average horse and clinical judgement is needed for a successful outcome.

How to Advise Diets for Specific Disciplines

Performance horses are expected to compete across a range of disciplines, speeds and duration; clearly diet has a part to play. Equally important is appropriate training for the horse's intended workload. Different training regimes upregulate different muscle fibres and metabolic pathways, ensuring the appropriate energy intake can be utilised during work. Clients need to feed appropriately for the metabolic pathways they are conditioning; thus diets can be tailored for discipline-specific adjustments based on the type of work expected of the horse.

Feeding the endurance horse

If you have the chance to vet at an endurance competition, your role is to make sure the horse stays sound, is not dehydrated and that their heart rate (HR) is acceptable. Endurance horses must obtain an HR below a certain limit (usually 64 beats/min (bpm)) to pass the vet inspection within 15 min of crossing the end line of each loop, with the exception of the final loop, and 64 bpm within 20 min of crossing the finish line of the final loop.

Each endurance race is split into loops (usually 30–40 km) with a vet gate at the end of each loop. Several clinicians will be involved in vetting the horse before the race and at the vet gates, where horses are offered water, hay and sometimes feed, as well as at the end of the gates. There are also crew stops every 10 km or so from the second loop where the horse can be offered water.

The end of the race is completed as sprint and the speed varies according to the length of the race (160 km: 14.4 km/h; 120 km:17.9 km/h; 90 km:17.6 km/h) (Le Moyec *et al*., 2019). You are unlikely to come across horses younger than 4 years or older than 15 years. When it comes to diet, there are some clear indicators as to the relationship between exercise and energy substrates. The longer the distance, the lower are the levels of post-race lipids and acetate (Table 12.19), showing that the horses use fat as an energy supply.

Blood glucose levels do not drop as much over longer distances, because fatty acids are used for muscular functioning. Horses should have higher levels of muscle and liver glycogen from training adaptations, so they use muscle and liver glycogenolysis more; they need this glucose for anaerobic metabolism when they sprint the last part of the race (Le Moyec *et al*., 2019).

Horses that race over a longer distance show signs of protein catabolism and most will show signs of dehydration related to bodyweight loss, muscle inflammation and have higher levels of total bilirubin but not liver damage, (Le Moyec *et al*., 2014). The speed at which the horse races will impact upon their energy metabolism, with some horses sustaining mean speeds of 24 km/h under desert conditions. Horses that finish fast races have increased heart rate, albumin (ALB), total bilirubin (BIL), lactate (LACT), and lactate dehydrogenase

Table 12.18 The effects of diets fed to horses suffering from RER

Number of horses and workload	Study design	High starch	High fat	Results/conclusion from authors	Reference	Comments
Four TB mares with RER	3 × 3 latin square Fit horses 10 w exercise regime, 2 rest days Exercise 4 min walk (1.8 m/s), 2 min trot (4 m/s) 2 min canter (7 m/s) for 20 min Fed diets for 5 days Unfit turned away for 3–6 months pasture, then fed diets for 5 days	10.8% protein 3.4% fat 48% non-structural CHOs (NSC) starch = 41% (5.8× higher)	12.5% protein 12.5% fat (3.6× higher) 10% NSC starch 7.1%	No differences in cortisol between diets No differences between diets in cortisol between fit RER horses or unfit horses Fit horses fed high starch had higher cortisol compared with unfit (sig dif. not provided) Might be due to increased insulin increasing tryptophan to brain	Finno *et al.* (2010)	Limited time for adaptation to diets Authors noted that fit TBs have > cortisol compared with unfit
Five RER TB mares, three control TB mares	Random and then cross over 6 w of treadmill 4–5 days/w ,30 min walk, trot and canter and gallop (11 m/s)	135% calories of low starch and high fat 38.6% NSC 4.2 kg/day 53% of E intake Fat 2.8% 0.3 kg /day 8% E intake	24.8% NSC 2.1 kg/day 34% E intake Fat 7.1% 0.6 kg/day 20% E intake	Horses on the higher energy diet gained 2.4% BW Trend but no sig diffs in HR during or after SET No sig diffs in any parameters including lactate, CK etc Some subjective observation of increased excitability on high CHOs	MacLeay *et al.* (1999)	Rations/diets not comparable. Were observers blinded to diets?
One stallion, five TB mares with RER	5 w for 5 days/w walk, trot and canter, last 2 w canter replaced with 2 min gallop (11 m/s) 6% incline, rested Sat/Sun, stabled Isolcalorie diets (120.5 MJ DE/day); hay 1.2% BW	Starch 40% DE Fat 5% DE	Starch 7% DE Fat 20% DE	Fat diet – increase plasma ionised Ca Starch diet– CK sig higher after exercise (7×) but dependent on individual horses CK higher on Mondays regardless of diet Resting HR waiting on treadmill lower on fat diets No HR diffs during/post-exercise Subjective observations on behaviour	McKenzie *et al.* (2003)	Behaviour needs objective measurements; observers need to be blinded to diets

Table 12.19 Effect of the distance raced by 40 endurance horses on their metabolites[a]. (Modified from Le Moyec *et al.*, 2019.)

Distance	Mean speed (km/h)	HR at finish (bpm)	Plasma post-race samples lower than pre-race	Plasma post-race samples higher than pre-race	Higher post-race samples of longer distance compared with shorter	Lower post-race samples of longer distance compared with shorter
90 km (16 horses)	16.8	54.9	Glucose, alanine and compounds including N-acetyl moieties, e.g. glucosamine in hyaluronic acid	Branched-chain amino acids (BCAAs), lactate, acetate, glutamine, glutamate, citrate, creatine, glycerol, and aromatic amino acids (AAAs)	Acetate, glutamate, glutamine, citrate, creatine and urea	Lactate, lipids and N-acetyl functional groups
120 km (15 horses)	17.8	55.1				
160 km (9 horses)	16.7	55.8				

[a]Blood samples taken before race and 30 min after completion. NMR and metabolomic analysis

(LDH) and decreased blood urea nitrogen (BUN) compared with horses that were eliminated, but there was no difference in dehydration status (Halama *et al.*, 2021), which might suggest energy metabolism is the limiting factor.

Metabolomics (quantifying 792 metabolites) has confirmed that the most significant shifts in energy metabolism are an accelerated lipid and protein catabolism, together with utilisation of fatty acids, but also of glucose showing anaerobic metabolism at these faster speeds; a greater disruption of red blood cells reflects the oxidation of fats (Halama *et al.*, 2021).

Typical diets are high in fat (see Chapters 5 and 13).

Feeding racehorses

Racehorses work at a high intensity for a short period of time, using anaerobic energy, and high blood glucose is typical during these short bouts of exercise (Geor *et al.*, 2000). Exercise is a stress and as part of this reaction, tissues that have adrenergic receptors accelerate heart rate, release triglycerides from adipose tissue (for energy for other organs) and glucose from the liver, increase blood flow and increase glucose uptake to the muscles (independently of insulin) (Dallner, 2008). Horses in fast work use 3× more CHO oxidation compared with horses in light work, although there is evidence that fats are also used as an energy source for fast work over a longer duration (30 min) (Geor *et al.*, 2000). Racehorses have > 50% type IIa muscle fibres, reflective of their anaerobic fuel use, which increase with training, with hindlimbs being typically glycolytic and forelimbs oxidative (Kawai *et al.*, 2009).

It is worth reminding clients that there is a positive correlation between successful racehorses and higher muscle mass plus lower reserves of body fat (Fonseca *et al.*, 2013). As workload increases, it is important to check the energy intake of these horses, as a decrease in energy intake results in a reduction in muscle mass.

Dietary advice is generally very standardised on a racing yard and your biggest challenge will be to ensure adequate fibre intake, encouraging warm-down as well as warm-up and gentle exercise on days off and minimising the impact of travelling on normal feeding routines.

Feeding sports horses

Different training regimes have differing effects on muscle development and energy substrates used (Table 12.20).

Dressage horses

There is limited evidence as to the workload of dressage horses. The mean and peak heart rates for warmblood and thoroughbred horses warming up for elementary level (British Dressage (BD)) were 91 and 146 bpm; and for medium level mean 91 bpm, peak 144 bpm. These increased during the test at elementary level to mean 102±13 and peak 132±20 bpm, and at medium level to 107±8 and peak 132±10 bpm (Williams *et al.*, 2009), meaning that they are working aerobically because their HR < 180 bpm (see Chapter 3).

Diet can be adjusted to provide the slow-release energy for dressage horses according to their fat score (see Chapter 5).

> **Top tip**
>
> Be aware of the dangers of the top dressage horse with a 'good topline' that goes footy when it stops working – exercise protects the horse from insulin resistance (IR) until that exercise stops.
>
> - Remind owners that breakdown of food into nutrients for energy causes molecular-level inflammation.
>   - This is not a problem; the horse has mechanisms in place to counteract the inflammation.
>   - But constant excess nutrients (expressed as a high neck fat score) over time will stop those mechanisms, resulting in IR and chronic inflammation.
> - If you have scored a horse at > 4/5 for 12 months on its neck, then you need to consider potential insulin resistance (see Chapter 15).

Polo ponies

Your biggest challenge in advising polo ponies is encouraging enough adaptation time when the ponies first start to be fed and persuading the trainers to provide hay during the winter when the ponies are turned away. Fortunately, the initial training tends to be light work, but when playing about 7 min/chukka, HR can increase above 90% HR max (HR ≈ 195–208 bpm), interspersed with 3 min ~68–89 % HR max (HR ≈ 150–195 bpm), and another ~3 min ridden within ~41–68 % HR max (HR ≈ 90–150 bpm) (moderate to very hard) (Chanda *et al.*, 2016).

Because polo utilises both aerobic and anaerobic energy, a standard competition mix can be advised with alfalfa chaff and, depending on BFS, an oil supplement whilst ensuring adequate forage intakes.

Showing

All clinicians should attend at least one show championship class at one of the bigger shows such as the Horse of the Year Show (HOYS) or Hickstead to experience at first hand the challenges these horses are put under. The continued fashion of 'needing more condition' without explaining that the judge means muscle, not fatter, and the placing of these 'over-conditioned' horses in the top three (Fig. 12.9) is a major health and welfare concern.

The fatter the horse (Table 12.21), the greater is the reduction in physiological fitness. Fat horses have higher locomotory asymmetry, heart rates, lactate, respiratory rate and rectal temperatures but lower plasma glucose and fatty acids and haematocrit compared with fitter horses (Jansson *et al.*, 2021).

When advising exhibitors on diet, much of Chapter 15 is directly relevant.

Most show horses work at heart rates less than 180 bpm and are in light work, except for working hunters. Show horses should be fed as leisure horses (see Chapter 11) but if the rider can be persuaded to work the horse hard enough to develop an outline from muscle rather than fat, then slow-release (fat/fibre) competition mixes would be appropriate.

To maintain client compliance, you might have to concur with feeding conditioning or show mix, most definitely at less than recommended amounts. Be sure to advise a balancer in proportion to provide micronutrients.

Eventers

Most eventers are fed a mix of aerobic and anaerobic energy sources and competitors are less concerned with feed effects on behaviour, mainly because they feed appropriately for workload. Slow release can be provided by adequate high-quality forage and additional oil in combination with a competition mix for anaerobic energy. Ensure that clients competing at lower levels do not overestimate workloads. For dietary advice, see Table 12.22.

Table 12.20 Relationship between training, muscle development and energy substrates used in sports horses

Exercise duration	V lactate[a]	Speed (m/s)	Heart rate (bpm)	Muscle development	Consequence	Performance consequence	Reference
[b]45 min Long, low intensity	1.5	3.1	164	Increased size of mitochondria and myofibrils Increased area of myofibrils	Increase in ATPase type IIA muscle fibres (aerobic) Reduce type IIx fibres (anaerobic)	Improvement in muscle strength and aerobic capacity, enhanced muscle glycogen	Lindner *et al.*, (2013)
[b]45 min Long, medium intensity	2.5	3.4	173	Increase size of mitochondria and myofibrils	Improved mitochondrial density by 26% Significant selective hypertrophy of type IIA fibres		
[b]25 min High, short intensity	4	3.8	180	Increase size of mitochondria and myofibrils Total mitochondrial area stayed greater after rest period		Less improvement in muscle strength and aerobic capacity but improvement maintained for longer	
[c]1600 m week 1; 4000 m week 9	4–8 mmol/l	8–10 84–97% VO_{2max}			No differences	Cardiorespiratory capacity increased rapidly with the onset of training in horses. At training intensities between 40 to 90% VO_{2max}, the responses to training were not dependent on the intensity of the training exercise when the horses performed the same training distance.	Eaton *et al.* (1999)
	< 2 mmol/l	4–5 49–53% VO_{2max}					
[d]Low	< 0.9		41 (19% HR_{max})				Chanda *et al.* (2016)
[d]Low to medium	1.1	6.7 km/h	144 (65.5% HR_{max})				
[d]Match plays	4 8	10–14 km/h	175–195 (80–88% HR_{max})	Type IIx decreased Increased type IIa and I muscle fibres	Increased succinate dehydrogenase-positive fibres, intramuscular lipids, no change in glycogen	Improved oxidative metabolism rather than glycolytic; muscle fibres transition from fast to slow phenotypes	
Showjumpers: see Chapter 3)							

[a]Blood lactate mM $V_{lactate}$ is used as a measure of fitness during standardised exercise regimes so that horses are exercised at a defined speed and time to produce set blood lactate levels
[b]2-year-old Haflingers for 6 weeks
[c]TB horses for 9 weeks
[d]Polo ponies L, LM 3 weeks each; matches 12 weeks

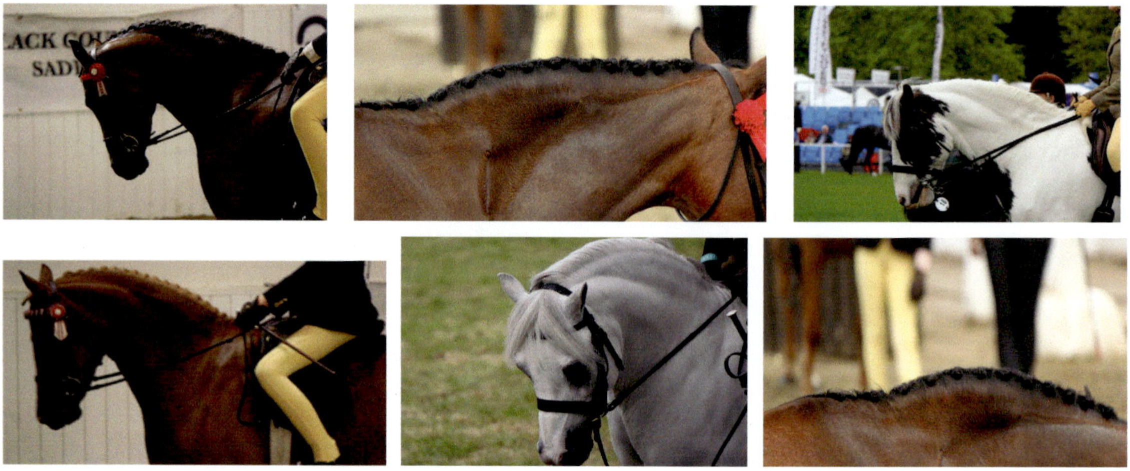

Fig. 12.9 Typical effects of 'over-conditioning' in show horses.

Showjumpers

The workload of showjumpers is generally anaerobic during jump-offs but aerobic in warm-up and first rounds (see Chapter 3: Table 3.5). The ration needs to be flexible, depending upon the individual horse and forage fed. Most SJ work for short durations compared with other disciplines. Muscle development is key for a successful jumper and leisure feeds will not provide the quality protein needed.

For dietary advice, see Table 12.23.

Summary

Nutrition, whilst frequently taken for granted until something goes wrong, plays an essential role in the preparation, competition and recovery of the horse, becoming more crucial the higher the level of performance. The support (nutrition, exercise programmes, fittening and recovery) varies according to discipline and must, to a point, be tailored to the individual horse.

1. **Always advise a minimum of 50% DMI as forage:**
    - Hay soaked for 30 min.
    - Split into multiple 'meals'.
    - Managed to allow foraging behaviour.
    - Chaff should be fed before concentrates.
    - Account for haylage DM.
    - Sugar beet fibre is a useful succulent.
    - Daily turnout is beneficial.
2. **Explain the time required for small intestine adaptation to starch digestion:**
    - Advise 1 g starch/kg BW/meal (small meals, fed more frequently).
    - Advise cooked starch:
        - To ensure hind gut health and maximise glycogen replenishment
        - Advise small meal within 1 h of exercise to replenish glycogen and protein.
    - Do not advise leisure feeds.
    - Advise competition feeds.
    - Good doers should be fed a performance balancer.
3. **Match the energy sources to the workload:**
    - Ensure the client conditions the horse for the final work required with appropriate exercise.
    - Fast anaerobic work should be supplied with starch-based calories.
    - Sustained aerobic work should be supplied with fibre and oil/fat calories.
    - Some disciplines need a mix of energy calories.
    - Use the labels to check ingredients and intakes.
4. **Teach clients to fat score:**
    - Horses should be muscled up to create 'top line' and bulk.
    - Do not accept a fat horse.
    - A crest is fat; there is no muscle above the nuchal ligament
    - Fat is a health and welfare issue.

Table 12.21 Parameters used to define fatness in relation to performance indices

Parameter	Measurement or score
Rump fat thickness (ultrasound)	12.8 mm
Fat (BF)	14.7 %
Fat mass (FM) (BW X BF%)	60 kg
Fat free mass (BW – FM)	348 kg
Neck score[a]	6.1
Back Score[a]	4.7
Rump score[a]	5.2
Tail head score[a]	5.9
Ribs score[a]	6.9
Shoulder blade[a]	7.6
Body condition score (Henneke see Chapter 3)	6.1
Cresty neck score (Ch 3)	2.3 cm

[a]as described in Jansson *et al.*, 2021

5. **Review rations seasonally and adjust accordingly:**
   - Use ration software when appropriate
   - Advise electrolytes strategically
   - Adapt but maintain feeding schedules during travel.

Every horse, competitor, supporting vet and nutritionist has a role in furthering the understanding of the relationship between nutrition, health and performance in the field, by keeping records. Simply quantifying and paying attention to the horse's diet and performance on a regular basis will provide (when collected alongside other records) clinical evidence that might make the difference between first and fifth, between health and disease, and between longevity and retirement.

Table 12.22 How to advise a diet for an eventer

Horse signalment	• 485 kg, 10 years old, mare • BFS 4.5/9 • Easy temperament • Loves her work • Competing at 2* moving up to 3*	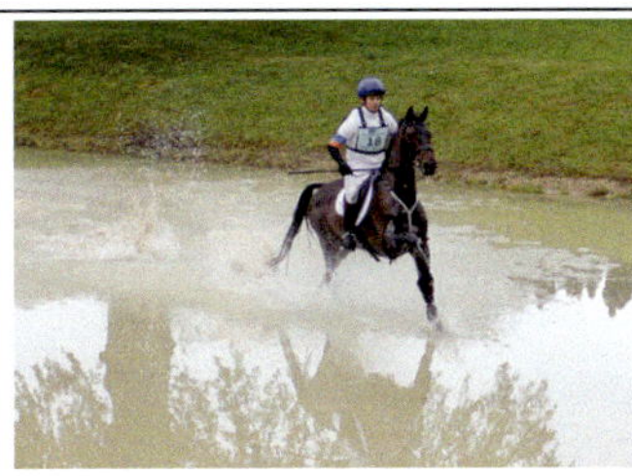
Horse history	• Easy to feed • Good and consistent appetite • Can put on weight easily • Client happy overall but wants a diet check as mare will be competing more at 3* level and what alterations should be made if mare starts to gain BFS.	
Workload	• Exercised 5 days per week for up to 1–1.5 h per day (with HRs 70–140 bpm) • Flat-work training session • Flat-work stretching • Hacking • Goes to the gallops once a week (HRmax 190) • Jumping session either at home or training show	
Current diet	• 10 kg hay • 3.0 Enduro Performance • 600 g lucerne chaff • 60 g salt • 60 g electrolyte supplement • Divided into 3 feeds	

Continued

Table 12.22 Continued.

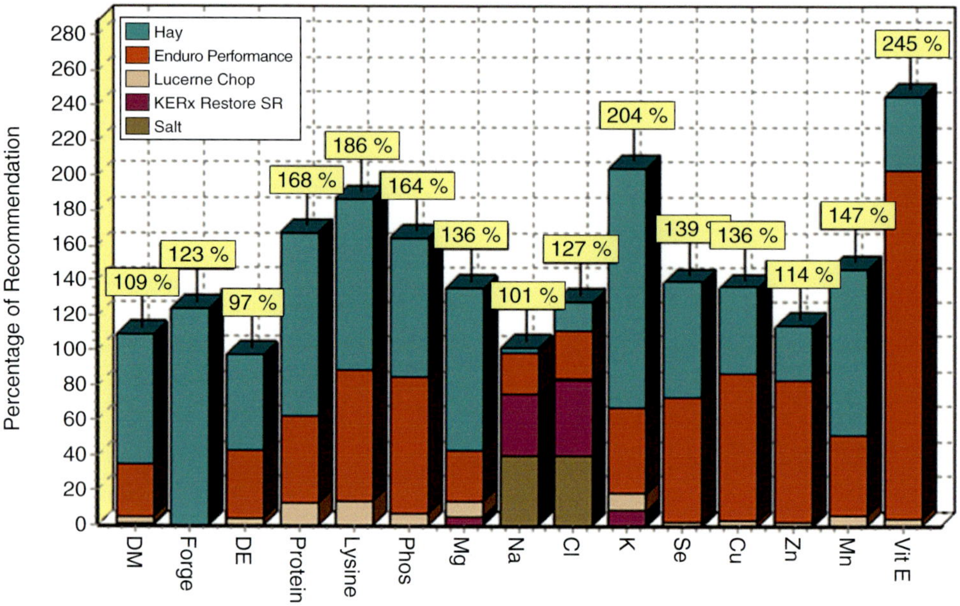

Current diet provides	• DE 131 MJ ○ The horse is currently maintaining a consistent BFS of 4.5, indicating that current calorie requirements are being met. • Concentrate feed ○ High fibre and oil mix (125 g fibre/kg and 100g oil/kg and 200g starch/kg), ○ Owner does not like to add additional oil to the feeds. • Diet provides: ○ enough starch for 'quickness of the leg and acceleration'; and ○ oil stamina for cross-country and multiple day competition.
Advice	• Diet is balanced and intake meets recommendations. • Encourage your client to continue with regular weighing and BFS processes. • If horse BFS increases: ○ The calorie content of the diet should be reduced while maintaining nutrient and total DM intake ○ Concentrate feed could be reduced by up to 1–1.5 kg to reduce DE intake to 110–118 MJ DE ○ Advise 400 g of a performance balancer added to ensure intake of micronutrients and protein ○ Hay could be soaked for up to 12 h ○ if this is not possible, discuss a low-calorie forage substitution.

Table 12.23 How to advise a diet for a showjumper

Horse signalment	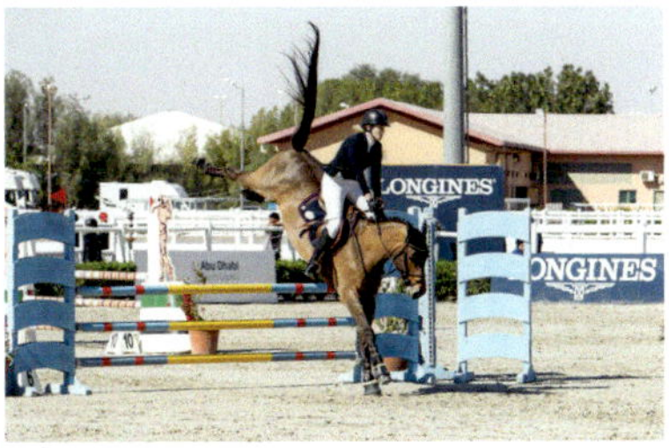	500 kg 12 years BFS 5.5/9
Horse history	• Easy to feed ◦ Has a good appetite ◦ Clears his feed and forage • Crib biter ◦ Sometimes distracted from eating forage ◦ Has led to a few colic episodes ◦ Tendency to drop condition	Excitable temperament Client happy with the current diet but wants to check that it is balanced
Workload	• Exercised 6 days per week. Worked for 30–45 min • 2 days flat work; • 1 jumping; • 2 days hacking with canter work on a gallop with 2 consecutive days off. • 2 h turnout – small, bare paddock. • Competition season: competes most weekends, at amateur affiliated level. ◦ Travelling for up to 3–4 h to an event.	
Current diet	Per day for each product: • 9 kg of grass hay (client describes as ad lib) • 2.5 kg of Competition Mix • 800 g of lucerne chaff • 1 cup of oil • 60 g of an electrolyte supplement Divided into three feeds. 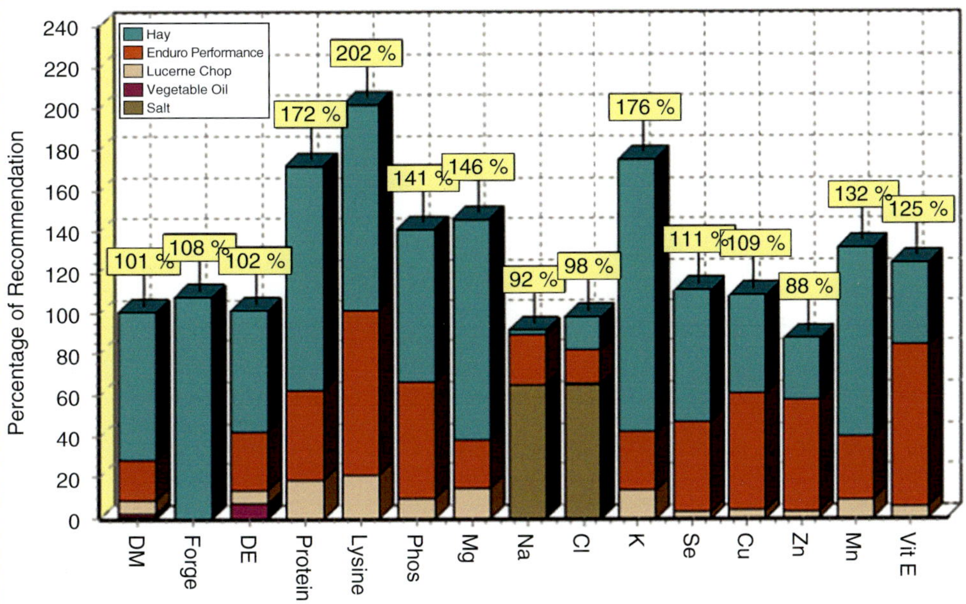	

Continued

Table 12.23 Continued

Advice	• **Current diet** provides 113 MJ DE ◦ DE_m = 75 (i.e. 15 × 5), ◦ DE light work = 90 MJ ◦ DE medium work = 105 MJ ▪ just maintaining fat cover; no need to decrease the energy intake. ◦ Check what the client means by 'drops condition' and teach them how to fat score • The client wanted the starch intake checked ◦ Mix contains 26% starch ◦ Feeding 2.5 kg providing only 0.65 kg starch/day. ◦ Fed in three meals: ▪ provides 0.21 kg starch/meal (216 g) ▪ only 0.43 g starch/kg BW/meal. • Sodium below requirements	
	Recommended diet • Feed more of both forage and concentrates if horse loses fat ◦ Concentrate intake and meal size can be increased to provide up to 1 g starch/kg BW/meal. ◦ Add 20 g salt. • Provide a variety of different forage sources ◦ Distract from the crib biting. ◦ Offer hay in different parts of the stable. • Offer some additional fibre sources to encourage chewing, improve protein intake and anaerobic calorie supply ◦ Sugar beet ◦ Alfalfa chaff ◦ Succulents. • Oil supplement could be added if client hesitant about increasing current feed. • Increase turnout if possible on better grazing. • Discuss timing of feed with relation to exercise.	

Notes

[i] https://cvm.msu.edu/research/faculty-research/comparative-medical-genetics/valberg-laboratory/type-2-polysaccharide-storage-myopathy

[ii] https://cvm.msu.edu/research/faculty-research/comparative-medical-genetics/valberg-laboratory/recurrent-exertional-rhabdomyolysis

Bibliography

Albright, J.D., Mohammed, H.O., Heleski, C.R., Wickens, C.L. and Houpt, K.A. (2009) Crib-biting in US horses: breed predispositions and owner perceptions of aetiology. *Equine Veterinary Journal* 41(5), 455–458.

Aldrich, K., Velez-Irizarry, D., Fenger, C., Schott, M. and Valberg, S.J. (2021) Pathways of calcium regulation, electron transport, and mitochondrial protein translation are molecular signatures of susceptibility to recurrent exertional rhabdomyolysis in Thoroughbred racehorses. *PLoS ONE* 16(2), e0244556. doi: 10.1371/journal.pone.0244556.

An, Y.H., Kim, J., Kim, H. J. and Lim, K. (2020) Effects of leucine-enriched essential amino acid supplementation on muscular fatigue and inflammatory cytokines in wheelchair basketball players. *Physical Activity and Nutrition* 24(2), 38–46. doi: 10.20463/pan.2020.0013.

Andrews, F.M., Buchanan, B.R., Smith, S.H., Elliott, S.B. and Saxton, A.M. (2006) *In vitro* effects of hydrochloric acid and various concentrations of acetic, propionic, butyric, or valeric acids on bioelectric properties of equine gastric squamous mucosa. *American Journal of Veterinary Research* 67(11), 1873–1882.

Archer, D.C., Pinchbeck, G.L., Proudman, C.J. and Clough, H.E. (2006) Is equine colic seasonal? Novel application of a model based approach. *BMC Veterinary Research* 2(1), 27.

Banse, H.E. and Andrews, F.M. (2019) Equine glandular gastric disease: prevalence, impact and management strategies. *Veterinary Medicine (Auckland, N.Z.)* 10, 69–76. doi: 10.2147/VMRR.S174427.

Banse, H.E., MacLeod, H., Crosby, C. and Windeyer, M.C. (2018) Prevalence of and risk factors for equine glandular and squamous gastric disease in polo horses. *The Canadian Veterinary Journal [La revue veterinaire canadienne]* 59(8), 880–884.

Bell, R.J., Mogg, T.D. and Kingston J.K. (2007) Equine gastric ulcer syndrome in adult horses: a review. *New Zealand Veterinary Journal* 55(1), 1–12.

Berschneider, H.M., Blikslager, A.T. and Roberts, M.C. (1999) Role of duodenal reflux in nonglandular gastric ulcer disease of the mature horse. *Equine Veterinary Journal* (Suppl. 29), 24–29.

Bonnefond, A., Yengo, L., Dechaume, A., Canouil, M., Castelain, M. *et al.* (2017) Relationship between salivary/pancreatic amylase and body mass index: a systems biology approach. *BMC Medicine* 15, 37. doi: 10.1186/s12916-017-0784-x.

Borgia, L.A., Valberg, S.J., McCue, M.E., Pagan, J.D. and Roe, C.R. (2010) Effect of dietary fats with odd or even numbers of carbon atoms on metabolic response and muscle damage with exercise in Quarter Horse-type horses with type 1 polysaccharide storage myopathy. *American Journal of Veterinary Research* 71(3), 326–336.

Borgia, L., Valberg, S., McCue, M., Watts, K. and Pagan, J. (2011) Glycaemic and insulinaemic responses to feeding hay with different non-structural carbohydrate content in control and polysaccharide storage myopathy-affected horses. *Journal of Animal Physiology and Animal Nutrition* 95, 798–807.

Boswinkel, M., Ellis, A.D. and Van Oldruitenborgh-oosterbaan, M.M.S. (2007) The influence of low versus high fibre haylage diets in combination with training or pasture rest on equine gastric ulceration syndrome (EGUS). *Pferdeheilkunde* 23, 123–129.

Bröjer, J.T., Essén-Gustavsson, B., Annandale, E.J. and Valberg, S.J. (2006) Proglycogen, macroglycogen, glucose, and glucose-6-phosphate concentrations in skeletal muscles of horses with polysaccharide storage myopathy performing light exercise. *American Journal of Veterinary Research* 67(9), 1589–1594.

Burke, L.M., Collier, G.R., Beasley, S.K. *et al.* (1995) Effect of coingestion of fat and protein with carbohydrate feedings on muscle glycogen storage. *Journal of Applied Physiology* 78, 2187–2192.

Camilleri, M. (2019) Gastrointestinal hormones and regulation of gastric emptying. *Current Opinion in Endocrinology, Diabetes, and Obesity* 26(1), 3–10.

Chanda, M., Srikuea, R., Cherdchutam, W. *et al.* (2016) Modulating effects of exercise training regimen on skeletal muscle properties in female polo ponies. *BMC Veterinary Research* 12, 245.

Cohen, N.D., Gibbs, P.G. and Woods A.M. (1999) Dietary and other management factors associated with colic in horses. *Journal of the American Veterinary Medical Association* 215, 53–60.

Cuddeford, D., Pearson, R.A., Archibald, R.F. and Muirhead, R.H (1995) Digestibility and gastrointestinal transit time of diets contained different proportions of alfalfa and oat straw given to Thoroughbred, Shetland ponies, Highland ponies and donkeys. *Animal Science* 61, 407–417.

Dallner, O. (2008) β-adrenergic regulation of glucose transporters. Doctoral thesis from the Department of Physiology, The Wenner-Gren Institute, Stockholm University, Stockholm, Sweden.

Damke, C., Snyder, A., Uhlig, A., Coenen, M. and Schusser, G.F. (2015) Impact of diet on 24-hour intragastric pH profile in healthy horses. *Berliner und Munchener tierarztliche Wochenschrift* 128(9–10), 345–349.

De Oliveira, E.P., Burini, R.C. and Jeukendrup, A.E. (2014) Gastrointestinal complaints during exercise: prevalence, etiology, and nutritional recommendations. *Sports Medicine* 44, S79–S85.

Dudgeon, W.D., Kelley, E.P. and Scheett, T.P. (2016) In a single-blind, matched group design: branched-chain amino acid supplementation and resistance training maintains lean body mass during a caloric restricted diet. *Journal of the International Society of Sports Nutrition* 13, 1. doi: 10.1186/s12970-015-0112-9.

Dukti, S.A., Perkins, S., Murphy, J., Barr, B., Boston, R. *et al.* (2006) Prevalence of gastric squamous ulceration in horses with abdominal pain. *Equine Veterinary Journal* 38(4), 347–349.

Dunstan, R.H., Macdonald, M.M., Thorn, B., Wood, D. and Roberts, T.K. (2020) Modelling of amino acid turnover in the horse during training and racing: a basis for developing a novel supplementation strategy. *PLoS ONE* 15(1), e0226988. doi: 10.1371/journal.

Dunstan, R.H., Macdonald, M.M., Murphy, G.R., Thorn, B. and Roberts, T.K. (2019) Modelling of protein turnover provides insight for metabolic demands on those specific amino acids utilised at disproportionately faster rates than other amino acids. *Amino Acids* 51(6), 945–959.

Dyer, J., Fernandez-Castaño Merediz, E., Salmon, K.S., Proudman, C.J., Edwards, G.B. *et al.* (2002) Molecular characterisation of carbohydrate digestion and absorption in equine small intestine. *Equine Veterinary Journal* 34(4), 349–358.

Dyer, J., Al-Rammahi, M., Waterfall, L., Salmon, K.S., Geor, R.J. *et al.* (2009) Adaptive response of equine intestinal Na+/glucose co-transporter (SGLT1) to an increase in dietary soluble carbohydrate. *Pflugers Archiv: European Journal of Physiology* 458(2), 419–430.

Eaton, M.D., Hodgson, D.R., Evans, D.L. and Rose, R.J. (1999) Effects of low- and moderate-intensity training on metabolic responses to exercise in Thoroughbreds. *Equine Veterinary Journal* (Suppl. 30), 521–527.

Escalona, E.E., Okell, C.N. and Archer, D.C. (2014) Prevalence of and risk factors for colic in horses that

display crib-biting behaviour. *BMC Veterinary Research* 10(1), 1–8.
Esmarck, B., Andersen, J.L., Olsen, S., Richter, E.A., Mizuno, M. and Kjaer, M. (2001) Timing of postexercise protein intake is important for muscle hypertrophy with resistance training in elderly humans. *The Journal of Physiology* 535(Pt 1), 301–311. doi: 10.1111/j.1469-7793.2001.00301.x.
Essén-Gustavsson, B., Blomstrand, E., Karlström, K., Lindholm, A. and Persson, S.G.B. (1991) Influence of diet on substrate metabolism during exercise. In: *Equine Exercise Physiology 3*. Proceedings of the 3rd International Conference on Equine Exercise Physiology, Uppsala, Sweden. ICEEP, Davis, California, pp. 288–298.
Eto, D., Yamano, S., Mukai, K. *et al.* (2004) Effect of high intensity training on anaerobic capacity of middle gluteal muscle in Thoroughbred horses. *Research in Veterinary Science* 76(2), 139–144. doi: 10.1016/j.rvsc.2003.08.010.
Faubladier, C., Chaucheyras-Durand, F., da Veiga, L. and Julliand, V (2013) Effect of transportation on fecal bacterial communities and fermentative activities in horses: impact of Saccharomyces cerevisiae CNCM I-1077 supplementation. *Journal of Animal Science* 91(4), 1736–1744. doi: 10.2527/jas.2012-5720.
Finno, C.J., McKenzie, E., Valberg, S.J. and Pagan, J. (2010) Effect of fitness on glucose, insulin and cortisol responses to diets varying in starch and fat content in Thoroughbred horses with recurrent exertional rhabdomyolysis. *Equine Veterinary Journal* (Suppl. 38), 323–328.
Firshman, A.M., Valberg, S.J., Karges, T.L., Benedict, L.E., Annandale, E.J. *et al.* (2005) Serum creatine kinase response to exercise during dexamethasone-induced insulin resistance in Quarter Horses with polysaccharide storage myopathy. *American Journal of Veterinary Research* 66(10), 1718–1723.
Fonseca, R.G., Kenny, D.A., Hill, E.W. and Katz, L.M. (2013) The relationship between body composition, training and race performance in a group of Thoroughbred flat racehorses. *Equine Veterinary Journal* 45(5), 552–557. doi: 10.1111/evj.12024.
Fritz, K.L., McCue, M.E., Valberg, S.J., Rendahl, A.K. and Mickelson, J.R. (2012) Genetic mapping of recurrent exertional rhabdomyolysis in a population of North American Thoroughbreds. *Animal Genetics* 43(6), 730–738. doi: 10.1111/j.1365-2052.2012.02351.x.
Geelen, S.N., Blázquez, C., Geelen, M.J., Sloet van Oldruitenborgh-Oosterbaan, M. M. and Beynen, A.C. (2001) High fat intake lowers hepatic fatty acid synthesis and raises fatty acid oxidation in aerobic muscle in Shetland ponies. *The British Journal of Nutrition* 86(1), 31–36.
Geor, R.J., Hinchcliff, K.W. and Sams, R.A. (2000) Beta-adrenergic blockade augments glucose utilization in horses during graded exercise. *Journal of Applied Physiology (Bethesda, MD: 1985)* 89(3), 1086–1098. doi: 10.1152/jappl.2000.89.3.108.
Geor, R.J., Larsen, L., Waterfall, H.L., Stewart-Hunt, L. and McCutcheon, L.J. (2006) Route of carbohydrate administration affects early post exercise muscle glycogen storage in horses. *Equine Veterinary Journal* (Suppl. 36), 590–595. doi: 10.1111/j.2042-3306.2006.tb05610.x.
Graham-Thiers, P.M. and Bowen, L.K. (2021) The effect of time of feeding on plasma amino acids during exercise and recovery in horses. *Translational Animal Science* 5(2), txab045. doi: 10.1093/tas/txab045.
Gunn H.M. (1987) Muscle, bone and fat proportions and muscle distribution of Thoroughbreds and other horses. In: *Equine Exercise Physiology 2*. Proceedings of the Second International Conference on Equine Exercise Physiology, San Diego, California, August 7–11, 1986. ICEEP, Davis, California, pp. 253–264.
Halama, A., Oliveira, J.M., Filho, S.A., Qasim, M., Achkar, I.W. *et al.* (2021) Metabolic predictors of equine performance in endurance racing. *Metabolites* 11(2), 82. doi: 10.3390/metabo11020082.
Harris, R.C., Hultman, E. and Nordesjö, L.O. (1974) Glycogen, glycolytic intermediates and high-energy phosphates determined in biopsy samples of musculus quadriceps femoris of man at rest. *Methods and Variance of Values, Scandinavian Journal of Clinical and Laboratory Investigation* 33(2), 109–120, doi: 10.1080/00365517409082477.
Hepburn, R.J. (2014) Endoscopic examination of the squamous and glandular gastric mucosa in sport and leisure horses: 684 horses (2005–2011), 2 [abstract]. *BMC Veterinary Research* 10(S1), 11.
Hewetson, M. (2006) Investigation of false colic in the horse. *In Practice* 28, 326–338.
Hillyer, M.H., Taylor, F.G. and French, N.P. (2001) A cross-sectional study of colic in horses on thoroughbred training premises in the British Isles in 1997. *Equine Veterinary Journal* 33(4), 380–385.
Hillyer, M.H., Taylor, F.G.R., Proudman, C.J., Edwards, G.B., Smith, J.E. *et al.* (2002) Case control study to identify risk factors for simple colonic obstruction and distension colic in horses. *Equine Veterinary Journal* 34(5), 455–463.
Hodgson, D.R., Rose, R.J. and Allen, J.R. (1983) Muscle glycogen depletion and repletion patterns in horses performing various distances of endurance exercise. *Equine Exercise Physiology* 7, 229–236.
Hodgson, D.R., Rose, R.J., Allen, J.R. and Dimauro, J. (1984) Glycogen depletion patterns in horses performing maximal exercise. *Research in Veterinary Science* 36(2), 169–173.
Hodgson, D.R., Rose, R.J., Allen, J.R. and Dimauro, J. (1985) Glycogen depletion patterns in horses competing in day 2 of a three day event. *The Cornell Veterinarian* 75(2), 366–374.

Houpt, K.A. (2012) A preliminary answer to the question of whether cribbing causes salivary secretion. *Journal of Veterinary Behavior* 7(5), 322–324.

Hudson, J.M., Cohen, N.D., Gibbs, P.G. and Thompson, J.A. (2001) Feeding practices associated with colic in horses. *Journal of the American Veterinary Medical Association* 219(10), 1419–1425.

Husted, L., Sanchez, L.C., Baptiste, K.E. and Olsen, S.N. (2009) Effect of a feed/fast protocol on pH in the proximal equine stomach. *Equine Veterinary Journal* 41, 658–662.

Hyyppä, S., Räsänen, L.A. and Pösö, A.R. (1997) Resynthesis of glycogen in skeletal muscle from standardbred trotters after repeated bouts of exercise. *American Journal of Veterinary Research* 58(2), 162–166.

Ivers, T. (2002) *Carbohydrates and glycogen loading*. In: *Proceedings of the First European Equine Nutrition & Health Congress*, Antwerp Zoo, Belgium.

Jansson, A., Harris, P., Davey, S.L., Luthersson, N., Ragnarsson, S. *et al*. (2021) Straw as an alternative to grass forage in horses—effects on post-prandial metabolic profile, energy intake, behaviour and gastric ulceration. *Animals* 11(8), 2197. doi: 10.3390/ani11082197.

Jansson, A., Gunnarsson, V., Ringmark, S., Ragnarsson, S., Söderroos, D. *et al*. (2021) Increased body fat content in horses alters metabolic and physiological exercise response, decreases performance, and increases locomotion asymmetry. *Physiological Reports* 9.

Jansson, A., Nyman, S., Lindholm, A. and Lindberg, J.E. (2002) Effects on exercise metabolism of varying dietary starch and sugar proportions. *Equine Veterinary Journal* (Suppl. 34), 17–21.

Jensen-Waern, M., Lindberg, Å., Johannisson, A., Gröndahl, G., Lindgren, J.Å. and Essén-Gustavsson, B. (1999) The effects of an endurance ride on metabolism and neutrophil function. *Equine Veterinary Journal* 31, 605–609.

Jeukendrup, A.E. (2003) Modulation of carbohydrate and fat utilization by diet, exercise and environment. *Biochemical Society Transactions* 31(Pt 6), 1270–1273.

Julliand, S., Martin, A. and Julliand, V. (2018) Effect of dehydrated alfalfa on equine gastric and faecal microbial ecosystems. *Livestock Science* 215, 16–20.

Kanter, M. (2018) High-quality carbohydrates and physical performance: expert panel report. *Nutrition Today* 53(1), 35–39. doi: 10.1097/NT.0000000000000238.

Kawai, M., Minami, Y., Sayama, Y., Kuwano, A., Hiraga, A. *et al*. (2009) Muscle fiber population and biochemical properties of whole body muscles in Thoroughbred horses. *Anatomical Record (Hoboken, N.J.: 2007)* 292(10), 1663–1669.

Kerksick, C., Harvey, T., Stout, J., Campbell, B., Wilborn, C. *et al*. (2008) International Society of Sports Nutrition position stand: nutrient timing. *Journal of the International Society of Sports Nutrition* 5(1), 1–12.

Kerksick, C.M., Arent, S., Schoenfeld, B.J., Stout, J.R., Campbell, B. *et al*. (2017) International Society of Sports Nutrition position stand: nutrient timing. *Journal of the International Society of Sports Nutrition* 14(1), 33.

Kienzle, E., Radicke, S., Landes, E., Kleffken, D., Illenseer, M. *et al*. (1994) Activity of amylase in gastrointestinal tract of horse. *Journal of Animal Physiology and Animal Nutrition* 72, 234–241.

Kline, K.H. and Albert, W.W. (1981) Investigation of a glycogen loading program for Standardbred Horses. In *Proceedings 7th Equine Nutrition and Physiology Symposium*, pp. 186–194.

Lacombe, V., Hinchcliff, K.W., Geor, R.J. *et al*. (1999) Exercise that induces substantial muscle glycogen depletion impairs subsequent anaerobic capacity. *Equine Veterinary Journal* (Suppl. 30), 293–297.

Lacombe, V., Hinchcliff, K.W., Geor, R.J. *et al*. (2001) Muscle glycogen depletion and subsequent replenishment affect anaerobic capacity of horses. *Journal of Applied Physiology* 91, 1782–1790.

Lacombe, V.A. and Hinchcliff, K.W. (2003) Interactions of substrate availability, exercise performance, and nutrition in muscle glycogen metabolism in horses. *JAVMA* 223, 1576–1585.

Lacombe, V., Hinchcliff, K.W., Kohn, C., Devor, S. and Taylor, L.E. (2004) Effects of feeding meals with various soluble carbohydrate content on muscle glycogen synthesis after exercise in horses. *American Journal of Veterinary Research* 65(7).

Lam, F.C., Khan, T.M., Faidah, H., Haseeb, A. and Khan, A.H. (2019) Effectiveness of whey protein supplements on the serum levels of amino acid, creatinine kinase and myoglobin of athletes: a systematic review and meta-analysis. *Systematic Reviews* 8(1), 1–12.

Le Moyec, L., Robert, C., Triba, M.N., Billat, V.L., Mata, X. *et al*. (2014) Protein catabolism and high lipid metabolism associated with long-distance exercise are revealed by plasma NMR metabolomics in endurance horses. *PLoS ONE* 9(3), e90730. doi: 10.1371/journal.pone.0090730.

Le Moyec, L., Robert, C., Triba, M.N., Bouchemal, N., Mach, N. *et al*. (2019) A first step toward unraveling the energy metabolism in endurance horses: comparison of plasma nuclear magnetic resonance metabolomic profiles before and after different endurance race distances. *Frontiers in Molecular Biosciences*, 6, 45. doi: 10.3389/fmolb.2019.00045.

Lindner, A., Dag Erginsoy, S., Kissenbeck, S., Mosen, H., Hetzel, U. *et al*. (2013) Effect of different blood-guided conditioning programmes on skeletal muscle ultrastructure and histochemistry of sport horses. *Journal of Animal Physiology and Animal Nutrition* 97, 374–386. doi: 10.1111/j.1439-0396.2012.01283.x.

Lorenzo-Figueras, M. and Merritt, A.M. (2002a) Effects of exercise on gastric volume and pH in the proximal portion of the stomach of horses. *American Journal of Veterinary Research* 63(11), 1481–1487. doi: 10.2460/ajvr.2002.63.1481.

Lorenzo-Figueras, M., Jones, G. and Merritt, A.M. (2002b) Effects of various diets on gastric tone in the proximal portion of the stomach of horses. *American Journal of Veterinary Research* 63(9), 1275–1278.

Luthersson, N., Nielsen, K.H., Harris, P. and Parkin, T.D. (2009) Risk factors associated with equine gastric ulceration syndrome (EGUS) in 201 horses in Denmark. *Equine Veterinary Journal* 41(7), 625–630.

MacLeay, J.M., Sorum, S.A., Valberg, S.J., Marsh, W.E. and Sorum, M.D. (1999) Epidemiologic analysis of factors influencing exertional rhabdomyolysis in Thoroughbreds. *American Journal of Veterinary Research* 60(12), 1562–1566.

MacLeay, J.M., Valberg, S.J., Pagan, J.D., Xue, J.L., De La Corte, F.D. *et al.* (2000) Effect of ration and exercise on plasma creatine kinase activity and lactate concentration in Thoroughbred horses with recurrent exertional rhabdomyolysis. *American Journal of Veterinary Research* 61(11), 1390–1395.

Malone, J.J., Hulton, A.T. and MacLaren, D. (2021) Exogenous carbohydrate and regulation of muscle carbohydrate utilisation during exercise. *European Journal of Applied Physiology* 121(5), 1255–1269.

Mata, F., Valenzuela, P.L., Gimenez, J., Tur, C., Ferreria, D. *et al.* (2019) Carbohydrate availability and physical performance: physiological overview and practical recommendations. *Nutrients* 11(5), 1084. doi: 10.3390/nu11051084.

Matsui, Y., Takayanagi, S., Ohira, T., Watanabe, M., Murano, H. *et al.* (2019) Effect of a leucine-enriched essential amino acids mixture on muscle recovery. *Journal of Physical Therapy Science* 31(1), 95–101. doi: 10.1589/jpts.31.95.

Maughan, R.J. (2005) The limits of human athletic performance. *Annals of Transplantation* 10(4), 52–54.

Mazzulla, M., Sawan, S.A., Williamson, E., Hannaian, S.J., Volterman, K.A. *et al.* (2020) Protein intake to maximize whole-body anabolism during postexercise recovery in resistance-trained men with high habitual intakes is severalfold greater than the current recommended dietary allowance. *The Journal of Nutrition*, 150(3), 505–511. doi: 10.1093/jn/nxz249.

McCue, M.E., Ribeiro, W.P. and Valberg, S.J. (2006) Prevalence of polysaccharide storage myopathy in horses with neuromuscular disorders. *Equine Veterinary Journal* (Suppl. 36), 340-344.

McCue, M.E., Valberg, S.J. and Mickelson, J.R. (2008a) Genetic approach to diagnosing polysaccharide storage myopathy. Research abstract, Vol. 54, *AAEP Proceedings*.

McCue, M.E., Valberg, S.J., Lucio, M. and Mickelson, J.R. (2008b) Glycogen synthase 1 (GYS1) mutation in diverse breeds with polysaccharide storage myopathy. *Journal of Veterinary Internal Medicine* 22(5), 1228–1233.

McCue, M.E., Valberg, S.J., Miller, M.B., Wade, C., DiMauro, S. *et al.* (2008c) Glycogen synthase (GYS1) mutation causes a novel skeletal muscle glycogenosis. *Genomics* 91(5), 458–466.

McCutcheon, L.J., Geor, R.J. and Hinchcliff, K.W. (2002) Changes in skeletal muscle GLUT-4 content and muscle membrane glucose transport following 6 weeks of exercise training. *Equine Veterinary Journal* (Suppl. 34), 199–204.

McGowan, C.M., Fordham, T. and Christley, R.M. (2002) Incidence and risk factors for exertional rhabdomyolysis in thoroughbred racehorses in the United Kingdom. *Veterinary Record* 151(21), 623–626.

McGowan, C.M., McGowan, T.M. and Patterson-Kane, J.C. (2009) Prevalence of equine polysaccharide storage myopathy and other myopathies in two equine populations in the United Kingdom. *The Veterinary Journal* 180(3), 330–336.

McKenzie, E.C., Valberg, S.J., Godden, S.M., Pagan, J.D., MacLeay, J.M. *et al.* (2003) Effect of dietary starch, fat, and bicarbonate content on exercise responses and serum creatine kinase activity in equine recurrent exertional rhabdomyolysis. *Journal of Veterinary Internal Medicine* 17(5), 693–701.

Mejía-Benítez, M.A., Bonnefond, A., Yengo, L., Huyvaert, M., Dechaume, A. *et al.* (2015) Beneficial effect of a high number of copies of salivary amylase AMY1 gene on obesity risk in Mexican children. *Diabetologia* 58(2), 290–294.

Mero, A. (1999) Leucine supplementation and intensive training. *Sports Medicine (Auckland, N.Z.)* 27(6), 347–358. doi: 10.2165/00007256-199927060-00001.

Merritt, A.M. (1999) The effect of a feed/fast protocol on the pH of the proximal stomach of horses. In: *Proceedings 42nd Congress*.

Merritt, A.M., Sanchez, L.C., Burrow, J.A., Church, M. and Ludzia, S. (2003) Effect of GastroGard and three compounded oral omeprazole preparations on 24 h intragastric pH in gastrically cannulated mature horses. *Equine Veterinary Journal* 35(7), 691–695.

Metayer, N., Lhŏte, M., Bahr, A., Cohen, N.D., Kim, I. *et al.* (2004) Meal size and starch content affect gastric emptying in horses. *Equine Veterinary Journal* 36(5), 436–440.

Muneyuki, T., Nakajima, K., Aoki, A., Yoshida, M., Fuchigami, H. *et al.* (2012) Latent associations of low serum amylase with decreased plasma insulin levels and insulin resistance in asymptomatic middle-aged adults. *Cardiovascular Diabetology* 11, 80. doi: 10.1186/1475-2840-11-80.

Murray, M.J. (1992) Gastric ulceration in horses: 91 cases (1987-1990). *Journal of the American Veterinary Medical Association* 201(1), 117–120.

Murray, B. and Rosenbloom, C. (2018) Fundamentals of glycogen metabolism for coaches and athletes. *Nutrition Reviews* 76(4), 243–259. doi: 10.1093/nutrit/nuy001.

Murray, M.J. and Eichorn, E.S. (1996) Effects of intermittent feed deprivation, intermittent feed deprivation with ranitidine administration, and stall confinement with ad libitum access to hay on gastric ulceration in horses. *American Journal of Veterinary Research* 57(11), 1599–1603.

Murray, M.J. and Schusser, G.F. (1993) Measurement of 24-h gastric pH using an indwelling pH electrode in horses unfed, fed and treated with ranitidine. *Equine Veterinary Journal* 25, 417–421.

Murray, M.J., Schusser, G.R., Pipers, F.S. and Gross, S.J. (1996) Factors associated with gastric lesions in Thoroughbred racehorses. *Equine Veterinary Journal* 28, 368–374. doi: 10.1111/j.2042-3306.1996.tb03107.x.

Nimmo, M.A. and Snow, D.H. (1983) Changes in muscle glycogen, lactate and pyruvate concentrations in the Thoroughbred horse following maximal exercise. *Equine Exercise Physiology*, 3, 237–244.

Nogueira, G.P. and Barnabe, R.C. (1997) Is the thoroughbred race-horse under chronic stress? *Brazilian Journal of Medical and Biological Research = Revista brasileira de pesquisas medicas e biologicas* 30(10), 1237–1239.

Nolazco Sassot, L., Villarino, N.F., Dasgupta, N., Morrison, J.J., Bayly, W.M. *et al.* (2019) The lipidome of Thoroughbred racehorses before and after supramaximal exercise. *Equine Veterinary Journal* 51, 696–700. doi: 10.1111/evj.13064.

Nostell, K.E., Essén-Gustavsson, B. and Bröjer, J.T. (2012) Repeated post-exercise administration with a mixture of leucine and glucose alters the plasma amino acid profile in Standardbred trotters. *Acta Veterinaria Scandinavica* 54(1), 7. doi: 10.1186/1751-0147-54-7.

NRC (National Research Council) (2007) *Nutrient Requirements of Horses: Sixth Revised Edition*. The National Academies Press, Washington, DC. doi: 10.17226/11653.

Padalino, B. and Raidal, S.L. (2020) Effects of transport conditions on behavioural and physiological responses of horses. *Animals: An Open Access Journal from MDPI* 10(1), 160. doi: 10.3390/ani10010160.

Padalino, B., Raidal, S.L., Carter, N., Celi, P., Muscatello, G. *et al.* (2017) Immunological, clinical, haematological and oxidative responses to long distance transportation in horses. *Research in Veterinary Science* 115, 78–87. doi: 10.1016/j.rvsc.2017.01.024.

Padalino, B., Davis, G. L. and Raidal, S.L. (2020) Effects of transportation on gastric pH and gastric ulceration in mares. *Journal of Veterinary Internal Medicine* 34(2), 922–932. doi: 10.1111/jvim.15698.

Palmgren Karlsson, C., Jansson, A., Essén-Gustavsson, B. and Lindberg, J.E. (2002) Effect of molassed sugar beet pulp on nutrient utilisation and metabolic parameters during exercise. *Equine Veterinary Journal* (Suppl. 34), 44–49. doi: 10.1111/j.2042-3306.2002.tb05390.

Pedersen, S.K., Cribb, A.E., Windeyer, M.C., Read, E.K., French, D. *et al.* (2018) Risk factors for equine glandular and squamous gastric disease in show jumping Warmbloods. *Equine Veterinary Journal* 50(6), 747–751. doi: 10.1111/evj.12949.

Perry, E., Cross, T.L., Francis, J.M., Holscher, H.D., Clark, S.D. *et al.* (2018) Effect of road transport on the equine cecal microbiota. *Journal of Equine Veterinary Science*, 68, 12–20. doi: 10.1016/j.jevs.2018.04.004.

Pierzynowski, S.G., Goncharova, K., Gregory, P.C., Westrom, B., Podpryatov, S.E. *et al.* (2017) Experiments suggesting extra-digestive effects of enteral pancreatic amylase and its peptides on glucose homeostasis in a pig model. *Scientific Reports* 7, 8628. doi: 10.1038/s41598-017-07387-2.

Pierzynowska, K., Oredsson, S. and Pierzynowski, S. (2020) Amylase-dependent regulation of glucose metabolism and insulin/glucagon secretion in the streptozotocin-induced diabetic pig model and in a rat pancreatic beta-cell line, BRIN-BD11. *Journal of Diabetes Research* 2148740. doi: 10.1155/2020/2148740.

Pratt, S.E., Geor, R.J. and McCutcheon, L.J. (2006) Effects of dietary energy source and physical conditioning on insulin sensitivity and glucose tolerance in standardbred horses. *Equine Veterinary Journal* (Suppl. 36), 579–584. doi: 10.1111/j.2042-3306.2006.tb05608.x.

Purdom, T., Kravitz, L., Dokladny, K. and Mermier, C. (2018) Understanding the factors that effect maximal fat oxidation. *Journal of the International Society of Sports Nutrition* 15, 3. doi: 10.1186/s12970-018-0207-1.

Rabuffo, T.S., Hackett, E.S., Grenager, N., Boston, R. and Orsini, J.A. (2009) Prevalence of gastric ulcerations in horses with colic. *Journal of Equine Veterinary Science* 29(6), 540–546.

Ribeiro, W.P., Valberg, S.J., Pagan, J.D. and Gustavsson, B.E. (2004) The effect of varying dietary starch and fat content on serum creatine kinase activity and substrate availability in equine polysaccharide storage myopathy. *Journal of Veterinary Internal Medicine/American College of Veterinary Internal Medicine* 18, 887–894.

Russell, M.A., Rodiek, A.V. and Lawrence, L.M. (1986) Effect of meal schedules and fasting on selected plasma free amino acids in horses. *Journal of Animal Science* 63(5), 1428–1431. doi: 10.2527/jas1986.6351428x.

Sandin, A., Girma, K., Sjöholm, B., Lindholm, A. and Nilsson, G. (1998) Effects of differently composed feeds and physical stress on plasma gastrin concentration in horses. *Acta Veterinaria Scandinavica* 39(2), 265–272.

Scantlebury, C.E., Archer, D.C., Proudman, C.J. and Pinchbeck, G.L. (2011) Recurrent colic in the horse:

incidence and risk factors for recurrence in the general practice population. *Equine Veterinary Journal* (Suppl. 39), 81–88. DOI: 10.1111/j.2042-3306.2011.00383.x.
Scantlebury, C.E., Archer, D.C., Proudman, C.J. and Pinchbeck, G.L. (2015) Management and horse-level risk factors for recurrent colic in the UK general equine practice population. *Equine Veterinary Journal* 47(2), 202–206. doi: 10.1111/evj.12276.
Schmidt, O., Deegen, E., Fuhrmann, H., Dühlmeier, R. and Sallmann, H.P. (2001) Effects of fat feeding and energy level on plasma metabolites and hormones in Shetland ponies. *Journal of Veterinary Medicine. A, Physiology, Pathology, Clinical Medicine* 48(1), 39–49.
Shirazi-Beechey S.P. (2008) Molecular insights into dietary induced colic in the horse. *Equine Veterinary Journal*, 40(4), 414–421. doi: 10.2746/042516408X 314075.
Smith, B.L., Jones, J.H., Hornof, W.J., Miles, J.A., Longworth, K.E. *et al.* (1996) Effects of road transport on indices of stress in horses. *Equine Veterinary Journal* 28(6), 446–454. doi: 10.1111/j.2042-3306.1996.tb01616.x.
Smyth, G.B., Young, D.W. and Hammond, L.S. (1988) Effects of diet and feeding on post-prandial serum gastrin and insulin concentrations in adult horses. *Equine Veterinary Journal* 7, 56–59.
Smyth, G.B., Young, D.W. and Schumacher, J. (1989) Postprandial serum gastrin concentration in normal foals. *Equine Veterinary Journal* 21, 285–287.
Snow, D. and Harris, R.C. (1991) Effects of daily exercise on muscle glycogen in TB horses. *Equine Exercise Physiology*, vol. 3. ICEEP, pp. 299–304.
Stewart-Hunt, L., Pratt-Phillips, S., McCutcheon, L.J. and Geor, R.J. (2010) Dietary energy source and physical conditioning affect insulin sensitivity and skeletal muscle glucose metabolism in horses. *Equine Veterinary Journal* (Suppl. 38), 355–360. doi: 10.1111/j.2042-3306.2010.00255.x.
Suthers, J.M., Pinchbeck, G.L., Proudman, C.J. and Archer, D.C. (2013) Risk factors for large colon volvulus in the UK. *Equine Veterinary Journal* 45, 558–563.
Sykes, B. and Jokisalo, J.M. (2015) Equine glandular gastric ulcer syndrome (EGGUS). *Equine Veterinary Education* 27, 372–375. doi: 10.1111/eve.12287.
Sykes, B.W., Bowen, M., Habershon-Butcher, J.L., Green, M. and Hallowell, G.D. (2019) Management factors and clinical implications of glandular and squamous gastric disease in horses. *Journal of Veterinary Internal Medicine* 33(1), 233–240. doi: 10.1111/jvim.15350.
Sykes, B.W., Hewetson, M., Hepburn, R.J., Luthersson, N. and Tamzali, Y. (2016) European College of Equine Internal Medicine Consensus Statement – Equine Gastric Ulcer Syndrome in Adult Horses. *Journal of Veterinary Internal Medicine* 29(5), 1288–1299. doi: 10.1111/jvim.13578.
Tateo, A., Padalino, B., Boccaccio, M., Maggiolino, A. and Centoducati, P. (2012) Transport stress in horses: effects of two different distances. *Journal of Veterinary Behavior* 7(1), 33–42.
Tinker, M.K., White, N.A., Lessard, P., Thatcher, C.D., Pelzer, K.D. *et al.* (1997) Prospective study of equine colic risk factors. *Equine Veterinary Journal* 29(6), 454–458.
Traub-Dargatz, J.L., George, J.L., Dargatz, D.A., Morley, P.S., Southwood, L.L. *et al.* (2002) Survey of complications and antimicrobial use in equine patients at veterinary teaching hospitals that underwent surgery because of colic. *Journal of the American Veterinary Medical Association*, 220(9), 1359–1365.
Treiber, K.H., Hess, T.M., Kronfeld, D.S., Boston, R.C., Geor, R.J. *et al.* (2006) Glucose dynamics during exercise: dietary energy sources affect minimal model parameters in trained Arabian geldings during endurance exercise. *Equine Veterinary Journal* (Suppl. 36), 631–636. doi: 10.1111/j.2042-3306.2006.tb05617.x.
Urschel, K., Geor, R.J., Waterfall, Shoveller and Mccutcheon (2010) Effects of leucine or whey protein addition to an oral glucose solution on serum insulin, plasma glucose and plasma amino acid responses in horses at rest and following exercise. *Equine Veterinary Journal* 42(Suppl. 38), 347–354.
Urschel, K.L., Escobar, J., McCutcheon, L.J. and Geor, R.J. (2011) Effect of feeding a high-protein diet following an 18-hour period of feed withholding on mammalian target of rapamycin-dependent signaling in skeletal muscle of mature horses. *American Journal of Veterinary Research* 72(2), 248–255.
Valberg, S. (1989) Glycogen depletion patterns in the muscle of Standardbred Trotters after exercise of varying intensities and durations. *Equine Veterinary Journal* 18, 479–484.
Valberg, S.J., Macleay, J.M., Billstrom, J.A., Hower-Moritz, M.A. and Mickelson, J.R. (1999) Skeletal muscle metabolic response to exercise in horses with 'tying-up' due to polysaccharide storage myopathy. *Equine Veterinary Journal* 31(1), 43–47.
Waran, N.K. (1993) The behaviour of horses during and after transport by road. *Equine Veterinary Education* 5, 129–132.
Waran, N.K., Robertson, V., Cuddeford, D., Kokoszko, A. and Marlin, D.J. (1996) Effects of transporting horses facing either forward or backward on their behavior and heart rate. *Veterinary Record* 139, 7–11.
Ward, S., Sykes, B.W., Brown, H., Bishop, A. and Penaluna, L.A. (2015) A comparison of the prevalence of gastric ulceration in feral and domesticated horses in the UK. *Equine Veterinary Education* 27, 655–657.
Waters, A.J., Nicol, C.J. and French, N.P. (2002) Factors influencing the development of stereotypic and redirected behaviours in young horses: findings of a four year prospective epidemiological study. *Equine Veterinary Journal* 34(6), 572–579.

Welsh, R.S., Davis, J.M., Burke, J.R. and Williams, H.G. (2002) Carbohydrates and physical/mental performance during intermittent exercise to fatigue. *Medicine and Science in Sports and Exercise* 723–731.

Whitfield-Cargile, C.M., Coleman, M.C., Cohen, N.D., Chaoun-Emanuelli, A.M., DeSolis, C.N. *et al*. (2021) Effects of phenylbutazone alone or in combination with a nutritional therapeutic on gastric ulcers, intestinal permeability, and fecal microbiota in horses. *Journal of Veterinary Internal Medicine* 35(2), 1121–1130. doi: 10.1111/jvim.16093.

Willard, J.G., Willard, J.C., Wolfram, S.A. and Baker, J.P. (1977) Effect of diet on cecal pH and feeding behavior of horses. *Journal of Animal Science* 45(1), 87–93.

Williams, R., Chandler, R. and Marlin, D. (2009) Heart rates of horses during competitive dressage. *Comparative Exercise Physiology* 6(1), 7–15. DOI: 10.1017/S1478061509303679.

Williams, S., Tucker, C.A., Green, M.J. and Freeman, S.L. (2011) Investigation of the effect of pasture and stable management on large intestinal motility in the horse, measured using transcutaneous ultrasonography. *Equine Veterinary Journal* 43, 93–97.

Williams, S., Tucker, C.A., Green, M.J. and Freeman, S.L. (2015) Water intake, faecal output and intestinal motility in horses moved from pasture to a stabled management regime with controlled exercise. *Equine Veterinary Journal* 47, 96–100.

Williams, Z.J., Bertels, M. and Valberg, S.J. (2018) Muscle glycogen concentrations and response to diet and exercise regimes in Warmblood horses with type 2 Polysaccharide Storage Myopathy. *PLoS ONE* 13(9), e0203467. doi: 10.1371/journal.pone.0203467.

Wllson, A.D., Badnell-Waters, A.J., Bice, R., Kelland, A., Harris, P.A. *et al*. (2007) The effects of diet on blood glucose, insulin, gastrin and the serum tryptophan: large neutral amino acid ratio in foals. *The Veterinary Journal* 174(1), 139–146.

13 Electrolytes

ROD FISHER

Abbey Equine Clinic, Abergavenny

Learning Objectives

LO1 Explain the role of electrolytes.
LO2 Explain thermoregulation, dehydration, its consequences and the role of water in rehydration.
LO3 Describe the composition of sweat and the implications of isotonic versus hypotonic versus hypertonic.
LO4 Compare and contrast sweat loss across different disciplines.
LO5 Describe the clinical conditions associated with electrolyte loss and management solutions.
LO6 Discuss management strategies to minimise the risk of dehydration.
LO7 Compare and contrast electrolyte supplements and explain what ingredients are necessary and which are fillers by using labels as an example.
LO8 Be able to choose the appropriate electrolyte regime according to discipline and workload.
LO9 Describe the content of electrolytes in common competition feeds and compare with requirements for electrolytes replacements.

At the end of this chapter, you will be able to provide specific advice on why, when and how to supplement electrolytes for performance horses.

Overview

Electrolytes are minerals that dissociate into ions and are responsible for maintaining plasma osmotic concentration and fluid balance as well as controlling thirst and drinking. It is essential to maintain electrolyte homeostasis in order to ensure normal cellular function, particularly important in nerve and muscle cells.

However, horses lose large quantities of electrolytes in their sweat, depending on workload and effort, and can become dehydrated. A number of clinical conditions are associated with electrolyte loss and dehydration; the amount of electrolytes lost should be estimated before deciding what electrolytes to advise. Electrolytes can be replenished in a variety of ways. The type and amount of electrolytes needed will depend upon the workload of the horse, its general management and the horse's diet.

> 'Cutaneous water and electrolyte losses are affected by thermoregulation, independent of hydration status and/or electrolyte homeostasis. The negative balance for water, Na, K and Cl may be a factor in limiting performance and impairing recovery. The strategy in caring for a horse before, during and after exercise involves improving hydration and electrolyte status and the use of NaCl in feed or in a watery solution (iso- or hypotonic).'
>
> (Coenen, 2005)

The Role of Electrolytes

Electrolytes are minerals (Na, K, Cl) that dissociate into ions in solutions with electrical charges in the plasma to maintain osmolarity of the plasma, and fluid balance. Body fluids and the electrolytes sodium (Na), potassium (K) and chloride (Cl) hold

  Evidence-based Equine Nutrition: A Practical Approach for Professionals (T. Hollands and L. Drury)
DOI: 10.1079/9781789245134.0013

a key position in the thermoregulation of sweating animals. The osmotic concentration (osmolality) of body fluids is important in preventing cell dehydration or cell swelling by controlling fluid shifts (McKeever, 2004) as well as controlling thirst and drinking. It is essential to maintain electrolyte homeostasis to maintain normal cellular function; this is particularly important in nerve and muscle cells. Ultimately the balance of body fluids affects arterial blood pressure and cardiovascular stability and the ability to perfuse tissues, modulated by splenic contraction in early exercise.

The electrolytes maintain fluid balance between the two body compartments: the intracellular (inside cells) fluid (ICF) and extracellular fluid (circulatory fluid – plasma volume and interstitial lymph fluid) (ECF). The amount of electrolytes in the two fluids differs; sodium (Na), a cation, is found in the highest concentration in the ECF and this is balanced by the two anions carbonate (HCO_3) and chloride (Cl). Of the body's exchangeable potassium (K), 95% is a cation found in the ICF together with magnesium; the anions in the ICF are phosphates and proteins.

The correct balance of body fluids is essential for optimal health and athletic performance (Kronfeld, 2001a) and is maintained by the intake and loss of electrolytes and the movement between the fluids at cellular level.

Water

To maintain hydration in a horse, it is vital that the horse has access to water; electrolytes should not be replenished after exercise without the horse drinking water (Coenen, 2005). Horses will drink 15–60 litres of water/day and will drink more if their diet is high in potassium and protein. Water accounts for 50–70% of bodyweight in the adult, so 250–350 kg in a 500 kg horse (Carlson, 1987), and 70–80% in foals (Rose, 1981; Frape, 1986), with 65–70% being in intracellular fluid and 30% (about 100 litres) in extracellular fluid (Tasker, 1967).

Diet has an impact on the amount of water and electrolytes a horse consumes. High-fibre diets, particularly those high in pectin, such as sugar beet, increase water consumption and plasma volume. The increase in water intake is reflected by an increase in bodyweight (Coenen *et al*, 1990).

The excretion of fluids via urine and faeces is related to intake to enable the horse to maintain the correct balance of water and electrolytes within its body. Water loss is normally accounted for as 18% lost in urine, 51% in faeces and 31% in insensible fluid loss (respiratory and cutaneous losses) (Tasker, 1967). In the large colon the water content of approximately 90% on entry is reduced to 60% in the faeces. Most Na and Cl (96%) and 75% K and phosphate entering the large colon from the ileum are absorbed (Frape, 1986). The large colon effectively acts as a reservoir of electrolytes

Control of Electrolyte and Water Balance

The amount of water and electrolytes lost in sweat is independent of diet and is only affected by workload and weather. Fluid requirement is dramatically increased by work (increasing in accordance with the severity of the work) and by increased loss in sweat and from the respiratory tract. Rise in environmental temperature increases water requirement so that a rise from 15°C to 20°C increases water requirement by 15–20%.

You need to know how and when to advise on electrolyte and water intake according to the workload, the temperature and the sweat loss of the horse. It is useful to understand how these factors interact, in order to provide the most appropriate advice.

Since sweat is hypertonic by the time that electrolyte replacement is required, it leads to hypotonic hypohydration, which inhibits thirst. Plasma hypotonicity is exacerbated by supplementing with water alone; it is necessary to correct the hypotonicity and its resultant alkalosis with electrolytes (Na, K and, particularly, Cl).

Inadequate intake or excessive loss of fluid or electrolytes results in disorders of fluid balance. It is essential that the client ensures that the fluids and electrolytes are in balance to maintain homeostasis and maintain normal physiology and normal cellular function. The correct balance of fluids, electrolytes and acid base have to be maintained within a narrow range in both the internal and external fluids.

Internal regulation

Key to maintaining the correct balance is the regulation of ECF osmolarity and the concentrations of the electrolytes. Although ICF and ECF have different ionic composition they are osmotically in equilibrium, with free water diffusing between.

Electrolytes move between the fluids both passively and by active transport. This results in an osmotic gradient and water diffuses down the concentration gradient across the cell membrane until hydrostatic pressure is sufficient to prevent the diffusion of further electrolyte particles. Active ion pumps (sodium/potassium, calcium/magnesium and calcium ATPase) in cell membranes fatigue during exercise (Kronfeld, 2001a). This affects the supply of metabolic substrate and the removal of waste products from cells.

As the horse loses water through sweat, the concentration of sodium in the blood will increase, stimulating the hypothalamus which in turn stimulates the pituitary to release antidiuretic hormone (ADH), resulting in the kidneys retaining water. As the horse loses sodium in the sweat, the adrenal cortex secretes aldosterone, which results in more sodium being retained by the kidneys.

The published range of normal plasma concentrations of electrolytes (Table 13.1) can vary quite widely, altering according to the state of hydration.

Effect of Exercise on Electrolyte Balance

Thermoregulation, dehydration, its consequences and the role of water in rehydration

Approximately 75–80% of fuel used in muscle contraction ends in heat production and an increase in the temperature of muscle cells. While this initially helps to improve muscle performance and is the purpose of 'warming up' before strenuous exercise, it soon becomes detrimental to muscle cell function.

Cells function most efficiently within a limited temperature range and so it is important that excess heat is removed.

Heat production and sweat loss depend on:

- intensity and duration of activity being undertaken;
- training state/acclimatisation;
- body fat and hair cover acting as insulation, thereby reducing heat loss;
- temperament: sweat rate is increased in excitable horses; and
- environmental conditions (ambient heat and humidity).

How does exercise affect electrolyte and water balance?

Initially fluid volume is redistributed to support the increased heart rate, followed by fluid and electrolytes for thermoregulation and sweat.

If these stores that are being lost through sweat are not replaced, then the horse will become dehydrated and suffer hyperthermia, cardiovascular instability and fatigue.

At the start of exercise, packed cell volume is increased by the splenic contraction but this decreases rapidly by 15–20% after only 4 min of incremental exercise (McKeever *et al.*, 1993). The movement of water and electrolytes to the interstitial space means they can be taken up by the muscles or used to produce sweat, resulting in a reduction in plasma volume (PV).

The reduction in PV is related to the loss of total body water due to sweating. In short-term exercise these changes are temporary and return to normal within about an hour after finishing work.

Sweating

Increased exercise is accompanied by an increase in sweating. The horse (unlike people) cannot conserve

Table 13.1 Normal plasma concentration of electrolytes (mEq/l)

Electrolyte	Frape (1986)	Rose and Hodgson (2000)	Kingston (2004)
Na^+	134–143	132–142	133–142
K^+	3.3–5.3	3.2–4.2	3.3–3.9
Cl^-	89–109	94–104	100–110
Phosphate PO_4	1.1–1.5	0.75–1.25	
Ca	2.7–3.9	2.7–3.3	2.7–3.3
Ionised Ca^{2+}			1.7
Mg^{2+}	0.62–1.1		
Bicarbonate HCO_3^-		26–34	25–28

sodium when it sweats but this means that it can move a greater amount of water to the skin surface and increase evaporation, improving cooling. This means that you need to be responsive to the potential large losses of electrolytes and water in the exercising horse (Table 13.2). Equine sweat is hypertonic to plasma and thus it is essential that electrolytes are replaced, specifically chloride – the loss of which will lead to metabolic alkalosis (McCutcheon and Geor, 1998).

Top tip

The amount of sweat a horse loses can be measured by weighing the horse before and after exercise – the kilograms lost equate to the litres of sweat lost.

The Composition of Sweat and the Implications of Isotonic versus Hypotonic versus Hypertonic

Sweat composition is affected by different thermal environmental conditions (McCutcheon *et al.*, 1995). Ionic composition and osmolality of sweat are lowest at the start of exercise and increase over the period of exercise (Table 13.3).

During prolonged sweating the concentration of sodium in plasma reduces, leading to conservation of sodium (McCutcheon and Geor, 2010). Further fluid and electrolyte losses occur during the recovery period, which is extended in humid conditions. The sweat rate during the recovery period is reduced where the horse is acclimatised to the environmental conditions, so that fluid loss is reduced (McCutcheon and Geor, 2010).

Dehydrated horses sweat less than euhydrated (normally hydrated) horses, probably due to reduced blood supply to the skin, so that fluid loss is greater in the earlier stages of sweating (Hodgson and Rose, 1994). However, the efficiency of thermoregulation is correspondingly compromised.

Effect of ambient relative humidity (RH) on water and electrolyte requirements

As humidity rises, the rate of heat loss progressively falls, due to reduced efficiency of evaporation since

Table 13.2 Electrolyte losses (g/day) in sweat[a] for a 500 kg horse

Electrolyte	5 litres	10 litres	25 litres	40 litres
Na	27	43	93	142
Cl	41	71	163	254
K	34	43	70	97
Mg	12	13	19	24

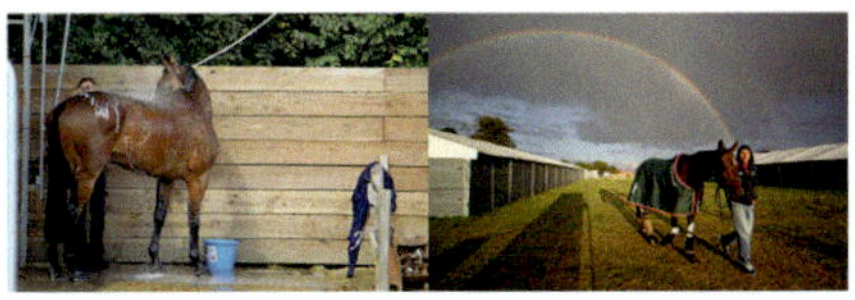

[a]At low-intensity exercise, horses lose 5–10 litres of sweat per hour, increasing to 15 l/h at high intensities

Table 13.3 Ionic composition of equine sweat and plasma (mmol/l). (Adapted from Lindinger and Ecker, 1995; McCutcheon *et al.*, 1995; McKeever, 2004.)

	Sodium (Na)	Potassium (K)	Chloride (Cl)
Plasma			
Pre-competition	140	3.8	100
Post-competition	133	3.2	84
Sweat			
Early	115–150	25–50	160
Prolonged	132–167	25–33	160–181
Human sweat	50	5	60

Top tip

The voluntary intake of saline alone is potentially hazardous for any horse at rest. If salt is supplemented in a feed or water, it is essential that plain water also be made available ad libitum.

It is also important that, after salt intake, sufficient time is allowed to give the horse the opportunity to drink an adequate quantity of water. Approximately 4 h before exercise would be appropriate (Coenen, 2005).

Do remind clients that rehydration involves both water and electrolytes.

the thermal gradient between skin temperature and environmental temperature reduces. Although there is progressive increase in the formation of drops of sweat on the coat, this conductive heat loss is approximately only 5–10% as efficient and does not compensate for the reduced evaporative heat loss (Hodgson and Rose, 1994).

Efficiency of heat loss depends on the ratio of body surface area to body mass. The best horses for endurance competition (where heat dissipation is paramount) are Arabian types (Fig. 13.1), while Warmbloods are very inefficient.

Hypohydration results in reduced peripheral blood flow to the skin and reduced efficiency of sweating. Efficiency of sweating can be increased by aggressive cooling, which increases the thermal gradient with the environmental temperature.

Initially sweat is hypotonic compared with equine plasma, but very much less hypotonic than human sweat. The ionic concentration rapidly increases as sweating continues, so that it rapidly becomes hypertonic compared with plasma (McCutcheon *et al.*, 1995). In particular, chloride and potassium concentrations increase. This leads to dehydration, hypokalaemia, hypochloraemia and metabolic alkalosis.

Potassium loss is disproportionately high, with loss predominantly from within the cells. Loss from skeletal muscle cells is of particular concern.

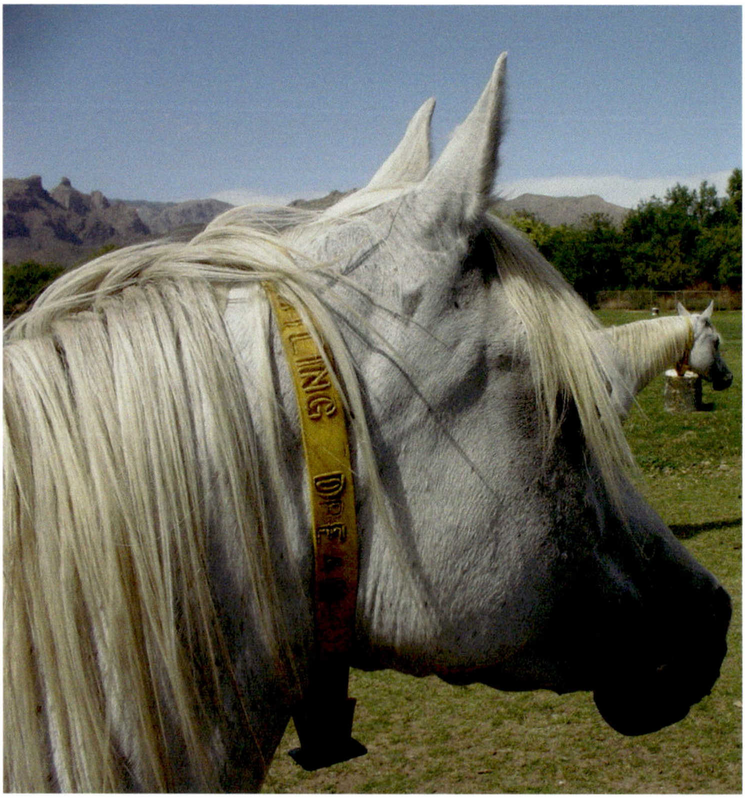

Fig. 13.1 Arabians are efficient at dissipating heat.

Endurance horses are susceptible to potassium deficiency (Fielding, 2015). Levels in plasma and extracellular fluid may remain relatively normal and so measurement of plasma potassium is not an accurate indication of total body potassium. However, sweat may account for up to 30% decrease in plasma potassium (Rose *et al.*, 1980). The Na:K ratio in plasma is 35:1; in sweat it is 3.5:1 (Rose *et al.*, 1980). Replacement of potassium losses must be undertaken with care.

Dehydration and Exhaustion

Dehydration results from fluid and electrolyte losses. It may be the result of inadequate dietary supply, excessive sweating during exercise or from losses from the alimentary tract, most commonly from diarrhoea. Fluid and electrolyte losses lead to fatigue, dehydration and exhaustion, sometimes called the 'exhausted horse syndrome' (Fig. 13.2).

This is exacerbated by hyperthermia and the depletion of energy stores. Clinically the horse has an increased temperature and heart and respiratory rates, severe depression and unwillingness to eat or drink. Potentially this can be fatal.

Dehydration is not clinically apparent until fluid loss exceeds 5% total bodyweight but is likely to be fatal at above 12%.

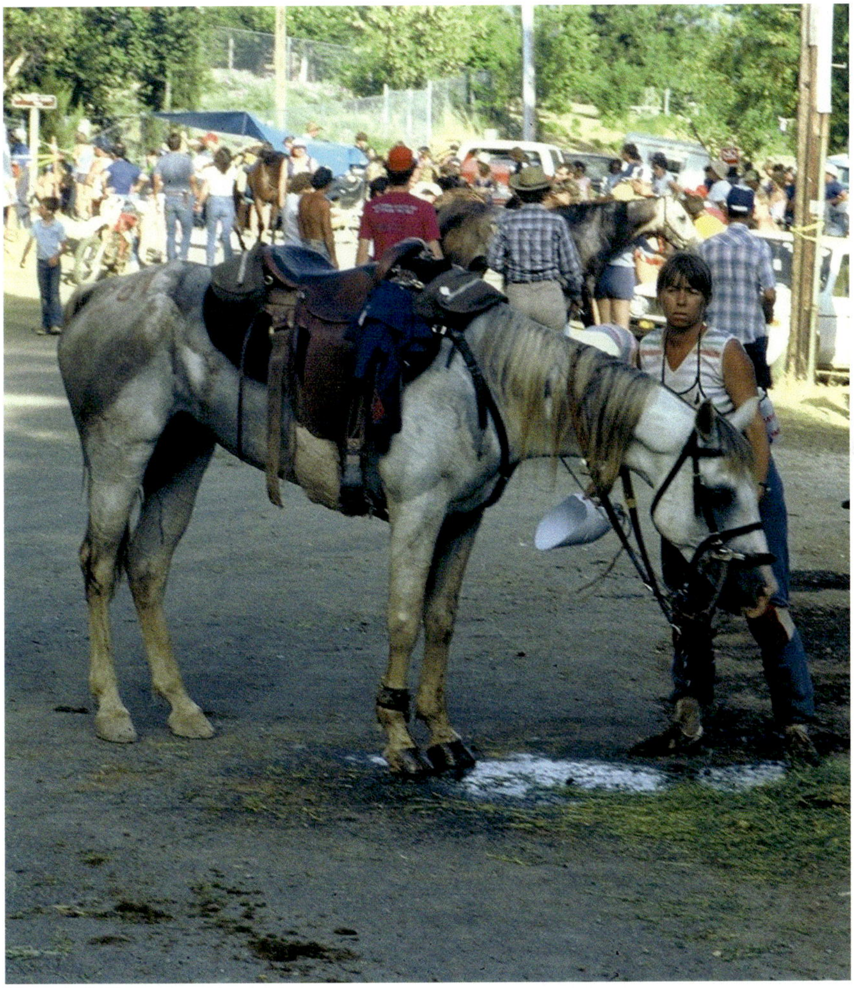

Fig. 13.2 An exhausted horse. Photo Rod Fisher.

Clinical signs of dehydration in the horse

- Increased heart rate, weak pulse due to reduced blood pressure from circulatory stress. Capillary refill time is increased.
- Increased respiratory rate. When the horse is hypothermic, panting respirations help to remove body heat.
- Reduced intestinal motility: the reduced blood volume is diverted to the vital organs. This may progress to colic.
- Extremities become cold.
- Congested mucous membranes and reduced capillary refill rate (the rate at which the mucous membrane returns to normal colour after applying pressure to the gum above the lateral incisor) due to haemoconcentration, refill taking up to 5 s. As dehydration increases the mucous membranes may become dry, dark and muddy.
- Reduced skin elasticity, sunken eyeballs, drooping eyelids and ears due to reduced subcutaneous fluid. If the skin is pinched into a tent (customarily over the point of the shoulder) and released, the more dehydrated the horse the longer the skin will remain tented before it returns to normal.
- As blood supply to the skin reduces further, there is absence of sweat and the skin dries quickly.
- Urine production is reduced and urine colour darkens, due to concentration.
- Loss of smoothness and fine coordination of movement (microklutz), muscle tremors.
- Gait becomes less precise, or wandering with reduced elasticity of gait.
- As dehydration increases the horse becomes increasingly reluctant to eat or drink, exacerbated by the loss of large concentrations of electrolytes in sweat.
- Bodyweight is reduced, mainly due to loss of fluid. A loss in bodyweight of 1 kg equates to 1 litre fluid loss. A weighbridge would be required before and after exercise to provide a sufficiently accurate assessment. This is usually not practical during exercise at home but the facility is usually provided at top competitions and you should encourage clients to use them.
- May become immobile or recumbent.

Top tip

A pilot study indicates that a weight tape, whilst not providing an accurate BW in competition horses, does measure the change in bodyweight loss as validated by a weighbridge, which gives an indication of fluid loss (Ellis and Hollands, 2001).

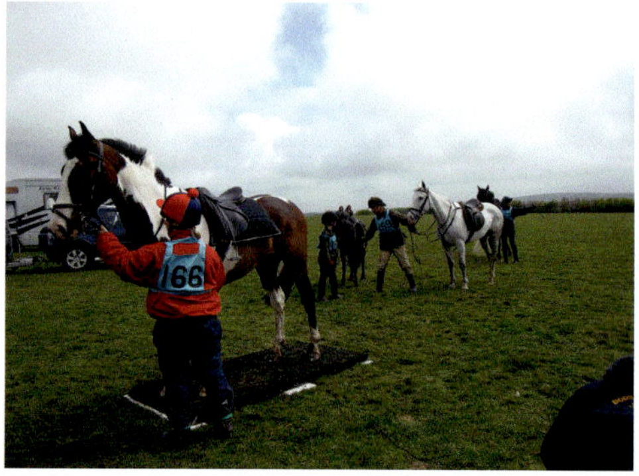

Laboratory changes resulting from dehydration include the following:

- Increased haematocrit/packed cell volume (PCV).
- Increased total serum protein (TSP). This can be easily and quickly measured using a hand-held veterinary refractometer.
- Serum phosphate increases.
- Neutrophilia, lymphopenia, eosinopenia.
- Blood glucose is reduced.
- Plasma creatinine is increased.
- Acid/base status is variable, depending on the cause of the dehydration.
- Urine specific gravity increases. Easily measured with a veterinary refractometer.

Management of dehydration and exhaustion

Correction of water deficit is the most essential consideration; the replacement of specific electrolytes is a secondary consideration. However, thirst is controlled by Na concentration of body fluids and so water alone reduces Na concentration, leading to reduction in thirst and increase in urinary loss.

- Employ aggressive treatment.
- The type of fluid given is relatively unimportant.

- Under field conditions, pulse rate +/– body temperature are good guides to effectiveness of treatment.
- Treatment should be continued until the heart rate falls below 50 bpm and the horse is willing to eat and drink voluntarily.

Sweat Loss Across Different Disciplines

Sweat loss provides a considerable challenge to water and electrolyte homeostasis. Sweat production increases in increasing ambient temperature and sweat loss reaches a maximum in hot dry conditions (McCutcheon *et al.*, 1995). The core temperature of a horse galloping 3.2 km (2 miles) would increase by 6.1°C; approximately 70% of the heat generated by muscle activity is lost by the evaporation of sweat, with further small amounts of heat lost by convection, conduction and radiation from the skin surface. Up to 30% of the remaining heat loss is via the respiratory tract (McCutcheon and Geor, 1998). Without this loss of heat the core temperature would rise dramatically. Unlike in humans, sweat composition in horses does not alter with increasing fitness (McConaghy *et al.*, 1995).

Endurance horses

An endurance horse (Fig. 13.3) travelling at 17 km/h sweats at 12.5 l/h, producing 30,000 BTUs (3.165×10^7 Joules) (Ridgeway, 1992, personal communication).

A similar quantity of sweat is produced hourly over the first several hours of moderate exercise (Jenkinson *et al.*, 2006). This equates with up to 50 ml/m^2 surface area/min. This compares with a maximum sweat loss of approximately 2 l/h (17 ml/m^2/min) in humans (Marlin and Nankervis, 2002a). Sweat rate varies depending on exercise intensity (McCutcheon and Geor, 1998).

It is sometimes falsely assumed that acidosis is a sequel to endurance exercise so that bicarbonate forms a major component of electrolyte mixtures. Since horses are usually alkalotic after prolonged exercise, the inclusion of bicarbonate is contraindicated.

Low-intensity prolonged exercise

- Electrolyte changes are associated with alterations in total body water, resulting predominantly from sweating.
- Plasma sodium levels may increase or decrease slightly or remain constant.
- Potassium is generally reduced but may remain normal or even be slightly increased.
- Considerable chloride loss in sweat leads to renal retention of bicarbonate and metabolic alkalosis (Hodgson and Rose, 1994).

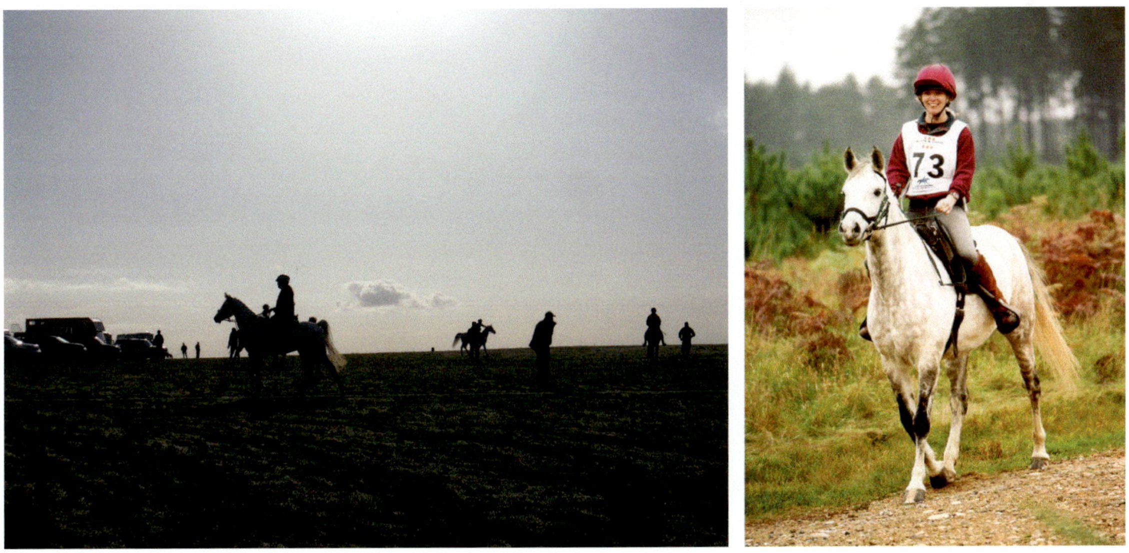

Fig. 13.3 Endurance horses.

Event horses

Event horses (Fig. 13.4) lose a significant amount of fluid during the endurance phase of an event. Andrews *et al.* (1993) measured an average loss of 18.4 l in 48 horses during the cross-country phase of a long-format three-day event.

Short-duration intense exercise

- Large transient changes in electrolyte levels.
- Sodium increase.
- Potassium transiently greatly increased.
- Chloride largely unchanged (as it exchanges with lactate across muscle cell membranes).
- HCO_{3-} is reduced and H^+ increases, causing metabolic acidosis (Hodgson and Rose, 1994).

Racehorses

Racehorses (Fig. 13.5) working at high speeds can lose 1–5 l in even a short period of time (Harris, 1998). However, the effect on the horse is minimal and there is rapid rebalance of fluid shift and fluid loss.

Bodyweight losses due to sweating

The loss of 3–4% bodyweight as sweat has a significant effect on metabolic efficiency, with significant reduction in circulatory volume.

In humans, 1% reduction in bodyweight due to fluid loss results in a 10% reduction in performance. The effect is less in horses because fluid in the hind gut acts, to some extent, as a compensatory reservoir.

During short-term exercise, changes in plasma sodium and chloride levels are minimal, but in prolonged exercise there is a disproportionate loss in chloride due to sweat loss. However, in short-term exercise, loss of plasma water results in an increase in potassium level.

The stimulus for exercise-induced sweat production is epinephrine (adrenaline), produced in the adrenal medulla and delivered to the periphery of the sweat gland. Sweat rate is modulated by variation in blood flow. Unlike in humans, the horse's sweat gland cannot conserve sodium and so sodium loss in sweat is greater and sweat composition is hypertonic (McCutcheon and Geor, 1998).

Clinical Conditions Associated with Electrolyte Loss and Management Solutions

Sporadic/extrinsic exertional rhabdomyolysis (ER)

Sporadic muscle damage is caused by extrinsic factors (Fig. 13.6) and it is important that clients appreciate

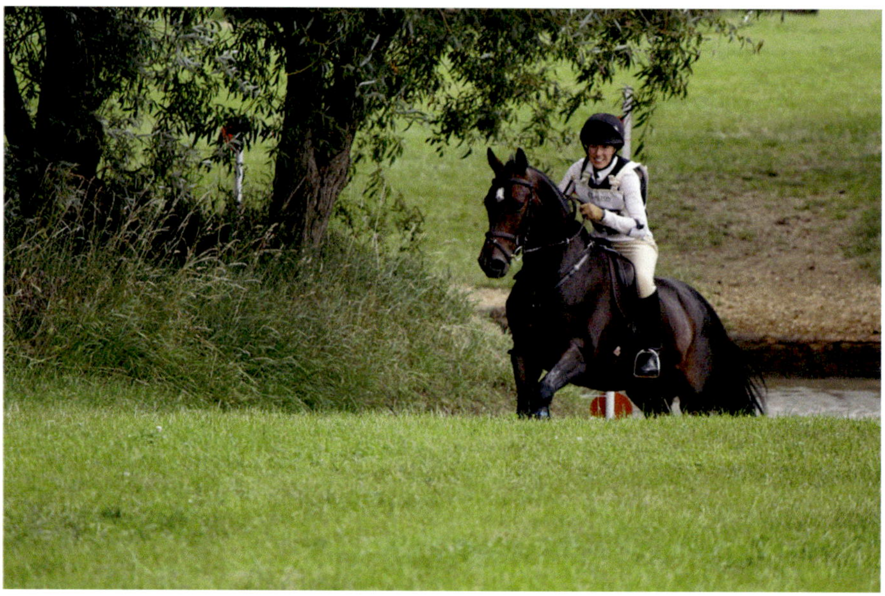

Fig. 13.4 Event horse.

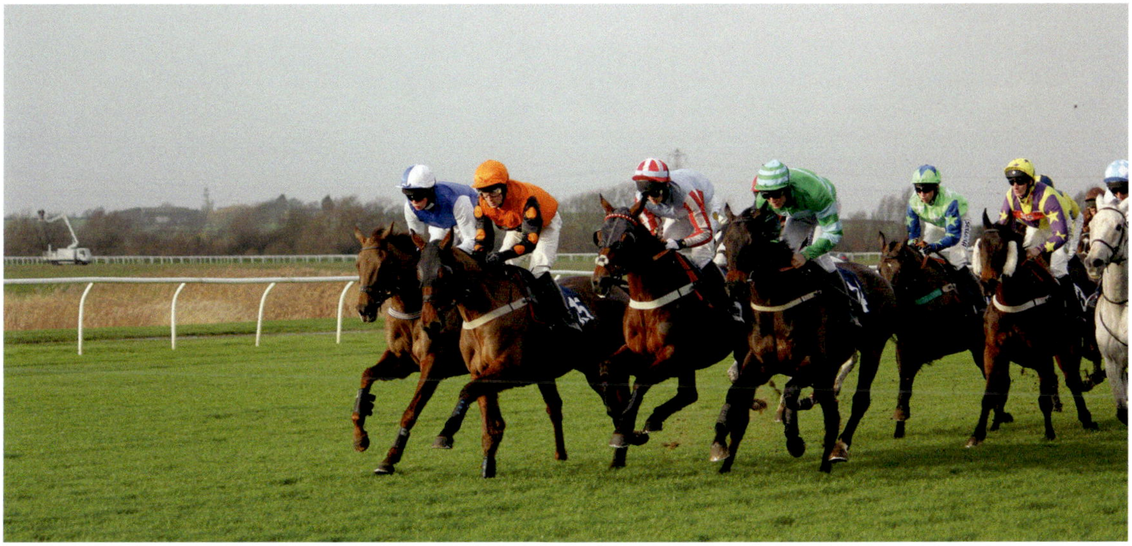

Fig. 13.5 Racehorses.

- Typically leisure or good doer performance horses
- Inadequate stretching and muscle fatigue
  - Owners often over-estimate fitness of horse
  - Children's ponies at the start of school holidays
  - Pleasure rides
  - Low level endurance riding
  - Little warm up and warm downs
- Inappropriate feeding
  - Little or no vit/min supplementation
  - Handful of competition mix
  - Low energy feeds at less than recommended intakes
  - Soaking hay depleting minerals

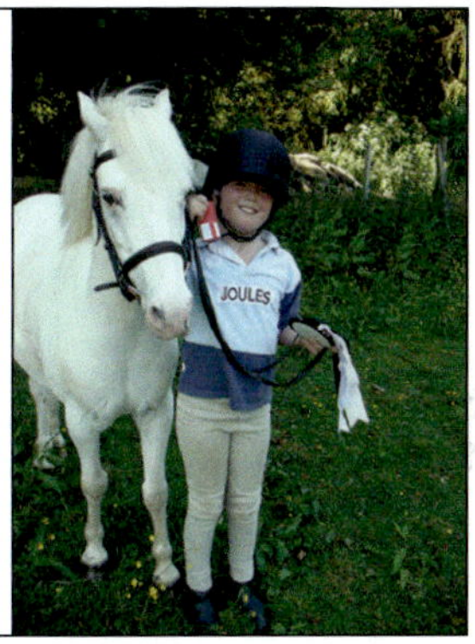

Fig. 13.6 Examples of risk factors and groups of horses typically at risk of sporadic exertional rhabdomyolysis.

that it has a different aetiology from myopathies caused by diseases. It is similar to delayed-onset muscle soreness (DOMS) in humans and is characterised by mild stiffness, shortened stride and profuse sweating, with possible increasing severity through to recumbency. Painful muscle cramps usually resolve in a matter of hours. Affected horses have dark urine, discoloured by myoglobin released from damaged muscle cells. Perversely, cases of sporadic ER may recur in isolated bouts following exertion.

The main pathology is muscle damage due to exercise in excess of the fitness of the horse, loss of electrolytes in sweat (Harris, 1991; Beech *et al.*, 1993), inflammation and swelling of the muscle (Liburt *et al.*, 2010).

Treatment of sporadic rhabdomyolysis is centred in the first instance on relief of pain, correction of fluid and electrolyte imbalances, increase of antioxidant nutrients and minimisation of renal damage caused by myoglobin.

Although lactic acidosis was thought to be an important contributory factor in this condition, many affected horses have metabolic alkalosis. In fact, this type of muscle damage is not associated with lactate. Lactic acidaemia is rarely, if ever, observed in either horses or humans. A metabolic alkalosis is the most common acid–base abnormality and is associated with hypochloraemia (Koterba and Carlson, 1982; Valberg *et al.*, 1993).

Long-term management depends on the underlying contributing causes and trigger factors, such as exercise, nutrition and correcting micronutrient imbalances, including electrolyte imbalances. A full ration evaluation is required (Harris *et al.*, 2013) (Table 13.4).

Horses carrying excess weight as well as not being fit also seem to be at increased risk of muscle damage. Horses that are carrying 25–30% above their 'ideal' weight (includes rider and tack) have higher creatine kinase (CK), increased muscle soreness and tightness and higher lactate after exercise compared with horses carrying 15–25% excess weight (Powell *et al.*, 2008).

Electrolyte imbalances may be due to inadequate or imbalanced intake or an individual problem with absorption or utilisation, about which there is little published data (Harris and Snow, 1991; McKenzie *et al.*, 2002).

In the first instance, simply check dietary adequacy; a simple ration adjustment plus some advice on workload should minimise the risk of a repeat episode.

Should you wish to investigate further, then electrolyte balance can be assessed by fractional urinary electrolyte clearance (Harris and Snow, 1991; Harris and Gray, 1992). Using the Urinary Fractional Excretion Test (UFET) (Box 13.1). it is possible to restore normal fractional excretion of individual electrolytes to within the expected reference range which, together with other management changes, may lead to a clinical improvement.

Anhidrosis

Anhidrosis is a condition of impaired thermoregulation found in some horses in hot environments. In such cases the ability to sweat is inadequate to control body temperature, particularly in TBs and Thoroughbred crosses (TBXs) (Mackay *et al.*, 2015). Clinically the horse shows exercise intolerance and prolonged recovery, leading to fatal heat stroke.

Problems associated with specific electrolytes

Many of the clinical conditions arising from electrolyte imbalances are multifactorial and cannot be attributed to one particular electrolyte. Consequently, the clinical pictures for several of the conditions described below overlap and the clinical picture becomes complex.

Sodium

The principal cation, nearly all in the ECF: 40% (Frape, 1986) to > 50% Coenen (2005) of total Na is in the skeleton. Electrolyte homeostasis and acid–base balance is centred on sodium The resting 500 kg horse requires 8–22 g/day, primarily as NaCl, and the requirement increases dramatically when the horse is sweating (Harris, 1998) Sodium is readily absorbed from the gut and excreted via the kidneys. The large intestine acts as a reservoir when large quantities are lost as sweat. However, an excess or deficiency of sodium can result in serious pathology (Table 13.5).

Potassium

While 98% of potassium is intracellular, the intracellular:extracellular ratio is critical to maintain membrane resting potential and action potential in nervous tissue. Therefore, mild imbalances in electrolyte levels may have potentially serious neurological consequences (Fielding, 2015). At speeds exceeding 4 m/s, hyperkalaemia is likely to be present and so supplementation with K would be contraindicated, since neuromuscular excitability would be induced. Since uptake of K^+ into cells is enhanced by glucose and insulin, low plasma glucose and insulin levels would also increase the hyperkalaemia. Consequently, there is a good argument for not including K in electrolyte supplements during competition. Potassium is important in the resynthesis of muscle glycogen using oral or IV glucose but only before, or after the end of (not during), the event. Potassium replacement should be carried out with care, particularly in IV administration (Table 13.6).

Table 13.4 Dietary advice for leisure horse out at grass with sporadic rhabdomyolysis

Horse signalment	12 y, 15 hh cob type gelding 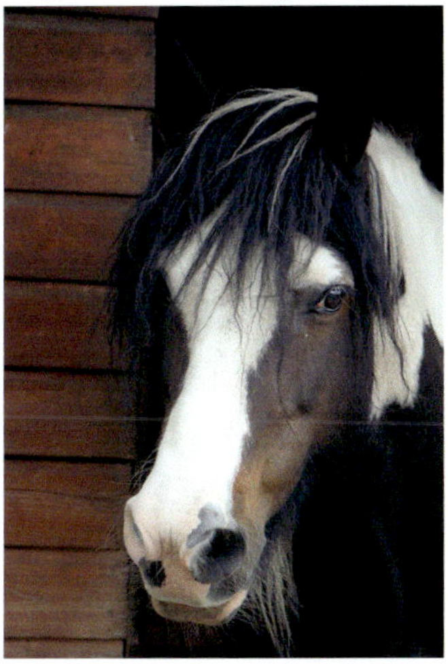	Breed tendency to put weight on easily – weight tape indicates 525 kg
Horse history	Generally light exercise, kept ticking over by mother; daughter broke up for Easter hols and took horse for 12-mile sponsored pleasure ride. Very stiff when got home and unloaded from trailer. 1 h later white frothy sweat on hind quarters and couldn't leave stable	Over-exertion – not fit for the workload
Differentials[a]	PCV; CK; AST	Extrinsic muscle damage
Results of any tests	BFS 4, 4, 4 Urine discoloration is a practical useful guide	High fat tissue % increased risk of increased CK and lactate after exercise
Current diet	Grazing 6 h/day; soaked hay – large haynet at night; ½ scoop horse and pony nuts	Grass intake varied – sparse and not managed, so feed value low; soaked hay leaches minerals, specifically electrolytes; quantity of feed not sufficient to provide daily requirements of any micronutrients
Advice	Overfed but undernourished – not fit enough for the work Provided a suggestion for fittening Use muzzle in field and increase turnout – improves fitness	Continue with soaking hay but increase to 6 kg. Sugar beet 0.5 kg dry weight then soaked to provide pectin and improve water within gut High-spec balancer fed at 100 g/100 kg BW so 525 g/day split into two feeds and 25 g salt in each feed

[a]CK levels rise quickly from normal of approx. 300 to 1000–5000 (stiffness) to above 10,000 in clinical cases of tying up. Severe cases can exceed 100,000. May not be correlation between CK levels and severity of clinical signs. Blood levels peak at approx. 6 h and return to normal in 3–4 days. AST levels rise more slowly, reaching lower maxima (but over 10,000) but levels decline slowly over approx. 3 weeks.

Box 13.1 Urinary fractional electrolyte excretion

Renal excretion of electrolytes is an indicator of their homeostatic level. The Fractional Electrolyte Excretion test allows a comparison between the serum electrolyte level and that expected from the urinary excretion level, taking into consideration the excretion level of a substance (creatinine) which accurately reflects the glomerular filtration rate in the kidneys. A free-flow urine sample and serum sample need to be taken concomitantly. This can be used to adjust the dietary intake of the electrolyte as necessary.

The test is completed following a suitable time interval to allow the electrolyte imbalance resulting from the episode of rhabdomyolysis to resolve, with the horse on the diet on which it suffered the attack of rhabdomyolysis, in order to identify any abnormality. The test is then repeated at least 2 weeks after any correctional dietary changes have been made in response to the results of the test, preferably with the horse on full feed and in full work. The response to restoration of balance is variable and the wide daily variation in fractional excretion of electrolytes makes the value of the technique limited for testing for specific electrolyte derangements (Naylor, 2015). Correction of electrolyte imbalances is unlikely to lead to improvement unless other management changes are made concurrently.

Table 13.5 A summary of low and high sodium levels and treatment options in the horse

Hyponatraemia	Hypernatraemia
Serum sodium concentration below 134 mmol/l results from acute water intoxication as a consequence of psychogenic polydipsia or the iatrogenic intravenous infusion of hypotonic solutions. Alternatively, the condition may be secondary to renal failure, ruptured bladder or diarrhoea. Potentially fatal oedema of the brain, particularly after rapid ingestion of large volumes of water following water deprivation, is manifested as apparent blindness, loss of menace response and seizures.	Hypernatraemia represents a deficit of water relative to Na concentration such that serum Na exceeds 144 mmol/l (Hurcombe, 2008). This condition can be secondary to either excess of salt intake, or severe dehydration due to illness or prolonged water deprivation. A sudden rise in serum [Na+] over a few hours, as in excessive oral supplementation during prolonged (endurance) exercise, predisposes the horse to hyperpnoea, muscle weakness, lethargy and marked thirst. There may be tremors of face, neck and shoulders.
Treatment	
Hypertonic saline must be given slowly in order to avoid seizures. Furosemide would also be helpful in cases where hyponatraemia is accompanied by volume overload.	Water orally, *or* hypotonic IV infusion, although the more hypotonic, the slower the infusion should be given, in order to avoid inducing cerebral oedema.

Chloride

Chloride is obtained by ingestion in feed and 84% is lost in urine and faeces (Groenendyke *et al.*, 1988). Most of the remainder is lost in sweat, as already discussed. Chloride is both absorbed and secreted in the GI system. Extracellular concentration of chloride is considerably higher than intracellular concentration (Table 13.7).

Calcium

Ninety-nine per cent of body calcium is stored in bone, 0.9% intracellularly and 0.1% extracellularly, of which 48% is free ionised Ca^{2+} (Aguilera-Tejero, 2015).

Changes in extracellular Ca levels are responsible for clinical disorders. Only ionised calcium is probably likely to be active and this constitutes approximately 50% of total calcium.

Calcium concentration is regulated by complex hormonal control of intestinal absorption and renal excretion. This involves parathyroid hormone (PTH), vitamin D and calcitonin. Large amounts of calcium are absorbed from the intestine and excreted through the kidneys. In addition, up to 500 mg/h may be lost in sweat and up to 1 g/l in the milk of a lactating mare.

Table 13.6 A summary of low and high potassium levels and treatment options in the horse

Hypokalaemia	Hyperkalaemia
A serum potassium concentration of below 3.5 mEq/l indicates hypokalaemia. However, this does not accurately reflect intracellular concentration, which may vary considerably from extracellular concentration. Measurement of intracellular concentration is not practical. Inadequate intake may result from food deprivation or anorexia. Fortunately there are generally high levels of potassium in feed, particularly alfalfa hay. • Relatively high levels in sweat mean that prolonged exercise may result in abnormal loss. • Hypokalaemia may be secondary to hypomagnesaemia. • Potassium loss is exacerbated by endotoxaemia, possibly diarrhoea and/or increased renal losses. The significance of acid/base imbalance is controversial. Loss of potassium results in muscle weakness and may cause cardiac dysrhythmias.	Hyperkalaemia results from a serum [K^+] in excess of 4.5 mEq/l.Small increases in plasma [K^+] as potassium is released from muscle cause local arteriolar vasodilation and increased blood flow to the muscle (Kronfeld, 2001b). However, larger increases are harmful and potentially fatal. **Causes of hyperkalaemia:** • Hyperkalaemia is linked to hyperkalaemic periodic paralysis (HYPP), an autosomal dominant condition of certain heavily muscled horses including Quarter Horses and Appaloosas (Aleman, 2008). The abnormality affects the skeletal muscle sodium channel gene, allowing excessive influx of sodium and outward flux of potassium, causing persistent depolarisation of muscle cells. • Other causes of anuria (urethral obstruction) have a similar effect. Potassium reduces the excitability of muscle, particularly cardiac muscle, so that the increased cardiac flaccidity reduces heart rate and cardiac output, leading to syncope in diastole. In foals, increasingly bizarre ECG findings may be seen. All of these signs are potentially life threatening. In addition, skeletal muscle may develop fasciculations and weakness.
Treatment	
Correction of hypokalaemia should be made with care. Potassium is highly digestible so that oral preparations (KCl (as Lite-salt) or KI) are most practical. Magnesium supplementation can increase the digestibility of potassium (Hintz and Schryver, 1976). Where IV infusion is necessary the required deficit to be replaced can be calculated using the formula: K^+ deficit = 0.3 × bodyweight (kg) × (4 – measured [K^+]) mEq. Rate of IV infusion should not exceed 0.5 mEq /kg/h (Hurcombe, 2008).	Hyperkalaemia is treated with IV 5% dextrose. Protamine Zinc Insulin can be used to promote potassium uptake into the cells. 23% Calcium borogluconate (0.5 ml/kg IV over 20 min) can provide protection against myocardial effects. It is preferable to give the calcium borogluconate diluted in 3–5 l isotonic saline intravenously. Bicarbonate solutions may be indicated but only as a secondary line of treatment and must not be given with calcium preparations.

Table 13.7 A summary of low and high chloride levels and treatment options in the horse

Hypochloraemia	Hyperchloraemia
May be physiologically normal but may follow increased loss due to: • renal or GI damage; • excessive sweating; • insufficient intake; or dilution effect of increased ECF (which may follow the administration of fluids with minimal or no electrolytes) or uroperitoneum, as may follow ruptured bladder.	Usually results from renal dysfunction and is associated with metabolic acidosis. Water deprivation may lead to a concentration effect of ECF. Clinical signs are associated with acidosis (depression, anorexia and polypnoea).
Treatment	
Hypochloraemia may not require specific treatment apart from correction of the metabolic alkalosis with which it is associated.	Treatment of hyperchloraemia is directed at correcting the underlying cause; where this is renal dysfunction, oral sodium bicarbonate is helpful.

Ionised calcium (iCa) increases the voltage required to open Na^+ channels in nerve fibres, so deficiency (iCa below 6 mg/dl) (Hurcombe, 2008) makes neuronal tissue more excitable. This leads to reduced gut motility, tetanic spasms and incoordination and skeletal muscle paresis (Table 13.8).

Magnesium

Magnesium plays a significant role in several physiological processes (Stewart, 2015), including:

- Glycolysis
- Oxidative phosphorylation
- Nucleic acid and protein synthesis
- Ion pump function.

Magnesium acts as a membrane stabiliser, regulating calcium channel activity. It impacts on function of smooth muscle and cardiomyocytes (Table 13.9).

Since 50–60% magnesium is in hydroxyapatite in bone and less than 1% is extracellular, serum levels are not a reliable indicator (Hurcombe, 2008).

Phosphorus

Phosphorus constitutes 1% total body weight, of which 85% is as hydroxyapatite in bone and < 1% is in ECF. In blood, 50% is ionised, bound to cations, the prevalent form being HPO_4^{2-}. The significance

Table 13.8 Clinical signs associated with low calcium levels and treatment options in the horse

Hypocalcaemia	
Seen in several clinical conditions of the horse • Exercise-induced hypocalcaemia • Eclampsia, particularly in overweight mares grazing lush pasture in late pregnancy, up to several days after weaning. • Transport tetany • Endotoxaemia, sepsis • Colic, gastrointestinal disease Occasionally in liver disease, acute renal failure, oxalate ingestion or secondary hyperparathyroidism resulting from excessive dietary phosphorus causing complexes that prevent absorption from the small intestine	Clinical signs of hypocalcaemia are generally non-specific but can include muscle fasciculations, difficulty in chewing and swallowing, involuntary lip and tongue movements and, in more advanced cases, seizures. Adults may show synchronous diaphragmatic flutter (SDF, 'Thumps') after exercise-induced hypocalcaemia, particularly where the horse has sweated excessively. However, it may also follow metabolic disturbances caused by diarrhoea or several of the other conditions above. It occurs secondary to excessive chloride loss causing hypochloraemic metabolic alkalosis and respiratory alkalosis. SDF is often associated with low calcium and magnesium levels. The common name of 'thumps' refers to the clinical manifestation of a rhythmic tic on the horse's flank, starting on the left flank before progressing to become bilateral. Right atrial depolarisation stimulates activity in the phrenic nerve as it crosses the surface of the heart, which in turn stimulates diaphragmatic contraction synchronous with the heart contraction. Usually the flutter starts once exercise has stopped. The heart rate is generally slower than expected for that state of dehydration, usually approximately 50 bpm.
Treatment Where there is high requirement (as in exercising or lactating horses) or anorexia it is good practice to supplement with calcium as a prophylactic precaution. Calcium carbonate (ground limestone) in feed is cheap and effective in most cases. However, check the dietary intake in the first instance and consider alfalfa as a source of Ca – it is more digestible and palatable compared with limestone (Cuddeford *et al.*, 1990)	Treatment is most effective with IV infusion of isotonic saline or Ringers solution to which 50 ml of 23% calcium gluconate has been added to a 5 l bag. Alternatively, 250–500 ml calcium gluconate can be given to a 500 kg horse by slow IV injection. Mares with lactation tetany can be given 250 ml/450 kg calcium and magnesium combined by slow IV injection while continuously monitoring cardiac rhythm

Table 13.9 Clinical signs associated with low and high magnesium levels and treatment options in the horse

Hypomagnesaemia	Hypermagnesaemia
Magnesium levels in lush green pasture are low and, in this situation, dietary intake may be low, unless the horse is being fed a compound feed or vitamins and mineral supplement. The magnesium requirement in early lactating mares is high. Even so, dietary deficiency in horses is very unlikely. Hypomagnesaemia causes acetyl choline to be released at the neuromuscular junction. Clinical manifestations are rare, but may be seen as restlessness, hypersensitivity, muscle weakness and fasciculations, leading to muscle spasms and cardiac dysrhythmias. A consequence of hypomagnesaemia may be hypokalaemia and concurrent hypocalcaemia, which causes tetany.	Hypermagnesaemia is not generally seen apart from when oral magnesium is used excessively in treatment of large colon impaction.
Treatment	
Treatment with $MgSO_4$ can be given as 15–150 mg/kg/day as a 5% solution in isotonic saline, but is more easily given as an oral supplement of 30–60g/horse daily.	Calcium gluconate is appropriate.

of abnormal plasma phosphorus levels is generally under-appreciated (Toribio, 2015).

In addition to bone mineralisation, phosphate is essential in muscle contraction, neurological functions, cell membrane integrity and numerous other functions (Table 13.10).

Increased phosphate stimulates parathyroid hormone (PTH) release, enhancing renal P excretion and promoting bone resorption. Vitamin D increases intestinal absorption and renal reabsorption, increasing bone formation and remodelling.

Practical Management to Minimise Risk of Dehydration or Exhaustion

Do make sure that your client is aware of the following preventative management tools that can be used to minimise the risk of dehydration and ensure that their horses can exercise hard.

1. Ensure that the horse is fit and not overweight.
2. Ensure that the horse is acclimatised to the environmental conditions.
   - Avoid pre-existing intercurrent infection.
3. Train the horse to drink; and offer water frequently.
   - Loss of hypertonic sweat results in hypotonic plasma, which inhibits voluntary water intake.
   - Horses drink water most readily when it is offered at between 10°C and 20°C.
     - However, Sosa Leon *et al.* (1995) showed no difference in absorption or elimination rates of fluids given at 5°C, 21°C and 37°C.
   - Most fluids are absorbed within 2 h of oral administration.
     - Cool drinking water should not be used to try to cool the horse's core temperature. Nerves in the mouth and throat suppress drinking of cold hypotonic solutions (McKeever, 1998).
   - Often there is a short time window immediately after stopping work when the horse is prepared to drink, after which water will not be consumed for 30 min or more.
     - When offered water the horse will often sip a small quantity then look around before returning to drink a much larger quantity; it is important to allow time for this second intake.
   - If the environment is quiet the horse is much more likely to drink.
     - Some horses are reluctant to drink water away from home; in this case it may be necessary to advise clients to bring water from home.
     - The addition of flavouring to disguise the taste of the water may be helpful provided that the horse has been trained to drink the flavoured water at home. Apple juice

Table 13.10 A summary of clinical signs associated with low and high phosphorus levels and treatment options in the horse

Hypophosphataemia	Hyperphosphataemia
Hypophosphataemia results from dietary insufficiency, vitamin D deficiency, reduced gut absorption through damaged gut wall or, more commonly in cases of acute deficiency, intracellular redistribution due to carbohydrate overload, hypoglycaemia, sepsis or respiratory alkalosis. Clinically, signs of skeletal and smooth muscle and neurological dysfunction are rare in cases where serum P fall below 1.0 mg/dl. Muscle weakness and fasciculations and cardiac arrhythmias may be present in acute cases. In chronic cases there may be weight loss, pica, bone mineral loss or lameness.	(Serum P > 5.0 g/dl) Hyperphosphataemia is rare, the result of secondary hyperparathyroidism, vitamin D intoxication, metabolic acidosis, cellular injury due to rhabdomyolysis or crush injury, bisphosphonate treatment or, rarely, renal failure. In acute cases clinical signs resemble those of hypocalcaemia (tetany, hyperexcitation, muscle fasciculations and cardiac arrhythmias). Chronic cases may show lameness or nutritional secondary parathyroidism (osteodystrophia fibrosa, 'bran disease', 'big head').
Treatment	
There are no approved products for treatment which is rarely necessary. However, cows that are recumbent due to hypophosphataemia are treated with 50 g sodium phosphate as a drench	Treatment is not usually necessary apart from dietary alterations, including phosphorus restrictions. Calcium carbonate can be fed as a phosphate binder

(at 5 ml/l water) or peppermint essence can be useful for this purpose.

- Horses need to be trained to consume water with electrolytes, starting with very dilute electrolyte solution and gradually increasing the concentration. As the horse becomes more dehydrated it becomes more amenable to drinking water containing electrolytes.

4. Employ aggressive cooling.
   - Hyperthermia resulting from short periods of intense exercise is more easily reduced than a temperature that has risen slowly over prolonged, less intensive exercise.
   - Aggressive cooling is most efficiently undertaken by pouring large quantities of cold water over the large muscle masses (areas of maximum blood flow).
   - Ice can be used to cool the water but should not be applied to the horse. Ice applied directly to the skin may damage the skin tissues.
     - There is no advantage in scraping the water from the skin. Contrary to traditional belief, there is no evidence that the application of cold water to muscle masses predisposes to rhabdomyolysis.
     - There is no evidence that the application of very cold water causes peripheral vasoconstriction, reducing blood flow to the skin and reducing the rate of heat loss, at least in the early stages of cooling (Marlin *et al.*, 1998).
   - The application of wet towels to parts of the body is effective in cooling for only the short period that they remain cool and wet; after that they serve to prevent heat loss.
   - Periods of gentle walking between applications of water improve blood flow to the skin and render cooling more efficient.
   - The use of fans may help to increase the rate of convective cooling.

5. Ensure that the horse is being fed an appropriate ration for their workload.
   - Horses working hard or competing should not be fed leisure rations.
   - Feeds for horses in light work have lower inclusion of electrolytes compared with competition feeds.
   - If the horse is a 'good doer', then advise a performance balancer rather than a conventional mix.
   - Ensure that electrolytes are fed to replace those lost during work.

Prevention and management of dehydration occurring during transport

Transport by road or air is stressful to horses (Leadon *et al.*, 1989; Marlin and Nankervis, 2002b). Travelling is equivalent to walking for the same period or twice that of standing in a stable. The stress is affected by the experience in travelling, including the space provided, orientation of the horse, temperature and humidity, temperament of the horse and the standard of driving.

Generally, less than 3 h travelling has a negligible effect on the horse's subsequent health and performance but long road journeys covering several days and long-haul flights, exacerbated by refuelling stops, quarantine checks, time spent loading and unloading, have a significant effect on weight loss, due in the main to dehydration (Marlin and Nankervis, 2002b).

Bodyweight changes were measured in a group of endurance horses travelling from the UK to Portugal (Fig. 13.7). In this case, inadequate recovery time was allowed between arrival and competition and between competition and the start of the return journey. Horses were unable to return to their home bodyweight and suffered significant fluid losses, which would not normally be recorded.

The best guide to dehydration is measurement of weight loss. In addition to faecal fluid loss, weight loss can result from: (i) reduced water intake; (ii) insufficient stops; or (iii) increased sweating, particularly in hot and humid conditions and/or where the horse has a nervous temperament. In all these situations both water and electrolytes are lost. Sweating can be reduced by maintaining: (i) environmental temperature of 15–17°C (facilitated by travelling at night); (ii) ventilation and air circulation within the partition; and (iii) avoiding over-rugging.

Recovery of bodyweight after travelling is slower than after strenuous exercise (where weight loss is usually replaced overnight) and slower after flying than after road transport (Marlin *et al.*, 2001). Where weight loss exceeds 4% bodyweight it is recommended that 8–10 l isotonic electrolyte solution be given by nasogastric tube; where weight loss exceeds 6% bodyweight, consider replacement with intravenous fluids.

Recovery from a long-haul flight will probably take approximately 5 days before acclimatisation starts. Until the horse recovers 50% of lost bodyweight, exercise should be restricted to in-hand or ridden walking.

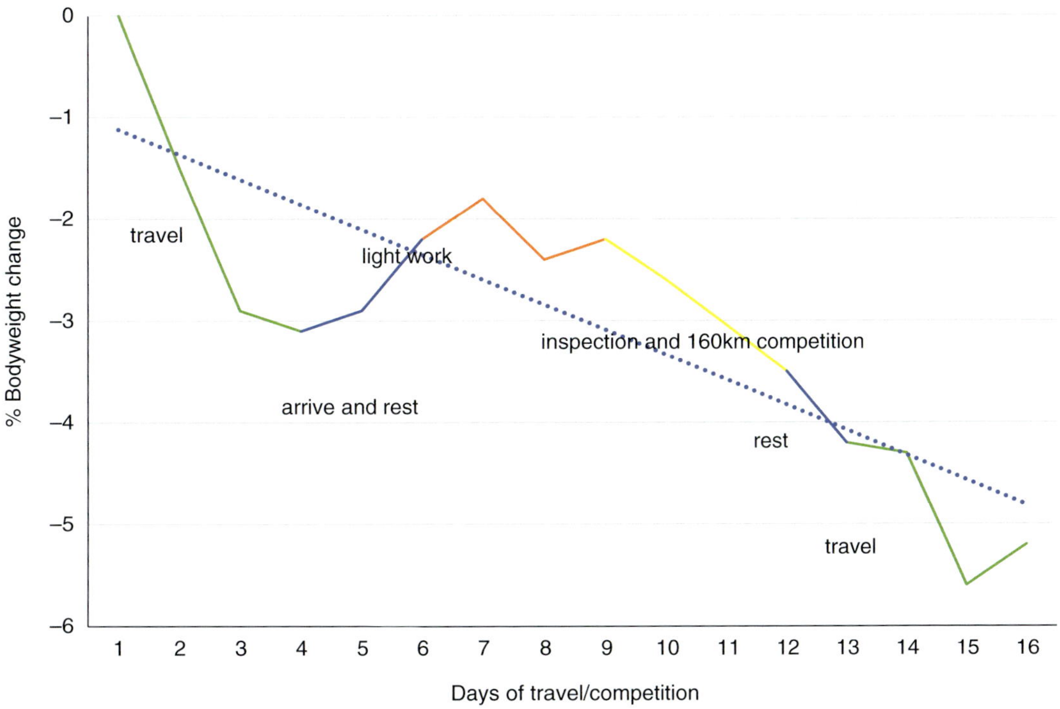

Fig. 13.7 Average weight changes of six horses travelling by road to Portugal to participate in a 160 km endurance race (Fisher, unpublished data).

Practical Management to Replace Electrolytes

Correcting fluid loss

Where the horse is drinking

- Encourage the horse to drink up to 5 l water/15 min.
- Flavouring water, adding sugar beet water, providing apples and other succulents aid rehydration.
- Electrolytes need to be provided to ensure that the fluid intake is isotonic so that the electrolyte concentration is the same as that in the plasma.
  - This is necessary for the horse to retain fluid, since a hypotonic solution reduces thirst and increases urinary loss.
- If the horse will not take water with electrolytes, offer water alone and supply balanced electrolytes in feed.
- High-fibre diets, specifically those that are high in pectin (sugar beet), are associated with an increased fluid and electrolyte reservoir (Meyer, 1987; Warren *et al.*, 1999) in the large colon acting as 'bowel ballast'.

Where the horse is not drinking but gut activity is audible on auscultation

- Give fluids by nasogastric tube
  - 10 l balanced electrolyte solution/h
- While water alone or hypotonic solutions restore PCV and TSP levels in the dehydrated horse, they result in hyponatraemia and delayed restoration of K and Cl (Monreal *et al.*, 1999).
  - An isotonic solution with electrolyte composition similar to sweat for oral rehydration of exercising horses causes the plasma volume to be restored faster, voluntary fluid intake higher and urine output lower (Jansson *et al.*, 1995). It promotes the thirst stimulus and retention of ingested fluid. Hypertonic fluids are not well absorbed from the small intestine.
- In humans, glucose +/– amino acids will enhance Na uptake from the gut, but this is not so in the horse. Although glucose in the electrolyte mixture helps to restore PCV and TSP levels, the hyponatraemia is reduced and the delayed K and Cl restoration is prolonged by glucose.
  - Glucose can aid palatability of some electrolyte supplements, specifically those that have high levels of electrolytes.

Where the horse is not drinking and gut activity is not detectable

- IV fluids should be given.
- Where dehydration results from excessive sweating, use physiological (normal) saline or Ringers solution. Solutions containing bicarbonate or lactate should be avoided.
  - Lactated solutions are indicated where dehydration results from diarrhoea.
  - Initially give 10 l, then reassess.
- KCl can be included at 1–3 g/l but should not exceed 9 g/h.
- Glucose may be helpful in assisting moving K^+ into cells but concurrent insulin would probably help the process.
- In severe cases hypertonic saline (7.2% NaCl) can be used at up to maximum 4 ml/kg but water should be available for oral consumption. Followed by balanced isotonic crystalloid fluids – its value in increasing PCV is superior to 0.9% saline (Magdesian, 2015).
- The replacement of fluids by rectal infusion may be considered as a safe, simple and cheaper practical alternative or adjunct to intravenous or nasogastric fluid administration, particularly when nasogastric administration is not possible (Khan *et al.*, 2019).
  - However, this method is most valuable for the replacement of water (tap water is suitable) only; the inclusion of electrolytes needs to be further evaluated.
  - Since infusion rate should be at maintenance or twice maintenance level, this technique is ideal for long-term fluid maintenance but would require supplementary (IV) therapy in more acute conditions.
- The horse should be rehydrated before the administration of NSAIDs is considered.

Maintaining Electrolyte Balance

Homeostasis can be helped in the competing horse by supplementation with water and electrolytes before, during and after work to counteract depletion and optimise performance. Unlike carbohydrate loading in the human athlete, it is not possible to pre-load with electrolytes, but merely to correct any existing deficits. Where electrolyte losses are expected and it is important that electrolyte levels are optimised in preparation, tapering of the workload for 2–3 days in advance may help this (Marlin and Nankervis, 2002b).

Some of the electrolyte requirements are obtained from natural food sources, but in the working horse these will need to be supplemented.

You can advise providing electrolytes, either in feed or water; based on alterations in plasma and sweat loss, choice often depends upon which the horse finds most palatable. Manufacturers might add Ca and Mg, P, glucose and other nutrients such as amino acids, vitamins and trace minerals.

Some clients like to provide a salt block, but this should not be relied upon and horses working hard will require broad-spectrum electrolyte supplementation.

- In the non-working horse, a broad-spectrum vitamin/mineral supplement is adequate.
- In the working horse, the level of supplementation required is dictated by the level at which the horse is working, their sweat loss (see Table 13.2, above) and the electrolytes provided by their compound ration (Table 13.11).

Because electrolyte replacement is most important in horses undergoing prolonged low-intensity exercise where there is likely to be a metabolic alkalosis, supplementation with bicarbonate in feed or fluids is contraindicated.

Electrolyte Levels in Horse Feeds

All compound feeds and forage sources contain electrolytes appropriate for the workload for which

Table 13.11 Declaration of electrolytes (g/kg as fed) in common feeds and feed ingredients for horses

Feed	Na	Cl	Mg	K	Ca	Recommended daily intake (kg) for a 500 kg horse in work
Competition-Fit Balancer	3.8	2.2	5.1	1.16	2.99	
Competition-Fit Mix	3.6	7.2	1.4	9.9	10.6	
Competition-Fit Cubes	4.2	7.9	2.3	10	10	
Enduro-Performance	2.4	5.3	1.4	13	12.3	
Re-Covery Mash	4.5	8.7	1.4	13	9.8	
Re-Leve	2.5	2.9	2.8	17	11.7	
Polo Pencils	4	7.3	2.2	10.5	10	
[a]Performance Concentrate Muesli	4.0	9.0	5.5	11.5	19	1.25–1.6
Competition Mix	3.5	8.5	4.0	10	10	2–5
Competition Cubes	3.3	7.5	3.0	9.0	10	2–5
Stay Power Muesli	3.6	8.5	3.7	11.5	11	2–5
Stay Power Cubes	3.4	9.0	3.7	10	12	2–5
Elite Sport Muesli	4	8	3.5	9.5	10	2–5
TopSpec Comprehensive Balancer	?	?	6	?	24	0.5
TopSpec Performance Lite Balancer	?	?	6	?	20	0.5
Baileys Performance Balancer	?	?	?	?	30	0.5
Baileys Ease & Excel	3	?	4	?	12	
Barley	0.1	1.4	1	4.7	0.6	
Beet pulp (unmolassed)	1	1	15	5	12	
Maize	0	0.6	1	3.3	0.3	
Molasses (cane)	2.1	15	3.5	35	7.4	
Naked oats	0.1	0.7	1.3	3.6	0.9	
Oatfeed	0.2	1	0.6	4	0.9	
Oats	0.1	0.7	1.2	3.6	1	
Peas	0.2	1	1.3	9.5	0.9	
Rice bran	0.1	0.9	6	14	16	
Soya hulls	0.2	0.3	2.3	12	5	
Soya (full fat)	0.2	0.4	2.3	17	2.2	
Wheat	0	0.9	1.4	4.1	0.4	
Hay (UK average)	1	0.1	1.8	17	3.5	6.25 kg fresh weight
Haylage (UK average)	1	0	1	20	3.5	10.9 kg fresh weight
Grass (UK average)	0.1	0	1.5	26	4	31 kg fresh weight out 6 h

[a]Correct as per datasheets version August 2021

they have been formulated (Table 13.11) but most will be deficient in sodium. Sodium attracts water and high levels of sodium in commercially available feeds would lead to an increase in spoilage, which is why sodium may be deficient in feed.

Top tip

The most basic supplement, common salt (NaCl), should be added at approximately 50 g daily if the horse is working.

There are differences between commercially prepared feeds as to which electrolytes are provided by the feed and in what quantities, depending on the brand that you recommend (Table 13.11).

Pasture and forage are generally high in potassium and can provide adequate levels of magnesium. However, chloride levels are variable and sodium tends to be low.

Many factors, including where the forage was grown, the soil quality and water condition during growing, will affect the electrolyte levels.

Top tip

If horses are eating adequate forage, they will always be eating excess potassium relative to requirements.

Cereals are deficient in electrolytes, and if being fed in large quantities you would need to advise additional supplementation of all micronutrients, including electrolytes. Manufacturers will provide information on electrolyte inclusion when asked, but this is meaningless unless you know the amount of food the horse is consuming (Table 13.12).

Top tip

If a horse loses 10 l of sweat and is on a balanced competition ration, you would normally be recommending additional salt to balance 5.5 g of sodium and 11 g of chloride. Remember that salt contains 40% sodium and 60% chloride, so the owner would need to add 18 g of salt to cover this loss.

Top tip

1 teaspoon of salt weighs 6 g and contains 3.6 g chloride and 2.4 g sodium.
To balance a 10 l sweat loss:

- the client would need to feed 3 teaspoons of salt in addition to the compound feed;
- or ½ dose of a well-formulated electrolyte supplement.

Clearly greater losses cannot be replenished immediately and can take up to 1 week of supplementation

If the horse is eating a well-formulated performance ration, then a comprehensive electrolyte supplement might not be needed until the horse starts to lose more than 2% of its bodyweight (Table 13.13).

Factors to consider when advising an electrolyte supplement

- Look at the percentage electrolyte inclusion.
- Look at the feeding rate.
- A properly formulated electrolyte balance will reflect the horse's requirements and replace electrolyte loss over a period of time.
- Although two supplements may appear to provide the same or similar level of electrolyte

Table 13.12. The amount of electrolytes (g/day) provided by a typical competition ration[a] for a 500 kg horse

Mineral	3 kg Concentrate (600 g/100 kg BW)	9 kg Hay[b]	Total
Na	21	24	45
Cl	51	41	92
K	60	127	187
Mg	24	10	34

[a]9 kg hay and 3 kg Dodson & Horrell Competition Mix (correct as per data sheet version August 2021)
[b]Variable according to hay type, growing and harvesting conditions

Table 13.13 Electrolytes needed by a horse relative to sweat loss in addition to the typical competition ration shown in Table 13.12

Minerals needed (g)	Sweat loss (litres)				
	Rest	5	10	25	40
Na	0	0	0	10	97
Cl	0	0	0	71	163
K	0	0	0	0	0
Mg	0	0	0	0	0

supplementation, one may have a higher feeding rate and will therefore provide a higher level of electrolytes.

- Check that the electrolyte supplement you are advising does not contain high levels of sugar (usually seen as dextrose on the label) at the detriment of electrolyte content. Do note, however, that sodium is absorbed via SLGT-1 at the same time as glucose and water (Dyer *et al.*, 2009), thus some glucose in electrolytes supplements is useful.

Oral supplementation

Choice of electrolytes is often driven by your client's preferences based on what they perceive as being most palatable for their horse.

Powders

Powders are mixed into feed. The composition can become increasingly complex, depending on the quantity of work required.

Sometimes your owner will want to make their own electrolyte supplement (Box 13.2). Do remind them that the provision of salt licks is inadequate; the horse will not lick the amount necessary to fulfil its requirements. The amount taken will depend on the palatability of the block, depending on the other constituents.

If they are using table salt, then this can be refined by adding ground limestone ($CaCO_3$) at 25 g daily. Calcium is more available from alfalfa and this quantity needs to be taken into consideration.

Solutions

Hypotonic and isotonic fluids are absorbed more rapidly than hypertonic fluids, and fluid and electrolyte excretion in urine is slower (Sosa Leon *et al.*, 1995).

Isotonic fluid intake is ideal and manufacturers should be able to confirm that their supplements meet these criteria when made up with the necessary quantity of water.

Isotonic fluids are not very palatable and so horses should be trained to drink balanced electrolytes in solution.

Box 13.2 Homemade electrolyte mix

1 part rock salt (NaCl)
1 part Lite Salt (Lo Salt), which is two parts NaCl and one part KCl
1 part ground limestone ($CaCO_3$)

or:

10 g NaCl
4 g KCl
0.5 g $CaCO_3$
0.25 g $MgCl_2$

9 g of electrolytes are lost in 1 l of sweat, so 90 g of electrolytes should be added to 10 l of water.

Top tip

- Start with dilute solution – increase until horse is drinking correct dilution.
- Flavourings might help.
  - Apple juice or peppermint essence.
  - Water in which sugar beet was soaked.

In humans, the addition of glucose in the oral replacement solution enhances fluid uptake (Schedl *et al.*, 1994) but this does not appear to be the case in the horse (Sosa Leon *et al.*, 1995). Indeed, in order to keep the solution isotonic, fewer electrolytes are given and so the solution is less effective.

Pastes

Hypertonic pastes can be a practical method of replacing electrolytes where a horse will not drink electrolytes in water voluntarily. Hypertonic fluids draw water into the intestinal lumen until the solution is isotonic, thus dehydrating the horse further, which should trigger the horse's thirst; therefore an unrestricted supply of water *must* be available at the same time.

Electrolyte preparations in the small intestine must become isotonic before they can be absorbed, so there may be some delay in the absorption of hypertonic pastes.

Concentrated pastes may come into contact with gastric ulcers in the stomach, causing a painful response similar to putting salt on an open wound, and colic signs may be evident. If it is intended to use concentrated electrolyte pastes, then the likelihood of the presence of gastric ulcers should be considered.

How to Advise an Appropriate Electrolyte Regime According to Discipline and Workload

It is clear that one solution does not fit all and it is important to adapt the electrolyte regime according to bodyweight, exercise level and duration and ambient temperatures. Some examples of how this is achieved are provided below.

Eventers

Remember that many horses lose weight due to dehydration during travelling, so advise clients to weigh their horses on arrival and ensure that they have been offering water during travelling or adding wet sugar beet into feeds.

Prolonged riding-in before dressage can result in as much bodyweight loss as after cross-country and thus most clients should be feeding electrolytes through the competition, after ensuring the horse has drunk (Table 13.14).

Endurance horses

It is important to remember that over-exertion in endurance horses (Table 13.15) results in alkalosis rather than acidosis, thus the dietary support should differ.

Feeding high dietary intakes of calcium prior to a race has the potential to exacerbate alkalosis, because it decreases the horse's ability to mobilise the calcium during extended exercise, with similar physiological mechanism to cows in early lactation. Remember to check for excess calcium intakes prior to racing.

However, once competing, extra calcium and magnesium can be supplemented, as uptake carrier molecules will be triggered to maximise absorption and increase ionised blood calcium.

All performance horses will have travelled to the event and it is important to advise clients to adjust watering, feeding and electrolyte supplementation based on the length of journey

Transport adaptations

Advise clients to train horses to drink water containing electrolytes from a bucket, as well as fresh water gradually, building up to isotonic concentration before travelling.

- Most clients find that horses do not drink for the first 6 h of travelling (personal communications).
  - Despite this, it is good practice to encourage clients to offer water 4 h after start of journey; some owners will syringe water.
- Although it is not possible to pre-load with electrolytes, remind clients to ensure that there are no electrolyte deficiencies at the start of travelling or strenuous work.
  - They should be feeding an electrolyte formulation best approximating to electrolyte distribution in plasma, using in-feed formulations.
- Encourage them to monitor fluid/electrolyte losses by weighing the horse regularly whenever practical.
- Teach horses to drink from a bucket at home.
  - Flavour water at home and continue to do so throughout travelling at competitions to encourage drinking.
  - Ensure water is neither too hot nor too cold.
- Feeding routine should be maintained (albeit smaller feeds); sugar beet is an excellent succulent

Summary

- Electrolytes are electrically charged inorganic salts which play a major role in maintaining osmotic pressure and fluid balance in tissues. They also help to maintain acid–base status.
- Changes in body fluids initially enhance and then limit cellular function and athletic performance.
- Primary cations are sodium and potassium; primary anions are chloride and phosphate.
- Calcium and magnesium play a supporting role.
- Fluid and electrolyte imbalances affect dehydration and exhaustion, gastrointestinal and renal function and play an important part in many other clinical conditions, including exertional rhabdomyolysis and anhidrosis.
- Clinical conditions often result from imbalances of multiple electrolytes.
- Exercise has considerable effects on electrolyte balance and total body water.

Table 13.14 Dietary advice for event horse with reduced water intake and observed reduced time to fatigue

Horse signalment	11 y, 16.2 hh Warmblood gelding 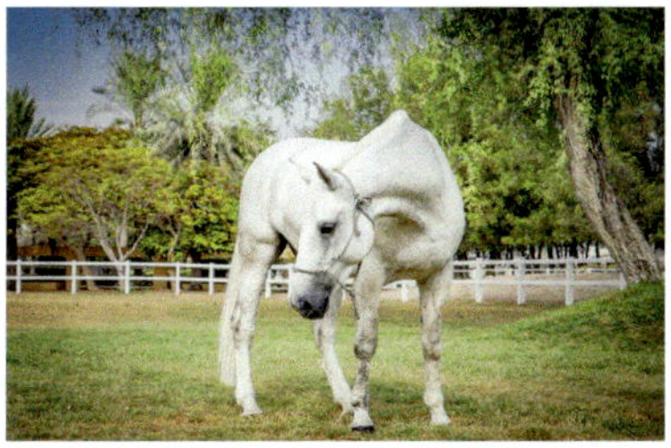	Horse maintains good weight and weight tape indicates 565 kg BFS 5/9
Horse history	Horse stepping up in fitness level in preparation to move up to the next competitive level and owner wants to make sure that her electrolyte programme is in line with increased work level. She has recently observed that the horse is drinking less, especially at competition, and this is causing early fatigue	Delayed capillary refill time
Differentials	Elevated haematocrit	Electrolyte imbalance, fatigue
Results of any tests	Urine discoloration is a practical useful guide	Ideal optimum BFS, water intake and electrolyte programme require review
Current diet	Grazing 1 h/day; haylage – two large haynets in the morning and at night – 3.0 kg of performance feed 30 g of table salt added, no salt block and no electrolyte supplement currently used.	Haylage on examination is wet and therefore compromising DM intake. May also account for reduced water intake. Automatic waterer currently in use. Sample of haylage has been taken for analysis. Feed is being fed at recommended intake.
Advice	Haylage is being underfed due to perception of increased calorie content and not currently being weighed. Work level has increased with more fast work incorporated	Continue with haylage but increase to 2% of BW per day[a]. Increased calorie intake from haylage may require calories from hard feed to be reduced. Ensure that you advise a competition feed balancer in proportion to the reduction in competition feed to maintain vitamin and mineral balance, e.g. 2 kg of performance feed plus 250 g balancer. Use 300 g of an unfortified low sugar and starch palatable soaked mash pre- and post-training and competition to aid water intake, e.g. Recovery Mash.
Electrolytes	Horse sweating more, therefore electrolyte supplement needs to be incorporated	Free access to a salt block. Add 60 g of a well-fortified electrolyte supplement divided over the two feeds, e.g. KER Restore Monitor actual water using a bucket until problem is resolved

[a]Show the client how to work this out on a DM basis based on the forage analysis; important that this is then calculated as fed % (see Chapter 9).

Table 13.15 Dietary advice for endurance horse experiencing sporadic exertional rhabdomyolysis

Horse signalment	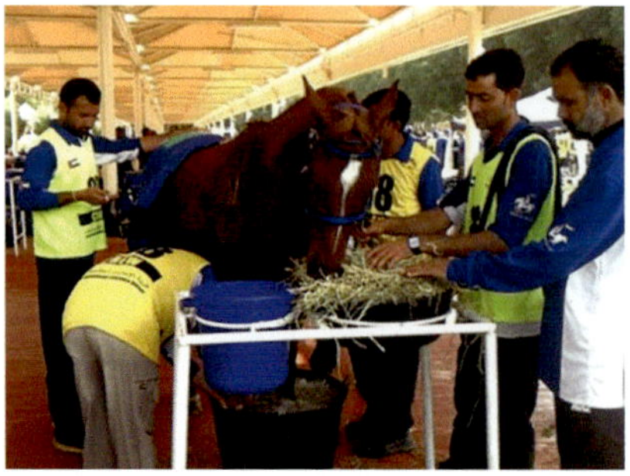	Arabian horse, 9 y old averages 401 kg on a weighbridge. Maintains a BFS of 4.5/ 9.

Horse history	• Water intake and appetite all good.
	• Mare had been in oestrus pre-competition.
	• Weighed weekly, pre- and post-endurance race.
	• Previously been working well through training in lead-up to competition.
	• Competing (championship level)
	  o completed first loop well (mean 15.4 kmph)
	  o passed vet inspection 10 min post-arrival.
	  o Continued observation showed HR remaining elevated at 64 bpm.
		• 20 min post-vet inspection, horse increased muscle stiffness
		  o Withdrawn from competition
		• 30 min post-arrival, HR still 64 bpm.
		  o Gluteal muscles hard to touch

Differentials	• Elevated
	  o temperature
	  o CK 58330 iu/ml
	  o AST 12845 iu/ml
	• Lowered blood calcium level 2.73 mmol/l
		Muscle rhabdomyolysis

Current diet	• Access to grazing and daily sand paddock turnout during wet weather.
	• Timothy hay 1% of BW/day
	  o in the morning and evening,
	  o although not weighed out.
	• 5 kg endurance feed
	  o fed over four feeds per day
	• 800 g of a hay/alfalfa blend chaff
	• 120 g of an electrolyte supplement added to two of the four feeds
	  o There is no access to a salt lick and additional salt is not added to the feed
		Feed is fully fortified, although will not provide adequate Na or Cl

Advice	• Hay is underfed
	  o perception of increased bulk and gut fill
	  o excess weight, and increased heat load
	  o observed to be very fine with a lot of leaf shatter.
	  o increase to 1.8% of BW/day, preferably 2%
	  o increase frequency of provision.
	• Adequate hay provision will help with potassium, calcium and magnesium intake.
	• Use software ration evaluation to illustrate nutrient intakes coming from 5 kg of feed alone.
	• Free access to a pure salt block and add 120–200 g of a well-fortified electrolyte supplement divided equally over the feeds.	

Continued

Table 13.15 Continued.

Ongoing husbandry	• Blood work suggests: o Increase calcium levels prior to competition to enhance availability of calcium during extended periods of exercise. o Advise feeding up to 1 kg of alfalfa pre-race to top up calcium reserves • Review electrolyte and feeding programme for maintenance of energy provision o Pre-competition and resume normal training. o Competition electrolyte supplements may differ from training o Additional provision of calcium and magnesium, administered at each vet gate and water stop. • Additional supplements are not required, as feed is well fortified and from a reputable brand and fed at recommended intake to meet calorie requirement.	

- Thermoregulation is vital to maintain optimal tissue function, achieved by sweat loss.
- Environmental temperature and relative humidity hugely affect sweat loss.
- Transport may contribute to dehydration and exhaustion.
- Fluid and electrolyte imbalance can be corrected by voluntary oral replacement or by administration via nasogastric tube or IV administration.
- Replacement of electrolytes is best achieved by supplementation in feed.
- Electrolyte levels in commercially available supplements should be examined carefully and matched to the horse's work requirement and insensible losses.

Bibliography

Aguilera-Tejero. (2015) Calcium haemostasis and derangements. In: Fielding, C.L. and Magdesian, K.G. *Equine Fluid Therapy*. John Wiley & Sons, Ames, Iowa, pp. 55–75.

Aleman, M. (2008) A review of equine muscle disorders. *Neuromuscular Disorders* 18, 277–287.

Andrews, F.M., Ralston, S.L., Sommardahl, C.S. *et al.* (1993) Weight loss, water loss and cation balance in horses competing in a 3-day event. In: *Proceedings Thirteenth Equine Nutrition & Physiology Society Symposium*, p. 203.

Beech, J., Lindborg, S. and Braund, K.G. (1993) Potassium concentrations in muscle, plasma and erythrocytes and urinary fractional excretion in normal horses and those with intermittent exercise-associated rhabdomyolysis. *Research in Veterinary Science* 55, 43–51.

Carlson, G.P. (1987) Haematology and body fluids in the equine athlete: a review. In: Gillespie, J.R. and Robinson, N.E. (eds) *Equine Exercise Physiology 2: Proceedings of the Second International Conference on Equine Exercise Physiology*. ICEEP, Davis, California, pp. 393–425.

Coenen, M. (2005) Exercise and stress: impact on adaptive processes involving water and electrolytes. *Livestock Production Science* 92, 131–145.

Coenen, M., Meyer, H. and Stadermann, B. (1990) Amount and composition of the GIT content according to type of feed and exercise. *Advances in Animal Physiology and Animal Nutrition* 21, 7–20.

Cuddeford, D., Woodhead, A. and Muirhead, R. (1990) Potential of alfalfa as a source of calcium for calcium deficient horses. *The Veterinary Record* 126(17), 425–429.

Dyer, J., Al-Rammahi, M., Waterfall, L., Salmon, K.S., Geor, R.J. *et al.* (2009) Adaptive response of equine intestinal Na+/glucose co-transporter (SGLT1) to an increase in dietary soluble carbohydrate. *Pflügers Archiv–European Journal of Physiology* 458(2), 419–430.

Ellis, J.M. and Hollands, T. (2001) A preliminary investigation into the use of weightapes for the detection of dehydration in the performance horse. In: Proceedings of the 40th British Equine Veterinary Association Annual Congress. Abstract, p. 221.

Fielding, C.L. (2015) Potassium homeostasis and derangements. In: Fielding, C.L. and Magdesian, K.G. (eds) *Equine Fluid Therapy*. J.D. Wiley & Sons Inc., Ames, Iowa, pp. 27–44.

Frape, D. (1986) *Equine Nutrition and Feeding*. Longman Scientific & Technical, London, pp. 49–63.

Groenendyk, S., English, P.B. and Abetz, I. (1988) External balance of water and electrolytes in the horse. *Equine Veterinary Journal* 20, 189–193.

Harris, P.A. (1991) The equine rhabdomyolysis syndrome in the United Kingdom: epidemiological and clinical descriptive information. *British Veterinary Journal* 147, 373–384.

Harris, P. (1998) Tied up with electrolytes – or not? In: Pagan, J.D. (ed) *Advances in Equine Nutrition*. Nottingham University Press, Nottingham, UK, pp. 513–530.

Harris, P.A., Coenen, M. and Geor, R.J. (2013) Controversial areas in equine nutrition and feeding management: the editors' views. In: Geor, R.J., Harris, P.A. and Coenen, M. (eds) *Equine Clinical and Applied Nutrition*. Saunders Elsevier, Edinburgh, pp. 443–454.

Harris, P.A. and Gray, J. (1992) The use of urinary fractional electrolyte excretion test to assess electrolyte status in the horse. *Equine Veterinary Education* 4, 162–166.

Harris, P.A. and Snow, D.H. (1991) Role of electrolyte imbalances in the pathophysiology of the equine rhabdomyolysis syndrome. *Equine Exercise Physiology* 3, 435.

Hintz, H.F. and Schryver, H.F. (1976) Potassium metabolism in ponies. *Journal of Animal Science* 42, 231–239.

Hodgson, D.R. and Rose, R.J. (1994) *The Athletic Horse: Principles and Practice of Equine Medicine*. W.B. Saunders Co., Philadelphia, Pennsylvania, pp. 71–72.

Hurcombe, S.D.A. (2008) Electrolytes and neurological dysfunction in horses. In: Furr, M. and Reed, S. (eds) *Equine Neurology*. Wiley-Blackwell Publishing, Hoboken, New Jersey, pp. 269–282.

Jansson, A., Nyman, S., Morgan, K., Palmgren-Karlsson, C., Lindholm, A. *et al*. (1995) The effect of ambient temperature and saline loading on changes in plasma and urine electrolytes (Na+ and K+) following exercise. *Equine Veterinary Journal* (Suppl. 20), 147–152.

Jenkinson, D.M., Elder, H.Y. and Bovell, D.L. (2006) Equine sweating and anhidrosis part I: equine sweating. *Veterinary Dermatology* 17, 361–392.

Khan, A., Hallowell, G.D., Underwood, C. and Van Eps, A.W. (2019) Continuous fluid infusion per rectum compared with intravenous and nasogastric fluid administration in horses. *Equine Veterinary Journal* 51(6), 767–773.

Kingston, J. (2004) Appendix 2 – References ranges for serum biochemical variables in athletic horses In: Hinchcliffe, K.W., Kaneps, A.J. and Geor, R.J. (eds) *Equine Sports Medicine & Surgery*. Saunders Elsevier, Oxford, pp. 1300–1301.

Koterba, A. and Carlson, G.P. (1982) Acid-base and electrolyte alterations in horses with exertional rhabdomyolysis. *Journal of the American Veterinary Medical Association* 180, 303–306.

Kronfeld, D.S. (2001a) Body fluids and exercise: physiological responses (Part I). *Journal of Equine Veterinary Science* 21, (7), 312–322.

Kronfeld, D.S. (2001b) Body fluids and exercise: Replacement strategies. *Journal of Equine Veterinary Science* 21(8), 368–375.

Leadon, D., Frank, C. and Backhouse, W. (1989) A preliminary report on studies on equine transit stress. *Journal of Equine Veterinary Science* 9(4), 200–202.

Liburt, N.R., Adams, A.A., Betancourt, A., Horohov, D.W. and McKeever, K.H. (2010) Exercise-induced increases in inflammatory cytokines in muscle and blood of horses. *Equine Veterinary Journal* (Suppl. 38), 280–288.

Lindinger, M.I. and Ecker, G.L. (1995) Ion and water losses from body fluids during a 163 km endurance ride. *Equine Veterinary Journal* (Suppl. 18), 314–322.

Mackay, R.J., Mallicote, M., Hernandez, J.A., Craft, W.F. and Conway, J.A. (2015) A review of anhidrosis in horses. *Equine Veterinary Education* 27(4), 192–199.

Magdesian, K.G. (2015) Replacement fluids therapy in horses. In: Fielding, C.L. and Magdesian, K.G. (eds) *Equine Fluid Therapy*. John Wiley and Sons Inc., Ames, Iowa, pp. 161–174.

Marlin, D.J. and Nankervis, K. (2002a) *Equine Exercise Physiology*. Blackwell Science Ltd, Oxford, pp. 127–150.

Marlin, D.J. and Nankervis, K. (2002b) *Equine Exercise Physiology*. Blackwell Science Ltd, Oxford, pp. 276–284.

Marlin, D.J., Scott, C.M., Roberts, C.A. *et al*. (1998) Post exercise changes in compartmental body temperature accompanying intermittent cold water cooling in the hyperthermic horse. *Equine Veterinary Journal* 30(1), 28–34.

Marlin, D.J., Schroter, R.C., White, S.L. *et al*. (2001) Recovery from transport and acclimatisation of competition horses in a hot humid environment. *Equine Veterinary Journal* 33, 371–379.

McConaghy, F.F., Hodgson, D.R., Evans, D.L. and Rose, R.J. (1995) Effect of two types of training on sweat composition. *Equine Veterinary Journal* (Suppl. 18) 285–288.

McCutcheon, L.J. and Geor, R.J. (1998) Sweating: fluid and ion losses and replacement. *Veterinary Clinics of North America: Equine Practice* 14, 75–95.

McCutcheon, L.J. and Geor, R.J. (2010) Effects of short term training on thermoregulatory and sweat responses during exercise in hot conditions. *Equine Veterinary Journal* 42(Suppl. 38), 135–41.

McCutcheon, L.J., Geor, R.J., Hare, M.J. *et al*. (1995) Sweating rate and sweat composition during exercise and recovery in ambient heat and humidity. *Equine Veterinary Journal* (Suppl. 20), 153–157.

McKeever, K.H. (1998) Effect of exercise on fluid balance and renal function in horses. *Veterinary Clinics of North America: Equine Practice* 14, 23–44.

McKeever, K.H. (2004) In: Hinchcliffe, K.W., Kaneps, A.J. and Geor, R.J. (eds) *Equine Sports Medicine & Surgery*. Saunders Elsevier, pp. 853–871.
McKeever, K.H., Hinchcliffe, K.W., Reed, S.W. *et al.* (1993) Role of decreased plasma volume in hematocrot alterations during incremental treadmill exercise in horses. *American Journal Physiology* 265, R404–R408.
McKenzie, E.C., Valberg, S.J., Pagan, J.D. *et al.* (2002) Electrolyte balance in Thoroughbred horses with recurrent exertional rhabdomyolysis consuming diets with varying dietary cation-anion balance. *American Journal of Veterinary Research* 63, 1053–1060.
Meyer, H.(1987). Nutrition of the equine athlete. In: Gillespie, J.R. and Robinson, N.E. (eds) *Equine Exercise Physiology 2*. ICEEP Publishing, Davis, California, pp. 644–673.
Meyer, H. (2015) Nutrition of the equine athlete. In: Gillespie, J.R. and Robinson, N.E. (eds) *Equine Exercise Physiology 2*. ICEEP, Davis, California, pp. 644–673.
Mickelson, J.R. and Valberg, S.J. (2015) The genetics of skeletal muscle disorders in horses. *Annual Review of Animal Biosciences* 3, 197–217.
Monreal, L., Garzon, N., Espada, Y., Ruiz-Gopegui, R. and Homedes, J. (1999) Electrolyte vs. glucose – electrolyte isotonic solutions for oral rehydration therapy in horses. *Equine Veterinary Journal* (Suppl. 30), 425–429.
Naylor, R.J. (2015) Exertional rhabdomyolysis: recent advances in knowledge. *Livestock* 20(5), 294–297.
Powell, D.M., Bennett-Wimbush, K., Peeples, A. and Duthie, M. (2008) Evaluation of indicators of weight-carrying ability of light riding horses. *Journal of Equine Veterinary Science* 28(1), 28–33.
Rose, R.J. (1981) A physiological approach to fluid and electrolyte therapy in the horse. *Equine Veterinary Journal* 13(1), 7–14.
Rose, R.J. and Hodgson, D.R. (eds) (2000) *Manual of Equine Practice*, 2nd edn. W.B. Saunders, Philadelphia, Pennsylvania, p. 769.
Rose, R.J., Arnold, K.S., Church, S. and Paris, R. (1980) Plasma & sweat electrolyte concentrations in the horse during long distance exercise. *Equine Veterinary Journal* 12, 19–22.
Schedl, H.P., Maughan, R.J. and Gisolvi, C.V. (1994) Intestinal absorption during rest and exercise: implications for formulating an oral rehydration solution (ORS). *Medicine and Science in Sports and Exercise* 26, 267–280.
Sosa Leon, L.A., Davie, A.J., Hodgson, D.R. and Rose R.J. (1995) The effects of tonicity, glucose concentration and temperature of an oral rehydration solution on its absorption and elimination. *Equine Veterinary Journal* (Suppl. 20), 140–146.
Stewart, A.J. (2015) Magnesium homeostasis and derangements In: Fielding, C.L. and Magdesian, K.G. (eds) *Equine Fluid Therapy*, 1st edn. John Wiley & Sons Inc., Ames, Iowa, pp. 76–87.
Tasker, J.B. (1967) Fluid and electrolyte studies in the horse III: intake and output of water, sodium and potassium in normal horses. *Cornell Veterinarian* 57, 649–657.
Toribio, R.E. (2015) Phosphorus homeostasis and derangements In: Fielding, C.I. and Magdesian, K.G. (eds) *Equine Fluid Therapy*, 1st edn. John Wiley & Sons Inc., Ames, Iowa, pp. 88–100.
Valberg, S., Häggendal, J. and Lindholm, A. (1993) Blood chemistry and skeletal muscle metabolic responses to exercise in horses with recurrent exertional rhabdomyolysis. *Equine Veterinary Journal* 25, 17–22.
Warren, L.K., Lawrence, L.M., Brewster-Barnes, T. and Powell, D.M. (1999) The effect of dietary fibre on hydration status after dehydration with frusemide. *Equine Veterinary Journal* (Suppl. 30), 508–513.

14 Feeding for Breeding

Louise Jones

Scout Farm

Learning Objectives

LO1 Describe and compare common feeding managements for the breeding horse.
- Understand the natural and artificial breeding seasons.
- Review the role of diet in reproductive efficiency.

LO2 Describe how to feed through 1st, 2nd and 3rd trimesters.
- Managing the broodmare who is a good doer.
- Feeding the broodmare with higher energy demand.

LO3 Explain how to feed through lactation.

LO4 Describe how to feed the foal from birth to weaning.
- Explain the importance of colostrum.
  - Discuss the nutritional options for orphaned foals.
- Foal management tips to minimise the risk of feed-related developmental orthopaedic disease (DOD).

LO5 Feeding the youngster from weaning to 2 years old.
- Recognise the value of monitoring body condition and growth rate in youngstock.

LO6 Discuss the nutritional requirements of stallions.

At the end of this chapter, you will be able to summarise the changes in nutrient requirements through the breeding cycle from conception through to weanling/yearling, so you can advise the client on the correct ration for the breeding horse to support the healthy development of the foetus through to yearling.

Introduction and Overview

It is acknowledged that only 25% of genetic differences is down to genetics, the remaining 75% is the interaction between our genes and our pre- and post-natal nutritional environment (Teh *et al.*, 2014). In people, suboptimum nutrition *in utero* (over- or underfeeding of energy, protein or micronutrients) reduces growth rate, increasing the risk of obesity in early childhood (Sharkey *et al.*, 2009) and obesity, diabetes and hypertension in offspring (Roseboom *et al.*, 2003, 2006; Fowden *et al.*, 2005; Gicquel *et al.*, 2008; Sathishkumar *et al.*, 2009). Gestating animals fed restricted protein and vitamins and minerals produce offspring that are born with insulin resistance (Moysten and Symonds, 2009), because the foetus adapts to maximise uptake of nutrients ensuring they are metabolically prepared to survive a low-nutrient diet, typical of native ponies.

Overnutrition during pregnancy has been linked to neonatal adiposity, obesity and metabolic issues in the offspring (Samuelsson *et al.*, 2008; Ford *et al.*, 2009).

Often mares are overweight and pass that adiposity on to their foals (Eriksson *et al.*, 2015). This does not mean that foals are not born fat but rather that they are born with a higher adiposity, i.e. have a higher fat:muscle cell ratio (Fall, 2011). This often results in a challenge for the owner, making these horses particularly challenging to manage. If diet meets a foal's metabolic capacity, then it will

DOI: 10.1079/9781789245134.0014

not become diseased; exceed that metabolic capacity and it is biologically disadvantaged.

There is a massive body of literature across all species, including horses, providing evidence that the uterine nutritional environment has a direct impact on the foetus's future metabolic capacity (Satterfield *et al.*, 2010; Coverdale *et al.*, 2015; Peugnet *et al.*, 2016; Fowden *et al.*, 2006).

Clearly the correct nutrition needs to start preconception and continue through pregnancy, lactation, growth and maturation, not forgetting the stallion of course.

Your nutritional advice is key for a successful pregnancy, for the health of the foal and its future offspring. Whilst clinicians dealing with studs are familiar with the intricacies of breeding, for many it is an unfamiliar subject as it happens infrequently. This chapter aims to provide enough detail for both the experienced and less experienced clinician.

Natural and Artificial Breeding Seasons

The horse is a seasonal breeder and mares experience anoestrus during the winter months, when there are fewer hours of daylight. During early spring, the mare's oestrus cycle begins to normalise. This 'transitional stage' lasts around 60–90 days, after which the normal 21-day oestrous cycles begin. Photoperiod, temperature and nutrition all play a part in 'switching on' the mare's oestrous cycle.

Natural breeding season

The natural breeding season is designed to coincide with seasonal changes in the nutritional value and availability of pasture (Fig. 14.1); grass is an important source of nutrients for horses breeding during the natural breeding season (Table 14.1). Most sports and leisure horses, those used in embryo transfer (ET) programmes or mares being bred by artificial insemination (AI) will be bred during the natural season.

Artificial breeding season

If your client is based in the northern hemisphere and breeding Thoroughbreds (TBs) destined for the racetrack, they will use the artificial breeding season, which declares 1 January as the official date of birth for all foals. Although natural covering is required, the artificial breeding season of the racing TB means that mares often enter their last trimester or early lactation during the winter months.

> **Top tip**
>
> In the racing industry, mares are typically re-bred annually, often on their first oestrous cycle after parturition, so are concurrently lactating and pregnant.

Mares will be placed under lights, or wear specifically designed light masks, to mimic the increasing

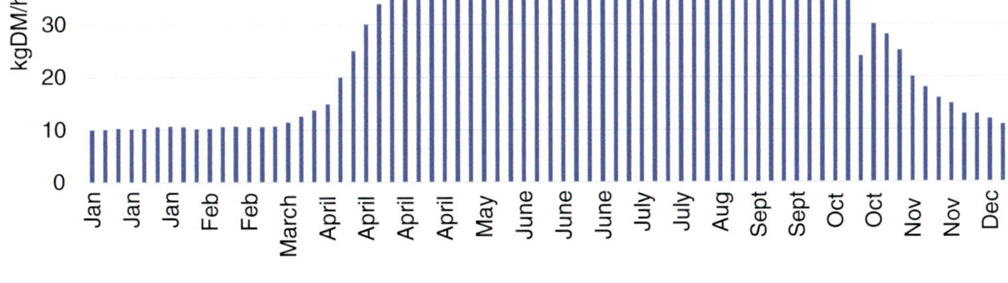

Fig. 14.1 Typical grass growth in the UK. (Adapted from Agriculture and Horticulture Development Board, 2019.)

Table 14.1 The relevance of grass availability to breeding stock during the natural breeding season

Season	Relevance of grass availability
Spring	The spring 'flush' of grass growth helps to: • provide a rising plane of nutrition prior to the breeding season; and • provide foals with access to good-quality forage during 'natural' weaning.
Summer	Continued good grazing during the summer months helps to: • ensure stallions maintain weight during the breeding season; • support condition and milk production in lactating mares; and • support growth in youngstock.
Autumn	The autumn 'flush' of grass growth helps to: • support continued milk production; • aid weight gain for horses that may have lost weight during the breeding season; and • support growth in youngstock.
Winter	Grass growth declines in the winter to coincide with, or contribute to: • decreased milk production; and • slowing of growth rate in youngstock.

day length that would occur naturally during the spring months. Most TB breeders prefer to have foals born early in the season (January–March), as they will be more mature when offered for sale or when racing as 2- or 3-year-olds, compared with foals born later in the season.

Feeding the Broodmare

Overview: implications of epigenetics

Whilst further research is required, current evidence suggests that maternal diet plays an important role in foetal programming, affecting the long-term health and athletic performance of the foal.

In horses, maternal overnutrition has been shown to alter the uterine environment and lipid profiles of embryos (Sessions-Bresnahan *et al.*, 2018); reducing colostrum immunoglobulin G (IgG) concentrations, impairing insulin sensitivity and increasing leptin concentrations in the foal (Ousey *et al.*, 2008; George *et al.*, 2009; Thorson *et al.*, 2010; Cavinder *et al.*, 2012).

Severe undernutrition of the mare during mid-pregnancy negatively affects *in utero* growth and birth weight (Wilsher and Allen, 2006). Foals born to undernourished mares have delayed testicular maturation, decreased insulin sensitivity and reduced cannon bone width (Robles *et al.*, 2017). Depending on the nutrient restriction, epigenetic changes occur (DNA methylation, histone post-translational modifications and non-coding RNA) which change gene expression for target genes, resulting in changes in fat deposition and energy homeostasis in the foal and up to three more generations, (van Dijk *et al.*, 2015).

Nutritional requirements

The nutritional requirements during pregnancy and lactation are well defined (NRC, 2007) (Table 14.2) and assume that the horse is in moderate condition. Energy intake may need to be adjusted for individuals that are over- or underweight.

Pre-pregnancy

Energy requirements

You should start talking to your clients several months before they plan to breed. The mare should be neither fat nor thin, because this will affect her reproductive efficiency (Sessions-Bresnahan *et al.*, 2016). Mares coming into the breeding season at BFS 3–3.5/5 start cycling earlier and have higher conception rates, whereas mares in low body condition (BFS < 2.5/5) require more cycles per conception, with an increased risk of early embryonic loss (Henneke *et al.*, 1984; Cavinder *et al.*, 2009).

Low body condition, or bodyweight loss, in the immediate pre-breeding period may alter leptin levels (Fitzgerald and McMannus, 2000; Fitzgerald *et al.*, 2002; Čebulj-Kadunc and Cestnik, 2008), reducing fertility by 66% (Fradinho *et al.*, 2014).

The overweight mare

Many mares have fat scores > 3.5, 3.5, 3.5 (> 7/9). Obesity is linked to reduced reproductive efficiency

Table 14.2 Daily nutrient requirements of 500 kg horse during pregnancy. (Made using data from NRC, 2007.)

	DE (MJ)	CP (g)	Vitamin A (iu)	Vitamin E (iu)	Calcium (g)	Phosphorus (g)	Magnesium (g)	Copper (mg)	Iodine (mg)	Zinc (mg)	Selenium (mg)
Maintenance											
Average	69.8	630	15,000	500	20	14	7.5	100	3.5	400	1
Month of pregnancy											
< 5	71.6	630	30,000	800	20	14	7.5	100	3.5	400	1
5	72.8	685									
6	74.9	704									
7	77	729			28	20	7.6				
8	80	759									
9	84.5	797			36	26.3	7.7	125	4.0		
10	89.6	841									
11	71.6	893									
Lactation											
1 month	132.7	1535	30,000	1000	59.1	38.3	11.2	125	4.4	500	1.25
2 months	132.7	1530			58.9	38.1	11.1				
3 months	128.	1468			55.9	36	10.9				
4 months	123	1398			41.7	26.6	10.5				
5 months	118	1330			39.5	24.7	10.2				
6 months	113.8	1265			37.4	23.2	8.7				

in the mare, including longer oestrous cycles, delayed anoestrus and increased risk of abnormal follicle maturation (Henneke *et al.*, 1984). It is also associated with insulin dysregulation and possibly leptin resistance (Table 14.3).

> **Top tip**
>
> Encourage your client to assess their mare's BW and BFS (see Chapter 3: 'Body fat scoring') well in advance of the breeding season, allowing sufficient time for any necessary weight gain or loss to be achieved.

Protein requirements

Protein provision is important for reproductive efficiency. Mares fed a diet low in quality protein develop a greater number of smaller follicles during the transitional period, ovulate later in the breeding season and are at greater risk of embryonic loss (van Niekerk and van Niekerk, 1997, 1998).

Vitamins and minerals

Vitamin and mineral deficiencies, or imbalances, have been linked to reproductive issues in several species (Stowe, 1967; Hidiroglou, 1979; Ingle *et al.*, 2017; Wilson *et al.*, 2018). Even well-maintained spring and summer pasture is deficient in some vitamins and minerals (Jones *et al.*, 2005).

Antioxidant intake is particularly important, because oxidative damage can have a detrimental effect on female fertility, causing low oocyte quality and reduced conception rates and increasing the risk of abortion (Vural *et al.*, 2000; Ruder *et al.*, 2009; Abuelo *et al.*, 2015; Wojsiat *et al.*, 2017). Omega-3 fatty acids could be beneficial for female fertility, by helping inhibit prostaglandin production, prolonging the maintenance of the corpus luteum (CL) (Lass and Belluzzi, 2019), aged mares fed a supplement containing a combination of antioxidants and omega-3 fatty acids had improved oocyte metabolic function and embryo development (Catandi *et al.*, 2020).

Dietary advice

The mare should be placed on a rising plane of nutrition 3–4 weeks prior to covering and should have a BFS of 3–3.5/5 at conception to maximise reproductive efficiency (challenging for mares that are overweight); advise maintaining current BFS but no further weight gain. Weight loss in the 4–8 weeks prior to the breeding season is not recommended and may negatively affect the onset of oestrus.

Access to grazing

Breeding in the natural breeding season means access to good-quality spring/summer pasture, which can provide the mare with excess energy and protein intake prior to covering, resulting in unwanted weight gain (Fig. 14.2).

Although fresh pasture is a good source of vitamin E, and α-linolenic acid, it will not supply optimal levels of other essential minerals such as copper and zinc (Table 14.4). You should recommend feeding a multivitamin and mineral supplement or a feed balancer for light work to rectify the deficiencies (Fig. 14.2).

Some clients like to feed a stud feed prior to conception, but there is no justification for this, because the grass is providing excess calories and they are likely to be feeding less than recommended quantities (Fig. 14.3). If grass is poor and additional calories are required to maintain condition, you would be better advising a leisure feed.

Limited or no access to good grazing

Access to good-quality pasture is likely to be limited for Thoroughbred mares breeding during the artificial breeding season.

Higher levels of hard feed will be required to balance energy, protein and micronutrient intake from conserved forages; a stud cube or muesli is recommended (Fig. 14.4).

> **Top tip**
>
> Balancing micronutrients:
>
> - If your client is feeding less that the recommended amount it will be necessary to 'top up' micronutrient intake.
> - Advise feeding a feed balancer or multivitamin and mineral supplement in proportion.
>   - If feeding half the recommended amount of Stud Cubes, recommend half the daily recommended amount of balancer or vitamin/mineral supplement.

Table 14.3 The effect of obesity on conception rates and foal health

Condition	Effect	Reference
Insulin resistance	• Increases the risk of problems such as laminitis. • Detrimental effect on reproductive efficiency. • Increased inter-ovulatory periods and greater numbers of subordinate follicles. • Vary depending on factors such as parity, BFS, age. • Pregnancy-induced IR in a mare with pre-existing IR, advise low NSC diet.	Prado, 2016 Seghieri *et al.*, 2005; Shalayel *et al.*, 2011; Rebholz *et al.*, 2012
Insulin sensitivity	Decreases slightly during pregnancy, limiting maternal glucose utilisation, shunting adequate supply to the foetus.	Fowden *et al.*, 1984; George *et al.*, 2011 Bell *et al.*, 1999
Mares with high fat score	Produce milk with a high fat and low protein content	Doreau *et al.*, 1993

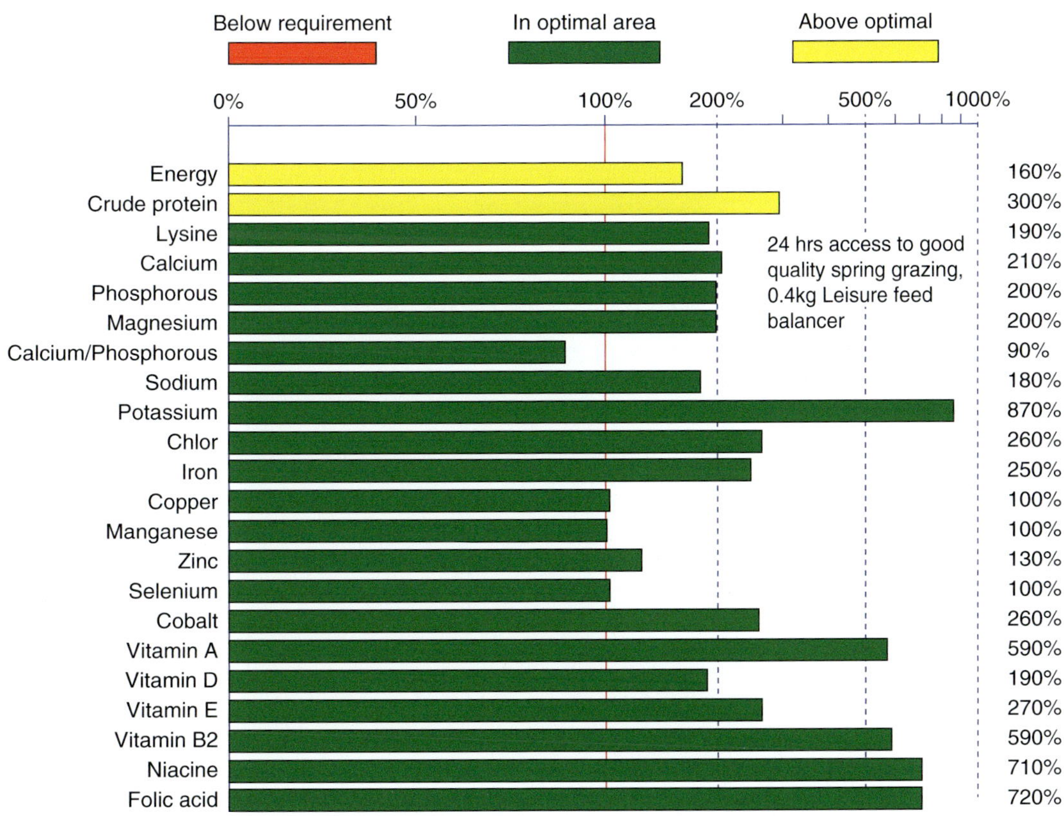

Fig. 14.2 Diet check for a 440 kg Connemara broodmare. The micronutrient content of the diet is within the optimal range but excess calories and protein. Access to pasture may need to be restricted and replaced with a suitable conserved forage to limit further weight gain (see Chapter 4) or advise a muzzle (see Chapter 9).

Table 14.4 Average mineral content of UK pasture, hay and haylage (Jones *et al.*, 2005; Jones, 2020, unpublished)

Mineral (/kg DM)	Summer pasture	Hay	Haylage	NRC (2007) requirements
Calcium (g/kg)	7.3	4.2	4.4	4.7[a]
Phosphorus (g/kg)	3.1	2.2	2.3	2.6[a]
Magnesium (g/kg)	1.6	1.1	1.2	0.7[a]
Zinc (mg/kg)	27.8	19.5	22.9	40[b]
Copper (mg/kg)	6.4	4.1	4.7	10[b]

[a]Based on a 12-month-old 500 kg mature weight horse, consuming 2.5% of bodyweight as DM.
[b]Based on all horses irrespective of physiological status.

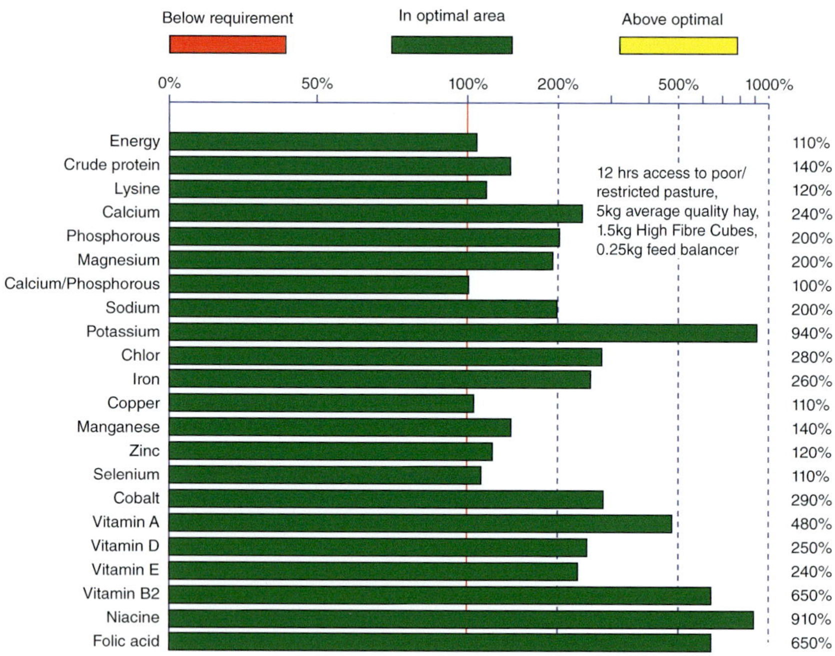

Fig. 14.3 Diet check for a 500 kg Irish Sports Horse broodmare. All nutrients are within the optimal range.

Gestation

Gestation is the period from conception to birth. In the mare it averages 340 days (range 320–370 days) divided into three trimesters (Table 14.5).

1st Trimester

Energy and protein

Mares must not be allowed to become obese during this period, but do not advise weight loss during the first trimester even if your client's mare is overweight.

If breeding in a natural cycle:

- Nutrient requirements are similar to horse at maintenance or in light work.
- Does not need extra energy/protein if good-quality grass available.

When bred out of season:

- Supplementary feed needs to balance hay/haylage.

Vitamins and minerals

The broodmare's mineral requirements do not increase in the first trimester of pregnancy (NRC,

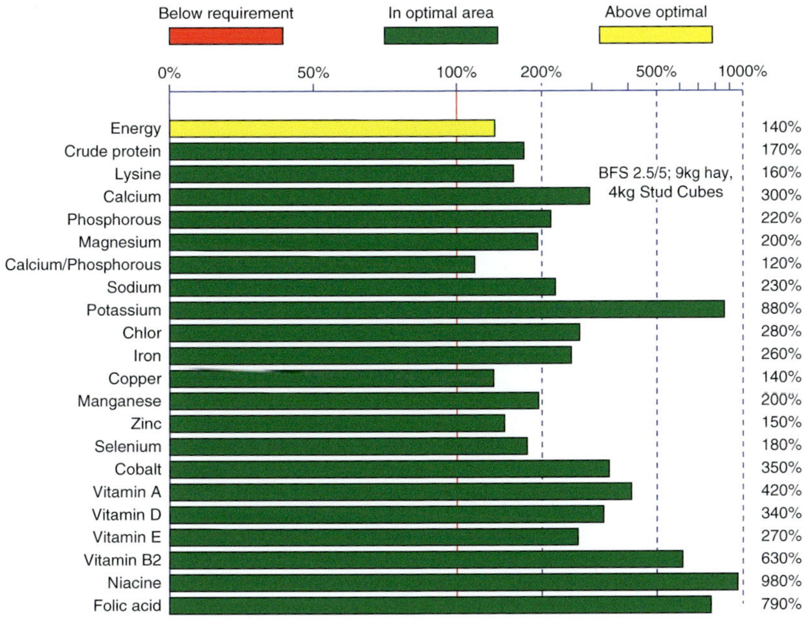

Fig. 14.4 Diet check for a 500 kg Thoroughbred brood mare. Energy intake is higher than basic requirements to facilitate weight gain. All other nutrients are within the optimal range.

Table 14.5 The pregnancy and lactation cycle

	1st trimester	2nd trimester	3rd trimester	Total	Lactation
Duration	0–113 4 months	114–226 4–8 months	227–340 8–12 months	320–365 11.4–12.8 months Mean 340 days / 11 months	6–8 months
Energy requirements	Maintenance (M)	Maintenance	1.1×M 9th month 1.13×M 10th month 1.2×M 11th month		Early 2×M Mid 1.4×M Late 1.2×M

2007) (Table 14.2). Based on foetal deposition data, requirements for vitamins A and E increase from conception (Meyer and Ahlswede, 1978; Lawrence, 2013) (Table 14.2).

Dietary advice

Natives and pleasure horses

- Leisure balancers 100 g/100 kg BW to provide micronutrients and protein (Fig. 14.5) unless losing fat, then a leisure feed (200–400 g/100 kg BW).

Sports horses

As per natives unless in work.

- Advise for current workload, no extra for pregnancy.

Thoroughbreds

If lactating:

- Stud ration at 0.8–1.2 kg/100 kg BW.
- No additional requirements for pregnancy.
- Use PCHorse to check.

If maiden:

- Feed for maintenance to balance forages.
- Often studs like to feed a stud ration.
- If feeding less than recommended, then advise a stud balancer.

2nd Trimester

Energy and protein

The mare's energy and protein requirements increase from the fifth month of pregnancy (Table 14.2).

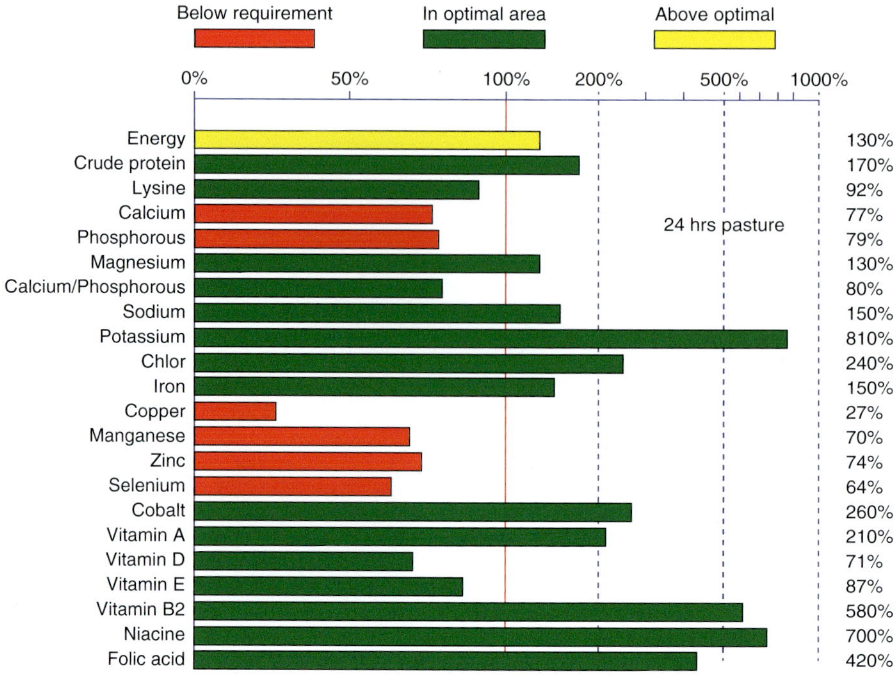

Fig. 14.5 Diet check for a 200 kg pony broodmare, early pregnancy, non-lactating. Calorie intake is above requirements but deficient in several micronutrients: advise a leisure balancer. Access to pasture may need to be restricted and replaced with a suitable conserved forage to limit further weight gain (see Chapter 4) or advise a muzzle.

Most weight gain is expected to occur during the final trimester, but the mare might gain significant weight (Lawrence *et al.*, 1992), providing a nutritional buffer should food sources become scarce during the later stage of pregnancy.

If weight loss is required, it is safer for your client to attempt this during the second trimester, but this must be carefully monitored, as sudden weight loss in mid-gestation detrimentally affects placental development, reducing foetal growth (Wilsher and Allen, 2006). Do not forget that foetal size will increase mare's BW; encourage clients to BFS.

Vitamins and minerals

Inadequate mineral intake is common during mid-gestation, potentially with significant effects on the developing foal. Your client may not appreciate that forage will not provide adequate levels of several minerals, particularly if their mare is maintaining or even gaining condition. Recommend that your client feeds a feed balancer or a multivitamin and mineral supplement (Fig. 14.6).

If individual feeding is not possible, a 'mineral bucket/lick' can be provided, although daily intake is likely to be unreliable.

Dietary advice

Natives and sports horses

- Advise clients to continue the same feeding as the 1st trimester but if grass is low quality or low availability or conserved forage, slowly move across to stud balancer.
- If the mare is gaining excessive weight on pasture, intake may need to be restricted and an alternative lower-calorie forage such as a late-cut hay provided.

Thoroughbreds

- Feed intake might need adjusting or changing depending on grass growth and if foal at foot was weaned early.
- If reducing stud feed, then substitute with same proportion of stud balancer to maintain vitamins and minerals.

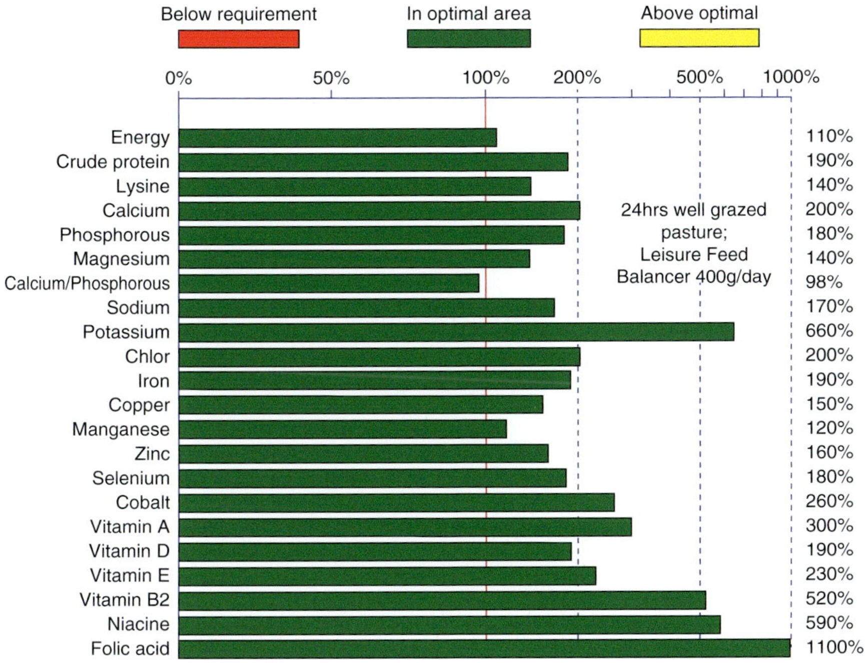

Fig. 14.6 Diet check for a 400 kg Arab mare, 5th month gestation. All nutrients are within the optimal range. All horses grazing will consume excess potassium.

3rd Trimester

Energy and protein

Over 60% of foetal growth takes place in late gestation and the mare's energy and protein requirements continue to increase (Table 14.2). Mares should be expected to gain around 12–15% BW throughout pregnancy; the majority of this happens during late gestation.

Moderate energy restriction during late pregnancy, though undesirable, does not appear to affect the foal's birth weight, although an increase in gestation length has been noted (Banach and Evans, 1981; Henneke *et al.*, 1984; Hines *et al.*, 1987). The effects of more severe energy deficits during the latter stages of gestation are currently unknown.

Excessive energy intake will result in increased adiposity and the risk of conditions such as laminitis, particularly in mares suffering from a pre-existing metabolic abnormality (Table 14.3).

Energy intake is inversely correlated with colostral IgG concentrations but does not appear to cause failure of passive transfer (FPT) (Coverdale *et al.*, 2015).

Vitamins and minerals

The requirements for calcium, phosphorus and magnesium increase from the seventh month (Table 14.2); deficiencies or imbalances in these minerals may result in skeletal weakness in the foal (Glade, 1993).

The mare's requirements for zinc and selenium do not increase during gestation; however, the selenium status of the neonatal foal depends on placental passage (Dill and Rebhun, 1985). Adequate selenium prevents white muscle disease (WMD) in newborn foals (Thorson *et al.*, 2010; McKenzie, 2018).

Requirements for copper (Cu), iodine and iron, and to a lesser degree sodium and chloride, increase from the 9th month of pregnancy (NRC, 2007). The mare's intake of Cu is correlated with liver copper concentrations in the foal ensuring foetal liver stores (Meyer and Ahlswede, 1978). Adequate supplementation of the mare is essential, as copper administration via injection does not influence foal copper status (Pearce *et al.*, 1998b). Copper status in the foal is related to maternal dietary intake during gestation but does not appear to be improved by supplementation of the mare post-partum (Pearce *et al.*, 1998a,b). Copper intake should be considered alongside the levels of antagonists such as zinc and iron.

Adequate vitamin E intake plays a key role in the immunoglobulin content of colostrum and transfer of passive immunity to the foal (Hoffman *et al.*, 1999); colostral IgG levels are improved with vitamin E (Janicki *et al.*, 2000; Thorson *et al.*, 2010).

Dietary advice

It is important to support foetal growth.

Natives, sports horses and leisure horses

Overnutrition is more likely to cause a problem than undernutrition.

- Inexperienced breeders think their mare requires a stud mix or cube in late gestation; these will provide too much energy (Fig. 14.7).
- Change from leisure balancer to stud balancer (100 g/100 kg BW).

Thoroughbred mares foaling in January–March

- Late gestation during the winter.
  - Nutritional value and availability of pasture low.
  - Reliant on conserved forage and hard feed to meet their nutritional needs.
- Advise stud mix or cube (0.6–1.2 kg/100 kg BW) (Fig 14.8).

Mares may back off their forage, especially conserved forage, and hard feed.

- Encourage clients to divide the mare's ration into several small meals.
- If intake falls appreciably below the manufacturer's recommended daily intake:
  - Advise proportional replacement with feed balancer.
- If mare is a maiden or has a history of poor colostrum quality:
  - Advise additional omega-3 fatty acids (e.g. fish oil, linseed oil) and vitamin E.

Lactation

Colostrum

Colostrum accumulates in the mare's teats ('waxing up') normally 1–4 days before parturition, but the mare can wax up and even drip colostrum for days before foaling. The 'running' of small amounts

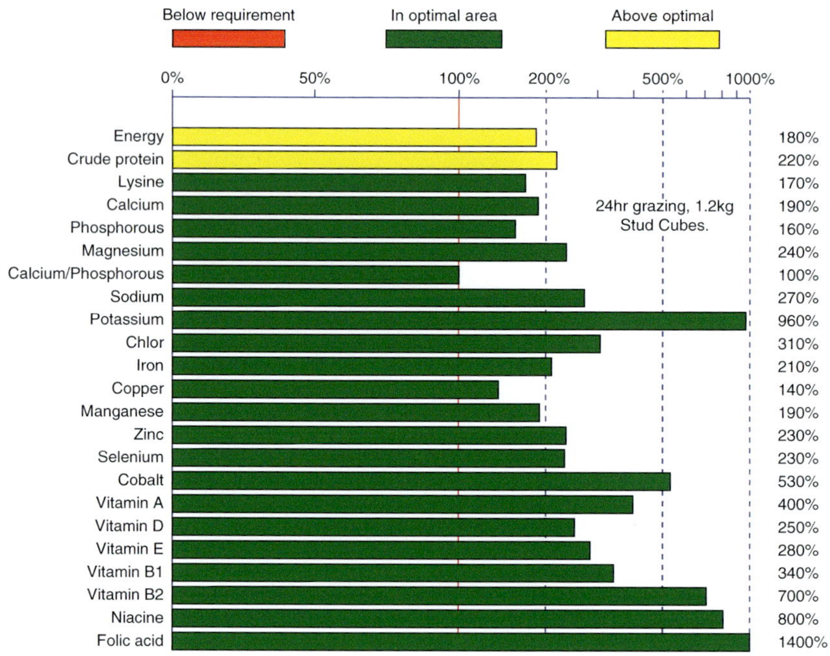

Fig. 14.7 Diet check for a 300 kg Dartmoor broodmare, late pregnancy. The energy and protein content of the diet is above requirements. Advise stud balancer at 100 g/100 kg BW and restrict grass intake, but maintain DMI.

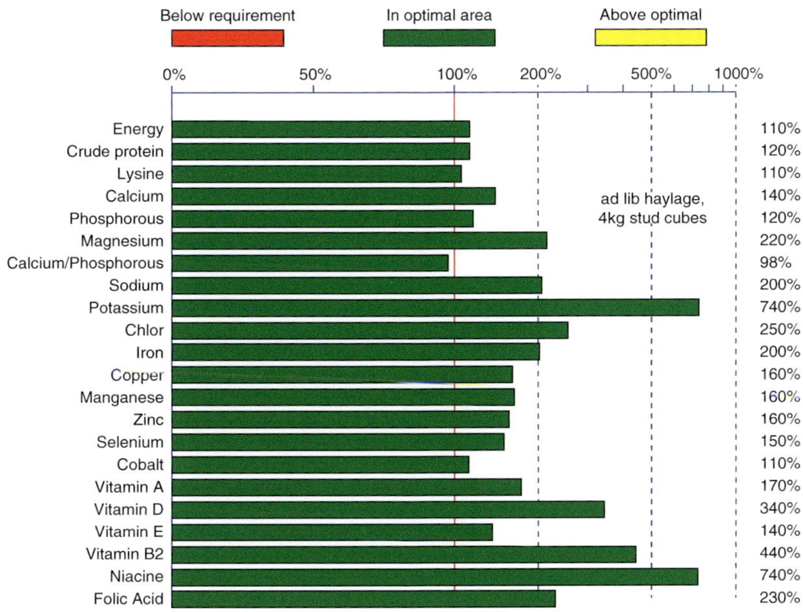

Fig. 14.8 Diet check for a 525 kg Thoroughbred broodmare, late pregnancy. All nutrients are within the optimal range.

of colostrum close to foaling is not uncommon, but premature lactation should be investigated as it often is associated with abortion.

> **Top tip**
>
> If large amounts of colostrum are lost the foal may need an alternative supply to ensure adequate passive transfer of immunoglobulins (Igs). It is vital for the mare to pass on protection to her foal via colostrum – proteins reduce by 20% and Igs by 40% after 24 h (Rouse and Ingram, 1970).

Requirements

Lactation is a period of substantial physiological stress for the broodmare. During this time, the mare must recover from parturition, potentially re-breed and produce milk. Milk production is estimated to be 3–4% BW during the first 2 months of lactation, after which it gradually declines to approximately 2% BW at 5 months post-foaling (Gibbs *et al.*, 1982; Santos and Silvestre, 2008). Lactation can be broadly divided into two stages: early lactation, which is from birth until 3 months; and late lactation, from 3 months after foaling until weaning

Energy

The mare's energy requirements are twice that of maintenance – higher than many racing TBs. Failure to provide adequate energy intake will result in weight loss and may decrease subsequent reproductive performance (Henneke *et al.*, 1984); this is particularly important for TB mares who are usually re-bred. The mare's diet can to some extent influence the nutritional value of milk. Certainly, severe or prolonged dietary deficiencies reduce both milk output and its nutritional content (Gibbs *et al.*, 1982; Martin *et al.*, 1991; Gentry *et al.*, 2002). However, provided that your client's mare is in good condition, moderate energy and protein restrictions do not appear to affect the volume or nutritional value of milk, because the mare mobilises her own body stores of energy, protein and minerals in order to meet the demands of milk production (Manso Filho *et al.*, 2008).

Mares fed excess energy produce milk that has a lower concentration of total solids, protein, fat and gross energy, although foal growth is unaffected, maybe because excess energy intake results in increased yields of less nutrient-dense milk (Pagan and Hintz, 1986; Doreau *et al.*, 1993).

The source of calories provided to the mare may also play a role in milk composition. Mares receiving proportionately higher amounts of energy from dietary fat had increased levels of certain fatty acids in the milk (Zeyner *et al.*, 1996; Hoffman *et al.*, 1998). The practical significance of these findings is unknown, but maybe beneficial for foal health.

Protein

Your client should also consider both the total amount and the quality of protein being fed. Specifically formulated feeds for broodmares will contain high-quality protein sources such as soyabean or alfalfa; check the label! The protein requirements are twice that of maintenance.

Vitamins and minerals

Requirements for most vitamins and minerals, particularly for the macrominerals calcium and phosphorus, which are found in large quantities in milk, increase during lactation (Table 14.2).

The mineral composition of mare's milk does not appear to be significantly affected by dietary intake (Breedveld *et al.*, 1988; Baucus et al., 1989). Research in humans has shown that the levels of certain minerals in breast milk such as B-vitamins and vitamins C and D are associated with maternal intake (Dror and Allen, 2018). Further research is required to establish the effect of maternal intake of vitamin concentrations in mare's milk

Dietary advice

The majority of owners will be aware of the mare's increased nutritional requirements and the lactating mare's appetite and feed intake will typically increase to approximately 3% BW.

Natives and sports horses

- If weight gain is not desired, and the mare is maintaining condition on grass, advise a stud feed balancer (Fig. 14.9).
- If grass quality drops, and the mare starts to lose weight just on balancer towards the end of lactation, advise product from a leisure range (unlikely to be fed at recommended intake) (Fig. 14.10).
  - Adjust stud balancer proportionately.

Thoroughbreds

- Ad libitum forage.
  - Conserved forage will not meet the lactating mare's micronutrient requirements.

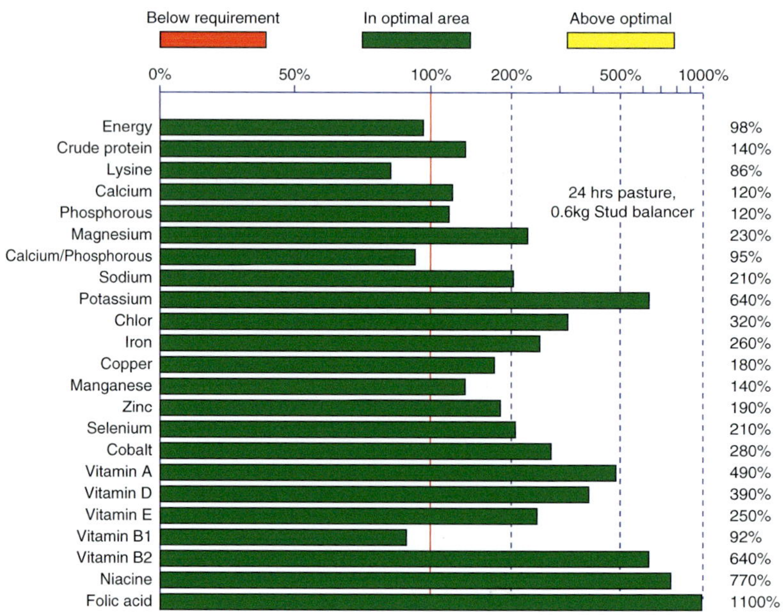

Fig. 14.9 Diet check for a 600 kg Warmblood broodmare, 2nd month lactation. All nutrients are within the optimal range. Advise monitoring fat score of mare and foal and add 0.5 kg alfalfa to improve lysine.

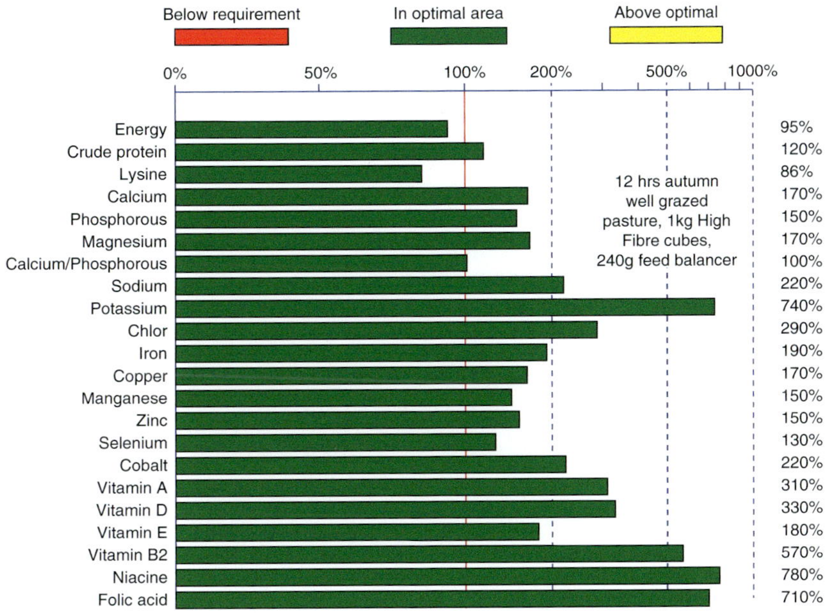

Fig. 14.10 Diet check for a 400 kg Connemara broodmare, 5th month lactation. All nutrients are within the optimal range.

- The amount of compound feed depends on forage quality and availability, stage of lactation, milk output and BFS.
- BFS the mare regularly and adjust her energy intake accordingly.
- Stud mix or cube is appropriate (0.6–1.4 kg/100 kg BW).
  - If feeding less than the manufacturer's recommended intake, advise a feed balancer in proportion (Fig. 14.11).
- Older nursing foals, if allowed by the mare, may consume significant amounts of the dam's feed.
  - Providing a suitable creep feed, in a way that does not allow the mare access, can help limit the foal's consumption of the mare's feed.

Drying off the mare prior to weaning

Despite a lack of evidence to support the practice, it is common for all hard feed to be removed from the mare to facilitate cessation of milk production, commonly referred to as 'drying off'. The author advises against this, particularly if it coincides with mid-gestation (i.e., if the mare has been re-bred).

Two weeks prior to weaning, advise gradual reduction of feed, which combined with the lack of suckling stimulus should be sufficient stop milk production. Maintain a balanced ration by advising a feed balancer or a multivitamin and mineral supplement.

> **Top tip**
>
> Remind your client to carefully observe the udder during the weaning period for any signs of problems (e.g. mastitis). It may also be necessary to explain that they should not milk the mare, even if she has a full bag, as this will only prolong milk production.

Feeding the Foal

At birth, the foal's BW is generally 10% of dam's BW, depending on the mare's age and parity (Wilsher and Allen, 2003; Meirelles *et al.*, 2017).

Neonates have a high metabolic rate and low glycogen reserves (Ousey, 2003; McKenzie and Geor, 2009) and if they fail to nurse they can rapidly become hypoglycaemic, hypovolaemic and hypothermic (Stoneham, 2016).

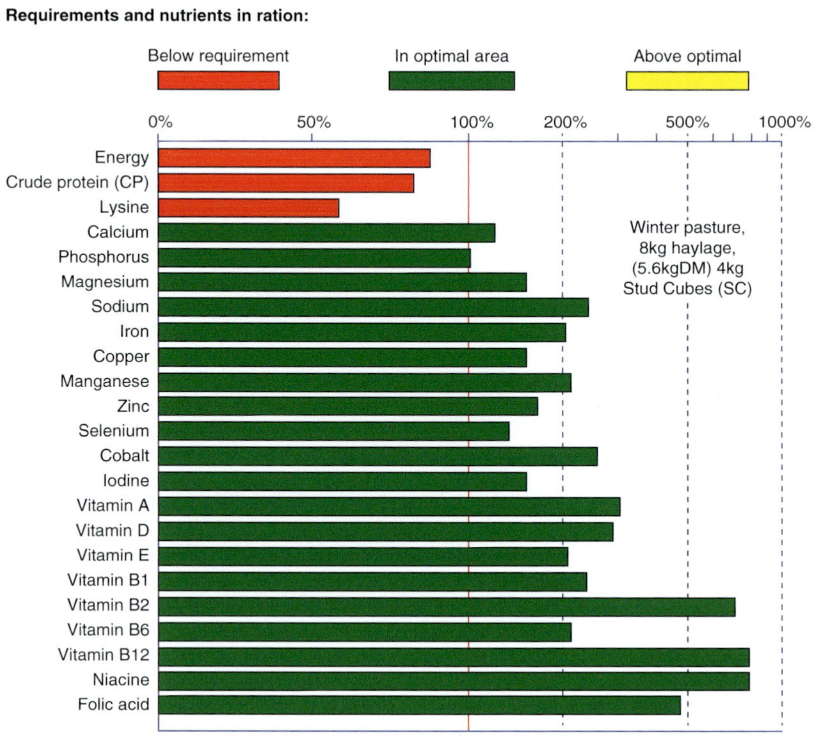

Fig. 14.11 Diet check for Thoroughbred broodmare, 600 kg, 2nd week lactation, foal at foot. Being fed the lowest recommended quantities (800 g/100 kg BW) of SC. Advise increasing, but check forage:conc ratio, currently 70% forage:30% ratio. Remember to ensure meal size does not provide more than 1g starch/kgBW/meal.

Colostrum

The ingestion of adequate amounts of good-quality colostrum (30–40 ml/kg BW) is essential for passive transfer of maternal derived immunoglobulins (IgG, IgA, IgM), lymphocytes and neutrophils needed for the development of the foal's immune system (Kohn *et al.*, 1989; Burns, 2007; Stoneham, 2016). Colostrum also contains growth factors (e.g. IGF-1 and IGF-2), enzymes and hormones (Burns, 2007). These non-nutrient components play an important role in preparing the gut for the digestion of enteral feed (Ousey, 2006).

Failure of passive transfer

Low IgG content of the colostrum, the foal not nursing or if the mare has 'run' colostrum can result in failure of passive transfer (FPT) or partial failure of passive transfer (PFPT), defined as serum IgG concentrations of < 400 mg/dl or 400–800 mg/dl, respectively, at 24 h (Tyler-McGowan *et al.*, 1997).

If FPT or PFPT has occurred and the foal is < 12 h old, colostrum should be provided orally or by nasogastric intubation. In foals > 12 h old, hyperimmune serum/plasma transfusion is often recommended (Freccero *et al.*, 2017; Nichola Reynolds, personal communication, 1 June 2020).

Top tips

Foals should ingest colostrum within 4 h of birth.

- Efficiency of absorption starts to decline after 6–8 h (Stoneham, 2013).
- Some foals may require assistance to stand and suckle.

Continued

Continued.

If the foal is unable to nurse, but the dam has plenty of colostrum, the mare should be milked, and the colostrum fed (5 ml/kg BW hourly) for 6–8 h using a bottle and suitable teat.

- The dam's own foal *must* nurse sufficiently before collection.
- Collect colostrum within 3–4 h of parturition.
- Amount taken will vary depending on the mare (250–500 ml for a 500 kg mare).
- Clean udder with warm water.
- A clean, preferably sterilised, container should be used to collect the colostrum.
- If necessary, colostrum can be administered via nasogastric intubation.

If the mare has inadequate or poor-quality colostrum, stored colostrum should be provided.

- Ideally, the IgG level should be tested; it needs to be, for example, direct assay – 1000 mg IgG/dl or a bioassay of 800 mg/dl in the foal's plasma.
- If your client does not already have one, you should encourage them to consider purchasing a Brix refractometer.
- If not using straight away:
  - Label with the mare's name, date and specific gravity (mg IgG/dl).
  - Store for up to 1 year in a household freezer.
  - Thaw at room temperature or slowly in water bath at 30–37.5°C.
  - Do not attempt to use direct heat or a microwave, which will lead to destruction of the immune proteins.

If your client has multiple mares, you should encourage them to collect and store good-quality colostrum. Colostrum should *not* be collected from:

- maiden mares;
- mares producing foals affected with neonatal isoerythrolysis (NI); or
- mares that have tested positive for red cell alloantibodies.

Milk (300–500 ml/day for a 500 kg mare) can also be collected and frozen for later use following the same principles. This should only be collected from a mare that appears to have large quantities and whose foal is strong and healthy.

Nursing Foals

Milk

The nursing foal will suckle up to 10 times an hour, with each bout lasting approximately 1 min, gradually decreasing to around twice per hour at 2–3 months of age (Smith-Funk and Crowell-Davis, 1992).

Normal physiological and physical parameters

The newborn foal should be monitored, where possible from a distance, for normal feeding behaviour (Table 14.6).

Table 14.6 Normal neonatal feeding behaviour (Kirsty McCann, personal communication, 5 January 2019)

Feeding behaviour	Time after parturition
Sternal recumbency	5 min
Attempt to stand	15 min
Suckle reflex	30 min
Standing	1–2 h
Suckling	2–3 h
Urination	6–10 h
Meconium passed	24 h

Creep feeding

Creep feeding minimises the risk of:

- gastrointestinal disturbances post-weaning;
- post-weaning depression in growth rates (Pugh and Williams, 1992) as the gut can adapt slowly;
- accelerated/compensatory growth, which may increase the risk of developmental orthopaedic disease (DOD); and
- the foal not wanting to eat an unfamiliar feed.

Monitoring growth rate (BW, height and BFS) is a useful guide as to when to advise creep feeding.

The month of birth may influence a foal's growth (Kocher and Staniar, 2013). Winter-born foals have slower growth rates than those born in the spring (Pagan *et al.*, 2006), which may be because of increased energy expenditure on thermoregulation rather than growth, although reduced nutrient intake in the lactating mare may also be a factor. Month of birth did not affect growth rate of UK Thoroughbreds for the first 200 days of age (Jones and Hollands, 2005). The considerable differences between Thoroughbred growth patterns around the world (Huntington *et al.*, 2007) are most likely a result of differences in seasonality, environment and feeding practices.

Top tip

Although foals will begin to consume non-milk carbohydrate sources from around 1 week of age, their ability to digest and utilise them may not be fully efficient until around 3–4 months of age.

Backward or weak foals

Backward or weak foals should be introduced to a suitable creep feed at 1–2 weeks old to increase their calorie intake.

Foals maintaining weight

There is no need to advise compound feed until 2–3 months of age, coinciding with a reduction in the nutritional value of milk. Various 'creep feeds' are available for feeding at 100–550 g/100 kg BW/day – check with the manufacturer as to the most suitable.

Dietary advice

Creep feeds are designed to be readily digested by young foals with immature hind-gut fermentative capacity and should contain a significant proportion of milk or other high-quality protein source, e.g. soyabean, fed at 1 kg/100 kg BW or 500 g/day/month of age.

Creep feeding systems

Creep feeding systems allow the foal, but not the mare, access to the feed. They vary from buckets with bars across the top, to feeding areas with openings only wide enough to allow the foal to enter (Fig. 14.12).

Top tip

- Make sure your client introduces creep feeding carefully, to accustom the foal over a few days or weeks.
- Ensure conserved forage, is hygienic and good quality.
  - Hay is preferable; haylage is more likely to induce diarrhoea in younger foals.

Orphan Foals

Orphan foals can be time consuming and emotional for amateur breeders. Do explain that it is not dissimilar to a baby insofar as the foal needs frequent nursing – often hourly to start.

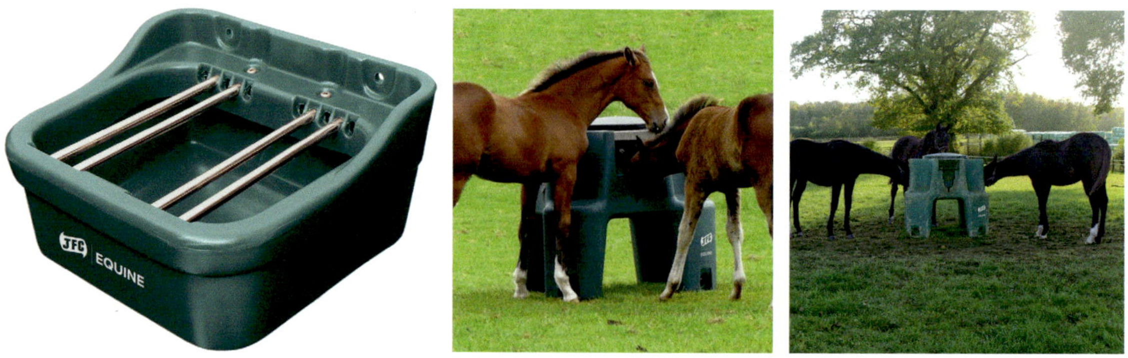

Fig. 14.12 Various creep feeding methods. (Images courtesy of JFC Equine.)

Foals > 3.5 months of age

Healthy foals orphaned at > 3.5 months of age do not necessarily require a milk-based diet, because the dietary requirements of these foals can be met through a combination of a suitable creep feed and ad libitum access to good-quality forage.

If a milk substitute is required for a very backward foal, advise feeding according to the manufacturer's instructions. Monitor average daily gain (ADG) to maintain constant growth rate; adjust feeding rates accordingly. Record daily intake of fresh, clean water.

Foals < 3.5 months of age

Younger foals will need a milk-based diet and if orphaned in the immediate post-partum period will also require adequate quantities of good-quality colostrum; IgG status should be tested to ensure that FPT or PFPT has not occurred.

Fostering

The TB foal should be fostered onto a suitable docile nurse or foster mare, which will take several days of intensive management. Using a scented blanket may assist with the fostering process (Kelly, 1999; Paradis, 2012a; Stoneham, 2013).

Foster mares should be matched as closely as possible for stage of lactation. If significant differences exist between the foal's age and the mare's stage of lactation, drench with commercial liquid vitamin and mineral supplement to compensate for the natural waning in the mineral content of milk (Stoneham, 2013).

Foster mares often produce large quantities of milk (Willard *et al.*, 2005). Monitor the foal closely, as increased ADG may result in developmental issues.

Milk replacers

If fostering is not possible, a specifically formulated mare's milk replacer should be fed. Milk pellets are not suitable as a replacement for 'liquid milk'.

> **Top tip**
>
> In an emergency, diluted goat's milk (75% milk to 25% water) or semi-skimmed (2% fat) cow's milk with 20 g of dextrose or glucose added per litre can be used. Sucrose should not be used, as young foals produce limited sucrase (Kevin Corley, personal communication, 19 August 2020; Wilson, 1987; Paradis, 2012a; Stoneham 2013)

Dietary advice: feeding schedule

Advise clients as follows.

- Foals 0–2 days of age are fed hourly.
- Foals from 3 to 14 days of age are fed every 2 h (Kevin Corley, personal communication, 19 August 2020; Ousey, 2003), gradually decreasing frequency and increasing volume (Table 14.7).
- Ad libitum access to a milk replacer is not recommended, as this can result in excessive ADG and increased risk of DOD.

> **Top tip**
>
> Recommend a more dilute solution to improve acceptability.
>
> - Use approximately 10–15% less milk powder than the manufacturer's recommendations.
> - Gradually increase, over 5–7 days, to recommended mixing strength.
>
> In the first few weeks, warming the milk to body temperature can increase acceptance

Advising feeding milk replacers

Your advice on feeding milk replacers will depend on your client's experience and commitment.

Bottle-feeding

Bottle-feeding is the most popular.

- Requires both patience and perseverance during first few days.
- Challenging to find a suitable teat.
  - Lamb teats are preferable.
- Those designed for calves are often too large and may lead to aspiration pneumonia, particularly in foals with perinatal asphyxia syndrome (Kevin Corley, personal communication, 19 August 2020).

Bottle-feeding may humanise the foal.

- To begin with your client may enjoy this.
- As the foal grows, often results in behavioural problems.

Transition to wide scoop or bucket

This should be encouraged as soon as possible.

- Transition from bottle to a wide scoop, then to bucket.
  - Reduces the amount of labour required.

Table 14.7 Milk replacer suggested feeding schedule and daily intakes

Age	Daily milk intake (ml/kg BW)	Number of milk feeds/day[a]	Creep feed[b] (g/kg BW/day)
Newborn	Colostrum		
1 day	100	24 (hourly)	0
2 days	200	24 (hourly)	0
3–14 days	200	12 (every 2 h)	0–5
2–3 weeks	200	7 (every 3 h, 5 h break overnight)	5–8
3–4 weeks	200	6 (every 3 h, 8 h break overnight)	5–8
4–14 weeks	150–200	6 (every 3 h, 8 h break overnight)	5–8
14+ weeks	Begin gradual weaning		8–15

[a]May need to be adjusted according to the individual
[b]Should be divided into 2–4 feeds/day so that meal size is no more than 4–5 g/100 kg BW/meal.

- Helps to maintain a dissociation between feeding and the handlers.
- Enables foal to consume smaller quantities at more frequent intervals compared with bottle-feeding.
- Reduces digestive upsets, 'pot-belly'.
- Advise client to place two clean fingers in the foal's mouth.
- When the foal starts to suck, lift the scoop to between the foal's elbow and shoulder height and slowly remove fingers.
- Once drinking from a scoop, the client can use a contrasting-colour bucket hung on a wall.
- The young foal can only distinguish between light and dark.

Diarrhoea and constipation

Diarrhoea and constipation are common in orphan foals and are related to feeding milk replacers, changes in the diet (e.g. introduction of creep feed) or consumption of large volumes of milk in a single meal.

Foals suffering from diarrhoea must be monitored carefully, as they can become dehydrated quickly.

Creep feeds for orphan foals

For foals receiving a milk replacer, 5–8 g/kg BW is considered typical, depending on BFS. Older orphan foals may require up to 15g/kg BW/day and can be introduced from around 1–2 weeks of age, although the foal may not consume significant quantities until they are around 4 weeks of age. Check manufacturer's intake recommendations. 'Weaning' usually occurs at around 3.5–5 months, provided that the foal is growing well, confidently grazing pasture and consuming a suitable creep ration.

Weanlings and Yearlings

In the wild, foals remain with their dams for extended periods and gradual weaning usually occurs at 8–12 months of age (Tyler 1972; Berger, 1986). In the domesticated horse, weaning is usually enforced at around 6 months of age, once the foal's digestive system is sufficiently mature.

Top tip

If constipation or scouring coincides with the introduction of a milk replacer or increase in the volume of milk per meal:

- Recommend feeding a more dilute solution, in more frequent meals.
  - Gradually reintroduced to a full-strength mix and slowly reduce feeding frequency.
- In foals older than 24 h, the use of pro- and prebiotics may be helpful.
- Discuss with your client the importance of maintaining high standards of hygiene.
  - Milk should be made immediately prior to feeding.
  - If necessary, the daily ration can be mixed ahead of time and kept covered in a refrigerator until it is used.
  - Any milk that is not used within 24 h should be discarded.
  - All utensils should be cleaned and sterilised after each use.
- Remind clients that it is common for foals reared on a milk replacer to have reduced muscle development and a more pot-bellied appeared. In most cases this is not a concern and will usually resolve by 4–6 months of age.

Energy requirements

Undersupply of dietary energy will result in poor body condition and reduced growth, whereas oversupply of calories will lead to rapid growth or excessive bodyweight, both of which are associated with DOD (Savage *et al.*, 1993a).

Growth rate and BFS need to be monitored to calculate energy requirements.

Monitoring energy intakes using growth rates

Advise clients to monitor and record the BW, using an equine weighbridge, and a height stick (Fig. 14.13).

If your client does not have access to a weighbridge, formulas can be used for estimating BW (Staniar *et al.*, 2004; Rodríguez *et al.*, 2007; Paradis, 2012a).

> **Top tip**
>
> Inexperience breeders may attempt to use a weight tape to assess BW, but these are not accurate for growing youngstock.

Estimating youngstock BW from predicted adult weight

If BW cannot be accurately assessed, then BW as a percentage of predicted adult BW can be used as a rough guide (Table 14.8).

BW can be plotted and compared with growth curves (GCs) (Fig. 14.14).

Most GCs are based on racing Thoroughbreds and may not be accurate for other breeds.

> **Top tips**
>
> - Growth curves, when combined with information of ADG, are useful to identify, and address, periods of reduced growth (e.g. post-weaning).
> - Growth curves should be specific to the horse's breed, month of birth and location.
>
> Body fat score for foals: currently no BFS system specifically for young horses.
>
> - Foals should be born with comparatively low levels of body fat.
> - Current recommendations are to use the lower end of the Henneke *et al.* (1983) BCS system when assessing young foals (Paradis *et al.*, 2012a).
> - Using the modified 0–5 scoring system (see Chapter 3) will help clients identify adiposity in the supra orbital fossa and above the nuchal ligament.

Protein

Adequate intake of quality protein is critical for growing youngstock; lysine is the first limiting

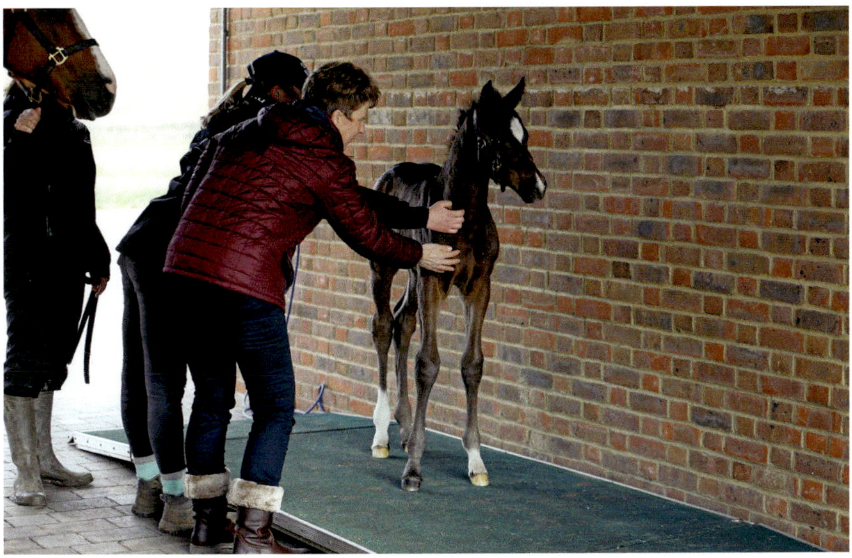

Fig. 14.13 Monitoring bodyweight of youngstock using a weighbridge. (Photo courtesy of Laura Green.)

Table 14.8 Estimated bodyweight and height as a percentage of mature BW and height. (Adapted from Jones *et al.*, 2005; NRC, 2007; Becvarova and Buechner-Maxwell, 2012.)

Age (months)	Estimated BW as a % of mature weight	Estimated height as a % of mature height
Birth	10%	61–64%
3	30–32%	70–73%
4	33–36%	75–78%
6	43–46%	80–82%
8	54–55%	84–85%
12	64–67%	85–90%
14	69–71%	90–92%
16	73–76%	92–94%
18	77–80%	94–96%
22	85–90%	96–98%

amino acid, followed by threonine and methionine (Graham *et al.*, 1994; Ott and Kivipelto, 2002). The total protein intake can be reduced if the intake of these limiting amino acids is adequate (Staniar *et al.*, 2001).

Top tip

- The levels of individual amino acids do not legally have to be declared.
  - Most feed companies will willingly provide details of the amino acid content of their products.
- In the absence of exact figures, check the list of ingredients.
  - High-quality protein sources (e.g. soyabean or alfalfa meal) should feature high on a descending list of ingredients.

Vitamins and minerals

The most critical minerals for healthy growth are calcium and phosphorus and the trace minerals copper and zinc. Check mineral balances; excessive levels of zinc and phosphorus reduce the absorption of copper and calcium, respectively, potentially resulting in increased risk of skeletal problems (NRC, 2007). The levels of other antagonists such as iron and molybdenum should also be considered.

Top tip

It is important that your clients are aware that even the best-quality pasture or conserved forage will not contain optimal levels of all the essential minerals needed to support optimal growth and development.

Although vitamins play a critical role in health, growth and development, the growing horse's requirements for several vitamins, including vitamin E and vitamin K, have not been well studied. Equally, toxicities for many vitamins have not been reported, or are extremely rare in horses.

Top tip

Over-supplementation is common:

- when youngstock are fed significantly higher than the recommended level of a commercial feed or supplement; or
- where several products are combined.

Weaning Methods

Ideally, the foal should be weaned into a group of other similarly aged weanlings to encourage normal psychological development.

Top tip

Recommend early weaning if:

- the foal is growing too rapidly;
- the foal is gaining excessive BW;
- the foal has signs of DOD; or
- the mare is becoming overly thin.

On the other hand, weaning may be delayed for foals that have been ill or are immature for their age.

Weaning methods will depend on:

- your client's individual circumstances;
- the availability of resources and facilities;

Gold Dust 2021 (Stud Farm 2021)

Sire: Silver Sun — Sex: Filly

Dam: Gold Dust — DOB: 13/02/2021

Foal Growth Data Compared With: reference file: Thoroughbred, Worldwide, Fillies

Weight Date	Age (days)	Foal BW (kg)	Ref. BW (kg)	BW % Ref	Foal ADG (kg/d)	Ref. ADG (kg/d)	Foal HT (cm)	Ref. HT (cm)	HT % Ref	WT Per-centile	HT Per-centile	ADG Per-centile
13/02/2021	1	58.0	52.2	+11%				102.3		78.0		
22/02/2021	10	72.0	67.8	+6%	1.6	1.7	106.0	106.1	0%	71.2	48.9	50.7
21/03/2021	37	110.0	105.2	+5%	1.4	1.4	114.0	113.3	+1%	65.9	56.6	49.5
20/04/2021	67	146.0	140.2	+4%	1.2	1.2	120.0	120.2	0%	65.4	48.5	51.5
26/05/2021	103	190.0	178.6	+6%	1.2	1.1	127.0	126.6	0%	75.1	53.8	63.4
28/06/2021	136	220.0	209.0	+5%	0.9	0.9	131.0	130.4	0%	72.8	56.0	41.8
25/07/2021	163	240.0	230.5	+4%	0.7	0.8	133.0	133.0	0%	68.4	50.0	33.5
26/08/2021	195	260.0	254.3	+2%	0.6	0.7	136.0	135.7	0%	60.8	53.1	29.6
26/09/2021	226	280.0	275.3	+2%	0.6	0.7	138.0	138.2	0%	58.2	47.3	33.2

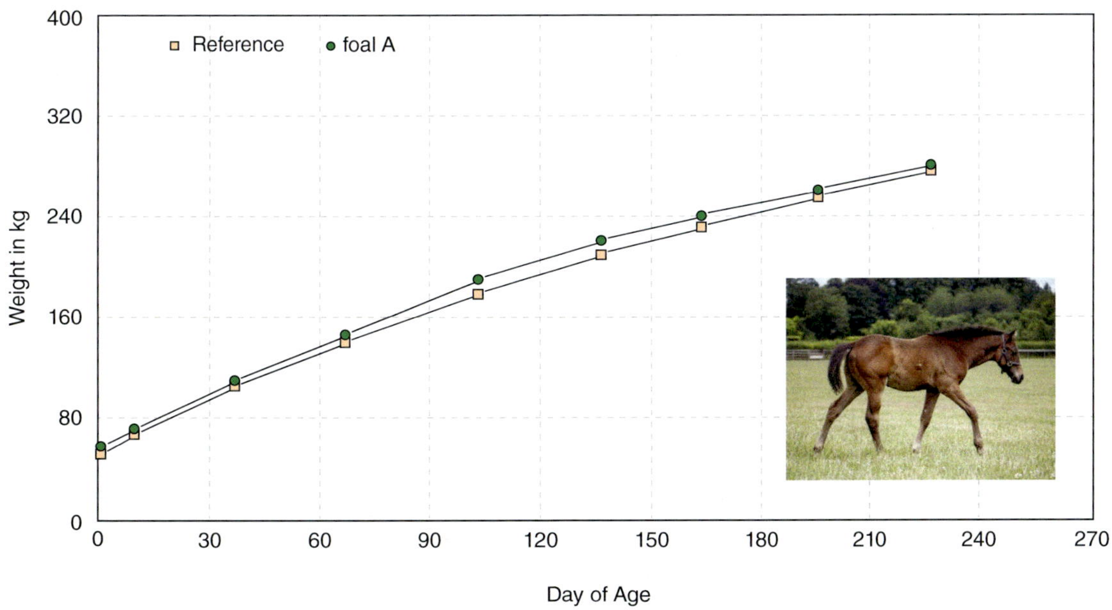

Fig. 14.14 Example growth curve. (Image courtesy of Polly Bonner. Produced by GroTrac.)

- individual stage of the foal's development;
- the strength of the mare and foal attachment; and
- the ability of the client to implement the chosen method effectively.

Pasture group weaning

Pasture group weaning is chosen by most larger studs.

- One or two individual mares are removed from the group.
- Leaves foal within an established group and in familiar surroundings.
- All mares gradually removed over a period of weeks.

Pros:

- Less stressful for the foal (Heleski *et al.*, 2002; Erber *et al.*, 2012).

Cons:

- Not possible for clients with only one mare.

Stable weaning

- Stable the foal.
  - Once settled and eating well, can be turned out with other weanlings or older horse.
- Turn the mare away in a distant field.

Pros:

- Relatively easy for breeders with 1–2 foals.

Cons:

- Care must be taken to ensure the foal does not injure itself when confined alone.
- Paired foals may form a close bond, can be counterproductive if separated.
- More stressful compared with gradual weaning (McCall *et al.*, 1985).

Gradual weaning

Separation of the mare and foal for gradually increasing lengths of time.
Pros:

- Mare and foal continue to be able to see, hear, smell and touch each other.
- Foal is unable to suckle.
- Foals have lower heart rates and blood cortisol levels, compared with those weaned abruptly (Hoffman *et al.*, 1995; Apter and Householder, 1996).

Cons:

- Prolonging gradual weaning process may increase anxiety in some individuals.
- Increases the risk of mastitis in the mare.

Impact of weaning on behaviour

Weaning can result in reduced growth rates, inappetence, oral stereotypies and/or mild diarrhoea equine gastric ulceration (EGUS) (Waters *et al.*, 2002; Erber *et al.*, 2012). Correct nutrition prior to, during and after weaning is essential to help minimise the risk of these problems.

Foals fed a 'fat-and-fibre' based diet had lower cortisol levels post-weaning, demonstrated reduced reactivity and lower levels of locomotion compared with those fed a 'starch-and-sugar' diet (Holland *et al.*, 1996). Be aware that research-based diets might contain considerably higher starch and sugar than that provided in a commercial creep feed (Nicol *et al.*, 2005).

There appears to be a link between the type of diet and development of stereotypies, but it is difficult to separate cause and effect from feeding management and environment. Stabled or barned weanlings are at significantly greater risk of wood-chewing compared with those weaned at pasture; and if fed concentrates they are at an increased risk of crib-biting; whereas concentrate feed post-weaning was associated with a reduced risk of wood-chewing (Waters *et al.*, 2002). Foals developing oral stereotypies post-weaning have greater suckling motivation and spend more time sucking and nuzzling the teat prior to weaning (Nicole and Badnell-Waters, 2005). The rank of the mare in the herd may also affect behaviour post-weaning (Waters *et al.*, 2002).

Weaning, whether abrupt or gradual, induces a physiological stress and alters the faecal microbiota (Jacquay *et al.*, 2019). A change in diet (i.e. transition from a milk-based diet) is a recognised primary cause of alterations to the foal's intestinal microflora (De La Torre *et al.*, 2019).

Your client may wish to feed a probiotic (see Chapter 6) during the weaning period. Products containing live bacteria (e.g. *Bifidobacterium*, *Lactobacillus*, *Streptococcus*, *Enterococcus* and *Lactococcus* species) are not currently licensed for use in equine feeds in the EU and UK.

Feeding Weanlings

If not already doing so, recommend that your client introduces the foal to the concentrate ration they intend to feed post-weaning at least 1 month prior to weaning, to ensure adaptation of the digestive system to digest hard feed; fed alongside ad libitum good-quality, forage. If fresh pasture is limited, high-quality conserved forage must be provided.

> **Top tip**
>
> Advise an early-cut hay to:
>
> - minimise the 'pot-bellied' appearance often associated with more mature hay; and
> - reduce loose droppings, which can be an issue for youngstock fed haylage, particularly if the dry matter (DM) is low.
>
> Test the forage (see Chapter 9).

Dietary advice

Weanlings that are too heavy or have early signs of DOD or are being weaned onto good-quality spring or early autumn pasture will not require large amounts of hard feed.

- Advise a low-calorie feed balancer for youngstock or a performance vitamin and mineral supplement to ensure adequate intake of essential amino acid, vitamins and minerals.

Foals being weaned in the late autumn, fed predominantly conserved forage, or individuals destined for the sales ring may require a more calorific feed.

- Advise a yearling cube/youngstock mix.
- If feeding less than the manufacturer's recommended amount, recommend a proportional quantity of feed balancer or vitamin and mineral supplement to guarantee adequate micronutrient intake.

Feeding Yearlings

The term 'yearling' applies to horses between the ages of 1–2 years, with the exception of racing Thoroughbreds, which in the Northern Hemisphere are declared as yearlings on 1 January of the year following their birth, regardless of date of birth.

Yearlings and 2-year-olds continue to grow. A Thoroughbred 'yearling' will typically gain 0.45–0.75 kg/day, decreasing to 0.2 kg/day by 24 months of age. Ideally, yearlings and 2-year-olds should be kept at fat score 2.5–3/5 on their ribs.

> **Top tip**
>
> It is not uncommon for yearlings and 2-year-olds to receive an unbalanced diet (Gibbs and Cohen, 2001).

> **Top tip**
>
> If your client's youngstock are maintaining optimal condition and growth on good-quality pasture they may not fully appreciate the need for supplementary feed.
>
> Forage alone will not provide adequate levels of all the essential minerals and this may increase the risk of issues including DOD and poor hoof quality.

Dietary advice

- Youngstock maintaining BW grazing good-quality pasture only require a low-intake nutrient-dense feed.
  - A feed balancer is ideal in these situations (Fig. 14.15).
- Winter months or for youngstock in exercise:
  - Forage alone is insufficient to meet energy/protein requirements.
  - Advise feeds specifically designed for youngstock.
- If feeding less than the recommended quantity:
  - Advise proportional quantity of feed balancer.

Sales Prepping

Thoroughbred youngstock are sold as either foals or yearlings. They are normally 'broken' at around 18 months of age and many 'flat' horses will then commence formal racehorse training when they are 2 years old.

Before sales they undergo a period of 'sales preparation', which usually lasts 8–12 weeks and includes a significant level of exercise:

- predominantly hand walking; or
- mechanical walker and lungeing (Bolwell *et al.*, 2012).

An increase in calorie intake will be required.

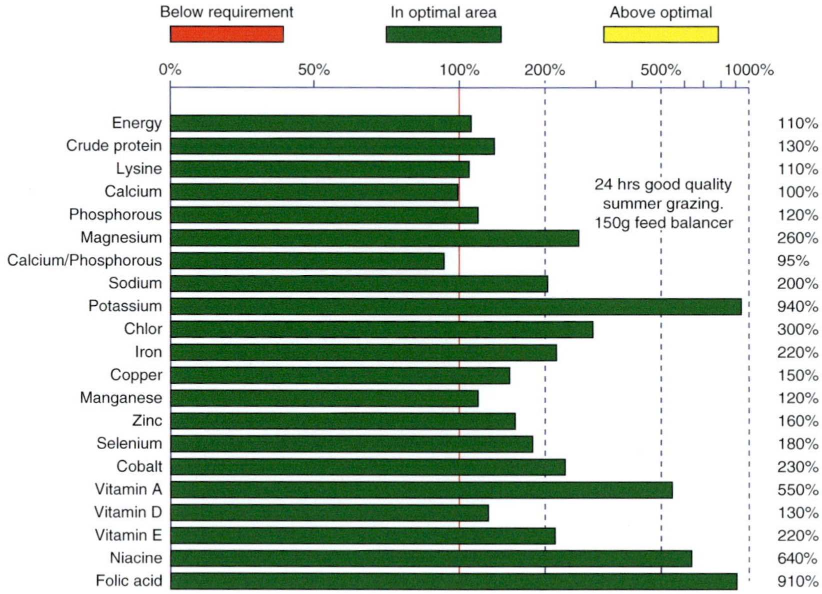

Fig. 14.15 Diet check for 12-month-old Dartmoor (125 kg). The energy and micronutrient content of the diet are within the optimal range. Advise fat scoring and monitor weight gain carefully, as eating 10% more energy than required (a horse only needs to eat 3.8–4.9 MJ DE to gain 1 kg fat) (NRC, 2007).

Dietary advice

There are several options when it comes to choosing a feed for 'sales prep'. Each breeder or consignor will have their own individual preference.

- Either stud cube/mix or a youngstock feed.
- Feed specifically designed for horses being prepared for the sales ring have become increasingly popular (Fig. 14.16).

Thoroughbred youngstock, particularly yearlings, being offered for sale at auction are required to appear well-muscled and have a slightly higher degree of body fatness, compared with their peers not being offered for sale. This allows for the slight loss of BW that is associated with transportation too, and stress whilst at the sales, but might predispose them to DOD.

Developmental Orthopaedic Disorders (DOD)

DOD affects the limbs of young horses, disrupting the normal development of the musculoskeletal system. The aetiology is complex and there is no single causative factor. Genetics, exercise, endocrine influences, environmental/management circumstances, trauma/injury and nutrition are all thought to play a role in DOD. Steps should be taken to minimise nutritional risk factors associated with DOD.

Energy

Excessive growth, including periods of compensatory growth potentially because of genetic predisposition or excess calorie consumption (Thompson *et al.*, 1988a,b), has been linked to DOD (Sandgren *et al.*, 1993; van Weeren *et al.*, 1999). Not all studies have found a link between energy intake, weight gain and DOD; several predisposing factors appear to coexist (Savage *et al.*, 1993a; Jelan *et al.*, 1996; Ott *et al.*, 2005).

Hormonal factors in a response to feeding non-structural carbohydrates (NSC) might be a cause of DOD (Ralston, 1996; Henson *et al.*, 1997; Staniar *et al.*, 2007). *In vivo*, elevated post-prandial glycaemic, and the resulting insulinaemic, responses directly affect growth factor/hormones (thyroxine (T4) and insulin-like growth factor-1 (IGF-1)) which are involved in cartilage formation (Henson *et al.*, 1997). Foals affected by osteochondrosis (OCD) had higher post-prandial glycaemic and insulinaemic responses (Ralston, 1996); other

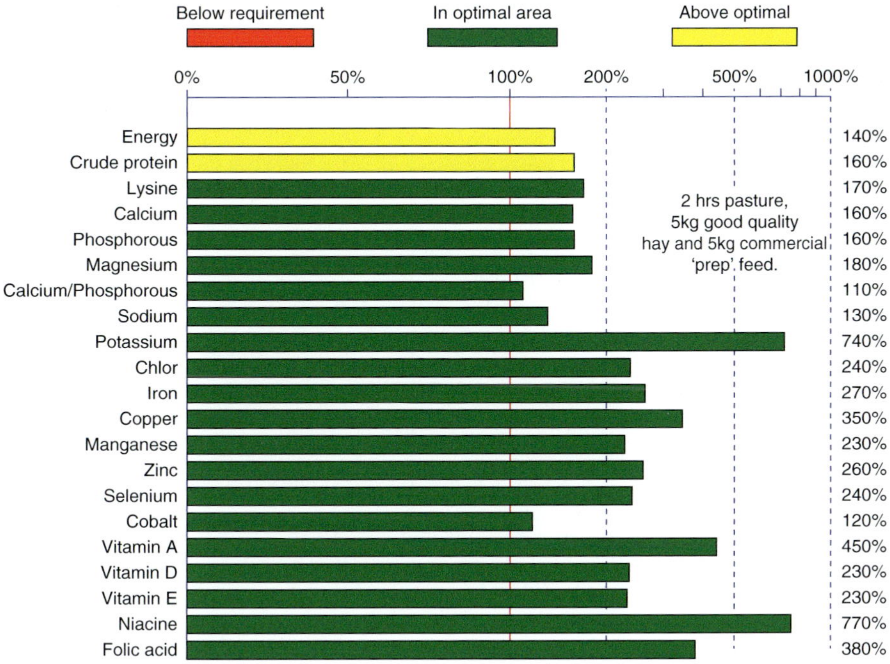

Fig. 14.16 Diet check for 16-month-old TB yearling in 'sales prep'. The energy and protein intake are above requirements. This is typical of diets fed during sales preparation.

researchers have not found differences in the glycaemic response of normal foals and those with OCD lesions (Pagan *et al.*, 2001).

Controlling glycaemic response

A number of factors influence a yearling's post-prandial glycaemic and insulinaemic response (see Chapter 5). Feeding yearlings their daily ration divided into four, rather than two, feeds/day decreases the post-prandial glycaemic peak (Steelman *et al.*, 2006).

Maternal nutrition and foetal programming may determine an individual's hormonal response to NSC intake (Coverdale *et al.*, 2015).

> **Top tip**
>
> For youngsters at high risk of this condition:
> - Advise feeding small, frequent meals.
> - Limit NSC intake to less than 1 g starch/kg BW/meal (see Chapter 5).

Balancing protein

Lowering protein intakes to help alleviate DOD has been a common recommendation in the equine industry. It is typically achieved by reducing the amount of hard feed, which inadvertently reduces energy intake, slowing weight gain and growth rate.

> **Top tip**
>
> Reducing protein intake (by reducing feed intake below the level recommended by the manufacturer):
> - may lead to reduced muscle development;
> - is not protective against developmental problems (Schryver *et al.*, 1987; Savage *et al.*, 1993a); and
> - can result in inadequate micronutrient intake, with detrimental effects on skeletal development.
>
> Reducing protein intake to below requirement is not recommended

Further work is needed to investigate the role of individual amino acids on skeletal problems in growing horses, particularly as there is increasing evidence to suggest that they may play a role in metabolic regulation (Harris *et al.*, 2005).

Minerals

Dietary cation–anion balance (DCAB)

DCAB of less than 130 meq/kg DM can cause increased calcium losses (Topliff *et al.*, 1989; Wall *et al.*, 1992) and prolonged consumption of a diet with a low DCAB may have the potential to lead to bone demineralisation.

Copper

Copper plays an important role in the enzymes lysyl-oxidase and superoxide dismutase (SOD), which are involved in cartilage formation and turnover (Prockop and Tuderman, 1982; Pearce *et al.*, 1998b; Gee *et al.*, 2004).

Foals whose dams were supplemented with copper and zinc have a reduction in physitis scores (Pearce *et al.*, 1998a); foals born with high liver copper content had improved repair of OCD lesions (van Weeren *et al.*, 2003); youngstock fed copper-deficient diet had increased OCD lesions (Knight *et al.*, 1990; Hurtig *et al.*, 1993).

The amount of copper provided from the ration should be assessed on an ongoing basis. Experience shows that copper intake of 20 mg/kg DM is beneficial for foals susceptible to DOD (NB: legal limit is 34 mg Cu/kg DM). High levels of dietary zinc may adversely affect copper absorption (McDowell, 2003); the zinc-to-copper ratio should be between 4:1 and 5:1 (Hintz, 1996). Excessively high iron intake may also inhibit copper absorption (NRC, 2007).

Vitamins

Several vitamins are required for optimal bone health. Vitamin A is involved in the development of osteoblasts, whilst vitamin D is needed for calcium absorption and vitamin K is a cofactor for the gamma-carboxylation of many proteins, including osteocalcin. For youngstock (> 3 months of age) with limited access to good-quality pasture, additional vitamin provision is recommended.

Make sure your client feeds a balanced ration, thereby reducing the risk of DOD (Box 14.1).

Box 14.1 Minimising the nutritional risks associated with DOD

- Maintain steady growth rates.
  - Regularly monitor ADG and BCS.
- Advise adequate, but not excessive, calorie intake.
  - Foals (3+ months) consuming excessive calories from milk may require early weaning.
- Test the nutrient and mineral content of any forage fed.
  - Adjust the hard feed/supplementation accordingly.
- Ensure that the mare receives optimal mineral intake.
  - Particularly calcium, phosphorus, copper and zinc during gestation.

Stallions

The nutritional requirements of breeding stallions depend on breeding frequency, level of exercise and temperament. Stallions covering only a handful of mares or those used for semen collection two or three times a season are unlikely to have increased nutrient requirements. Thoroughbred stallions can undertake up to four natural coverings daily during the peak breeding season – their nutritional requirements may be up to 50% greater than that of a horse at maintenance.

Your client's stallion may be in regular exercise or may find it difficult to 'relax' during the covering season, expending additional energy in activities such as pacing along a fence line when turned out.

There is limited research as to the specific nutrient requirements for stallions; most is extrapolated from other species.

Energy

Obesity negatively affects libido and fertility in humans (Ruby *et al.*, 2007; Hammoud *et al.*, 2008). The effects of low body condition on fertility are less well documented, but severely underweight stallions are likely to have reduced fertility and poor breeding performance.

Polyunsaturated fats and antioxidants

Studies in several species have indicated that diet plays a role in semen health (Lopez *et al.*, 2017;

Table 14.9 Supplementation of nutrients that improve semen health of stallions

Animals	Supplementation	Results	Reference
15 Thoroughbred, Arabian and Quarter Horse stallions, 7–26 y	Vitamin E 3000 iu /day	Supplementation improved motility in cooled semen at 48 h but motility of 24 h cooled or frozen semen was not affected	Gee *et al.*, 2008
7 Andalusian stallions	Ubiquinol (CoQ10) 1 gv	Supplementation improved motility and viability following cooling or freezing in stallions with suboptimum motility	Ruiz *et al.*, 2021
12 stallions, 3–12 y	Docosahexaenoic acid (DHA) 15 g, vitamin E 1000 iu, selenium 2 mg	Supplementation improved total and progressive motility in fresh and cooled semen	Goedde *et al.*, 2015
6 stallions	DHA 30 g	Supplementation increased sperm per ejaculate, motility and decreased sperm abnormalities	Elhordoy *et al.*, 2008
8 stallions	DHA-enriched nutraceutical 250 g/day	Supplementation increased in total, progressive and rapid motility in cooled semen	Brinsko *et al.*, 2005
Shetland pony stallions	Supplemented with tocopherol 300 mg/day; ascorbic acid 300 mg/day; L-carnitin 4000 mg/day; folic acid 12 mg/day	No pronounced effects on semen quality	Deichsel *et al.*, 2008
Warmblood stallions	Linseed oil 100 ml/day, combined with antioxidants	Supplementation attenuated a decline in motility and membrane integrity of cooled–stored semen	Lausigk *et al.*, 2014
Light-horse breeds	L-carnitine 20 g/day	Increase in progressive motility in stallions with low sperm motility	Stradaioli *et al.*, 2000

Efrat *et al.*, 2018). In stallions, the effects of various different supplementations on sperm health have been investigated (Table 14.9).

Minerals

Mineral supplementation may also influence fertility. In humans and other species, iodine and zinc have been highlighted as being particularly important for male fertility (Kumar *et al.*, 2006; Fallah *et al.*, 2018; Sun *et al.*, 2020).

Dietary advice

Stallions should have ad libitum access to forage to minimise risk of developing self-mutilating behaviours.

Stallions that maintain weight well on forage alone will not require large amounts of hard feed (Fig. 14.17).

Advise that pasture intake may need to be restricted and replaced with an appropriate low-calorie forage (see Chapter 4) and a balancer for stallions prone to excessive weight gain (Fig. 14.18); monitor BFS.

Busy, active stallions and those prone to weight loss will require a more energy-dense ration. Advise a cereal-based commercial stud cube/mix (0.6–1.1 kg/100 kg BW) (Fig. 14.19).

And do not forget to advise a balancer if stud mix is being fed at less than recommended requirements (Fig. 14.20)

Stallions with poor fertility, particularly those whose semen will be cooled or frozen, may benefit from omega-3 fatty acid supplementation (see Table 14.9). If your client is feeding a significant amount of oil, advise 100 iu vitamin E/100 ml of additional oil (Harris, 1999).

Several commercial supplements aimed at supporting stallion fertility are available. If your client chooses to use such a product you should advise them to start ideally 2 months prior to the breeding season, as the stallion's spermatogenic cycle is approximately 57 days (Johnson *et al.*, 1997). Joint supplements are also very popular with stallion owners, as repeated covering places additional

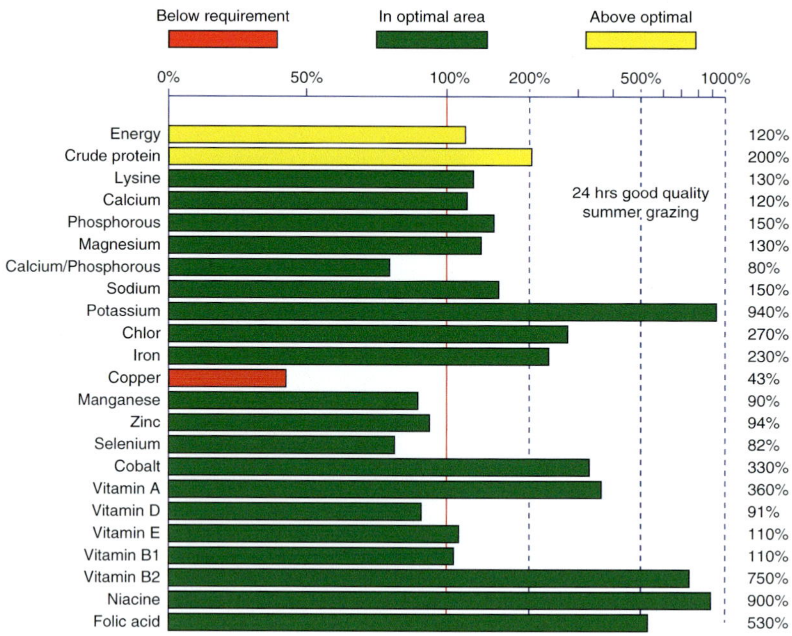

Fig. 14.17 Diet check for pony stallion, 300 kg. Above requirements for calories and protein, which may result in excessive weight gain. The levels of certain minerals are insufficient or lower than optimal.

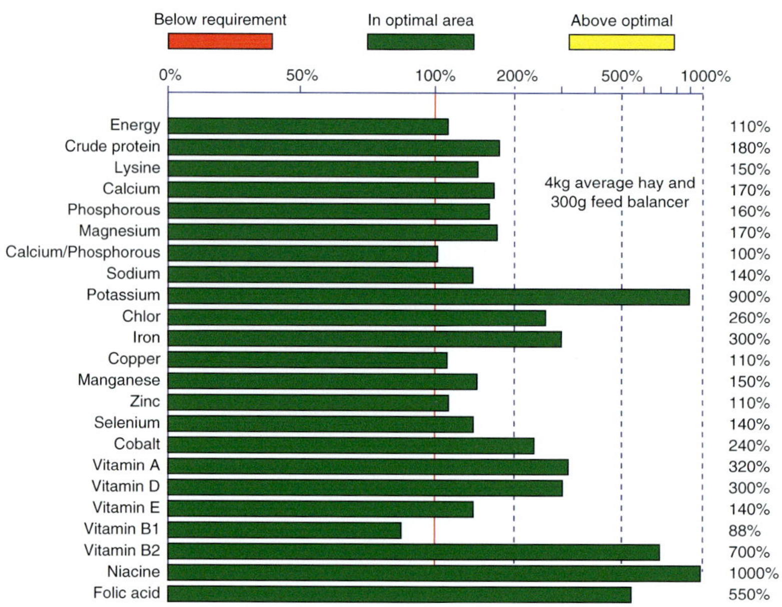

Fig. 14.18 Diet check for pony stallion, 300 kg, 12 h restricted grazing. The energy and micronutrient content of the diet are within the optimal range.

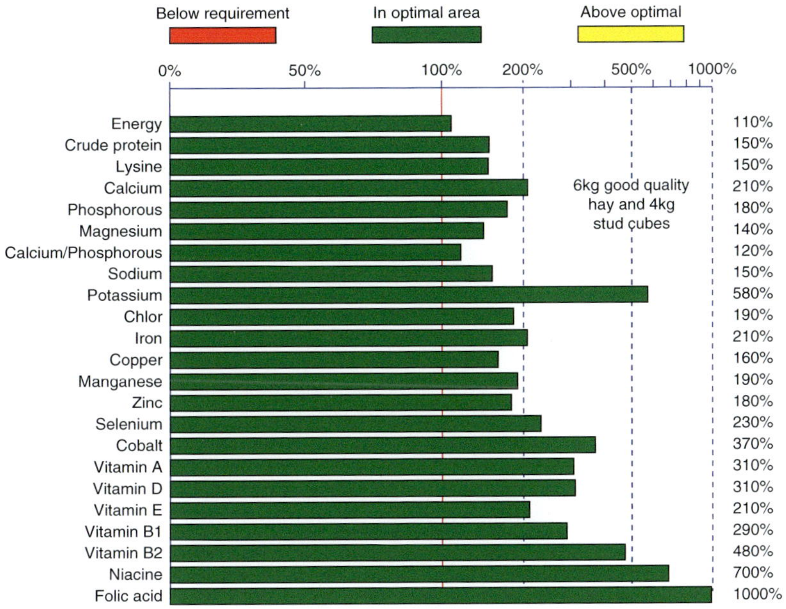

Fig. 14.19 Diet check for Thoroughbred stallion, 500 kg. The energy and micronutrient content of the diet are within the optimal range.

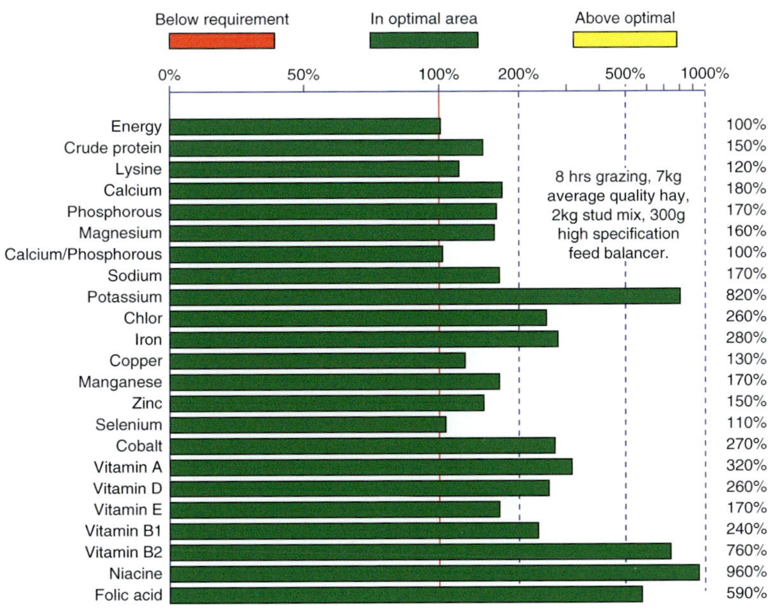

Fig. 14.20 Diet check for Warmblood stallion, 600 kg. The energy and micronutrient content of the diet are within the optimal range.

strain on the joints, especially in the hind limbs, and any joint pain may limit a stallion's willingness to breed.

Other Nutrition-related Issues in Breeding Stock

A complete review of all metabolic, nutritional, or gastrointestinal related issues in breeding stock is beyond the scope of this chapter.

Coprophagy

Coprophagy is normal and should not be seen as a concern in the young foal (Francis-Smith and Wood-Gush, 1977; Crowell-Davis and Houpt, 1985). It is believed that the ingestion of faeces plays an important role in populating the hind gut with beneficial microbes and you can reassure your client that in young foals it is not indicative of a nutritional deficiency.

Foal heat diarrhoea

Foal heat diarrhoea results from normal changes in the foal's gastrointestinal microflora due to introduction of feed (Kuhl *et al.*, 2010) and affects 80–95% of foals, usually occurring at around 5–15 days of age, coinciding with the occurrence of the mare's first heat following parturition. For less experienced breeders it can cause a great deal of concern. Originally thought to occur because of hormonal changes in the mare's milk, there is no correlation between foal heat in the mare and the onset of diarrhoea in foals (Johnston *et al.*, 1970); incidence is common in orphan foals that have no exposure to maternal hormones (Magdesian, 2005). It is usually mild and self-limiting, rarely requiring treatment, but your client will need to monitor the foal carefully.

Gastric ulcers

Prevalence of ulcers in foals is between 25% and 57%, although healthy foals are generally not examined endoscopically for ulcers (Murray *et al.*, 1990; Sanchez *et al.*, 1998; Murray, 1999; Elfenbein and Sanchez, 2012). Gastric ulcers do not appear to develop *in utero* and have not been found in aborted foetuses or foals that have died due to dystocia (Lewis, 2003). Most cases occur in foals > 2 days of age and common clinical signs include anorexia, bruxism, ptyalism, dorsal recumbency and colic (Stoneham, 1996; Murray, 1999).

A variety of factors can cause EGUS in foals, including nonsteroidal anti-inflammatory drugs (NSAIDs), stress, infection, delayed gastric emptying, infrequent feeding, long-distance transportation and prolonged recumbency (Breuhaus *et al.*, 1999; Murray, 1999). Stressful periods such as weaning have been shown to increase the incidences of EGUS (Vondran *et al.*, 2016). The incidence of EGUS in broodmares at pasture can be as high as 70% (Le Jeune *et al.*, 2009) and may be due to lack of dietary fibre (see Chapter 12).

Laminitis

Broodmares, due to a pregnancy-associated natural decline in insulin sensitivity, may be at particular risk of endocrinopathic laminitis (George *et al.*, 2011).

Mares that are overweight or those that have been diagnosed with insulin resistance (IR) pre-pregnancy will need to be managed carefully, particularly during the last trimester. Any calorie restriction during pregnancy should be carefully considered, because of the need to support foetal growth. Breeding from overweight mares and stallions with a history or at risk of endocrine laminitis should not be encouraged. Laminitis can also occur post-foaling, commonly associated with issues such as retained placenta or metritis (Warnakulasooriya *et al.*, 2018).

White muscle disease

White muscle disease is a nutritional myopathy caused by low selenium in foals (Gabbedy and Richards, 1970) and to a lesser degree vitamin E intake (Streeter *et al.*, 2012). Cases are typically geographically restricted to areas of low soil selenium content, but not all foals in these areas develop the disease (Delesalle *et al.*, 2017). If your client's land is thought to have low soil selenium content, or they have purchased conserved forage that may have been grown in a suspected low selenium area, soil and forage analysis is recommended

Conclusion and Summary

Your client will have many different reasons as to why they want to breed, whether that be commercially as part of their business or to carry on the bloodlines of a successful competition horse who is also a much-loved mare. They will have considered the significant financial costs and time implications, but every breeder, however large or small, will need to rely on their veterinarian as their best resource for help and advice.

TB studs breeding out of the natural season will rely on stud feeds fed in large quantities to balance conserved forages, whereas natives and sports horses are more likely to need balancers and lower-intake feeds to balance available grass.

Both groups should be fed for the 'work' they are doing in their first two trimesters and diet matched to nutrient requirements that increase in 3rd trimester and lactation. Most people overfeed energy before and during early pregnancy but underestimate energy needs for lactation.

Ensure that you communicate with your client on a regular basis and have become proficient in gathering essential and required horse and management information (Box 14.2) to support your client. In some cases, you might enlist the help of a qualified equine nutritionist who will liaise directly with your client to ensure correct and balanced nutrition through gestation, lactation and weaning. Equine nutritionists will also be able to provide guidance in relation to selecting high-quality and suitable feeds (see Chapter 8: 'Suitably qualified nutritionists').

A newborn healthy foal never fails to bring a smile and an amazing sense of satisfaction – may that feeling never leave you.

Box 14.2 Check list

1. Why are they breeding (e.g. racing, sales or grading prep, sports, as a 'pet' or long-term investment)?
2. Age of mare/foal/youngster.
3. Is this her first foal?
4. When is she due to foal (last service date)?
5. How is she managed, with respect to day-to-day management, and how will this change pre- and post-foaling?
6. Bodyweight and fat score.
7. Current diet of forage (hay/haylage) and concentrate feed.
8. Grazing availability and quality
9. Does she normally hold good body condition?
10. Does she eat well?
11. Is the mare in foal again?
12. Does she eat well during pregnancy and post-foaling?
13. If she has had a foal before, does she foal easily and is lactation good?
14. Any relevant foaling history – does she go to full term or is often over her due date?
15. Previous colostrum quality.
16. Have previous foals needed IgG infusions?
17. Have past progeny had very light or very heavy birthweights?
18. Have any of her offspring had orthopaedic problems, DOD issues or surgical procedures?
19. If you need to restrict the foal or mare for any reason, are there the facilities to do this?
20. Do you have the facility to track growth rates in foals (e.g. weighbridge, height stick)?
21. Any history of colic or digestive health disorders?
22. Any fertility issues?

Bibliography

Abuelo, A., Hernandez, J., Benedito J.L. *et al.* (2015) The importance of the oxidative status of dairy cattle in the periparturient period: revisiting antioxidant supplementation. *Journal of Animal Physiology and Animal Nutrition* 99, 1003–1016.

Agriculture and Horticulture Development Board (2019). Available at: https://ahdb.org.uk/dairy (accessed 1 January 2020).

Allen, W.R., Wilsher, S., Tiplady, C. *et al.* (2004) The influence of maternal size on pre- and postnatal growth in the horse: III Postnatal growth. *Reproduction* 127(67–77).

Apter, R.C. and Householder, D.D. (1996) Weaning and weaning management of foals: a review and some recommendations. *Journal of Equine Veterinary Science* 16, 428–435.

Bailey, S.R. and Bamford, N.J. (2013) Metabolic responses of horses and ponies to high and low glycaemic feeds: implications for laminitis. *Animal Production Science* 53, 1182–1187.

Banach, M.A. and Evans, J.W. (1981) Effects of inadequate energy during gestation and lactation on the estrous cycle and conception rate of mares and on their foal weights. In: *Proceedings of the 7th Equine Nutrition and Physiology Symposium*, Warrenton, Virginia, pp. 97–100.

Baucus, K.L., Ralston, S.L., Rich, G.A. and Squires, E.L. (1989) The effect of copper and zinc supplementation on mineral content of mares' milk. *Journal of Equine Veterinary Science* 9(4), 206–209.

Becvarova, I. and Buechner-Maxwell, V. (2012) Feeding the foal for immediate and long-term health. *Equine Veterinary Journal* 44, 149–156.

Bell, A.W., Hay, W.W. Jr and Ehrhardt, R.A. (1999) Placental transport of nutrients and its implications for fetal growth. *Journal of Reproduction and Fertility* 54, 401–410.

Berger, J. (1986) *Wild Horses of the Great Basin*. University of Chicago Press, Chicago and London.

Bolwell, C.F., Rogers, C.W., French, N.P. and Firth, E.C. (2012) Exercise in Thoroughbred yearlings during sales preparation: a cohort study. *Equine Veterinary Journal* 44(1), 20–24.

Boy, V. and Duncan, P. (1979) Time budgets of Camargue horses. 1. Developmental changes in the time budgets of foals. *Behaviour* 21, 187–201.

Breedveld, L., Jackson, S.G. and Baker, J.P. (1988) The determination of a relationship between the copper, zinc and selenium levels in mares and those in their foals. *Journal of Equine Veterinary Science* 8(5), 378–382.

Breuhaus, B.A., DeGraves, F.J., Honore, E.K. *et al.* (1999) Pharmacokinetics of ibuprofen after intravenous and oral administration and assessment of safety of administration to healthy foals. *American Journal of Veterinary Research* 60, 1066–1073.

Brinsko, S.P., Varner, D.D., Love, C.C., Blanchard, T.L., Day, B.C. *et al.* (2005) Effect of feeding a DHA-enriched nutriceutical on the quality of fresh, cooled and frozen stallion semen. *Theriogenology* 63(5), 1519–1527.

Buff, P.R., Dodds, A.C., Morrison, C.D., Whitley, N.C., McFadin, E.L. *et al.* (2002) Leptin in horses: tissue localization and relationship between peripheral concentrations of leptin and body condition. *Journal of Animal Science* 80(11), 2942–2948.

Burns, T. (2007) *Current Therapy in Equine Reproduction*. W.B. Saunders, St Louis, Missouri, pp. 452–453.

Carroll, C.L. and Huntington, P.J. (1988) Body condition scoring and weight estimation of horses. *Equine Veterinary Journal* 20, 41–45.

Carlsten, J., Sandgren, B. and Dalin, G. (1993) Development of osteochondrosis in the tarsocrural joint and osteochondral fragments in the fetlock joints of Standardbred trotters. I. A radiological survey. *Equine Veterinary Journal* 25(S16), 42–47.

Catandi, C., Obeidat, Y. and Stokes, J. (2020) Maternal diet can alter oocyte mitochondrial number and function. *Journal of Equine Veterinary Science* 89 (Abstract).

Cavinder, C.A., Vogelsang, M.M., Gibbs, P.G., Forrest, D.W. and Schmitz, D.G. (2009) Variances in reproductive efficiency of mares in fat and moderate body conditions following parturition. *The Professional Animal Scientist* 25(3), 250–255.

Cavinder, C.A., Burns, S.A., Coverdale, J. *et al.* (2012) Late gestational nutrition of the mare and potential effects on endocrine profiles and adrenal function of the offspring. *The Professional Animal Scientist* 28, 344–350.

Čebulj-Kadunc, N. and Cestnik, V. (2008) The influence of season and age on circulating melatonin and leptin concentrations in Lipizzan fillies. *Acta Veterinaria* 58, 25–31.

Clabough, D.L., Levine, J.F., Grant, G.L. and Conboy, H.S. (1991) Factors associated with failure of passive transfer of colostral antibodies in Standardbred foals. *Journal of Veterinary Internal Medicine* 5(6), 335–340.

Cohen, N.D., Matejka, P.L., Honnas, C.M. *et al.* (1995) Case-control study of the association between various management factors and development of colic in horses. *Journal of the American Veterinary Medical Association* 206, 667–673.

Coverdale, J.A., Hammer, C.J. and Walter, K.W. (2015) Horse species symposium: nutritional programming and the impact on mare and foal performance. *Journal of Animal Science* 93, 3261–3267.

Crowell-Davis, S.L. and Houpt, K.A. (1985) Coprophagy by foals: effect of age and possible functions. *Equine Veterinary Journal* 17(1), 17–19.

Csapo, J., Stefler, J., Martin, T.G., Makray, S. and Csapó-Kiss, Z. (1995) Composition of mares' colostrum and milk. Fat content, fatty acid composition and vitamin content. *International Dairy Journal* 5(4), 393–402.

Cymbaluk, N.F. (1990) Cold housing effects on growth and nutrient demand on young horses. *Journal of Animal Science* 68, 3152–3162.

De La Torre, U., Henderson, J.D., Furtado, K.L., Pedroja, M., Elenamarie, O.M. *et al.* (2019) Utilizing the fecal microbiota to understand foal gut transitions from birth to weaning. *PLoS ONE* 14(4), e0216211.

Deichsel, K., Palm, F., Koblischke, P. *et al.* (2008) Effect of a dietary antioxidant supplement on semen quality in pony stallions. *Theriogenology* 69, 940–945.

Delesalle, C., de Bruijn, M., Wilmink, S. *et al.* (2017) White muscle disease in foals: focus on selenium soil content. *A case series. BMC Veterinary Research* 13, 121.

Dill, S.G. and Rebhun, W.C. (1985) White muscle disease in foals. *Compendium on Continuing Education for the Practicing Veterinarian* 7, 627–635.

Doreau, M., Boulot, S. and Chilliard, Y. (1993) Yield and composition of milk from lactating mares: effect of body condition at foaling. *Journal of Dairy Research* 60(4), 457–466.

Dorn, C.R., Garner, H.E., Coffman, J.R., Hahn, A.W. and Tritschler, L.G. (1975) Castration and other factors affecting the risk of equine laminitis. *The Cornell Veterinarian* 65(1), 57–64.

Dror, D.K. and Allen, L.H. (2018) Overview of nutrients in human milk. *Advances in Nutrition* 1 (9), 278–294.

Duncan, P., Harvey, P.H. and Wells, S.M. (1984) On lactation and associated behaviour in a natural herd of horses. *Animal Behaviour* 32, 255–263.

Durham, A. and McGowan, C. (2012) Notes from the Boehringer Ingelheim webinar 04 September 2012. Current thoughts of where we are with PPID diagnostics. Available at: https://www.thelaminitissite.org/articles/current-thoughts-of-where-we-are-with-PPID-diagnostics-Andy-Durham (accessed 24 January 2023).

Efrat, M., Stein, A., Pinkas, H., Unger, R. and Birk, R. (2018) Dietary patterns are positively associated with semen quality. *Fertility and Sterility* 109(5), 809–816.

Elfenbein, J.R. and Sanchez, L.C. (2012) Prevalence of gastric and duodenal ulceration in 691 nonsurviving foals (1995–2006). *Equine Veterinary Journal* 44, 76–79.

Elhordoy, D.M., Cazales, N., Costa, G. and Estévez, J. (2008) Effect of dietary supplementation with DHA on the quality of fresh, cooled and frozen stallion semen. *Animal Reproduction Science* 3(107), 319.

Erber, R., Wulf, M., Rose-Meierhöfer, S., Becker-Birck, M., Möstl, E. *et al*. (2012) Behavioral and physiological responses of young horses to different weaning protocols: a pilot study. *Stress* 15(2), 184–194.

Eriksson, J.G., Sandboge, S., Salonen, M., Kajantie, E. and Osmond, C. (2015) Maternal weight in pregnancy and offspring body composition in late adulthood: findings from the Helsinki Birth Cohort Study (HBCS). *Annals of Medicine* 47(2), 94–99. doi: 10.3109/07853890.2015.1004360.

Fall, C.H. (2011) Evidence for the intra-uterine programming of adiposity in later life. *Annals of Human Biology* 38(4), 410–428. doi: 10.3109/03014460.2011.592513.

Fallah, A., Mohammad-Hasani, A. and Colagar, A.H. (2018) Zinc is an essential element for male fertility: a review of Zn roles in men's health, germination, sperm quality, and fertilization. *Journal of Reproduction & Infertility* 19(2), 69–81.

Fitzgerald, B.P. and McManus, C. (2000) Photoperiodic versus metabolic signals as determinants of seasonal anestrus in the mare. *Biology of Reproduction* 63, 335–340.

Fitzgerald, B.P., Reedy, S.E., Sessions, D.R., Powell, D.M. and McManus, C.J. (2002) Potential signals mediating the maintenance of reproductive activity during the non-breeding season of the mare. *Reproduction-Cambridge-Supplement* 59, 115–129.

Ford, S.P., Zhang, L., Zhu, M., Miller, M.M., Smith, D.T. *et al*. (2009) Maternal obesity accelerates fetal pancreatic β-cell but not α-cell development in sheep: prenatal consequences. *American Journal of Physiology-Regulatory, Integrative and Comparative Physiology* 297(3), R835–R843.

Fowden, A.L., Comline, R.S. and Silver, M. (1984) Insulin secretion and carbohydrate metabolism during pregnancy in the mare. *Equine Veterinary Journal* 16, 239–246.

Fowden, A.L., Giussani, D.A. and Forhead, A.J. (2005) Endocrine and metabolic programming during intrauterine development. *Early Human Development* 81, 723–734.

Fowden, A.L., Giussani, D.A. and Forhead, A.J. (2006) Intrauterine programming of physiological systems: causes and consequences. *Physiology (Bethesda)* 21, 29–37.

Fradinho, M.J., Correia, M.J., Grácio, V., Bliebernicht, M., Farrim, A. *et al*. (2014) Effects of body condition and leptin on the reproductive performance of Lusitano mares on extensive systems. *Theriogenology* 81(9), 1214–1222.

Francis-Smith, K. and Wood-Gush, D.G. (1977) Coprophagia as seen in thoroughbred foals. *Equine Veterinary Journal* 9(3), 155–157.

Freccero, F., Jole, M., Aliai, L., Chiara, C. and Carolina, C. (2017) Efficacy and safety of a commercial fresh-frozen hyperimmune plasma in foals with failure of passive transfer of immunity. *Journal of Equine Veterinary Science* 48, 174–181.

Gabbedy, B.J. and Richards, R.B. (1970) White muscle disease in a foal. *Australian Veterinary Journal* 46, 111–112.

Gee, E.K., Morel, P.C.H., Mogg, T.D., Firth, E.C., Grace, N.D. *et al*. (2004) Liver copper kinetics in Thoroughbred foals at pasture from birth to 160 days of age. *New Zealand Journal of Agricultural Research* 47(2), 109–118.

Gee, E.K., Bruemmer, J.E., Siciliano, P.D., McCue, P.M. and Squires, E.L. (2008) Effects of dietary vitamin E supplementation on spermatozoal quality in stallions with suboptimal post-thaw motility. *Animal Reproduction Science* 3(107), 324–325.

Gentry, L.R., Thompson, D.L. Jr and Gentry, G.T. Jr (2002) The relationship between body condition, leptin, and reproductive and hormonal characteristics of mares during the seasonal anovulatory period. *Journal of Animal Science* 80(10), 2695–2703.

George, L.A., Staniar, W.B., Treiber, K.H., Harris, P.A. and Geor, R.J. (2009) Insulin sensitivity and glucose dynamics during pre-weaning foal development and in response to maternal diet composition. *Domestic Animal Endocrinology* 37(1), 23–29.

George, L.A., Staniar, W.B., Cubitt, T.A., Treiber, K.H., Harris, P.A. *et al*. (2011) Evaluation of the effects of pregnancy on insulin sensitivity, insulin secretion, and glucose dynamics in Thoroughbred mares. *American Journal of Veterinary Research* 72(5), 666–674.

Gibbs, P.G. and Cohen, N.D. (2001) Early management of race-bred weanlings and yearlings on farms. *Journal of Equine Veterinary Science* 21(6), 279–283.

Gibbs, P.G., Potter, G.D., Blake, R.W. and McMullan, W.C. (1982) Milk production of quarter horse mares during 150 days of lactation. *Journal of Animal Science* 54(3), 496–499.

Gicquel, C., El-Osta, A. and Le Bouc, Y. (2008) Epigenetic regulation and fetal programming. *Best Practice & Research Clinical Endocrinology & Metabolism* 22(1), 1–16.

Glade, M.J. (1993) Effects of gestation, lactation, and maternal calcium intake on mechanical strength of equine bone. *Journal of the American College of Nutrition* 12(4), 372–377.

Goedde, L.D., Brennan, K.M., Ball, B.A., Lawrence, L.M., Troedsson, M.H. *et al.* (2015) 129 Effects of feeding a yeast-based supplement containing selenized yeast, vitamin E and A DHA-rich microalgae on sperm motion characteristics. *Journal of Equine Veterinary Science* 5(35), 438.

Grace, N.D., Pearce, S.G., Firth, E.C. and Fennessy, P.F. (1999) Concentrations of macro-and micro-elements in the milk of pasture-fed Thoroughbred mares. *Australian Veterinary Journal* 77(3), 177–180.

Graham, P.M., Ott, E.A., Brendemuhl, J.H. and TenBroeck, S.H. (1994) The effect of supplemental lysine and threonine on growth and development of yearling horses. *Journal of Animal Science* 72(2), 380–386.

Hammoud, A.O., Wilde, N., Gibson, M., Parks, A., Carrell, D.T. *et al.* (2008) Male obesity and alteration in sperm parameters. *Fertility and Sterility* 90(6), 2222–2225.

Harris, P.A. (1999) Feeding and management advice for tying up. In: *Proceedings of the BEVA Specialist Meeting on Nutrition and Behaviour*. Mars Inc, Waltham, UK, pp. 100–104.

Harris, P.A., Staniar, W. and Ellis, A.D. (2005) Effects of exercise and diet on the incidence of DOD. In: Juliand, V. and Martin-Roset (eds) *The Growing Horse: Nutrition and Prevention of Growth Disorders*. EAAP, Dijon, France, p. 114.

Heleski, C.R., Shelle, A.C., Nielsen, B.D. and Zanella, A.J. (2002) Influence of housing on weanling horse behavior and subsequent welfare. *Applied Animal Behaviour Science* 78(2–4), 291–302.

Henneke, D.R., Potter, G.D., Kreider, J.L. and Yeates, B.F. (1983) Relationship between condition score, physical measurements and body fat percentage in mares. *Equine Veterinary Journal* 15(4) 371–372.

Henneke, D.R., Potter, G.D. and Kreider, J.L. (1984) Body condition during pregnancy and lactation and reproductive efficiency of mares. *Theriogenology* 21(6), 897–909.

Henson, F.M., Davenport, C., Butler, L., Moran, I., Shingleton, W.D. *et al.* (1997) Effects of insulin and insulin-like growth factors I and II on the growth of equine fetal and neonatal chondrocytes. *Equine Veterinary Journal* 29(6), 441–447.

Hidiroglou, M. (1979) Trace element deficiencies and fertility in ruminants: a review. *Journal of Dairy Science* 62(8), 1195–1206.

Hines, K.K., Hodge, S.L., Kreider, J.L., Potter, G.D. and Harms, P.G. (1987) Relationship between body condition and levels of serum luteinizing hormone in postpartum mares. *Theriogenology* 28(6) 815–825.

Hintz, H.F. (1996) Mineral requirements of growing horses. *Pferdeheilkunde* 12(3), 303–306.

Hoffman, R.M., Kronfeld, D.S., Holland, J.L. and Greiwe-Crandell, K.M. (1995) Preweaning diet and stall weaning method influences on stress response in foals. *Journal of Animal Science* 73(10) 2922–2930.

Hoffman, R.M., Kronfeld, D.S., Herbein, J.H., Swecker, W.S., Cooper, W.L. *et al.* (1998) Dietary carbohydrates and fat influence milk composition and fatty acid profile of mare's milk. *The Journal of Nutrition* 128(12), 2708S–2711S.

Hoffman, R.M., Morgan, K.L., Lynch, M.P., Zinn, S.A., Faustman, C. and Harris, P.A. (1999) Dietary vitamin E supplemented in the periparturient period influences immunoglobulins in equine colostrums and passive transfer in foals. In *Proceedings of the 16th Equine Nutrition and Physiology Society Symposium*, pp. 96–97.

Holland, J.L., Kronfeld, D.S., Hoffman, R.M., Greiwe-Crandell, K.M., Boyd, T.L. *et al.* (1996) Weaning stress is affected by nutrition and weaning methods. *Pferdeheilkunde* 12, 257–260.

Holmes, A.D., McKey, B.V. and Wertz, A.W. (1946) The vitamin content of mare's milk. *Journal of Dairy Science* 29(3), 163–171.

Hudson, J.M., Cohen, N.D. and Gibbs, P.G. (2001) Feeding practices associated with colic in horses. *Journal of the American Veterinary Medical Association* 219(1), 419–425.

Huntington, P.J., Brown-Douglas, C.G. and Pagan, J.D. (2007) Growth of Australian thoroughbreds compared with horses in New Zealand, America, *England and India. Australian Equine Veterinarian* 26(1), 80–92.

Hurtig, M., Green, S.L., Dobson, H., Mikuni-Takagaki, Y. and Choi, J.J.E.V.J. (1993) Correlative study of defective cartilage and bone growth in foals fed a lowcopper diet. *Equine Veterinary Journal* 25(S16), 66–73.

Ingle, M.E., Bloom, M.S., Parsons, P.J., Steuerwald, A.J., Kruger, P. *et al.* (2017) Associations between IVF outcomes and essential trace elements measured in follicular fluid and urine: a pilot study. *Journal of Assisted Reproduction and Genetics* 34(2), 253–261.

Jacquay, E.T., Zeglin, L.H., Lillich, J.D., Sinclair, C.D., Jones, E.S. *et al.* (2019) Composition of the foal fecal microbiota in response to gradual and abrupt weaning. *Journal of Equine Veterinary Science* 76, 39–40.

Janicki, K.M. (2001) Effect of dietary selenium source and level on broodmares and their foals. *The Horse.* Available at: https://thehorse.com/118005/effects-of-selenium-source-on-mares-and-foals/ (accessed 11 May 2022).

Janicki, K.M., Lawrence, L.M. and Barnes T. (2000) The effect of dietary selenium source and level on broodmares and their foals. *Journal of Animal Science* 83 (Suppl. 1), 172.

Jelan, Z.A., Jeffoott, L.B., Lundeheim, N. and Osborne, M. (1996) Growth rates in Thoroughbred foals. *Pferdeheilkunde* 12, 291–295.

Johnson, L., Blanchard, T.L., Varner, D.D. and Scrutchfield, W.L. (1997) Factors affecting spermatogenesis in the stallion. *Theriogenology* 48(7), 1199–1216.

Johnston, R.H., Kamstra, L.D. and Kohler, P.H. (1970) Mares' milk composition as related to 'foal heat' scours. *Journal Animal Science* 31, 549–553.

Jones, L. and Hollands, T. (2005) Estimation of growth rates in UK thoroughbreds. *Pferdeheilkunde* 21, 121–123.

Jones, L., Lax, J. and Hollands, T. (2005) The mineral content of spring and summer pasture grazed by young growing Thoroughbred in the UK. *Pferdeheilkunde* 21, 21–23.

Katz, L., O'Dwyer, S. and Pollock, P. (2009) Nutritional muscular dystrophy in a four-day-old Connemara foal. *Irish Veterinary Journal* 62, 119–124.

Kelly, A.J. (1999) Practical tips on fostering. In: Harris, P.A., Gomershall, G.M., Davidson, H.P.B. and Green, R.E. (eds) *Proceedings of the BEVA Specialist Days on Behaviour and Nutrition*. Equine Veterinary Journals Ltd, BEVA, Ely, Cambridge, UK.

Klewitz, J., Struebing, C., Rohn, K., Goergens, A., Martinsson, G. *et al.* (2015) Effects of age, parity, and pregnancy abnormalities on foal birth weight and uterine blood flow in the mare. *Theriogenology* 83(4), 721–729.

Knight, D.A., Weisbrode, S.E., Schmall, L.M., Reed, S.M., Gabel, A.A. *et al.* (1990) The effects of copper supplementation on the prevalence of cartilage lesions in foals. *Equine Veterinary Journal* 22(6), 426–432.

Knight, D.A., Gabel, A.A., Reed, S.M., Embertson, R.M., Tyznik, W.J. and Bramlage, L.R. (1985) Correlation of dietary minerals to incidence and severity of metabolic bone disease in Ohio and Kentucky. *Proceedings of the Annual Convention of the American Association of Equine Practitioners* 31, 445–461.

Kocher, A. and Staniar, W.B. (2013) The pattern of thoroughbred growth is affected by a foal's birthdate. *Livestock Science* 154, 204–214.

Kohn, C.W., Knight, D., Hueston, W., Jacobs, R. and Reed, S.M. (1989) Colostral and serum IgG, IgA, and IgM concentrations in Standardbred mares and their foals at parturition. *Journal of the American Veterinary Medical Association* 195(1), 64–68.

Kruglik, V.L., Kouba, J.M., Hill, C.M., Skjolaas-Wilson, K.A., Armendariz, C. *et al.* (2005) Effect of feeding protected n-3 polyunsaturated fatty acids on plasma and milk fatty acid levels and IgG concentrations in mares and foals. In: *Proceedings of the 19th Equine Science Society Symposium,* Tucson, Arizona, pp. 135–136.

Kuhl, J., Winterhoff, N. and Wulf, M. (2010) Changes in fecal bacteria and occurrence of diarrhea during the first 6 weeks of life in foals born to mares supplemented with oral β-carotene. *Animal Reproduction Science* 121, 371–373.

Kumar, N., Verma, R.P., Singh, L.P., Varshney, V.P. and Dass, R.S. (2006) Effect of different levels and sources of zinc supplementation on quantitative and qualitative semen attributes and serum testosterone level in crossbred cattle (*Bos indicus* × *Bos taurus*) bulls. *Reproduction Nutrition Development* 46(6), 663–675.

Lass, A. and Belluzzi, A. (2019) Omega-3 polyunsaturated fatty acids and IVF treatment. *Reproductive BioMedicine* 38(1), 95–99.

Lausigk, Y.S. and Aurich, C. (2014) Influences of a diet supplemented with linseed oil and antioxidants on quality of equine semen after cooling and cryopreservation during winter. *Theriogenology* 81, 966–973.

Lawrence, L.M. (2013) Feeding stallions and broodmares. In: Geor, R., Harris, P. and Coenen, M. (eds) *Equine Applied and Clinical Nutrition. Health, Welfare and Performance.* Saunders Elsevier, Edinburgh, UK, pp. 231–242.

Lawrence, L. and Lawrence, T. (2009) Development of the equine gastrointestinal tract. In: Pagan, J.D. (ed.) *Advances in Equine Nutrition IV*. KER, Versailles, Kentucky, USA. Nottingham University Press, Nottingham, UK, pp. 173–183.

Lawrence, L.M., DiPietro, J., Ewert, K., Parrett, D., Moser, L. *et al.* (1992) Changes in body weight and condition of gestating mares. *Journal of Equine Veterinary Science* 12(6), 355–358.

Le Jeune, S.S., Nieto, J.E., Dechant, J.E. and Snyder, J.R. (2009) Prevalence of gastric ulcers in Thoroughbred broodmares in pasture: a preliminary report. *The Veterinary Journal* 181(3), 251–255.

Lepeule, J., Bareille, N., Robert, C., Ezanno, P., Valette, J.P. *et al.* (2009) Association of growth, feeding practices and exercise conditions with the prevalence of Developmental Orthopaedic Disease in limbs of French foals at weaning. *Preventive Veterinary Medicine* 89(3–4), 167–177.

Lewis, S. (2003) Gastric ulceration in an equine neonate. *Canadian Veterinary Journal* 44(5), 420–421.

Lopez, R.A., Van Soom, A., Arsenakis, I. *et al.* (2017) Boar management and semen handling factors affect the quality of boar extended semen. *Porcine Health Management* 3, 15.

Luthersson, N., Nielsen, K.H., Harris, P. and Parkin, T.D.H. (2009) Risk factors associated with equine gastric ulceration syndrome (EGUS) in 201 horses in Denmark. *Equine Veterinary Journal* 41(7), 625–630.

Madigan, J.E. and Aleman, M. (2015) *Colic in the neonatal foal.* In: *Manual of Equine Neonatal Medicine.* Available at: https://www.ivis.org/library/manual-of-equine-neonatal-medicine/colic-neonatal-foal (accessed 25 August 2020).

Magdesian, K.G. (2005) Neonatal foal diarrhea. *Veterinary Clinics: Equine Practice* 21, 295–312.

Manso Filho, H.C., McKeever, K.H., Gordon, M.E., Costa, H.E.C., Lagakos, W.S. *et al.* (2008) Changes in glutamine metabolism indicate a mild catabolic state in the transition mare. *Journal of Animal Science* 86(12), 3424–3431.

Martin, R.G., McMeniman, N.P. and Dowsett, K.F. (1991) Effects of a protein deficient diet and urea supplementation on lactating mares. *Journal of Reproduction and Fertility* 44, 543–550.

McCall, C.A., Potter, G.D. and Kreider, J.L. (1985) Locomotor, vocal and other behavioural responses to varying methods of weaning in foals. *Applied Animal Behaviour Science* 14, 27–35.

McDonnell, S.M. (2008) Practical review of self-mutilation in horses. *Animal Reproductive Science* 107, 219–228.

McDowell, L.R. (2003) *Minerals in Animal and Human Nutrition*. 2nd edn. Elsevier Science, Netherlands.

McFarlane, D. (2011) Equine pituitary pars intermedia dysfunction. *Veterinary Clinics of North America: Equine Practice* 27, 93–113.

McKenzie, H.C. III (2018) Disorders of foals. In: Reed, S.M. Bayly, W.M. and Sellon, D.C. (eds) *Equine Internal Medicine*, 4th edn. Elsevier, St Louis, Missouri, pp. 1365–1459.

McKenzie, H.C. 3rd and Geor, R.J. (2009) Feeding management of sick neonatal foals. *Veterinary Clinics of North America: Equine Practice*, 25(1).

Meirelles, M.G., Veras, M.M., Alonso, M.A., de Fátima Guimarães, C., Nichi, M. *et al.* (2017) Influence of maternal age and parity on placental structure and foal characteristics from birth up to 2 years of age. *Journal of Equine Veterinary Science* 56, 68–79.

Meyer, H. and Ahlswede, L. (1978) The intra-uterine growth and body composition of foals and the nutrient requirements of pregnant mares. *Animal Research & Development* 8, 86–111.

Moysten, A. and Symonds, M.E. (2009) Early programming of adipose tissue function: a large-animal perspective. *The Proceedings of the Nutrition Society* 68(4), 393–400. doi: 10.1017/S002966510999022X.

Murray, M.J. (1999) Gastroduodenal ulceration in foals. *Equine Veterinary Education* 11, 199–207.

Murray, M.J., Murray, C.M., Sweeney, H.J., Weld, J., Digby, N.W. *et al.* (1990) Prevalence of gastric lesions in foals without signs of gastric disease: an endoscopic survey. *Equine Veterinary Journal* 22(1), 6–8.

Nery, J., Schelino, G., O'Sullivan, J.A., Perona, G. and Bergero, D. (2006) DOD incidence in thoroughbred foals between 23 and 45 weeks of age–growth, nutrition and genetic factors. *Animal Research* 55(6), 591–601.

Nguyen, R.H., Wilcox, A.J., Skjærven, R. and Baird, D.D. (2007) Men's body mass index and infertility. *Human Reproduction* 22(9), 2488–2493.

Nicol, C. (1999) Understanding equine stereotypies. *Equine Veterinary Journal* 31, 20–25.

Nicol, C.J. and Badnell-Waters, A.J. (2005) Suckling behaviour in domestic foals and the development of abnormal oral behaviour. *Animal Behaviour* 70(1), 21–29.

Nicol, C.J., Badnell-Waters, A.J., Bice, R., Kelland, A., Wilson, A.D. *et al.* (2005) The effects of diet and weaning method on the behaviour of young horses. *Applied Animal Behaviour Science* 95(3–4), 205–221.

NRC (National Research Council) (2007) *Nutrient Requirements of Horses*, 6th edn. The National Academies Press, Washington, DC.

O'Donohue, D.D., Smith F.H. and Strickland, K.L. (1992) The incidence of abnormal limb development in the Irish Thoroughbred from birth to 18 months. *Equine Veterinary Journal* 24(4), 305–309.

Ott, E.A. and Asquith, R.L. (1986) Influence of level of feeding and nutrient content of the concentrate on growth and development of yearling horses. *Journal of Animal Science* 62(2), 290–299.

Ott, E.A. and Asquith, R.L. (1989) The influence of mineral supplementation on growth and skeletal development of yearling horses. *Journal of Animal Science* 67(11), 2831–2840.

Ott, E.A. and Kivipelto, J. (2002) Growth and development of yearling horses fed either alfalfa or coastal Bermudagrass: hay and a concentrate formulated for Bermudagrass hay. *Journal of Equine Veterinary Science* 22, 311–322.

Ott, E.A., Brown, M.P., Roberts, G.D. and Kivipelto, J. (2005) Influence of starch intake on growth and skeletal development of weanling horses. *Journal of Animal Science* 83(5), 1033–1043.

Ousey, J.C. (2003) Feeding the newborn foal in health and disease. *Equine Veterinary Education* 6, 50–54.

Ousey, J. (2006) Physiology and metabolism in the newborn foal with reference to orphaned or sick foals. *Nutrition and Feeding of the Broodmare* 120, 187–202.

Ousey, J.C., Fowden, A.L., Wilsher, S. and Allen, W.R. (2008) The effects of maternal health and body condition on the endocrine responses of neonatal foals. *Equine Veterinary Journal* 40(7), 673–679.

Pagan, J.D. (1994) Nutrient digestibility in horses. Feeding the performance horse. In: *Proceedings KER Short Course for Feed Manufacturers*, Lexington, Kentucky, pp. 127–136.

Pagan, J.D. and Hintz, H.F. (1986) Composition of milk from pony mares fed various levels of digestible energy. *The Cornell Veterinarian* 76(2), 139–148.

Pagan, J.D., Geor, R.J., Caddel, S.E., Pryor, P.B. and Hoekstra, K.E. (2001) The relationship between glycemic response and the incidence of OCD in Thoroughbred weanlings: a field study. *In: 47th Annual American Association of Equine Practitioners Convention*, San Diego, California, pp. 433-437 322–325.

Pagan, J.D., Geor, R.J., Caddel, S.E., Pryor, P.B. and Hoekstra, K.E. (2005) The relationship between glycemic response and the incidence of OCD in Thoroughbred weanlings: a field study. In: *Advances in Equine Nutrition III*. Kentucky Equine Research, Versailles, Kentucky, p. 433.

Pagan, J.D., Brown-Douglas, C.G. and Caddel, S. (2006) Body weight and condition of Kentucky Thoroughbred mares and their foals as influenced by month of foaling, season, and gender. In: *Nutrition and Feeding of the Broodmare*. European Association for Animal Production publication. Wageningen Academic Publishers, Wageningen, The Netherlands, pp. 245–252.

Palmer, P., Peugnet, P. and Robles M. (2017) Developmental programming in equine species: relevance for the horse industry. *Animal Frontiers* 7(3), 48–54. doi: 10.2527/af.2017-0128.

Paradis, M.R. (2012a) Feeding the orphan foal. In: *Proceedings of the 58th American Association of Equine Practitioners Convention*, pp. 402–406.

Paradis, M.R. (2012b) Normal foal nutrition. In: *Proceedings of the 58th American Association of Equine Practitioners Convention*, pp. 399–401.

Pearce, S.G., Grace, N.D., Firth, E.C., Wichtel, J.J., Holle, S.A. and Fennessy, P.F. (1998a)Effect of copper supplementation on the copper status of pasture-fed young Thoroughbreds. *Equine Veterinary Journal* 30(3), 204–210.

Pearce, S.G., Grace, N.D., Wichtel, J.J., Firth, E.C. and Fennessy, P.F. (1998b) Effect of copper supplementation on copper status of pregnant mares and foals. *Equine Veterinary Journal* 30(3), 200–203.

Peugnet, P., Wimel, L., Duchamp, G., Sandersen, C., Camous, S. *et al*. (2016) Enhanced or reduced fetal growth induced by embryo transfer into smaller or larger breeds alters post-natal growth and metabolism in pre-weaning horses. *PLoS ONE* 9(7), e102044.

Polzer, J. and Slater, M.R. (1997) Age, breed, sex and seasonality as risk factors for equine laminitis. *Preventive Veterinary Medicine* 29(3), 179–184.

Prado, J.C. (2016) Follicular dynamics in insulin resistant mares. Master's thesis, University of Tennessee, Knoxville. Tennessee Research and Creative Exchange. Available at: https://trace.tennessee.edu/utkgradthes/4303 (accessed 14 Aug 2020).

Prockop, D.J. and Tuderman, L. (1982) Posttranslational enzymes in the biosynthesis of collagen: extracellular enzymes. *Methods in Enzymology* 82, 305–319.

Pugh, D.G. and Williams, M.A. (1992) Feeding considerations for the neonatal foal. *Compendium on Continuing Education for Practising Veterinarian* 14(4), 526–530.

Ralston, S.L. (1996) Hyperglycemia/hyperinsulinemia after feeding a meat of grain to young horses with osteochondritis dissecans (OCD) lesions. *Pferdeheilkunde* 12, 320–322.

Rebholz, S.L., Jones, T., Burke, K.T., Jaeschke, A., Tso, P. *et al*. (2012) Multiparity leads to obesity and inflammation in mothers and obesity in male offspring. *American Journal of Physiology-Endocrinology and Metabolism* 302(4), E449–E457.

Redondo, A., Carranza, J. and Pablo T. (2009) Fat diet reduces stress and intensity of startle reaction in horses. *Applied Animal Behaviour Science* 118, 69–75.

Roberts, M.C., Kidder, D.E. and Hill, F.W.G. (1973) Small intestinal beta-galactosidase activity in the horse. *Gut* 14, 535–540.

Robles, M., Gautier, C., Mendoza, L., Peugnet, P., Dubois, C. *et al*. (2017) Maternal nutrition during pregnancy affects testicular and bone development, glucose metabolism and response to overnutrition in weaned horses up to two years. *PLoS ONE* 12(1), e0169295.

Robles, M., Peugnet, P.M., Valentino, S.A., Dubois, C., Dahirel, M. *et al*. (2018) Placental structure and function in different breeds in horses. *Theriogenology* 108, 136–145.

Rodríguez, C., Muñoz, L., Rojas, H. and Briones, M. (2007) New formula for bodyweight estimation of thoroughbred foals. *Veterinary Record* 161(5), 165.

Rodriguez, A.L., Van Soom, A., Arsenakis, I. and Maes, D. (2017) Boar management and semen handling factors affect the quality of boar extended semen. *Porcine Health Management* 3(1), 1–12.

Roseboom, T.J., Van Der Meulen, J.H., Ravelli, A.C., Osmond, C., Barker, D.J. *et al*. (2003) Perceived health of adults after prenatal exposure to the Dutch famine. *Paediatric and Perinatal Epidemiology* 17(4), 391–397.

Roseboom, T., de Rooij, S. and Painter, R. (2006) The Dutch famine and its long-term consequences for adult health. *Early Human Development* 82, 485–491.

Rouse, B.T. and Ingram, D.G. (1970) The total protein and immunoglobulin profile of equine colostrum and milk. *Immunology* 19, 901–907.

Ruby, H.N., Nguyen, A.J., Wilcox, R. *et al*. (2007) Men's body mass index and infertility. *Human Reproduction* 22(9), 2488–2493.

Ruder, E.H., Hartman, T.J. and Goldman, M.B. (2009) Impact of oxidative stress on female fertility. *Current Opinion in Obstetrics and Gynecology* 21(3), 219–222.

Ruiz, A.J., Tibary, A., Heaton, R.A., Hargreaves, I.P., Leadon, D.P. and Bayly, W.M. (2021) Effects of feeding coenzyme Q10-ubiquinol on plasma coenzyme Q10 concentrations and semen quality in stallions. *Journal of Equine Veterinary Science* 96, 103303.

Samuelsson, A.M., Matthews, P.A., Argenton, M., Christie, M.R., McConnell, J.M. *et al*. (2008) Diet-induced obesity in female mice leads to offspring hyperphagia, adiposity, hypertension, and insulin resistance: a novel murine model of developmental programming. *Hypertension* 51(2), 383–392.

Sanchez, L.C., Lester, G.D. and Merritt, A.M. (1998) Effect of ranitidine on intragastric pH in clinically normal neonatal foals. *Journal of the American Veterinary Medical Association* 212

Sandgren, B., Dalin, G. and Carlsten, J. (1993) Osteochondrosis in the tarsocrural joint and osteochondral fragments in the fetlock joints in

Standardbred trotters. *I. Epidemiology. Equine Veterinary Journal* 25(S16), 31–37.

Santos, A.S. and Silvestre, A.M. (2008) A study of Lusitano mare lactation curve with Wood's model. *Journal of Dairy Science* 91(2), 760–766.

Sathishkumar, K., Elkins, R., Yallampalli, U. and Yallampalli, C. (2009) Protein restriction during pregnancy induces hypertension and impairs endothelium-dependent vascular function in adult female offspring. *Journal of Vascular Research* 46(3), 229–239.

Satterfield, M.C., Coverdale, J.A. and Wu, G. (2010) *Review of fetal programming: implications to horse health*. In *Proceedings of the Annual Convention of the AAEP,* Baltimore, Maryland, December, pp. 207–214.

Savage, C.J., McCarthy, R.N. and Jeffcott, L.B. (1993a) Effects of dietary energy and protein on induction of dyschondroplasia in foals. *Equine Veterinary Journal* 16, 74–79.

Savage, C.J., McCarthy, R.N. and Jeffcott, L.B. (1993b) Effects of dietary phosphorus and calcium on induction of dyschondroplasia in foals. *Equine Veterinary Journal* 16, 80–83.

Schoster, A., Staempfli, H.R., Abrahams, M., Jalali, M., Weese, J.S. *et al*. (2015) Effect of a probiotic on prevention of diarrhea and *Clostridium difficile* and *Clostridium perfringens* shedding in foals. *Journal of Veterinary Internal Medicine* 29(3), 925–931.

Schryver, H.F., Nintz, H.F. and Lowe, J.E. (1971) Calcium and phosphorus inter-relationships in horse nutrition. *Equine Veterinary Journal* 3(3), 102–109.

Schryver, H.F., Meakim, D.W. and Lowe, J.E. (1987) Growth and calcium metabolism in horses fed varying levels of protein. *Equine Veterinary Journal* 19(4), 280–287.

Seghieri, G., De Bellis, A., Anichini, R. *et al*. (2005) Does parity increase insulin resistance during pregnancy? *Diabetic Medicine* 22, 1574–1580.

Sessions-Bresnahan, D.R., Schauer, K.L., Heuberger, A.L. and Carnevale, E.M. (2016) Effect of obesity on the preovulatory follicle and lipid fingerprint of equine oocytes. *Biology of Reproduction*, 94(1), 15.

Sessions-Bresnahan, D.R., Heuberger, A.L. and Carnevale, E.M. (2018) Obesity in mares promotes uterine inflammation and alters embryo lipid fingerprints and homeostasis. *Biology of Reproduction* 99(4), 761–772.

Shalayel, M., Al-Noaemi, M. and Salahaldein, A. (2011) Insulin resistance in the third trimester of pregnancy suffering from gestational diabetes mellitus or impaired glucose tolerance. In: Radenkovic, M. (ed.) *Gestational Diabetes*. IntechOpen, London, pp. 169–182.

Sharkey, D., Gardner, D.S., Fainberg, H.P., Sebert, S., Bos, P., Wilson, V., Bell, R., Symonds, M.E. and Budge, H. (2009) Maternal nutrient restriction during pregnancy differentially alters the unfolded protein response in adipose and renal tissue of obese juvenile offspring. *The FASEB Journal* 23(5), 1314–1324.

Smith-Funk, E.D. and Crowell-Davis, S.L. (1992) Maternal behavior of draft mares (*Equus caballus*) with mule foals (*Equus asinus* x *Equus caballus*). *Applied Animal Behaviour Science* 33, 93–119.

Smyth, G.B. (1988) Effects of age, sex and post mortem interval on intestinal lengths of horses during development. *Equine Veterinary Journal* 20, 104–108.

Staniar, W.B., Kronfeld, D.S., Wilson, J.A., Lawrence, L.A., Cooper, W.L. *et al*. (2001) Growth of thoroughbreds fed a low-protein supplement fortified with lysine and threonine. *Journal of Animal Science* 79(8), 2143–2151.

Staniar, W.B., Kronfeld, D.S., Hoffman, R.M., Wilson, J.A. and Harris, P.A. (2004) Weight prediction from linear measures of growing Thoroughbreds. *Equine Veterinary Journal* 36(2), 149–154.

Staniar, W.B., Kronfeld, D.S., Akers, R.M. and Harris, P.A. (2007) Insulin-like growth factor I in growing thoroughbreds. *Journal of Animal Physiology and Animal Nutrition* 91(9–10), 390–399.

Steelman, S.M., Michael-Eller, E.M., Gibbs, P.G. and Potter, G.D. (2006) Meal size and feeding frequency influence serum leptin concentration in yearling horses. *Journal of Animal Science* 84(9), 2391–2398.

Stelzleni, E.L., Warren, L. and Kivipelto, J. (2006) Effect of dietary n-3 fatty acid supplementation on plasma and milk composition and immune status of mares and foals. *Journal of Animal Science* 84, 392–393.

Stoneham, S.J. (1996) Practical aspects of diarrhoea in the foal with particular reference to rotavirus and gastroduodenal ulceration. *Equine Veterinary Education* 8, 84–90.

Stoneham, S.J. (2013) Feeding orphan and sick foals. In: Geor, R.J., Harris, P.A. and Coenen, M. (eds) *Equine Applied and Clinical Nutrition*, Saunders Elsevier, London, pp. 618–627.

Stoneham, S.J. (2016) Feeding orphan and sick foals. Available at: https://veteriankey.com/feeding-orphan-and-sick-foals/ (accessed 28 July 2020).

Stowe, H.D. (1967) Reproductive performance of barren mares following vitamin A and E supplementation. In: *Proceedings 13th AAEP New Orleans, LA*. AAEP, Lexington, Kentucky, p. 81.

Stradaioli, G., Sylla, L., Zelli, R., Supplizi, A.V., Chiodi, P. *et al*. (2000) Seminal carnitine and acetylcarnitine content and carnitine acetyltransferase activity in young Maremmano stallions. *Animal Reproduction Science* 64(3–4), 233–245.

Streeter, R.M., Divers, T.J., Mittel, L., Korn, A.E. and Wakshlag, J.J. (2012) Selenium deficiency associations with gender, breed, serum vitamin E and creatine kinase, clinical signs and diagnoses in horses of different age groups: a retrospective examination 1996–2011. *Equine Veterinary Journal* 44, 31–35.

Sun, Y., Chen, C., Liu, G.G., Wang, M., Shi, C. *et al.* (2020) The association between iodine intake and semen quality among fertile men in China. *BMC Public Health* 20(1), 1–8.
Suthers, J.M., Pinchbeck, G.L., Proudman, C.J. and Archer, D.C. (2013) Risk factors for large colon volvulus in the UK. *Equine Veterinary Journal* 45(5), 558–563.
Teh A.L., Pan, H., Chen, L., Ong, M.-L., Dogra, S. *et al.* (2014) The effect of genotype and in utero environment on inter individual variation in neonate DNA methylomes. *Genome Research* 24(7), 1064–1074.
Thakur, A.S., Littarru, G.P., Funahashi, I., Painkara, U.S., Dange, N.S. *et al.* (2015) Effect of ubiquinol therapy on sperm parameters and serum testosterone levels in oligoasthenozoospermic infertile men. *Journal of Clinical and Diagnostic Research* 9(9), BC01.
Thompson, K.N., Baker, J.P. and Jackson, S.G. (1988a) The influence of high dietary intakes of energy and protein on third metacarpal characteristics of weanling ponies. *Journal of Equine Veterinary Science* 8, 391–394.
Thompson, K.N., Jackson, S.G. and Rooney, J.R. (1988b) The effect of above average weight gains on the incidence of radiographic bone aberrations and epiphysitis in growing horses. *Journal of Equine Veterinary Science* 8, 383–385.
Thorson, J.F., Karren, B.J., Cavinder, C.A., Hammer, C.J. and Coverdale, J.A. (2010) Effect of selenium supplementation and plane of nutrition on mares and their foals: selenium concentrations and glutathione peroxidase. *Journal of Animal Science* 88(3), 991–997.
Tinker, M.K., White, N.A., Lessard, P., Thatcher, C.D., Pelzer, K.D. *et al.* (1997) Prospective study of equine colic risk factors. *Equine Veterinary Journal* 29(6), 454–458.
Tischner, M. (1985) Embryo recovery from Polish-pony mares and preliminary observations on foal size after transfer of embryos to large mares. *Equine Veterinary Journal*, 3(Suppl.), 96–98.
Topliff, D.R., Kennerly, M.A. and Freeman, D.W. (1989) Changes in urinary and serum calcium and chloride concentrations in exercising horses fed varying cation-anion balances. In: *Proceedings of the 11th Equine Nutrition and Physiology Society Symposium*, Stillwater, Oklahoma, pp. 1–2.
Tyler, S.J. (1972) The behaviour and social organization of the New Forest ponies. *Animal Behaviour Monographs* 5, 85–196.
Tyler-McGowan, C.M., Hodgson, J.L. and Hodgson, D.R. (1997) Failure of passive transfer in foals: incidence and outcome on four studs in New South Wales. *Australian Veterinary Journal* 75(1), 56–59.
Satterfield, M., Coverdale, J., Wu, G. and Moyer, W. (2010) Review of fetal programming: implications to horse health. In: *AAEP Proceedings*, vol. 56, pp. 217–214.
Sharkey, D., Gardner, D.S., Fainberg, H.P., Sebert, S., Bos, P. *et al.* (2009) Maternal nutrient restriction during pregnancy differentially alters the unfolded protein response in adipose and renal tissue of obese juvenile offspring. *The FASEB Journal* 23, 1314–1324. doi: 10.1096/fj.08-114330.
Ullrey, D.E., Struthers, R.D., Hendricks, D.G. and Brent, B.E. (1966) Composition of mare's milk. *Journal of Animal Science* 25(1), 217–222.
Ullrey, D.E., Ely, W.T. and Covert, R.L. (1974) Iron, zinc and copper in mare's milk. *Journal Animal Science* 38, 1276–1277.
van Dijk, S.J., Tellam, R.L., Morrison, J.L., Muhlhausler, B.S. and Molloy, P.L. (2015) Recent developments on the role of epigenetics in obesity and metabolic disease. *Clinical Epigenetics* 7, 66.
van Niekerk, F.E. and van Niekerk, C.H. (1997) The effect of dietary protein on reproduction in the mare. III. Ovarian and uterine changes during the anovulatory, transitional and ovulatory periods in the non-pregnant mare. *Journal of the South African Veterinary Association* 68(3), 86–92.
van Niekerk, F.E. and van Niekerk, C.H. (1998) The effect of dietary protein on reproduction in the mare. VII. Embryonic development, early embryonic death, foetal losses and their relationship with serum progestogen. *Journal of the South African Veterinary Association* 69(4), 143–149.
van Weeren, P.R., Sloet van Oldruitenborgh-Oosterbaan, M.M. and Barneveld, A. (1999) The influence of birth weight, rate of gain and final achieved height and sex on the development of osteochondrotic lesions in a population of genetically predisposed Warmblood foals. *Equine Veterinary Journal* (Suppl. 31), 26–30.
van Weeren, P., Knaap, J. and Firth, E. (2003) Influence of liver copper status of mare and newborn foal on the development of osteochondrotic lesions. *Equine Veterinary Journal* 35, 67–71.
Vervuert, I., Voigt, K., Brussow, N., Hollands, T., Cuddeford, D. and Coenen, M. (2005) Insulinaemic and glycaemic responses following changes in the order of feeding oats and chopped alfalfa to horses. *Pferdeheilkunde* 21, 89.
Vondran, S., Venner, M. and Vervuert, I. (2016) Effects of two alfalfa preparations with different particle sizes on the gastric mucosa in weanlings: alfalfa chaff versus alfalfa pellets. *BMC Veterinary Research* 12, 110.
Vural, P., Akgül, C., Yildirim, A. and Canbaz, M. (2000) Antioxidant defence in recurrent abortion. *Clinica Chimica Acta* 295(1–2), 169–177.
Wall, D.L., Topliff, D.R., Freeman, D.W., Wagner, D.G., Breazile, J.W. *et al.* (1992) Effect of dietary cation-anion balance on urinary mineral excretion in exercised horses. *Journal of Equine Veterinary Science* 12(3), 168–171.
Warnakulasooriya, D.N., Marth, C.D., McLeod, J.A., Hanlon, D.W. and Krekeler, N. (2018) Treatment of

retained fetal membranes in the mare—a practitioner survey. *Frontiers in Veterinary Science* 5, 128.

Waters, A., Nicol, C. and French, N. (2002) Factors influencing the development of stereotypic and redirected behaviours in young horses: findings of a four year prospective epidemiological study. *Equine Veterinary Journal* 34(6), 572–579.

Willard, J.G., Williams, J.L., Willard, J.C., Greene, J.R. and Knapp, E.A. (2005) The effect of age of dam on birth weight and growth rate of Thoroughbred foals. *The Growing Horse: Nutrition and Prevention of Growth Disorders* 114, 65.

Wilsher, S. and Allen, W.R. (2003) The effects of maternal age and parity on placental and fetal development in the mare. *Equine Veterinary Journal* 35(5), 476–483.

Wilsher, S. and Allen, W.R. (2006) Effects of a *Streptococcus equi* infection—mediated nutritional insult during midgestation in primiparous Thoroughbred fillies. Part 1: placental and fetal development. *Equine Veterinary Journal* 38, 549–557.

Wilson, J.H. (1987) Feeding considerations for neonatal foals. In: *Proceedings 24th American Association of Equine Practitioners Convention*, p. 823.

Wilson, R.L., Bianco-Miotto, T., Leemaqz, S.Y., Grzeskowiak, L.E., Dekker, G.A. *et al.* (2018) Early pregnancy maternal trace mineral status and the association with adverse pregnancy outcome in a cohort of Australian women. *Journal of Trace Elements in Medicine and Biology* 46, 103–109.

Winkelsett, S., Vervuert, I., Granel, M., Borchers, A. and Coenen, M. (2005) Feeding practice in warmblood mares and foals and the incidence to osteochondrosis. *Pferdeheilkunde* 21, 124–126.

Wojsiat, J., Korczyński, J., Borowiecka, M. and Żbikowska, H.M. (2017) Udział stresu oksydacyjnego w niepłodności żeńskiej oraz w zapłodnieniu metodą in vitro. *Advances in Hygiene & Experimental Medicine/Postepy Higieny i Medycyny Doswiadczalnej* 71.

Zeyner, A., Geißler, C., Peschke, I., Kny, G. and Jope, R. (1996) Beitrag zum Fettsäurenmuster in der Stutenmilch. *Pferdeheilkunde* 12, 213–219.

Zeyner, A. Bessert, J. and Gropp, J.M. (2002) Effects of feeding exercised horses on high-starch or high-fat diets for 390 days. *Equine Veterinary Journal* (Suppl. 34), 50–57.

15 The Chronically Inflamed (Obese) Horse: Understanding Adipose Biology

TERESA HOLLANDS

School of Veterinary Medicine, University of Surrey

Learning Objectives

LO1 Communicate the welfare issues associated with fatness by explaining the underlying adipose biology
LO2 Explain evidence that supports an underlying chronic inflammation in fat horses and its relationship with disease
LO3 Summarise factors including management and feeding practices that increase the risk of obesity in horses
LO4 Describe how to reduce the risk of obesity in horses
Measuring and communicating fatness
LO5 Make dietary recommendations for the obese horse and the prevention of weight gain
Controlling calories
Maintaining bulk
Balancing micronutrients
Exercise and lifelong management changes

At the end of this chapter, you will be able to provide evidence for dietary recommendations for managing and minimising obesity in horses based on your understanding of adipose biology.

An Overview of Obesity in Horses

Estimates of obese/overweight horses in the UK vary from 45% (Wyse *et al.*, 2008) to 54% of leisure horses (Stephenson *et al.*,2011). There is a greater incidence in ponies – 41% of ponies versus 26% of horses (Robin *et al.*, 2013), with 29% being hyperinsulinaemic (Morgan *et al.*, 2014). This undoubtedly reflects what you see on a daily basis.

Due to its prominence in the media, clients might understand the relationship between adiposity and health, but the effect on the horse (and human) is often delayed; thus clients find it difficult to accept the seriousness of their horses 'looking well'. Your clients are unaware that adipose tissue produces cytokines which totally compromise the way their horse can metabolise its food. They relate insulin resistance to the feeding of concentrates, although most leisure horses are only on low intakes of low-starch concentrates. Owners are unaware of the epigenetic risks – breeding fatness into breeds (see Chapter 14: 'Introduction and overview') – but they do associate fatness with a potential risk of laminitis.

Your clients need to know that their horses are suffering from chronic low-grade inflammatory disease, which:

- reduces their horse's immune response (Millner and Beck, 2012; Wood *et al.*, 2018); and
- reduces the efficacy of vaccinations (Horohov *et al.*, 2010; Honce and Schultz-Cherry, 2019).

It also increases the risk of:

- respiratory disease in humans (Zammit *et al.*, 2010) and potentially in horses (Bond *et al.*, 2018);

 Evidence-based Equine Nutrition: A Practical Approach for Professionals (T. Hollands and L. Drury)
DOI: 10.1079/9781789245134.0015

- dermatological conditions (Nedoszytko *et al.*, 2014);
- poor wound healing and infection (in humans) (Fasol *et al.*, 1992); and
- osteoarthritis (Salonen *et al.*, 2009).

All of these are positively correlated with increased fat mass, duration of fat mass and ageing.

Despite the health risks, only 4.5% of owners defined their horse as obese (Morrison *et al.*, 2017). This inability to recognise fatness is similar to human medicine and is attributed to the upward shift in what is considered normal body size (Burke *et al.*, 2010).

This normalisation (Harker *et al.*, 2011; Owers and Chubbock, 2013) means that 'fatness' or 'comfortably cuddly' is acceptable to most owners. In fact, one of the biggest risk factors of a horse being fat is being on a yard with other overweight horses (Salonen *et al.*, 2009) – a behaviour recognised as social reinforcement where an individual's decision is based on the collective decision (Mann, 2018), in this case the other livery owners (and an acceptability of this normality in the photos used in the media). This is a challenge that is recognisable to anyone who works with horse owners.

If clients do not recognise fatness, then the responsibility to educate the owner falls to you, other professionals and para-professions – in fact anyone with any interaction with the horse. The success of that communication depends in part on the language used, the trust and relationship that the client has with you, the support of the other para-professionals and an understanding of the factors that increase the risk of the horse getting fat.

- Various factors increase the risk of horses getting fat.
- Clients need to recognise fatness in their horses.
- You need to fat score the horse at every visit, so it becomes something that is normal, not accusatory, teaching the client to use the technique.
- Clients underestimate the calories from forage and would rather blame a handful of hard feed whilst at the same time overestimating their horse's workload.
- Clients fail to grasp the fact that they need to make lifelong lifestyle changes to keep their horses fit, including feeding, management and exercise; complicated by the fact that they think feeding excess calories to the good doer will make them more energetic.

Helping clients understand by providing them with a good evidence base to support your advice will empower them in the decision making, improving the health and welfare of all horses in your care. This will require the following:

- Appreciation that the dysregulation of their horse's fat tissue might have started before they owned them.
- An understanding of exactly what the fat cells are doing to their horses.
- Ongoing support:
  - over several visits; and
  - transitioning from fat to fit – in lots of small steps.

The Biology of Fat Cells

Because fatness or obesity is so prevalent in society, with many sensitive to 'sizeism', the seriousness and the complexity of the 'disease' is often overlooked. The effect of a dysfunctional adipose mass is varied across a spectrum; different cytokines are involved and, depending on the timing of sampling, results are variable. An ability to talk to clients about the underlying biology moves us from telling to showing the serious consequences.

Adipose tissue and cytokines

Adipose tissue (AT) (adipocytes, pre-adipocytes and macrophages) is the largest endocrine organ in the body secreting hormones, cytokines, metabolites and adipokines.

Adipokines function as hormones, impacting horses' regulation of their (and our) immune, metabolic and vascular systems (Zhang *et al.*, 1994; Kershaw and Flier, 2004), affecting the brain, liver, muscle systems and feedback to adipose tissue.

Top tip

In response to chronic overnutrition:

- Adipose tissue can become dysfunctional.
- Adipose tissue is remodelled.
- Dysregulation of the adipose cytokines and metabolites is induced, leading to metabolic dysfunction (Choe *et al.*, 2016).

The detrimental effect of obesity takes time

Metabolic dysregulation appears to be progressive; the number of macrophages 'entering' the fat cells increases in line with fat mass (Sun *et al.*, 2011), causing progressive increases in oxidative stress, production and secretion of proinflammatory adipokines, insulin resistance, and impaired microvascular function (Rutkowski *et al.*, 2009). This inflammation becomes pathological, affecting the whole body (horse or human) with an increase in plasma biomarkers and inflammatory cells (Table 15.1) (Rogero, and Calder, 2018), depending upon the amount of fat tissue (subcutaneous and visceral) and duration of the fatness.

Top Tip

Explain to the client that their horse has a dysfunctional adipose mass causing their horse to suffer from chronic low-grade inflammatory disease.

The fat mass of people and other animals varies. Fat as a percentage of total body mass varies between humans from 6% to 41% (Levenhagen *et al.*, 1999), to 27% of a dog's body mass (mean BCS 5/9) measured by dual-energy X-ray absorptiometry (DEXA) and computerised tomography (CT) (Turner *et al.*, 2020) but only 5% of the body mass of swine, camels, deer and bovines (Pond, 1978).

In horses, the dissected fat content varied from 1.7% (white adipose tissue) (BFS 1/9) to 30% in seven ponies (BFS > 5/9) (Dugdale *et al.*, 2011a,b). Dissected fat mass from 5-month-old foals varied from 5% to 13% and fillies were fatter than colts (Gee *et al.*, 2003). Other papers measured similar body fat % in mixed-age horses and ponies (Robb *et al.*, 1972; Schryver *et al.*, 1974; Westervelt *et al.*, 1976).

Why does excess adipose tissue change metabolism?

Insulin is the primary regulator of carbohydrate, fat, and protein metabolism, protecting against nutrient fluctuations by:

- increasing lipogenesis (the synthesis of fatty acids activated by high carbohydrate availability) in the adipose tissue;
- inhibiting lipolysis (breakdown) of stored fat in the adipose tissue;
- increasing:
  - synthesis of glycogen in the muscle;
  - protein synthesis;
  - the translocation of the GLUT-4 protein increasing muscle glucose;
  - gene expression of proteins required for the optimal cellular function, cellular repair, and growth; and
- suppressing glucose production and release from the liver, ensuring the metabolic availability of various fuels to the brain (Sears and Perry, 2015).

This metabolic control becomes compromised in obesity and fat cells stop insulin working properly.

Explaining to the client

There is a limit to how much extra nutrition cells can store. When they are full, the trouble starts.

In an overfed horse, the amount of glucose stored in the muscle and liver is exceeded, and the cells switch off to insulin. Normally, 80% of glucose should go to muscle cells (Vargas *et al.*, 2020); instead, the pancreas releases more insulin, which talks to the fat cells, sending blood glucose to the fat cells, which start to fill up (lipogenesis).

The extra insulin brings the blood glucose levels down and the fat cells 'mop up' the glucose. If the pancreas has continued exposure to excess calories, it ends up shouting at the fat cells by releasing even more insulin. The cells take notice but after a while they stop listening, so the pancreas shouts louder and releases even more insulin. High levels of insulin stop the fat cells releasing fat, sealing the extra calories in the fat cells, which increase in size.

Eventually the fat cells cannot hear insulin at all; they have switched off to the constant shouting and even a small amount of carbohydrate elicits a large response from the pancreas. Plasma insulin concentrations are elevated (hyperinsulinaemia) in horses with obesity-associated insulin resistance (Suagee *et al.*, 2011). Infusing glucose into normal non-obese ponies to maintain hyperinsulinaemia (serum insulin 1100 mU/l) results in laminitis (Asplin *et al.*, 2007).

Insulin resistance

> 'Insulin resistance (IR) is positively correlated with obesity in all species and is a pathophysiological state where cells display reduced responsiveness to the glucose-lowering activity of insulin' (Fazakerley *et al.*, 2019).

Insulin should stimulate GLUT to transport glucose from the blood. Exercise is protective, stimulating the movement (translocation) of vesicles containing glucose transporter proteins (GLUT-4) to the plasma membrane with an increase in plasma glucose (Suagee *et al.*, 2011).

Table 15.1 Adipokines[a] and their roles[b]

Adipokine/cytokine	Effects	Energy expenditure	Insulin sensitivity	Fatty acid oxidation	Appetite	Fat accumulation	Lipolysis	GLUT 4	Other roles
Leptin is secreted in response to food intake and inhibits appetite by regulating neural circuits located in the brain	Secreted by adipocytes in direct proportion to fat mass: 'leptin may be a marker of adipocyte hypertrophy and not just adiposity per se' (Reynolds *et al.*, 2019)	Increases	Improves	Increases	Decreases	Decreases	Increases and reduces muscle, liver and pancreatic intracellular lipid		Alters endothelial cell and microvascular function via: impaired insulin-mediated nitric oxide synthesis, increased ET-1 production, induction of oxidative stress, up-regulation of adhesion molecules
Tumour necrosis factor (TNF alpha) increased in the obese adipose tissue	Blocks adiponectin Increases adhesion molecules on endothelial cells		Decreases – inhibits insulin receptor signalling in adipose tissue and skeletal muscle		Decreases		Increases	Decreases	TNF is known to suppress genes involved in uptake and storage of fatty acids and glucose, as well as adipogenesis (Ruan *et al.*, 2002; Clement *et al.*, 2004a; de Luca and Olefsky, 2008)
Interleukin 6	Correlate with intolerance to CHOs. Inhibits adiponectin	Increases	Decreases		Decreases	Increases			
Adiponectin: exerts anti-obesity and anti-diabetic effects and alleviates insulin resistance by stimulating lipid oxidation and anti-inflammatory responses	Anti-inflammatory inhibits ROS, increases NO	Increases	Improves	Increases		Decreases			Secreted by mature adipocytes
Chemokine ligand 2 (CCL2)			Decreases insulin signalling in muscle cells						Attracts monocytes and basophils to the adipose cells. Molecular link in the negative cross-talk between adipose tissue and skeletal muscle
Interleukin 1-B (Mann *et al.*, 2016)	Positively associated with increase in fat tissue Increases inflammatory cytokines	IL-1β promotes metabolic dysfunction							Produced in the cytoplasm of cells, including monocytes, neutrophils, hepatocytes, but they are mostly synthesised by macrophages. One of the major cytokines found in the plasma

[a]Adipose tissue produces several adipokines and their production is regulated by insulin, catecholamines and adiposity
[b]Adipokines exert metabolic effects, both in central and in peripheral tissues

But in horses with IR, GLUT translocation to muscle and fat cell membranes is altered, which researchers suggest might indicate early pathogenic factors in disease development (Waller *et al.*, 2012).

IR reduces or stops both glycogenolysis and gluconeogenesis in the liver – less glucose is released and insulin-stimulated glucose uptake and utilisation in muscle and adipose tissues is reduced (Czech, 2020).

Insulin essential for life

It is important that owners appreciate that an increase in insulin within normal physiological limits is essential for life. In fact, there are times when animals become naturally insulin resistant for short periods of time, ensuring that blood glucose is diverted to the brain and other key organs. Do remind clients about IR in pregnancy (see Chapter 14: 'Gestation'), sepsis and starvation.

Long-term IR and metabolic compromise

This threatens the welfare of horses. Increased cellular inflammation alters insulin's function by increasing the phosphorylation of the insulin receptor substrate (IRS-1), reducing the strength of insulin's signal (Sears and Perry, 2015).

IR, cortisol and FAs

In people, a transporter at the blood–brain barrier responds to increased free fatty acids produced in the liver, activating the hypothalamus axis to release cortisol, triggering insulin resistance (Sears and Perry, 2015). Some of this response is due to the type of fatty acid (omega-6 versus omega-3), which is less relevant for your clients' horses: it is the increase in diacylglycerols (DAG) that seems to do the most damage (Sears and Perry, 2015). DAG is elevated in the serum of both vaccinated and infected horses and is a 'sensitive indicator of immune activation' (Wood *et al.*, 2018).

The relationship with IR, adiposity and fatty acids

The more fat on the outside, the more fat there is in the horse's bloodstream.

Horses with a high fat score (Dugdale *et al.*, 2011a,b; Pleasant *et al.*, 2013) or equine metabolic syndrome (EMS) (Elzinga *et al.*, 2016) have higher levels of plasma triglycerides (TGs) compared with lean horses, as do overweight people compared with their lean counterparts (Boden, 2008), generating IR in the muscles.

Clients often forget that, in turn, insulin plays a role in regulating the levels of fat in the blood. Explain to them that IR horses find it harder to lower serum free fatty acids (Czech, 2020); the more fat they can palpate on their horse, the more fat there is in the blood stream.

Plasma free fatty acids

As fat cells increase in size, cellular inflammation and insulin resistance develop increasing plasma free fatty acids (FFA). The problem with this is that free fatty acids:

- increase plasma chemokine (monocyte chemoattractant protein-1) (MCP-1), increasing migration and infiltration of monocytes/macrophages into adipose tissue;
- induce IR at cellular level by interacting with glucose transporter systems and phosphorylation, reducing glucose-6-phosphate and glycogen synthesis (Simon *et al.*, 2013); and
- cause IR and inflammation in skeletal muscle, liver and endothelial cells.

High FA in dogs increases IR *in vivo*, 'impairing hepatic insulin extraction which might contribute to the peripheral hyperinsulinaemia of obesity' (Wiesenthal *et al.*, 1999). Fat horses with increased free TGs had plasma insulin levels that exceeded published values (209±53 mIU/l) compared with non-obese ponies (Dugdale *et al.*, 2011a,b).

Intramuscular fat

The more fat they can feel, the more fat is stored in their horse's muscles.

Insulin increases the amount of fat stored in muscles. Lean insulin-sensitive horses infused with insulin had reduced adipose but increased skeletal muscle lipid transporters and fatty acid transporter proteins (Suagee *et al.*, 2013).

Increased intermuscular fat increases cytokine production because it acts like an ectopic fat depot similar to visceral adipose tissue (VAT) (Addison *et al.*, 2014). Fat horses have increased intermuscular adipose tissue and intramuscular fat (Fig. 15.1) (Dugdale *et al.*, 2011a,b).

Top tip

When a horse is fat, its metabolism is altered. The horse cannot prevent toxic lipid accumulation in the liver and skeletal muscle, which:

- increases pro-inflammatory cytokines; and
- stimulates lipolysis in adipocytes;

leading to lipotoxicity in the brain, liver, skeletal muscle, pancreatic islets, or other tissues (Yu *et al.*, 2002; Choe *et al.*, 2016), which changes whole-body glucose tolerance and insulin sensitivity (Czech, 2020).

Fat storage

Skeletal muscle fat (SMF) is the 'last resort' for excess fat (Table 15.2). SMF in people deregulates insulin signalling, resulting in insulin resistance (Feijóo-Bandín *et al.*, 2020).

Fat cell size

To store the extra fat, the visceral and mesenteric adipocytes increase in size (hypertrophy) (Joe *et al.*, 2009). An increase in fat cell size results in local adipose tissue micro-hypoxia (Trayhurn and Wood, 2004) which upregulates inflammatory cytokines (Hosogai *et al.*, 2007), resulting in the death of the fat cells. Compared with lean horses, obese horses with EMS have adipocyte hypertrophy (Fig. 15.2), increased inflammation and chemokine (C-C motif) ligand 2 (CCL2) expression in their intra-abdominal adipose tissue depots (peri-renal and retroperitoneal adipose tissue) (Reynolds *et al.*, 2019).

Increased visceral fat increases liver FFAs via the portal vein, decreasing hepatic clearance of insulin from the pancreas, which may cause increased peripheral levels of insulin and glucose (Bojsen-Møller *et al.*, 2018).

- Compared with controls, Equine Metabolic Syndrome (EMS) horses had:
  - significantly increased plasma triacylglycerides, diacylglycerides, monoacylglycerides and ceramide;
  - significantly lower plasma sphingomyelins, sulfatide and choline ether lipids/plasmalogens; and
  - positive correlation between plasma triglycerides and non-esterified fatty acids (NEFA), and body fat/condition score (Elzinga *et al.*, 2016).

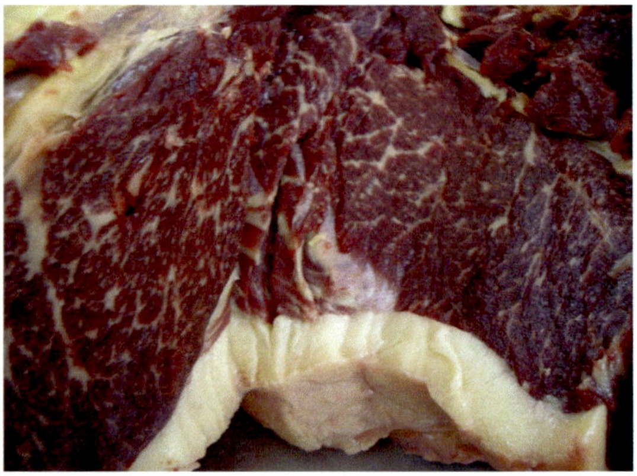

Fig. 15.1 Subcutaneous and intramuscular fat of a 250 kg pony (fat score 4, 4, 4). (Photo used with permission from Professor Derek Knottenbelt.)

Table 15.2 Fat storage depots

Fat storage depots	Order in which excess calories are stored
Subcutaneous (SAT)	1
Visceral (VAT)	2
Intermuscular (INTMF)	3
Intramuscular (IMF)	4
Skeletal muscle fat (SMF)	5

- Fat horses have higher fasting plasma triglyceride and NEFA regardless of whether they have EMS (Suagee *et al.*, 2013).

Regional Fat Deposition and IR

Regardless of the species, the longer the animal (including humans) is fat, the more fat is redistributed to several distinct anatomical areas within the body. The effect of adiposity (sometimes without obesity) on associated metabolic abnormalities seems to differ according to the anatomical distribution, and the functional peculiarities of the fat tissue. Whether this storage is the cause of insulin resistance or a consequence of it is under investigation

You will be familiar with the change in regional accumulation of fat characterising horses with EMS or pituitary pars intermedia dysfunction (PPID) (Fig. 15.3).

'Apple-shaped' people store visceral fat around the abdomen/stomach, historically associated with an increased risk of disease compared with 'pear storage'/subcutaneous (hips and bottom) (Fig. 15.4).

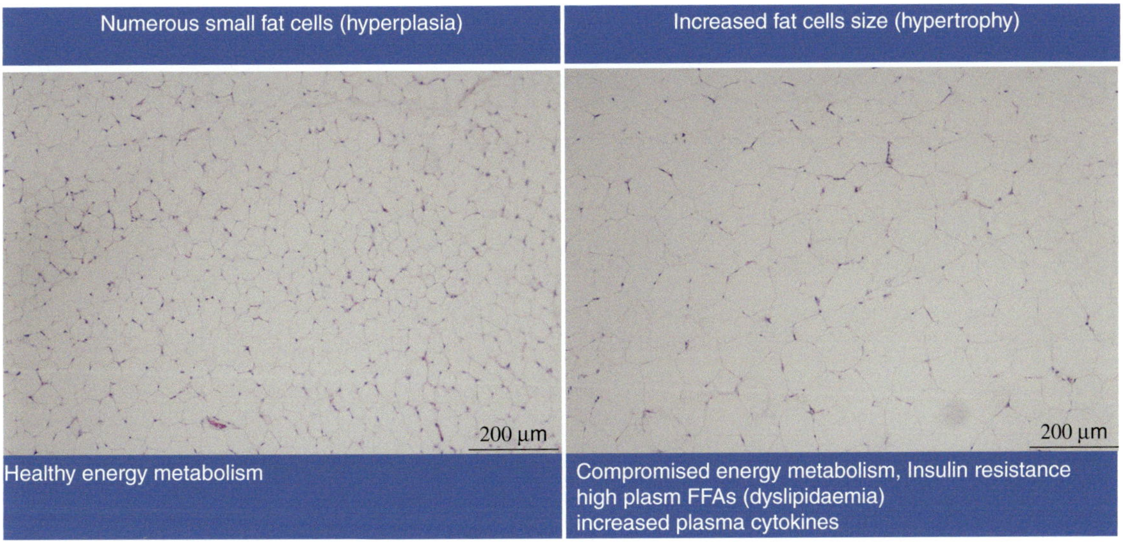

Fig. 15.2 A comparison of fat cell sizes between horses with EMS (exhibiting hypertrophy) and control horses (hyperplasia) (Reynolds *et al.*, 2019). (Photos copyright Dr Ruth Morgan, Royal Dick School of Veterinary Medicine, University of Edinburgh.)

Visceral or abdominal white adipose tissue correlates with insulin resistance and cardiovascular disease in humans (Feijóo-Bandín *et al.*, 2020), dogs (Mazaki-Tovi *et al.*, 2016) and cats (Okada *et al.*, 2017, 2019) compared with subcutaneous fat stores. Subcutaneous fat (manually palpated to allocate the horse a fat score) was thought to have little effect on metabolism, because fat cells under the skin increase in number (hyperplasia) to store the extra fat rather than increase in size (hypertrophy).

Body fat scoring

Body condition score (BCS) measures the amount of subcutaneous fat (subcutaneous adipose tissue: SAT) which increases in proportion to visceral fat (visceral adipose tissue: VAT) (Turner *et al.*, 2020). It may be that the anatomical position rather than 'fat type' is an indicator rather than the cause of IR. Mouse adipocyte size in both visceral and subcutaneous fat deposits is positively correlated with frequency of adipocyte death and macrophage numbers (Hosogai *et al.*, 2007).

Regional versus fat cell type

Human researchers have measured visceral and subcutaneous fat (Kang *et al.*, 2011; Samsell *et al.*, 2014; Karpe and Pinnick 2015) in the upper body (android or central) and lower body (gynoid or peripheral) area (Kang *et al.*, 2011) to categorise truncal fat by anatomical distribution rather than cell type.

Regional fat distribution (android–gynoid fat ratio), combined with lean tissue mass, is more predictive of long-term metabolic health compared with just total body fat or intra-abdominal compartmentalisation of fat (Okosun *et al.*, 2015). Upper-body SAT promotes inflammation (McLaughlin *et al.*, 2010) even in 'normal weight' people (Samsell *et al.*, 2014; Min and Min, 2015; Okosun *et al.*, 2015), although the risk differs between men and women (Lu *et al.*, 2019); whereas lower-fat distribution around the thighs decreases the risk of disease (Snijder *et al.*, 2005).

Regional distribution of fat

Regional distribution rather than the 'type' of fat might aid understanding of the subgroup of people clinically defined as metabolically healthy obesity (MHO) (Karpe and Pinnick, 2015; Blüher, 2020). MHO people (BMIs over 30 kg/m^2) are insulin sensitive, exhibit normal blood glucose, lipid levels and plasma inflammatory markers, with lower number of immune cells and higher proportions of

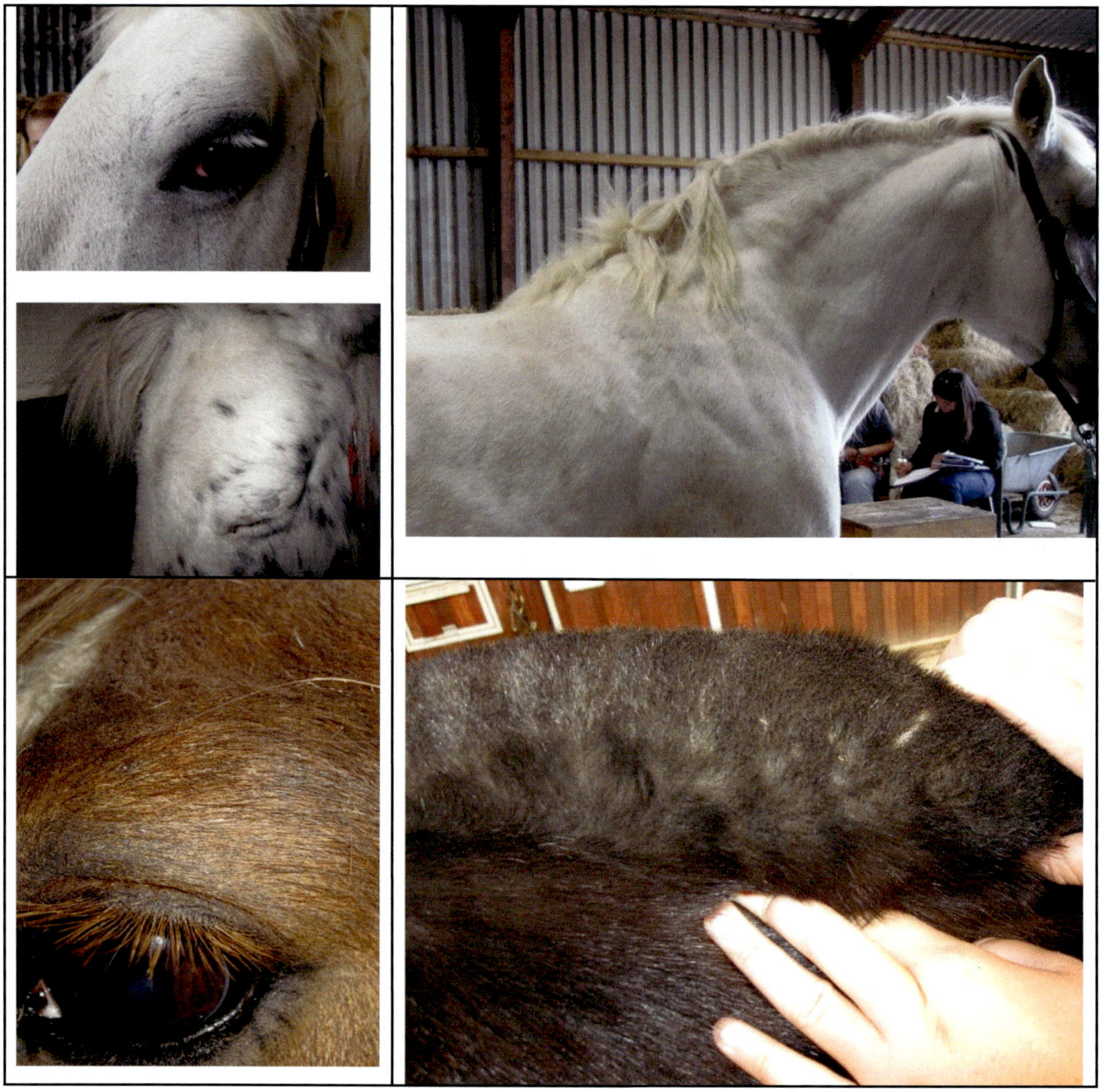

Fig. 15.3 Fat depots in the chronic inflammation horse. Metabolism changes where the horse stores its fat either in supraorbital fossa or as a cresty neck.

relatively small adipocytes in adipose tissues (Choe *et al.*, 2016).

It is only when the fat tissue is associated with an increased risk of disease that the medical term of obesity is used to describe this fat mass in people (Zdrojewicz *et al.*, 2017).

There are regional differences in gene expression and triglyceride (TG) turnover rate between upper-body and lower-body adipose tissue depots (similar to that between visceral and subcutaneous fat tissue (topography)) (Joe *et al.*, 2009; Karpe and Pinnick, 2015), but differences in gene expression are not recorded by all researchers (Pinnick *et al.*, 2014).

- There is a positive correlation between regional fat deposition and fat scoring in horses: as fat scores increased, dissected quantities of intermuscular white adipose tissue increased (Dugdale *et al.*, 2011a,b).

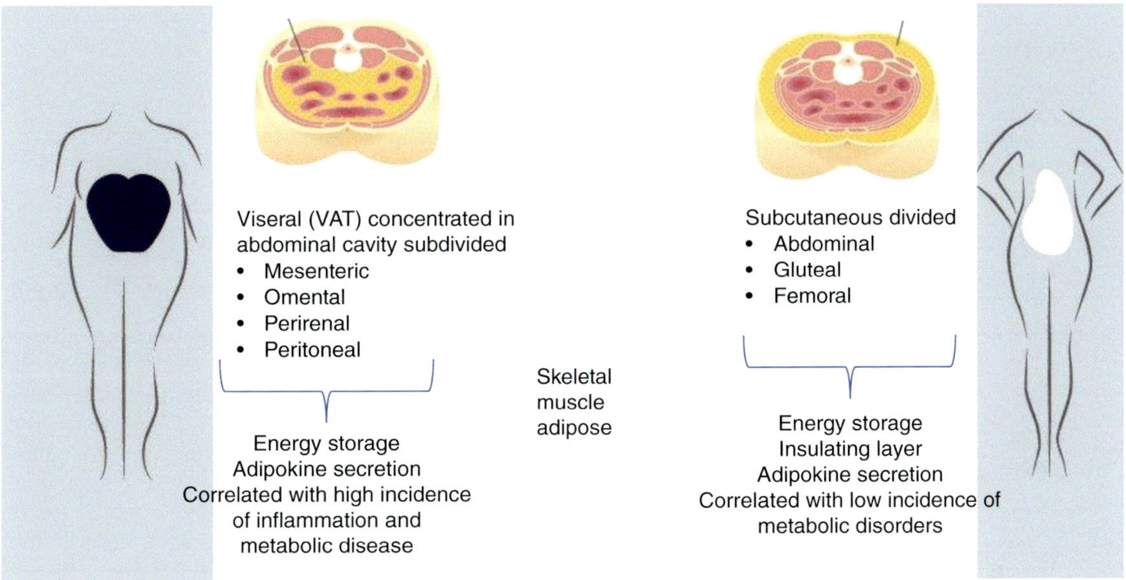

Fig. 15.4 Fat depots in humans.

- But horses with and without EMS have similar concentrations of cytokine gene expression, circulating cytokine and acute-phase proteins concentrations (Zak *et al.*, 2020a,b).

Maybe it is time to re-categorise fat deposits in horses.

Re-categorising upper and lower fat in horses

Specific subcutaneous deposits (nuchal ligament) in horses are correlated with an increase in insulin resistance (Fitzgerald *et al.*, 2019) and higher concentrations of mRNA coding for IL-1b and IL-6 (Burns *et al.*, 2010). Because this relationship was established with subcutaneous rather than visceral deposits, some researchers argue that adiposity in horses is not an inflammatory disease.

If fat distribution is re-categorised to upper and lower body (to include both visceral and subcutaneous in these areas), then the correlations might be better reflective of the chronic inflammation.

- Horses increasing in fat over a 2-year period had 'pro-inflammatory cytokine mRNA IL-1β, IL-6 and TNFα levels that were higher in subcutaneous depots compared to abdominal depots after body weight gain' (Blaue *et al.*, 2020).
- High levels of cortisol in people leads to a depletion of lower body fat and redistribution to upper body fat (similar to that seen in PPID and EMS).

The cresty neck

The cresty neck score could be used as measure of subcutaneous, intramuscular and possibly visceral fat deposit, i.e. a topographical indicator of inflammation in horses.

Cresty neck scores (Carter *et al.*, 2009b) have been validated through diagnosis and subsequent dissection (Briceño *et al.*, 2017).

Fat accumulated above the nuchal ligament (subcutaneous) and infiltrated into the muscle made it difficult to distinguish structures: 'Ultrastructural study of muscle fibre biopsies from the cresty neck revealed the presence of lipid droplets within the muscle fibres.' 'Grade 4-degree abundant fat vacuoles in the space inter myofibrillar tendency to coalesce and fatty infiltration in muscle tissue (marked lipomatosis)' (Briceño *et al.*, 2017).

Top tip

- Regional fat distribution can be measured in your clients' horses by teaching them the modified fat score index that allocates a score to the nuchal ligament as part of fat scoring the neck (see Chapter 3: 'How to cresty neck score').
- Higher nuchal AT is correlated with increased IL-6 mRNA and IL-6 and IL-1β expression, indicating increased gene expression of pro-inflammatory markers (Bruynsteen *et al.*, 2013).

As a crest gets bigger, clients will report that it has 'gone hard'. This might be because of crown-like structures.

Crown-like structures

These are found around dead adipocytes, thought to be resorbing the lipid remnants of these cells. They are more numerous in visceral than in subcutaneous fat; maybe because visceral fat cells die at a smaller size compared with SAT, which contain significantly larger depots (Murano *et al.*, 2008). In obese humans and mice, 90% of all adipose tissue macrophages form crown-like structures (CLS) (Murano *et al.*, 2008).

CLS have been found in various fat tissues in horses (Fig. 15.5)

Get clients to imagine the inflammatory response to these 'dying cells' and to consider that maybe CLS is only found in long-term crests, being a reflection of obesity duration, which is positively correlated with inflammation.

What Is Chronic Inflammatory Disease?

Because the pancreas does not become exhausted in the horse and there are mixed results in the literature, the question still remains as to whether horse obesity is a chronic inflammatory disease or whether it differs from other species. The debate in the equine literature might be an artefact of study design, small population numbers, artificially induced insulin resistance and short duration of obesity and it would be remiss to ignore the wider literature.

> 'Inflammation at the systemic and/or tissue levels has now been shown to be associated with all the main types of laminitis, from endotoxemic to endocrinopathic' (Eades, 2010).

The ever-increasing volume of research into equine obesity, whether the pathophysiology or aetiology of the disease, raises more questions than answers (as it does in other species too) but the similarities between the physiology, the biochemistry and diseases associated with obesity across all

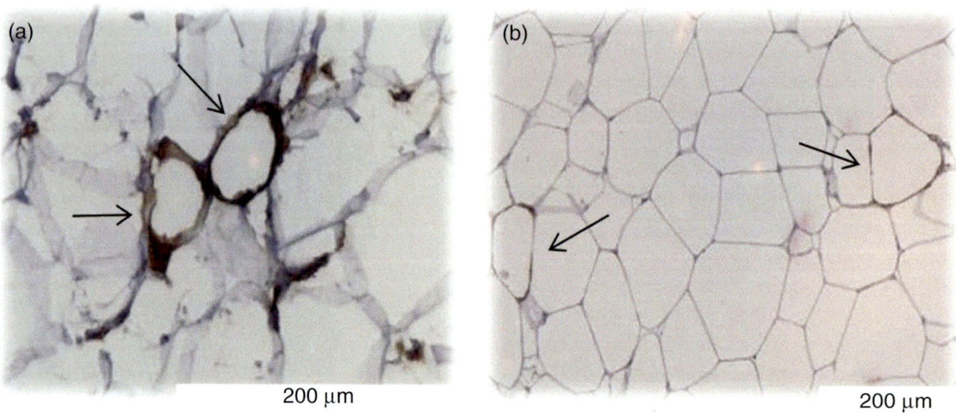

Fig. 15.5 Capping or crown-like structures (CLS) in fat tissue from the horse: (a) loin adipose tissue; (b) neck tissue. Arrows show the capping. This capping was found in multiple fat tissues in the horse (Adapted from Bruynsteen *et al.*, 2013.).

species is stark and clear. Factors associated with inflammation across all species include neutrophils, macrophages, tumour necrosis factor (TNF), suppressors of cytokine signalling (SOCS) proteins, interleukins, the hormones leptin and adiponectin, as well as free radicals, age and duration of obesity.

Why is dysfunctional fat inflammatory?

- Healthy subcutaneous adipose tissue produces anti-inflammatory adipokines (adiponectin, interleukin 10 (IL-10), or nitric oxide (NO)), which promote insulin sensitivity.
- Dysfunctional adipose tissue produces pro-inflammatory cytokines (leptin, TNF and interleukins 6 and 1b) (Feijóo-Bandín *et al*., 2020) causing activated macrophages to infiltrate the adipose tissue, promoting insulin resistance.

White blood cells (WBCs)/leukocytes (monocytes, lymphocytes, neutrophils, basophils and eosinophils)

Plasma free fatty acids increase infiltration of monocytes into adipose tissue.

- The WBC monocytes differentiate into macrophages, which become the most abundant cell type among adipose tissue, comprising nearly 50% of the total immune cells (Carvalheira *et al*., 2013).
- The number of macrophages 'entering' the fat cells increases in line with fat mass (Sun *et al*., 2011), increasing:
  - oxidative stress;
  - production and secretion of proinflammatory adipokines, as part of the immune response;
  - insulin resistance; and
  - impaired microvascular function (Rutkowski *et al*., 2009).
- The proportion of adipose tissue macrophages (ATMs) in fat cells increases from 18% in lean humans and mice to 40% in obese humans and mice.
- The increase in ATM is proportional to increased bodyweight correlating with insulin resistance (Lumeng *et al*., 2007).
- ATMs differentiate differently in obese people, producing different cytokines compared with lean people.
  - In lean people and mice, ATMs produce more arginase, supressing nitric oxide and IL-10 and improving insulin sensitivity by protecting the fat cells from TNF.
  - In fat people, monocytes differentiate into ATMs generating cytokines, including TNF, NO and IL-6 (Lumeng *et al*., 2007).
- EMS horses exhibit differences in ATM compared with lean controls (Fig. 15.6)
- The fatter the horse, the more WBCs in the fat and the more cytokines are produced.

Getting your head around the cytokines helps explain the danger of excess adipose tissue.

Cytokines produced by dysfunctional fat

Tumour necrosis factor (TNF)

Macrophages produce TNF, which:

- increases insulin resistance, by inhibiting adipose tissue and skeletal muscle insulin receptors;
- activates and recruits inflammatory cells, suppressing genes involved in uptake and storage of fatty acids, glucose and adipogenesis (Clark, 2007); and
- regulates macrophage function – key players in the pathogenesis of obesity (Parameswaran and Patial, 2011).

All fat animals with insulin resistance (IR) have higher levels of TNF mRNA and protein compared with the leaner controls (Hotamisligil *et al*., 1993) and horses are no exception.

> 'TNFα has been shown to play a pivotal role in orchestrating the cytokine cascade in many inflammatory diseases and because of this role as a "master-regulator" of inflammatory cytokine production' (Parameswaran and Patial, 2011).

Obese horses have higher blood TNF-α expression compared with lean controls, correlated with body fat scores (Vick *et al*., 2007).

- Laminitis-prone ponies have higher TNF-serum levels (Treiber *et al*., 2009).
- Increased serum TNF is an independent risk for IR (Vick *et al*., 2007).
- Fat (6.6–7.2/9) insulin-resistant horses have higher VAT TNF but no differences in SAT TNF compared with controls (Waller *et al*., 2012).

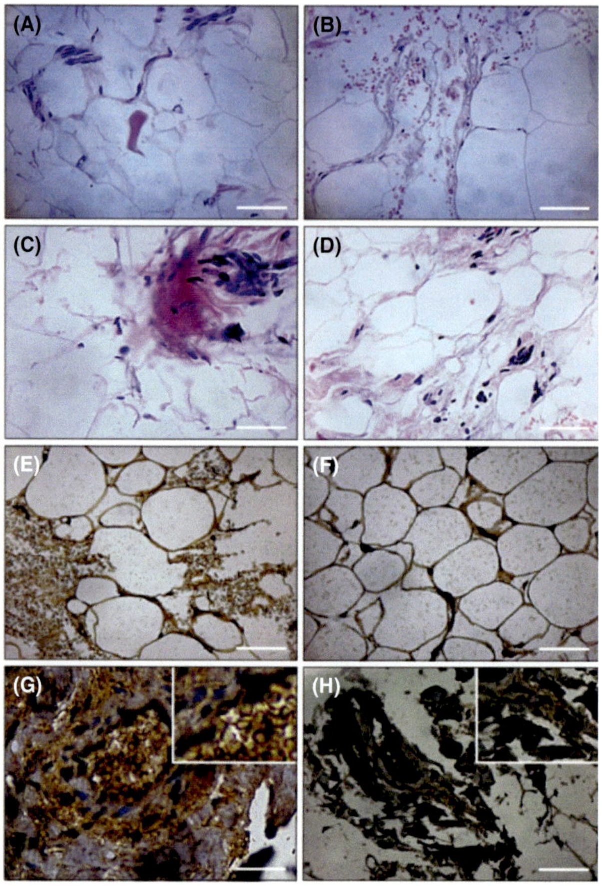

Fig. 15.6 Adipose tissue macrophages of equine metabolic (EMS) ponies (left-hand column) compared with lean ponies (right-hand column). Scale bar: 60 μm, 40× magnification. (Adapted from Basinska *et al*., 2015.)

- TNF is higher in:
  - both visceral and subcutaneous fat of EMS horses (peri-renal adipose tissue and retroperitoneal adipose tissue), compared with healthy horses (Reynolds *et al*., 2019)
  - serum (1.970 μg/ml), despite similar adipocyte TNF levels compared with controls (1.250 μg /ml) ($p = 0.0007$) (Basinska *et al*., 2015).

The length of time the horse has been fat, and thus the amount of adipocyte hypertrophy, might explain the differences in visceral and subcutaneous TNF levels.

And it is not just TNF.

Top tip

Clients need to understand that the longer their horse has been fat, then the more likely the 'engorgement of adipocytes with excess lipid, leading to dysfunction of the adipose tissue which can contribute to whole body insulin dysregulation through release of free fatty acids' (Reynolds *et al*., 2019).

Toll-like receptor-4 protein (TLR4)

IR horses have higher levels of both TLR4 and TNF in skeletal muscle and visceral fat tissue compared with normal horses (Waller *et al*., 2012).

TLR4 in insulin target tissues triggers the release of TNF from macrophages, activating the obesity-induced inflammatory pathway (Rogero and Calder, 2018) and pro-inflammatory kinases; and impairing insulin signal transduction, thereby causing insulin resistance and inflammation in the muscle (Kim and Sears, 2010).

Top Tip

- Because TLR4 is the trigger, it might be a better biomarker of early inflammation and laminitis compared with TNF (Waller *et al.*, 2012).
- TLR4 is triggered by a high omega-6:3 ratio.
- The main source of omega-3 in a horse's diet is fresh grass, which for overweight horses is often restricted or replaced by hay (low in omega-3), increasing omega-6:3 ratios.
- Advise a balancer

Interleukin-1β (IL-1)

TNF stimulates IL-1 production from macrophages, endothelial and epithelial cells.

- IL-1 is a pro-inflammatory cytokine controlling a variety of innate immune processes and involved in host-defence responses to infection and injury (Lopez-Castejon and Brough, 2011).
- IL-1 stimulates the hypothalamus, increasing the release of ACTH (Jung *et al.*, 2010).
- Circulating levels of IL-1 are lower in obese adolescents (Jung *et al.*, 2010) compared with obese adults.
  - Differences in levels might be related to strength of the inflammatory stimulus and the target tissue (Lopez-Castejon and Brough, 2011).
- Obese horses have higher blood TNF-α and IL-1β mRNA expression but lower IL-6 compared with non-obese horses, suggesting an independent risk for IR in obese horses (Vick *et al.*, 2007).
- Endogenous IL-1 gene expression is significantly decreased in hyperinsulinaemic obese horses compared with normal-weight horses (Holbrook *et al.*, 2012).

Interleukin 6 (IL-6)

- IL-6 is a pleiotropic cytokine secreted by and acting on a wide variety of tissues and cells.
- IL-6 has both pro- and anti-inflammatory properties:
  - regulating the synthesis of pro-inflammatory cytokines; and
  - promoting the synthesis of anti-inflammatory cytokines (Sarvas *et al.*, 2013).
- IL-6 levels are correlated with sex: obese women have higher IL-6 concentration compared with controls, but obese males do not (Popko *et al.*, 2010). This might be another reason why there are apparent conflicting results in the equine literature (see Table 15.3).
- Compared with a control group, EMS ponies have:
  - higher subcutaneous adipose tissue expression of IL-6; and
  - significantly elevated levels of serum IL-6 and TNF (Basinska *et al.*, 2015).
- ILP-6 and TNF are higher in mares, compared with geldings and stallions (Suagee *et al.*, 2012).

If Basinska *et al.* (2015) only studied geldings, they might have not measured differences. Researchers need to detail the sex of horses when comparing results.

The inflammatory response is also controlled by certain proteins that 'interact' with cytokines. TNF is the main cytokine responsible for hepatic production of acute-phase proteins (APRs) in several obese species (Popko *et al.*, 2010).

Proteins involved in cytokine responses

Acute-phase protein responses (APR)

By increasing insulin resistance causing hyperglycaemia and hypertriglyceridemia (Faty *et al.*, 2012), APR increases the delivery of nutrients to inflammatory and immune cells.

- In horses, the acute-phase protein (e.g. C-reactive protein, serum amyloid A (SAA)) appears to be the principal component of the response
  - SAA in humans is associated with diabetes and impaired glucose tolerance (Muhammad *et al.*, 2016).
- SAA reduces the storage capacity of adipocytes during APR.
  - It releases free fatty acids and reduces glucose transporter GLUT4, potentially resulting in adipose tissue insulin resistance (Faty *et al.*, 2012).

Plasma concentration of SAA protein increases 1000-fold within 24–48 h following inflammation, to protect cells from further damage (Faty *et al.*, 2012). Although increased serum SAA should increase the antioxidant ability of high-density lipoproteins (HDL) (Sato *et al.*, 2016) there is only a modest increase of SAA from enlarged adipocytes linked to inflammatory diseases (Faty *et al.*, 2012).

Likewise in horses, there is mixed evidence as to whether SAA indicates inflammation.

- Lipopolysaccharides, administered to horses as an inflammatory stimulus, increase SAA 236-fold above basal (Suagee *et al.*, 2013).
  - Although fat horses had no increase in SAA over a 2-year period (Blaue *et al.*, 2020) (see Table 15.3), there is a positive association of SAA with BCS and insulin (Suagee *et al.*, 2013) and exercise and diet (presumably resulting in fat loss) which, compared with diet alone, decreases serum SAA in fat horses (Bamford *et al.*, 2019).

You may have read that, because these results are inconclusive, equine obesity is not inflammatory, but that is not the conclusion of human research.

TNF also increases adipose levels of a group of proteins called suppressors of cytokine signalling, in the β-cell (Rønn *et al.*, 2007).

Cytokine signalling proteins (SOCSs)

SOCSs are tissue-specific signalling proteins which mediate cytokine-induced insulin resistance in adipocytes (Shi *et al.*, 2004), yet again emphasising how dangerous fat is for the horse. They do this by:

- downregulating cytokine signalling (Shi *et al.*, 2004);
- binding to the leptin receptor, preventing leptin action; and
- binding to the insulin receptor, impairing insulin action (Carow and Rottenberg, 2014);

all of which have the potential to exacerbate dysfunctional fat accumulation.

Obese/diabetic mice have high adipose levels of SOCS (Shi *et al.*, 2004), but SOCS levels drop if they are protected from insulin resistance (Palanivel *et al.*, 2012).

- IR horses have higher levels of SOCS3 in visceral and muscle tissue, compared with healthy horses.
- Higher levels of SOCS are positively correlated with TLR4 protein content in insulin-sensitive tissue in horses (remember that TLR4 increases IR).
- Maybe TLR4 indirectly regulates glucose homeostasis by downregulating insulin signalling and causing IR in the equine foot (Waller *et al.*, 2012).

Increased SOCS3 expression triggers the inhibitory effects of IL-6 on insulin signalling and glucose uptake; and sadly obesity/chronic low-grade inflammation is associated with increased levels of IL-6 (Sarvas *et al.*, 2013). Of course, this is related to duration of obesity; we know that as horses get fatter (over 2 years) there is an increase in their intra-abdominal macrophages (ATMs) (Blaue *et al.*, 2020). In people this obesity-correlated increase is stimulated by leptin both *in vitro* (Wilson *et al.*, 1997) and *in vivo* (Mabuchi *et al.*, 2005).

Hormones

Leptin

- Leptin is a polypeptide hormone.
- It regulates the storage, balance and energy use by the body.
  - Leptin is secreted by fat cells (adipocytes).
  - Levels are correlated with the degree of obesity.
- Circulating leptin binds to a receptor in the brain, in proportion to increased triglyceride (TG) content, to:
  - increase energy use; and
  - decrease food intake and bodyweight (Pérez-Pérez *et al.*, 2020).
- Leptin levels drop quickly in starvation or fasting, triggering overfeeding and decreasing energy expenditure (Ahima, 2008).

Top tip

- Weight loss during fasting or starvation is often unsuccessful because leptin triggers metabolic adaptations conserving energy.
- High levels of administrated leptin (as produced by a fat horse), and calorie restriction in people, increase inflammatory markers, platelet aggregation, vasoconstriction and nitric oxide deficiency (Canavan *et al.*, 2005).
- These are some of the reasons why you should advise owners of fat horses to decrease calories but maintain dry matter intake.

Leptin and obesity

Leptin acts as a pro-inflammatory adipokine, maintaining a chronic inflammatory state of obesity.

- Leptin signalling is impaired by increased inflammatory signals in the hypothalamus in obese animals (Meyers *et al.*, 2010), producing hyperleptinaemia (Pérez-Pérez *et al.*, 2020).

Table 15.3 A summary of current evidence that investigates the relationship between adiposity and inflammatory disease in the horse. Only significant results from the literature have been tabulated – for more detail see the cited papers. Available at: https://www.cabidigitallibrary.org/doi/book/10.1079/9781789245134.0000#suppl

- Initial high fasting serum leptin independent of baseline BMI/fat mass could predict increases in BMI and fat mass over time (Fleisch *et al.*, 2007).
  - Leptin might be a useful biomarker for susceptibility to chronic inflammation.
- High doses of leptin have no effect on appetite or bodyweight loss of obese humans (Bluher and Mantzoros, 2009; Pérez-Pérez *et al.*, 2020).
- Obese people are considered leptin resistant (Pérez-Pérez *et al.*, 2020), not leptin deficient (Ahima, 2008).
- Blocking the inflammatory signals with pharmaceuticals stops the impairment (Meyers *et al.*, 2010).

Leptin, appetite and obesity in ponies

There is a relationship between fatness and appetite in ponies. Non-obese ponies gaining weight for the first 4 weeks through the summer had increased appetites but after 7 weeks, as body fat score increased, appetite decreased to 79% of their original intake (Dugdale *et al.*, 2011a,b), maybe in response to leptin levels, which were not measured.

Obese ponies that ate less in the summer compared with non-obese ponies showed no changes in bodyweight or appetite over time, although fat mass increased.

The role of leptin is still to be fully elucidated in humans, but there is strong evidence that once obesity becomes established, an upward setting of leptin and other cascades defends the higher levels of body fat (Meyers *et al.*, 2010) together with a decrease in adiponectin levels.

If the ponies' fatness is maintained because of access to palatable food, then leptin will rise and eventually reduce, creating a new steady state but with higher adiposity.

Alternatively, was the food/energy intake low enough to trigger an increase in leptin to conserve energy expenditure or were they leptin resistant?

When the palatable diet is replaced by a less palatable diet, and intake is reduced, cellular leptin resistance in humans and other animals is not sufficient to maintain the full obesity phenotype (Meyers *et al.*, 2010), reducing diet-induced obesity (DIO). Maybe that is why straw is a useful forage for obese horses?

- As old horses get fatter, serum levels of leptin increase (Buff *et al.*, 2002).
- Leptin mRNA expression is significantly higher in the horse's neck compared with the mesenteric AT (Bruynsteen *et al.*, 2013).

Top tip

To minimise the upward setting of leptin:

- Body fat score every time you see a horse.
  - Write it down.
  - Teach the client to use the system every fortnight.
- Place fat horses at the bottom of the show placings.
  - Point out to dressage riders that the topline is fat, not muscle.
- Support the farrier in their sometimes forthright communication of fatness (Lynden *et al.*, 2018).
- Explain the epigenetic implications of breeding from fat animals (see Chapter 14: 'Feeding the broodmare').
- Do not tell the owner that their horse needs starving

Adiponectin

Adiponectin increases insulin sensitivity and reduces inflammation and is often studied at the same time as leptin.

- Human adiponectin:leptin ratio is negatively correlated with systemic inflammation and positively correlated with insulin resistance (Frühbeck *et al.*, 2017).
- Seasonal increases in ponies' subcutaneous body fat (measured by ultrasound) decreases adiponectin and increases leptin (Staub *et al.*, 2019).
- Decreases in ponies' weight and fat lowered leptin and increased adiponectin (Bamford *et al.*, 2019).
- EMS ponies have higher levels of leptin compared with controls, but no differences in adiponectin (Reynolds *et al.*, 2019).
  - This may be because adiponectin levels in horses were better predicted by higher cresty neck scores compared with higher body fat score (Fitzgerald *et al.*, 2019).

Another argument against equine obesity being inflammatory and causing insulin resistance is that the clearest relationship has only been recorded in old horses.

Ageing and Obesity

It is widely acknowledged that, as an animal or person ages, they become more chronically inflamed (inflammaging). The human literature discusses and explores the conundrum as to whether systemic inflammation in the ageing person is a cumulative negative effect of both obesity and ageing (Erskine *et al.*, 2017) or because of a loss of muscle mass.

- IL-6 is positively correlated with BMI, total body fat and % body fat in young and old people (Erskine *et al.*, 2017).
- When controlled for fat mass, TNF is positively correlated with older muscle size and strength (in muscle cells TNF stimulates protein synthesis during muscle remodelling) (Moore *et al.*, 2020).
- In ageing and obesity, WBC immune cell responses are dysregulated (Frasca and Blomberg, 2016).
    - This creates a pro-inflammatory microenvironment resulting in increased systemic inflammation and decreased longevity (Trim *et al.*, 2018).

Multispecies researchers:

- recognise that 'accumulation of predominantly pro-inflammatory immune cells in obese adipose tissue exacerbates the immunometabolic dysfunction of the tissue and might act as a potent stimulus for accelerating ageing in obesity' (Trim *et al.*, 2018); and
- acknowledge that ageing causes changes in adipose dysfunction irrespective of the amount of fat the animal carries.

The relationship between ageing and inflammation in horses may be complicated by the fact that the majority of older horses are fat or overweight (Ireland *et al.*, 2011), possibly in the early stages of EMS or PPID, confounding results.

- Aged healthy horses do *not* have higher levels of inflammatory cytokines compared with adult horses.
- Aged horses with PPID do have higher levels of inflammatory cytokines (Zak *et al.*, 2020a).
- Adult horses with EMS do not have higher levels of cytokines compared with matched controls but did have a strong correlation between the basal insulin and IL-6 serum concentrations (Zak *et al.*, 2020b).
- Old horses have higher levels of TNF compared with young, but when the older horses lost weight, then serum TNF also decreased (Adam *et al.*, 2009).

The results in old horses most probably are reflective of the obese horse. In human medicine, obesity is considered an accelerated model of ageing (Pérez *et al.*, 2016; Trim *et al.*, 2018). Remember: **the only scientific validated intervention for healthy longevity is the maintenance of lean body mass** (Adams *et al.*, 2016).

> **Top Tip**
>
> - Remind clients that human medicine shows that age-related increases in fat tissue increase pro-inflammatory cytokine levels that interfere with the insulin action (Park *et al.*, 2014).
> - Controlling the accumulation of visceral or upper body fat (crests) in their horses from an early age reduces chronic inflammation and the disease risk associated with the pathophysiology.

Linking the puzzle

Researchers are still attempting to elucidate the biology behind the inflammatory response; it is highly likely that relationships between obesity, cytokines and physiology will vary depending on numerous confounding and uncontrollable factors.

When considering if obesity is inflammatory, think why levels of cytokines relative to equine obesity are inconsistent in the literature.

- Are researchers taking samples from different tissues? We know that:
    - nuchal ligament, plasma and serum cytokine IL-1β mRNA expressions are significantly lower in the horse's loin AT compared with the mesenteric and peri-renal AT (Bruynsteen *et al.*, 2013); and
    - IL-1β, IL-6 and TNFα levels are higher in subcutaneous depots compared with abdominal depots after 2 years of weight gain (Blaue *et al.*, 2020).
- Are they measuring different cytokines (Table 15.1)?
- Are studies carried out on ponies or on horses with an induced form of hyperinasulinaemia, so straight comparisons are challenging (Elzinga *et al.*, 2016)?

- Are they studying horses that have been obese for different lengths of time?
- Are they taking measurements of isolated cytokines, adipose depots and depths so results are not always comparable?
  - Data should be expressed as g/adipose tissue to improve comparison (Trim *et al.*, 2018).

In horses, information that is missing includes:

- a full history as to length of obesity:
  - whether the horse has lost weight in the winter;
  - exercise levels (exercise is protective against IR, but also upregulates IL-6, which induces IR (Spangenburg, 2007));
  - breed of horse;
- the diet history:
  - feeding management.

Sampling relative to mealtimes will impact on the metabolite; sampling methods differ.

You can help work out the puzzle by:

- measuring and monitoring acute versus long-term effects;
- being pragmatic, recognising that 'adiposity is a heterogeneous and multifaceted disorder in which subgroups of obese subjects present varying cardiometabolic profiles' (Okosun *et al.*, 2015); and
- being pragmatic:
  - metabolically healthy obese people have high body fat and favourable lipid profiles, are highly insulin sensitive and do not suffer from diabetes or hypertension; and
  - metabolically unhealthy obese people are at a high risk of cardiometabolic disease.

Maybe we are trying to oversimplify obesity and horses should be grouped into these subgroups.

It is unlikely (but possible) that the horse is unique and their obesity is not related to chronic inflammation; however, there is enough evidence for you to support clients in understanding the effect that excess fat has on the long-term health and welfare of their horses, even if you do not want to call it chronic low-grade inflammatory disease!

Summarising the relationships between fat and the horse's health for clients might be the first step to discussing the advantages of their horse being fighting fit rather than fighting the fat (Box 15.1).

Factors Increasing the Risk of Chronic Low-grade Inflammation (Fatness/Obesity) in Horses

There are several factors that increase the risk of obesity in horses, some directly related to nutrition and many related to clients' personal views and perceptions and the social normalisation of obesity (Burke *et al.*, 2010).

- Clients tend not to recognise fatness in their own horses.
- They think that a handful of hard feed causes laminitis; they don't feed their horse – it gets fat on fresh air.
- They perceive that feeding will help their laid-back horse feel more energetic.
- They breed from horses winning in the show ring.

This is challenging for you, as it takes time for clients to accept evidence-based science.

Failure to recognise obesity

This is not restricted to horses. Children's risk of becoming overweight is positively correlated with parental overweight and obesity (Danielzik *et al.*, 2002) and closely reflects the BMI of the mother rather than the father.

The association between the fatness of the mother and child is likely linked to the fact that cooking and feeding a family is strongly associated with a caring maternal role (DeVault, 1991 – 'cooking as caring', cited in Cairns *et al.*, 2010). UK leisure horse owners report that feeding their horse reflects their caring and 'in fact building or reinforcing their relationship with it' (Furtado *et al.*, 2020). The emotional attachment of owners to their horses contributes to a lack of recognition of obesity in their horses; 60% of Dutch horse owners (who were predominantly female) considered their horses to be 'like a parent or child to them' (Visser and Van Wijk-Jansen, 2012).

There is a positive correlation between obesity in dogs and their owners (Nijland *et al.*, 2010). Dog and cat owners fail to recognise obesity in their pets, rationalising or justifying the problem as caring, because they have humanised the pet and consider feeding as caring (Larson and Villaverde, 2016). Underestimation of body condition by New Zealand's cat owners was the single most important risk factor for obesity (Loftus and Wakshlag, 2014); 27% of dog owners underestimate their dog's body condition score by 2 points, which is the same as 20–30% excess body fat (Singh *et al.*, 2002).

Box 15.1 Communicating adipose biology to clients

- Not all fat tissue is the same.
  - Some fat tissue is simply a store of excess calories.
  - Some fat tissue is dysfunctional.
- Dysfunctional fat tissue is metabolically active.
  - It secretes metabolites and hormones, called cytokines and adipocytokines.
- Dysfunctional fat increases the speed at which horses and humans age.
  - The horse will have a shortened lifespan.
- Dysfunctional fat changes the way the horse can handle its food at cell level.
  - It increases or causes insulin resistance.
  - It affects the lining of the blood vessels and changes blood flow.
  - It increases or causes chronic low-grade inflammation (CLI).
  - It reduces the effectiveness of the horse's immune system.
- The substances secreted by the dysfunctional fat change, depending upon where the horse stores its fat.
- In obesity, fat is redistributed:
  - to the nuchal ligament (topline);
  - above the eyes (supraorbital fossa);
  - around the organs (visceral) in the intestine; and
  - in the muscles.
    - If you see fat in these areas, it means that the horse's metabolism has changed.
    - Fat in the nuchal ligament is a warning that the horse is likely to be insulin resistant.
- Dysfunctional fat attracts white blood cells (macrophages) into fat tissue to mop up the damaged fat cells – they increase inflammation when they do this.
- The more fat the horse has and the longer it is fat, the greater is the dysfunction.
  - It is normal for the horse to get fatter in the spring and summer, especially if it is not working very hard.
  - But it is vital that the horse loses that fat in the winter.
    - If the horse is not working or in light work or young, then it is good if you can just see the ribs at the end of the winter.
- Exercise reduces the amount of damage the fat can do to the horse even before it starts to lose the fat
- Reducing the amount of food the horse eats makes its body think it is starving and so it hangs onto its fat more and resets its metabolism (leptin levels).
  - It is important to control or reduce calories but maintain bulk (dry matter intake).
- The effects of chronic, low-grade inflammatory disease or dysfunctional fat are not immediate – they can take years.
  - That is why not all fat horses have problems.
  - Think of fat as a stealth fat – it creeps up on the horse and you do not realise things are going wrong, until it is too late.
- Chronic low-grade inflammatory disease is poor welfare and bad for the horse's health.
- The more fat you can palpate:
  - the more fat there is inside the horse's body, wrapped around and within the organs; and
  - the more free fatty acids there are in its bloodstream.
  - This fat is secreting chemicals that are changing the horse's metabolism and killing it from the inside out – over time, slowly but surely.
- Reducing chronic low-grade inflammation reduces the horse's risk of:
  - osteoarthritis;
  - non-allergic skin conditions (e.g. sweet itch);
  - respiratory problems;
  - equine metabolic syndrome (EMS);
  - pituitary pars intermedia dysfunction (PPID)/Cushings;
  - laminitis;
  - unhealthy ageing; and
  - poor reactions to vaccinations.
- Fighting fit = healthy longevity (chronological and performance)

Even in Brazil, a country not known for overweight dogs, 68% of clients with obese dogs underestimated their dog's body condition score and 8% of those owners disagreed that obesity was a health risk (Porsani *et al.*, 2020a,b); in the UK, where 50% of dogs are overweight, 70% of UK dog owners feel other problems are more serious than obesity (PFMA, 2019).

What about your clients? Daily, you will be only too familiar with the above concepts and your experience is supported by the evidence: 60% of companion and casual riding horses are classed as obese (Furtado *et al.*, 2020) but only 4.5% of owners perceive their horse to be obese (Morrison *et al.*, 2017b), reinforcing the challenges you face.

Normalisation of obesity

Fatness in horses is normalised and socially acceptable (Burke *et al.*, 2010), reinforced by the persistent placing of obese horses in the show ring (and dogs at Crufts) subsequently featured in the media as examples of success (Fig. 15.7)

Despite this normalisation, pet owners are aware of the increased risk of diseases associated with obesity, as are horse owners (Furtado *et al.*, 2020), but the incidence of obesity continues to rise. Is there a lack of clarity in owners' understanding of 'obesity', which with other factors influences recognition and acceptance of weight-related discussions (Bland *et al.*, 2009; PDSA, 2020)?

> **Top tip**
>
> One of the factors affecting owners' lack of clarity on obesity can be resolved very easily: ensure that a body fat score (BFS) is recorded at every visit.

Intermittent body fat scoring in practice

Small animal vets (UK) rarely assign a body condition score (BCS) to dogs; only one consult out of 1899 had a BCS recorded, although 43 had a descriptive note as to 'overweight, underweight, fat or thin' (German and Morgan, 2008). In Canada, 89.6% of small animal consults in Ontario used and noted BCS and 44–68% of vets took a BCS monthly, 68% using the 5-point system compared with 38% using the 9-point score (Santarossa *et al.*, 2018).

The reasons cited by UK vets as to why they did not use BCS included the following.

- The dog was not overweight.
- Time constraints.
- Fear of causing offence (Cairns-Haylor and Fordyce, 2017).
- Or simply failure to record it on the system (even though 70% recorded bodyweight) (German and Morgan, 2008).
- If a dog is not overweight or obese, it is not necessary to record or raise awareness to owners (Cairns-Haylor and Fordyce, 2017).

> **Top tip**
>
> - Fat score the horse at every visit.
>   - Tell the owner the result and record the numbers.
> - Fat score at all or any routine consults.
>   - Becoming part of a regular routine means it is no longer a difficult discussion to conduct
>   - Negative connotations will no longer be linked to the task.
> - Provide numbers and charts (see Chapter 3: 'Why body fat scoring?') enabling clients to come to their own understanding.
> - Consider communication style.
>   - Dietitians and medical doctors avoid 'obese' or 'overweight' (Swift *et al.*, 2013)
>   - Human patients prefer to be told that 'your weight may be damaging your health' (Swift *et al.*, 2013).

Confusing body fat with bodyweight and condition

Bodyweight

Of horse owners who said that they BCS frequently, 46% actually used a weight tape (Murray *et al.*, 2015), which only provides information on the body mass (kg)of the horse. This highlights misunderstanding around the whole topic.

- Bodyweight does not provide information on body composition (fat:muscle).
- When speaking about fatness, it does not help that people talk about 'overweight' or 'too heavy', which in most clients' minds alludes to bodyweight (kg).
- A horse might be an ideal bodyweight based on breed and weight charts, but the horse could have a BFS of 4,4,4, indicating that the body mass contains too much fat.

It is important to achieve a disconnect between bodyweight and body composition. You need to change the owner's perception that a heavy horse is a muscly horse (discourage visual appraisal of fat cover – they need to palpate) and that muscle weighs more than fat. It does not (Fig. 15.8).

Have you come across the perception that a horse needs to put on 'weight' (fat) at the start of the competition season? (Ever heard of a human athlete who eats as much as they can and gets fat before they start a fittening regime? Very much doubt it.)

So why do clients want their horses to be fat before they start work? Because they can burn off the fat and change it to muscle as the horse starts to work – which, as you know, is physiologically impossible. Fat and muscle are two different tissues. Do make sure your clients understand the difference.

Condition

The term condition is used to describe body fat in production animals and is well understood. In horses, condition is a complimentary adjective that is used variously to describe a horse that:

- is well muscled;
- is fit;
- has a healthy coat;
- has good feet;
- has a rounded outline; and
- is not thin.

In most clients' minds, what 'condition' does not describe is fatness. Thus, when you condition score a horse, they think that you are checking if their horse is fit for purpose and that 'very good condition' is complimentary.

Consider the impact of changing the words 'body condition scoring' to 'body fat score' and provide them with a body fat index. Suddenly, it is very clear which tissue you are palpating and that the

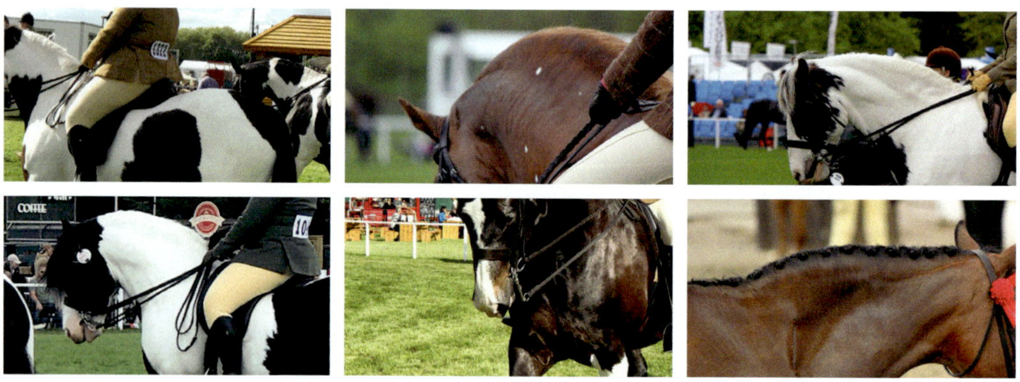

Fig. 15.7 The normalisation of obesity in the show ring. Note the crests, the lack of shoulder bone, hips or rib definition; none of the predetermined skeletal areas are palpable.

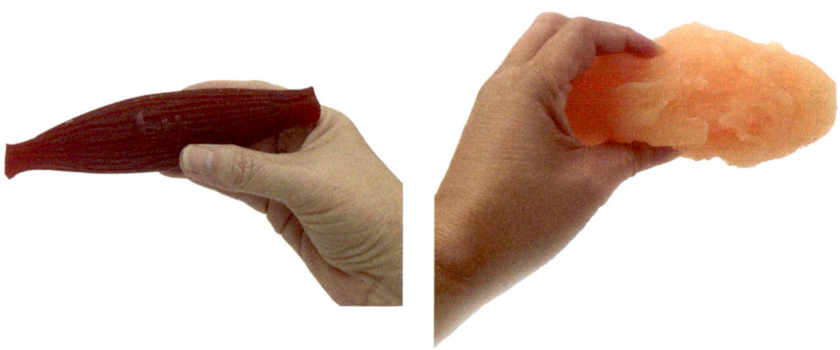

Fig. 15.8 A visual comparison of the same weight (450 g) of muscle (left) and fat (right). The same weights of fat and muscle have different bulk density and take up different volumes. Pictures with permission WRS group (www.healthedco.co.uk)

higher the number, the more fat there is on and in their horse's body.

Perception that horses get fat on fresh air

Higher fat scores are associated with the absence of feeding concentrates (Salonen *et al.*, 2009). Clearly, we need to contextualise that statement, but it does help to question the incorrect assumption that the reason horses are fat is because owners feed them too much hard feed. It took years before research validated data recorded by ambulatory nutritionists – that 90% of obese horses are fed < 1 scoop of feed (Salonen *et al.*,2009) (Fig. 15.9). Maybe the perception of feeding is based on surveyed horse owners (n = 506) who recorded that 90% of horses were being fed concentrate feed; no details on quantities were recorded (Stephenson *et al.*, 2011). Often owners will note chaff as a concentrate feed.

Horses that were at ideal fat score were more likely to be in work and thus clearly had a need for more concentrates. The feed that horses are getting fat by eating it is in fact forage – grass or hay.

Top Tip

- Remember to take quantitative information on the ration when taking a dietary history.
  - Most leisure horses should be on a high forage diet, so record the forage's contribution to the calorie intake.
- Hay provides a horse at maintenance with excess calories.
- A horse consuming 2.5% bodyweight (BW) grass dry matter (DM) eats nearly twice their calorie requirement (Fig. 15.10).

Alarmingly, horses can eat up to 5% of their bodyweight as dry matter (mean DMI 3.74, range 3.3–5.2% BW) (Smith *et al.*, 2007a,b).

Epigenetics

Long-term overfeeding takes on an even more serious note in breeding horses that pass on the genetic predisposition to adiposity, which can affect two to three generations (see Chapter 14: 'Feeding for breeding'). Photographic comparisons between the 1960s and 2000s highlight the differences: when did a massive crest on a Highland pony become acceptable?

Top Tip

- Horses do not get fat on fresh air.
  - Please remind clients that grass contains 9–11 MJ DE/kg DM.
- A 250 kg pony eating just 2.5% BW can eat 56–69 MJ DE/day or 3.3 MJ/h.
  - But the DE maintenance is only 32 MJ for maintenance and 39 MJ for light work (see Chapter 11: 'Feeding the leisure horse').

It is clearly vital that everything that the horse eats is accounted for, not just the 'bucket food'.

How to Increase Understanding of Obesity

If one of the biggest risk factors of animals being overweight is an owner's inability to recognise fatness, then a simple solution is to teach them a technique that measures the fat cover on their horse.

A simple palpation of fat on scientifically validated areas on the horse's skeleton provides a body fat score and it does not really matter which score you use; just teach them one of the techniques (see Chapter 3: Table 3.7).

Teaching fat scoring

Based on the statistics on horse fatness, it is highly likely that you are about to tell a client that their horse is fat. They are quite likely to disagree with you. At best, you start a conversation; at worst, they do not want you as their vet.

Start with a general discussion around the various signalment and history that you are taking – including the fact that you are going to fat score (they might recognise the technique as condition scoring).

- Ask them if they have heard of or used body fat/condition scoring.
  - Find out which system they know about.
- Explain that you would like to teach them the scoring system and that you would like them to score their horse on a fortnightly basis.
  - Monitoring and recording the numbers, together with photos (from the same perspective and distance each time), helps with compliance.

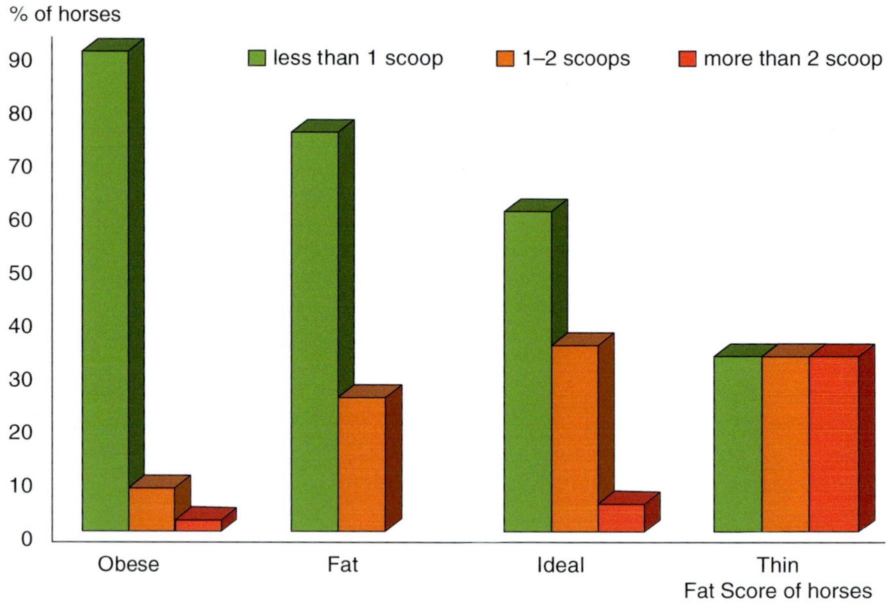

Fig. 15.9 A comparison between the fat score of horses and the number of scoops of hard feed being fed

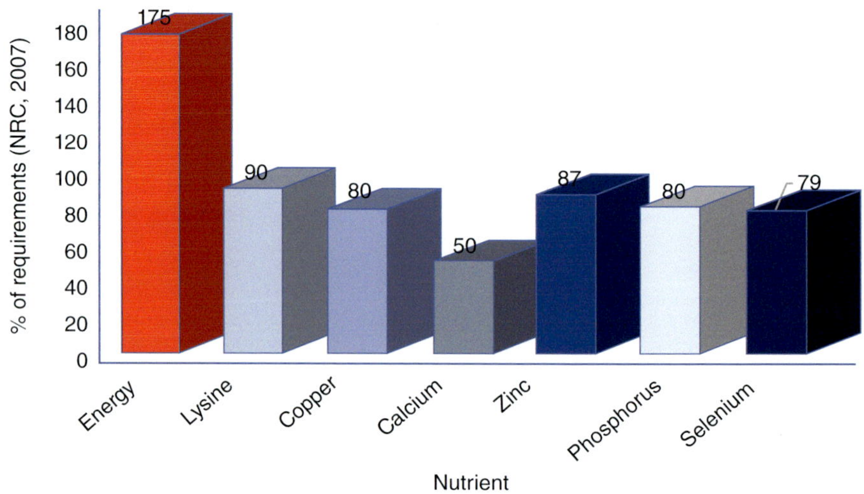

Fig. 15.10 The percentage of nutrients consumed by a horse in good grazing in 24 h compared with requirements. (NRC, 2007). Grass provides excess calories; horse eats 2.5% BW; excess calories (energy column) nearly double requirements; deficient in some minerals; sub-optimal nutrition.

- Ask to see the numbers when you check in with them.
- Provide them with a copy of the scoring system that you are going to use, so that you work together on obtaining the score, rather than you being the instructor.
- Work through their questions and queries (see Chapter 3: 'Horse Information required to check dietary adequacy as part of a dietary history').
- Remind them that fat tends to redistribute during a fat loss programme, so compare areas; do not average the score.

Table 15.4 Everyday memorable language and tools to describe fat scores

Area scoring	Everyday memorable language and tools to describe fat scores		
Neck – eye 'socket' (Supraorbital fossa) *Horses do not store fat above their eye unless their metabolism is compromised*	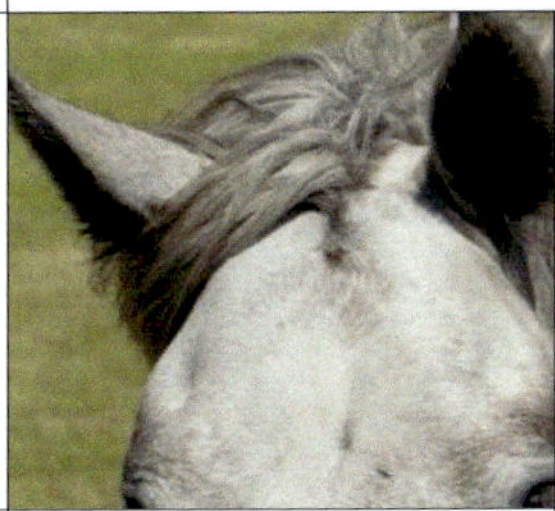	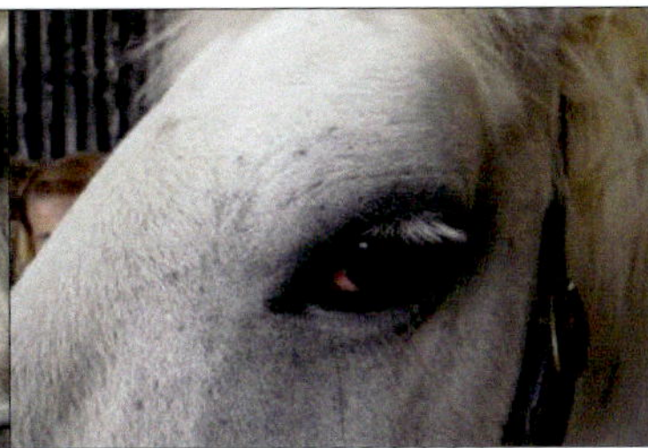	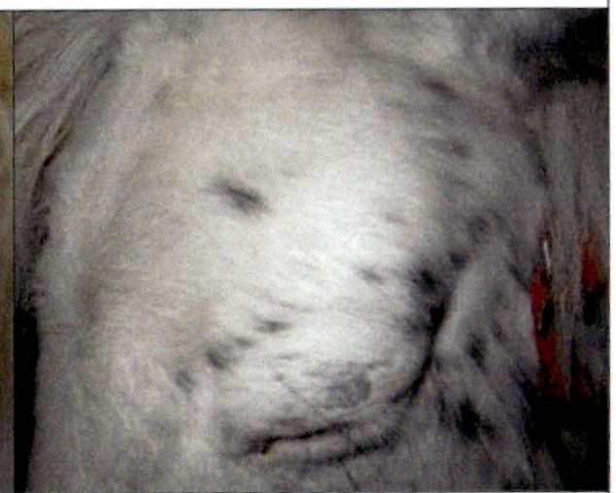
	Grade 1 Soft tissue above eye is concave to surrounding bone – *hollow above eye*	Grade 2 soft tissue is level with surrounding bone-*flat above eye*	Grade 3 soft tissue is convex with surrounding bone - *bulge above eye, spongy* *At risk from EMS (Carslake et al., 2021)*
Neck nuchal ligament *topline*	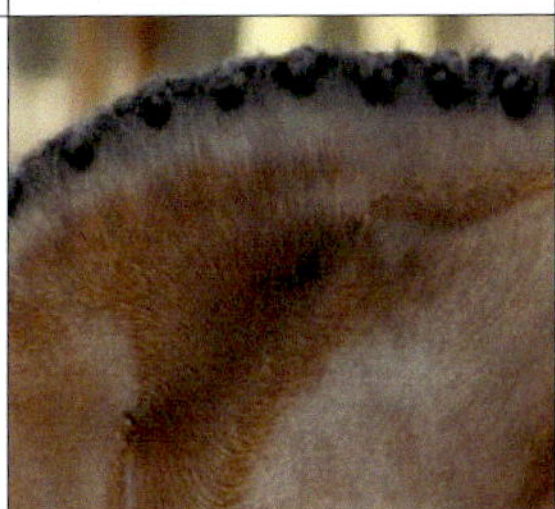	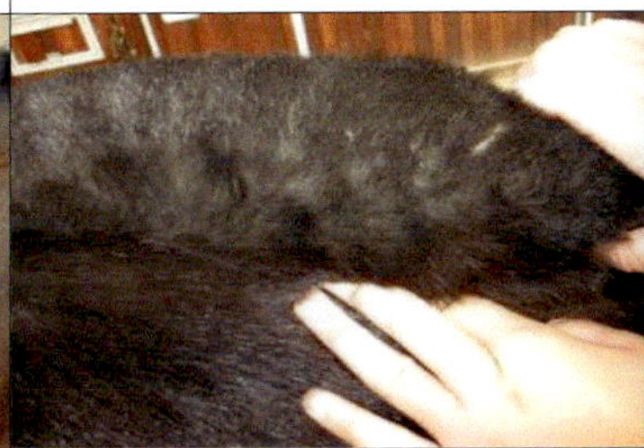	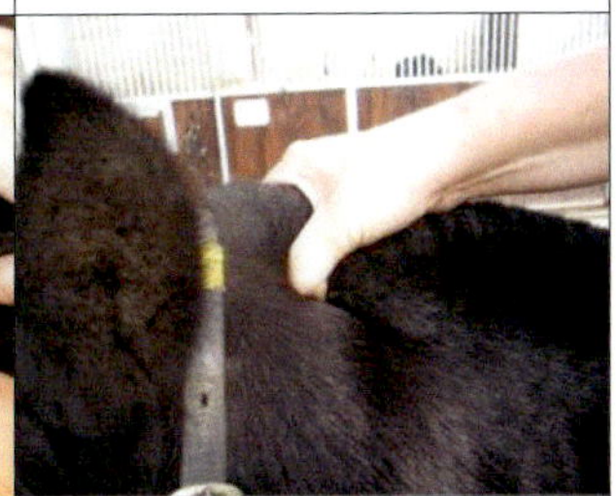
	Nuchal ligament is sensitive to 'pinch' >3cm above ligament (fat score 4/5)	often corrugation of fat tissue on neck when bend head (fat score 5/5)	>6cm fat above ligament (fat score 5/5)
Neck – *shoulder*	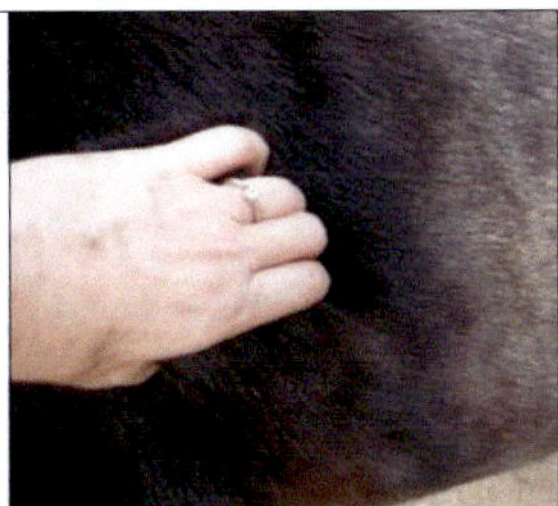	Can pinch an inch behind shoulder blade (fat score 4/5) Cellulytic fat lumps and skin stretched behind shoulder (fat score 5/5)	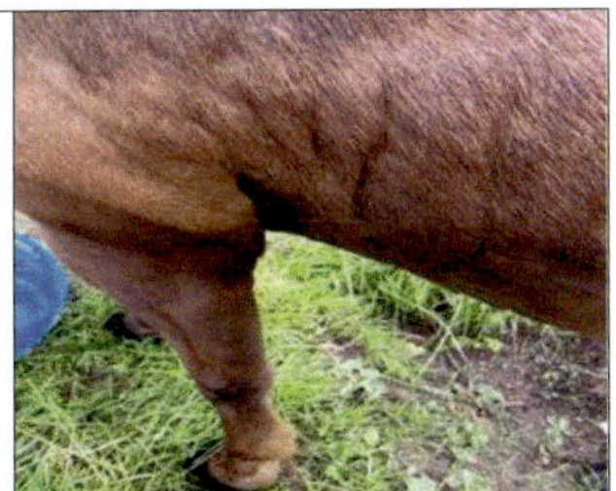
Back – *back bone* *Use various tools to emphasise the flat back*	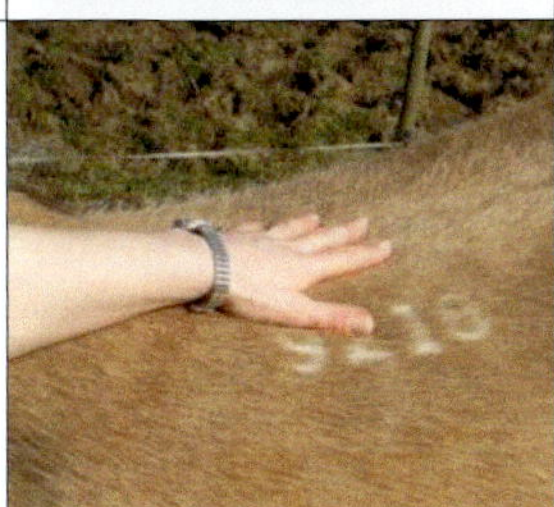	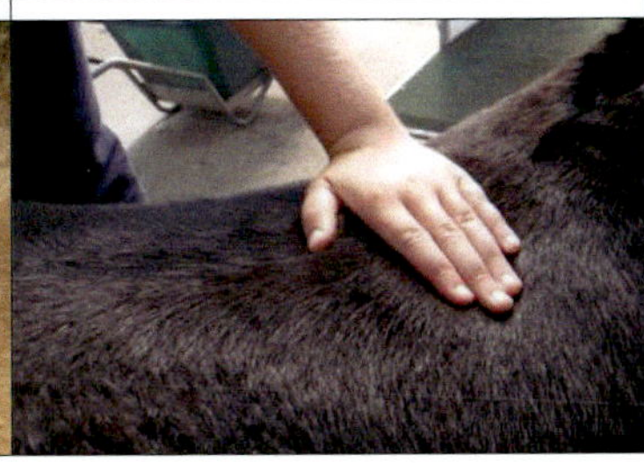	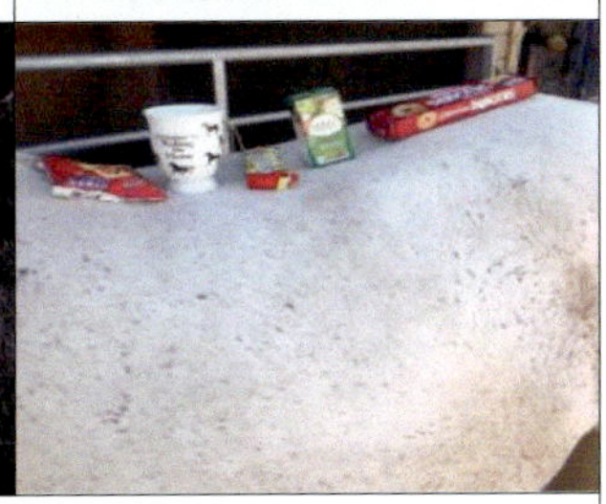
	Hand flat on back, back bone completely covered in fat (fat score 4/5)		

Continued

Table 15.4 Continued.

	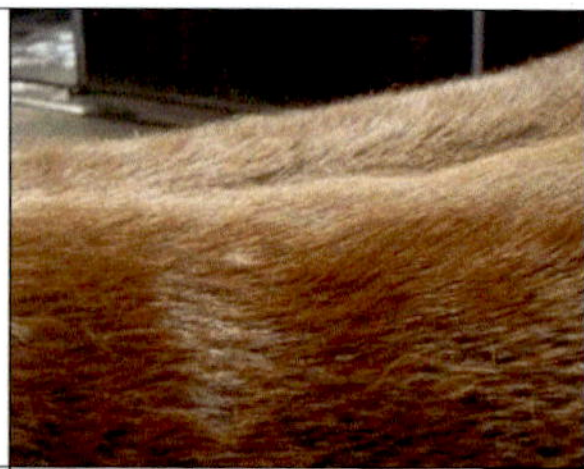	Hand flat on back but back bone buried in gutter (fat score 5/5)	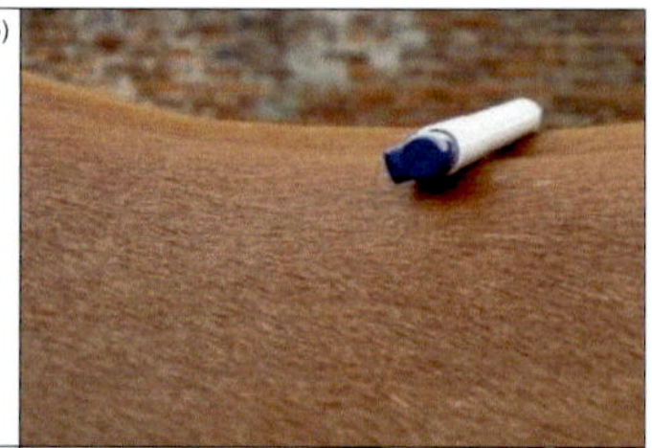
Bottom – pelvis and hips	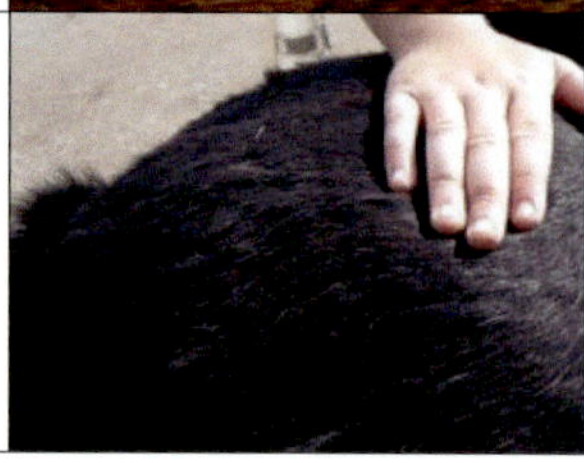	Any bones? fat totally covering hip and pelvis bones-finger tips not allowed- flat hand only! (fat score 4 _5/5)	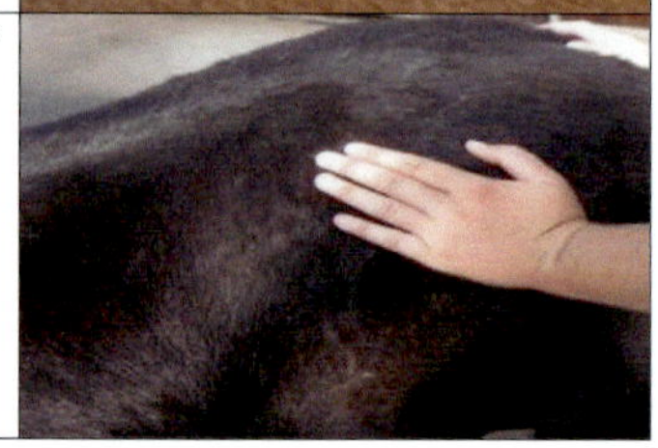

- Ask them to describe their horse to you (Table 15.4) and find out if the farrier has had a conversation with them.
  - Farriers seem to have the ability to be franker with the client than you might want to be (Lynden *et al.*, 2018, 2020).

How to Increase Compliance

Patience and persistence are required to turn the obesity tide and maybe we need to think carefully how we communicate the solutions.

Do not use the word 'diet'

For most horse owners (females), diet is a four-letter word associated with restriction and misery – the opposite to the caring persona associated with owning their own horse (Furtado *et al.*, 2020).

- You are providing a nutritional prescription and developing a healthy feeding plan.
- Support clients to make lifelong changes that will improve the health, longevity, welfare and performance of their horse by starting a new regime for their horse that reduces its risk of long-term, low-grade inflammatory disease.

Provide them with four target areas:

1. Count calories.
2. Maintain dry matter intake (bulk/forage).
3. Balance micronutrients.
4. Lifelong lifestyle changes.

Discuss and summarise the evidence behind your advice to encourage client understanding and help compliance (see Chapter 11: 'Feeding the leisure horse').

Control calorie intake

Losing fat tissue:

- improves insulin sensitivity and reduces insulin resistance;
- reduces chronic inflammation, the risk of numerous diseases; and
- improves health.

An overweight horse needs fewer calories compared with a lean horse (see Chapter 3: Table 3.1); but this decrease must be planned gradually.

- Weight loss will take months or years rather than weeks, otherwise you will be defeated by leptin and other diseases.
  - Do not expect to reduce fat scores by 0.5 (0–5 scale) within 2 months (Table 15.5).
- There is little or no evidence base for successful weight loss for a horse, but calculations have been adapted from calorie changes for weight gain (NRC, 2007) incorporating evidence for safe weight losses in other species.
- A reduction of 0.5 fat score over each part of the body requires a BW loss of about 16–20 kg for horses weighing 480–580 kg (3–3.5% BW loss).
  - The horse needs to eat 3.8–4.9 MJ DE less per 1 kg fat loss (NRC, 2007).

Top Tip

Soaking the daily hay ration (2.5% BW DMI) (see Chapter 9: Table 9.6) will reduce calories by 16–20%.

Maintain dry matter (bulk) intake

Owners know that horses are ad lib feeders and need to eat fibre. Remind them that all horses need to eat 2.5% of their bodyweight to reduce cortisol levels, minimise insulin resistance, reduce the risk of gastric ulcers, colic and stereotypies, but reduce calorie intakes (see Chapter 11: 'How to advise the correct compound feed').

Restricting bulk in short term for fat loss

Overweight ponies kept in stables with limited or no exercise successfully lost 1% BW/week when their intake was restricted to 1.5% BW (Dugdale *et al.*, 2011a,b) but ate up to 3 kg of wood shavings/day (Fig. 15.11) to satisfy their appetite and chewing behaviours (Curtis *et al.*, 2011); the authors did not report any colic. This is a useful short-term regime to reduce insulin resistance if ponies are confined to box rest because of laminitis, under your supervision. But long-term food restriction has several disadvantages, increasing leptin and insulin resistance as the metabolism adjusts to 'starvation' rations.

Fibre restriction, insulin resistance and cortisol levels

Obese sheep have an increase in cortisol in response to feeding compared with lean sheep (Challis and Brookes, 1989; Gardner *et al.*, 2005); reducing feeding frequency (even while maintaining energy intake) in numerous species increases cortisol levels (Amdi *et al.*, 2013; Manu *et al.*, 2020). Clients should be aware that prolonged exposure to high cortisol eventually leads to exhaustion of the tissue that secretes cortisol; high cortisol is correlated with insulin resistance (Rizza *et al.*, 1982).

Food restriction stimulates cortisol release (Kenny *et al.*, 2014); stereotypy behaviours are associated with an increase in cortisol (Vaz *et al.*, 2017) in many species. Restricting fibre in horses increases stereotypy behaviours, but researchers

Table 15.5 Duration[a] of calorie reduction to reduce horse's fat score by 0.5 (0–5) (adapted from NRC 2007 guide to weight gain)

Time period Days (months)	[b]Daily digestible energy reduction below maintenance[c] (MJ/day)	Daily % decrease in DE_m requirements
60 (2)	22–28	32–41
90 (3)	14.8–18.6	22–27
120 (4)	11.6–13.9	16–21
150 (5)	8.9–11.1	13–16
180 (6)	7.4–9.3	11–14

[a]Takes months or years, not weeks; apply right-hand column for all BWs
[b]Total decrease of 1344–1674 MJ DE over whole period
[c]DE_m = 63 MJ for 500 kg horse

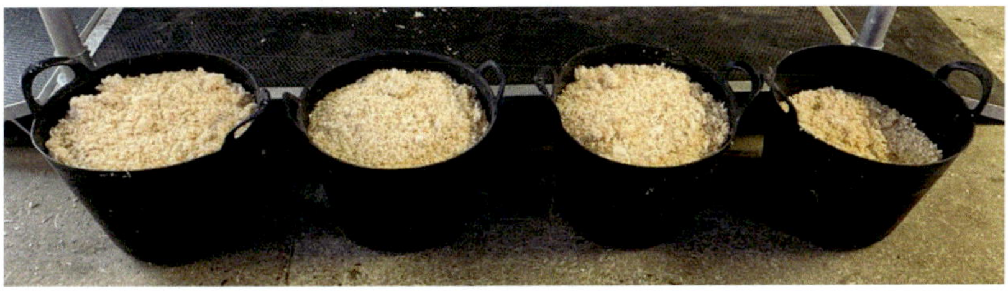

Fig. 15.11 The quantity of wood shavings equivalent to 3% BW of 500 kg horse.

have not shown a similar increase in cortisol with stereotypy behaviours (Fureix *et al.*, 2013).

In people, short-term decreases in food intake increases insulin resistance (Duska *et al.*, 2005). This is simply a survival mechanism: the thrifty gene ensures that available glucose stays in the blood and is used by the brain.

Weight loss reduces insulin resistance, but this must not be achieved by a drastic reduction in food intake.

Balance micronutrients

Clients are always delighted to be advised that they can feed their obese horse; it is essential that they are not undernourished in vitamins, minerals and protein. Recommend a balancer (see Chapter 11: 'How to advise the correct compound feed').

Lifetime commitment to management

Like all things in life, this is not a quick fix; your clients need support for as long as they have this horse. The changes that they make will take time to take effect and once they have seen the weight loss, they need to stay committed to the changes.

Rugging

Tell them to 'take it off' or, if being turned out, swap thick rugs for a lightweight waterproof rug, ensuring that they have a dry back for riding. Horses do not need a rug in the stable unless they have a full clip. Horses use 80% of their feed energy to stay warm. Rugging means feed energy goes on their back as fat. Cows and sheep are not rugged; horses have their own coats!

Regular exercise

Exercise has been shown to reduce insulin resistance even before fat loss. If the horse is sound, then 30 min riding 7 days/week in addition to turnout, covering 2 miles daily, increased their horse's heart rate to 80 bpm. Exercise plus calorie reduction improved insulin sensitivity and decreased serum amyloid A compared with horses that were 'just dieted' (Bamford *et al.*, 2019).

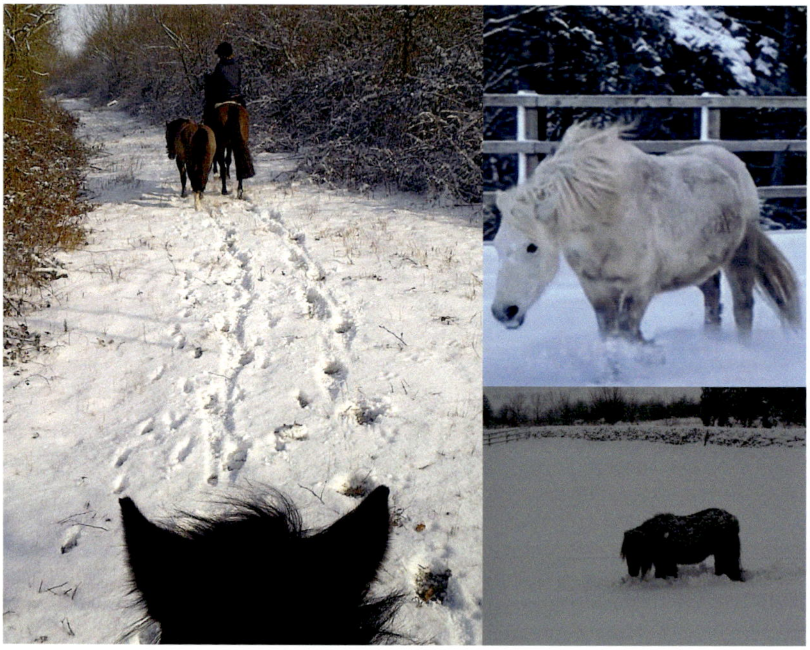

Fig. 15.12 Exercise should not be compromised in the winter.

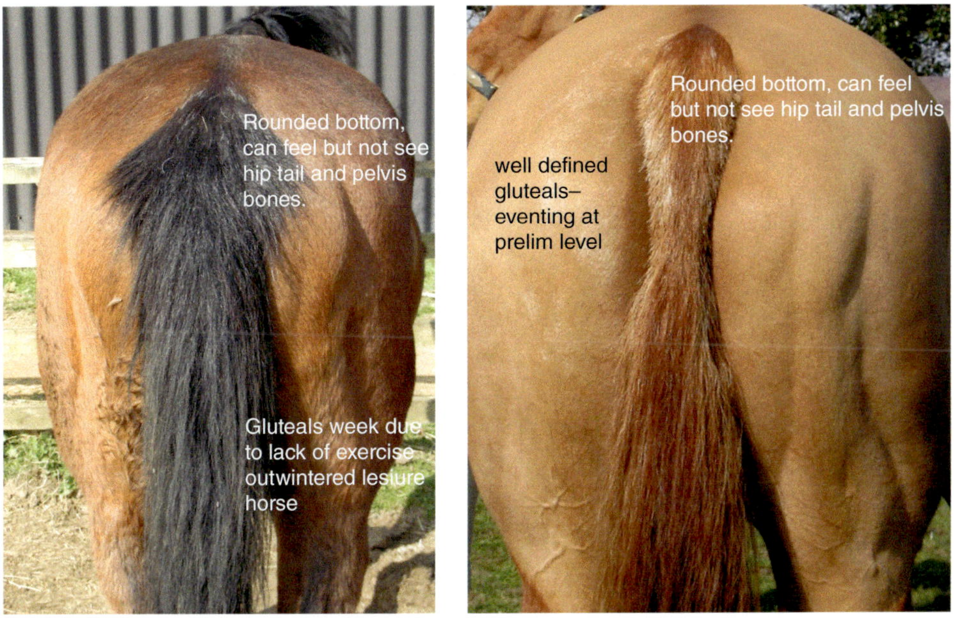

Fig. 15.13 Fat cover and condition of outwintered unridden horse compared with a competition horse. Both horses have an ideal fat score. The horse on the left (an outwintered TB type) has lost muscle; it is in poor condition but has good fat cover (fat score 3 on its bottom); it cannot be ridden for long. The horse on the right is prelim eventing; it is well muscled, in good condition and carrying the correct amount of fat (fat score 3 on its bottom). The difference between the two horses is muscle.

Encourage winter fat loss

Many clients are unable to commit to daily riding in the winter; their horses will lose muscle and they must not replace this muscle with fat. Daily turnout is a form of exercise (Fig. 15.12) which, if the livery yard allows, should be encouraged.

Stabled horses lose fitness compared with those at pasture (Graham-Thiers and Bowen, 2013), with an increased risk of colic (Williams *et al.*, 2011, 2014). As long as owners can feel but not see the ribs, shoulder blade etc, the horse has enough fat regardless of whether its bottom or neck is looking weak (Fig. 15.13).

Please encourage clients to see winter fat loss in unexercised (or weekend-exercised) horses as being a key part of healthy horse management. Undomesticated horses are biologically programmed to put on fat through the spring and summer, losing it in the winter, thus rarely exceeding their metabolic capacity. Wild horses will lose 8% fat tissue resulting in weight loss over the winter (500 kg horse loses 40 kg; 250 kg pony loses 20 kg), which they regain in the summer (Scheibe and Streich, 2003).

It is possible to manage and minimise the risk of horse obesity, but owners need support in realising they are changing the biology of the horse: the nutritional management is for life and will never be a short-term fix (Tables 15.6 and 15.7).

Summary

- Set up Facebook/Instagram and Well/Fit horse clinics to provide clients with ongoing support. What about:
  - photo walls of successful long-term fat loss;
  - monthly blog from clients and link to their Instagram of successful stories.
- Utilise yard visits by feed companies (ask them to bring a weighbridge/do a diet analysis).
- Every visit, body fat score every horse, record and teach the client.
- Remember that no owner knowingly has an overfat horse.
  - We are all responsible for equine obesity.

Continued p. 385.

Table 15.6 Dietary advice for Cob in show condition

Horse signalment	15 hh cob in show condition, 600 kg Fat score 5, 5, 5	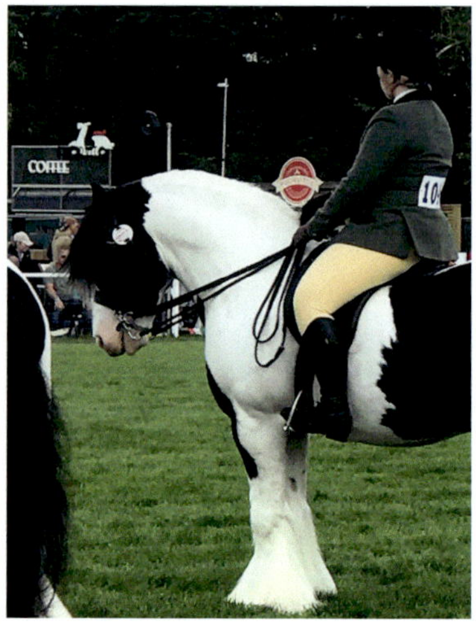
Horse history	Being placed in heavy horse classes – client had to self-isolate and horse was not ridden for 2 weeks	
Workload/exercise	Was daily schooling – 30 min walk and trot with occasional canter, 1 × 1 h hack/week at walk; client described as medium work but this is light work. Energy requirements for light work = M × 1.2= 76 × 1.2 = 91.2 MJ DE/day. Clearly this is excess calories for this horse.	
Results of any tests	Went lame. Farrier described it as footy with increased digital pulse, but X-rays did not show any change to pedal bone	
Current diet	Show improver mix (RI 0.5–0.58 kg/100 kg BW), Hay 1 slice morning, 1 slice lunchtime, 3 slices evening 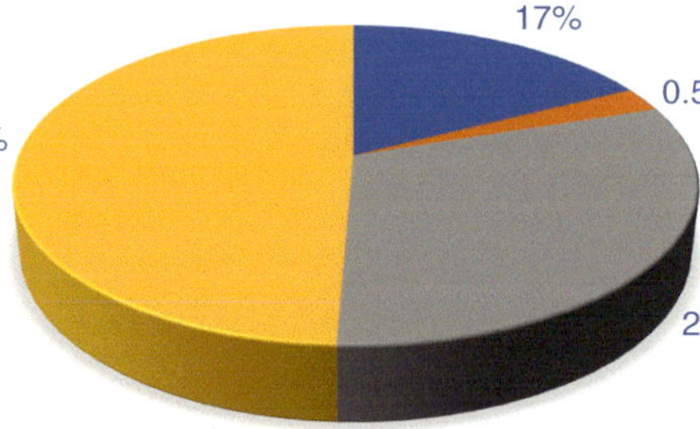	
Advice	Indicative dry matter and energy requirements are adjusted according to workload and bodyweight. Diet changed monthly (Table 15.7) but in week 4 of each month the quantities should be reduced for the start of the following month	

Continued

Table 15.6 Continued.

Solution	i. Oat straw
	• Satisfy appetite
	  ◦ Low calories
	  ◦ Less dusty than hay
	• Feed in multiple haynets or slow feeders
	  ◦ Divided into several smaller meals throughout day and evening
	ii. Soaked hay
	• Soak for minimum of 12 h
	  ◦ Place in separate haygrid to straw to encourage foraging
	  ◦ Needs to be analysed or should be last year's meadow/timothy hay, *not* ryegrass, so as low in calories as possible.
	iii. Hard feed
	• Balancer fed at 100 g/100 kg BW to provide vitamins/minerals and extra lysine as straw is deficient in all these – do check the label to ensure the nutrients are adequate.
	  ◦ Split into two or three small feeds but make sure client has container that holds exactly the correct amount
	• Add 100 g Hi Fi Lite to each 'meal' to encourage chewing and provide a visually bigger feed to help client compliance
	iv. Grazing
	• Use muzzle or front-and-back strip grazing to control grass intake
	• Get client to compare with grass availability outside of grazing paddock
	• Ensure predominantly meadow grass; preferably no ryegrass/clover

Special considerations	• 1 kg straw provides about 20% less calories than soaked hay equivalent, depending upon hay calorie content. Varying proportions according to workload and fat loss.
	• Ensure good dentition – teeth need checking regularly as straw is a 'tougher' fibre.
	• Get clients to keep an eye on fibre length in droppings:
	  ◦ Number and consistency of droppings to monitor risk of gut stasis and hydration.
	• If any concerns, change straw to soaked hay and lengthen timescale to achieve weight loss.
	• Encourage time in paddock, as increases movement and energy expenditure.
	  ◦ Clients need to do the supermarket bag and droppings tests weekly (see Chapter 11: 'Measuring grass in the field').
	• Exercise levels when sound need to be quantified – duration, speed and distance.
	• All advice needs to come with the caveat that feeding will need adjusting according to exercise, BW and fat score.
	• Be clear with client the time it takes to reduce the fat score.

Table 15.7 Indicative bodyweight loss[a] of an obese horse over 6 months

Time	Bodyweight (kg) at beginning of month	Weekly weight (wt) loss (kg)	Weekly BW loss (%)	Monthly wt loss (kg)	Monthly BW loss %	Monthly accumulated wt loss (kg)	Monthly accumulated BW loss %	Potential change in BFS	Calorie requirement[b] MJ DE/day (Tables 15.5 and 15.6) light work = M × 1.1	Indicative ration
Month 1	600	2	0.33	8	1.32	8	1.32	5,5,5	66.7	2 kg hay then soaked for 12 h (10 MJ) mixed with 12 kg (48 MJ) straw 600 g balancer (5.7 MJ) 300 g Hi Fi Lite (2.2 MJ)
Month 2	592	3	0.5	12	2	20	3.32	4.5, 4.5, 4.5	66	As above
Month 3	580	2.9	0.5	11.6	2	31.6	5.32	4.5, 4.5, 4.5	72 Ensure client is recording exercise duration and distance	6 kg hay then soaked (30 MJ) 4 kg straw (16 MJ) Limited grazing 4 h (3.6 kg dry wt, 12 kg fresh wt) (18 MJ) 600 g balancer (5.7 MJ) 0.2 kg alfalfa chaff (2 MJ)
Month 4	569	2.8	0.5	11.2	2	42.8	7.32	4,4,4	68[c]	5 kg hay then soaked (25 MJ) 5.8 kg straw (23.2 MJ) Limited grazing 3 h (2.6 kg dry wt, 8.8 kg fresh wt) (13 MJ) 600 g balancer (5.7 MJ) 0.2 kg alfalfa chaff (2 MJ)
Month 5	558	1.7	0.3	6.8	1.2	49.6	8.5	4,4,4	66	Limited grazing for 6 h (5.2 kg DM), 17 kg fresh wt (26 MJ); 600 g balancer (5.7 MJ) 300 g Hi Fi Lite (2.25 MJ) 8 kg straw (32 MJ)
Month 6	551	1	0.2	4	0.8	53.6kg	9.32	4,4,4	64	Limited grazing for 6 h (5.2 kg DM), 17 kg fresh wt (26 MJ); 600 g balancer (5.7 MJ) 200 g Hi Fi Lite (1.5 MJ) 7.5kg straw (30MJ)

[a]Ideal weight 535 kg (510–550kg) – initial plan to lose 50 kg (8.3% BW loss); [b]Assumes no work for first 2 months, then light work at 1.1 × M; [c]From week 4, calories reduced by 14% as becomes more difficult to shift weight with time.

- The single most effective, evidence-based intervention for health longevity (Adams *et al.*, 2016, 2018) is:
  - maintenance of a healthy body mass;
  - reduce adiposity, increase muscle; and
  - reduce chronic inflammation, improving robustness and resilience to disease.

A useful resource for clients is available at: https://www.liverpool.ac.uk/media/livacuk/equine/documents/Equine,Weight,Management.pdf (accessed 6 January 2023).

- Persistence and perseverance.
- Involve other professionals.
- Do not place fat show horses.
- Fail clearly obese horses in vettings.
- Do not use photographs of fat horses in any media.
- Provide long term support.
- Good luck.

Tips for clients

- **A**lways take nutrition into account.
- **B**alance vitamins and minerals.
- **C**ontrol calories but maintain bulk.
- **D**o fat score and weight tape fortnightly.
- **E**xercise is vital for longevity.
- **F**orage should be the foundation of all nutritional support.
- **G**ot rid of fat.
- **H**elp each other.
- **I**nsulin check regularly.

Bibliography

Abu Abed, M., Himmel, W., Vormfelde, S. and Koschack, J. (2014) Video-assisted patient education to modify behavior: a systematic review. *Patient Education and Counseling* 97(1), 16–22. doi: 10.1016/j.pec.2014.06.015.

Adam, A.A., Katepalli, M.P., Kohler, K., Ready, S., Stilz, J. *et al.* (2009) Effect of body condition, body weight and adiposity on inflammatory cytokine responses in old horses. *Veterinary Immunology and Immunopathology* 127(3–4), 286–294.

Adams, V.J., Watson, P., Carmichael, S., Gerry, S., Penell, J. and Morgan, D.M. (2016) Exceptional longevity and potential determinants of successful ageing in a cohort of 39 Labrador retrievers: results of a prospective longitudinal study. *Acta Veterinaria Scandinavica* 58(1), 1–14. doi: 10.1186/s13028-016-0206.

Adams, V.J., Ceccarelli, K., Watson, P., Carmichael, S., Penell, J. *et al.* (2018) Evidence of longer life; a cohort of 39 labrador retrievers. *The Veterinary Record* 182(14), 408. doi: 10.1136/vr.104167.

Addison, O., Marcus, R., LaStayo, P. and Ryan, S.A. (2014) Intermuscular fat: a review of the consequences and causes. *International Journal of Endocrinology* 2014, Article ID 309570, 11 pages, doi: 10.1155/2014/309570.

Ahima, R.S. (2008) Revisiting leptin's role in obesity and weight loss. *The Journal of Clinical Investigation* 118(7), 2380–2383. doi: 10.1172/JCI36284.

Amdi, C., Giblin, L., Hennessy, A.A., Ryan, T., Stanton, C. *et al.* (2013) Feed allowance and maternal backfat levels during gestation influence maternal cortisol levels, milk fat composition and offspring growth. *Journal of Nutritional Science* 2, e1.

Andreassen, S.M., Vinther, A., Nielsen, S.S., Andersen, P.H., Tnibar, A. *et al.* (2017) Changes in concentrations of haemostatic and inflammatory biomarkers in synovial fluid after intra-articular injection of lipopolysaccharide in horses. *BMC Veterinary Research* 13(1), 182. doi: 10.1186/s12917-017-1089-1.

Argo, C.M., Curtis, G.C., Grove-White, D., Dugdale, A.H., Barfoot, C.F. *et al.* (2012) Weight loss resistance: a further consideration for the nutritional management of obese Equidae. *Veterinary Journal* 194(2), 179–188. doi: 10.1016/j.tvjl.2012.09.020.

Asplin, K.E., Sillence, M.N., Pollitt, C.C. and McGowan, C.M. (2007) Induction of laminitis by prolonged hyperinsulinaemia in clinically normal ponies. *The Veterinary Journal* 174(3), 530–535.

Astrup, A. and Bügel, S. (2010) Micronutrient deficiency in the aetiology of obesity. *International Journal of Obesity* 34, 947–948.

Backhed, F., Ding, H., Wang, T., Hooper, L.V., Koh, G.Y. *et al.* (2004) The gut microbiota as an environmental factor that regulates fat storage. *Proceedings of the National Academy of Sciences* 101, 15718–15723. doi: 10.1073/pnas.0407076101.

Baker, L.A., Burrows, A.M., Nonella, K.J., Pipkin, J.L., Holmes, L.D. *et al.* (2020) Relationship between live body condition score and carcass fat measures in equine. *Translational Animal Science* 4(4), 1508–1515.

Bamford, N.J., Potter, S.J., Harris, P.A. and Bailey, S.R. (2016) Effect of increased adiposity on insulin sensitivity and adipokine concentrations in horses and ponies fed a high fat diet, with or without a once daily high glycaemic meal. *Equine Veterinary Journal* 48, 368–373.

Bamford, N.J., Potter, S.J., Baskerville, C.L., Harris, P.A. and Bailey, S.R. (2019) Influence of dietary restriction and low-intensity exercise on weight loss and insulin sensitivity in obese equids. *Journal of Veterinary Internal Medicine* 33, 280–286. doi: 10.1111/jvim.15374

Banse, H.E., Holbrook, T.C., Frank, N. and McFarlane, D. (2016) Relationship of skeletal muscle inflammation with obesity and obesity-associated hyperinsulinemia in horses. *Canadian Journal of Veterinary Research [Revue canadienne de recherche veterinaire]* 80(3), 217–224.

Basinska, K., Marycz, K., Śieszek, A. and Nicpoń, J. (2015) The production and distribution of IL-6 and TNF-a in subcutaneous adipose tissue and their correlation with serum concentrations in Welsh ponies with equine metabolic syndrome. *Journal of Veterinary Science* 16(1), 113–120.

Bertin, F.R., Taylor, S.D., Bianco, A.W. and Sojka-Kritchevsky, J.E. (2016) The effect of fasting duration on baseline blood glucose concentration, blood insulin concentration, glucose/insulin ratio, oral sugar test, and insulin response test results in horses. *Journal of Veterinary Internal Medicine* 30(5), 1726–1731. doi: 10.1111/jvim.14529.

Bland, I.M., Guthrie-Jones, A., Taylor, R.D. and Hill, J. (2009) Dog obesity: owner attitudes and behaviour. *Preventive Veterinary Medicine* 92, 333–340. doi: 10.1016/j.prevetmed.2009.08.016.

Blaue, D., Schedlbauer, C., Starzonek, J. *et al.* (2020) The influence of equine body weight gain on inflammatory cytokine expressions of adipose tissue in response to endotoxin challenge. *Acta Veterinaria Scandinavica* 62, 17. doi: 10.1186/s13028-020-0051.

Block, S.S., Butler, W.R., Ehrhardt, R.A., Bell, A.W., Van Amburgh, M.E. *et al.* (2001) Decreased concentration of plasma leptin in periparturient dairy cows is caused by negative energy balance. *The Journal of Endocrinology* 171(2), 339–348. doi: 10.1677/joe.0.1710339.

Blüher, M. (2020) Metabolically healthy obesity. *Endocrine Reviews* 41(3), 405–420. doi: 10.1210/endrev/bnaa004.

Bluher, S. and Mantzoros, C.S. (2009) Leptin in humans: lessons from translational research. *The American Journal of Clinical Nutrition* 89, 991S–997S.

Boden, G. (2008) Obesity and free fatty acids. *Endocrinology and Metabolism Clinics of North America* 37(3), 635–ix. doi: 10.1016/j.ecl.2008.06.007.

Bojsen-Møller, K.N., Lundsgaard, A.M., Madsbad, S., Kiens, B. and Holst, J.J. (2018) Hepatic insulin clearance in regulation of systemic insulin concentrations-role of carbohydrate and energy availability. *Diabetes* 67(11), 2129–2136. doi: 10.2337/db18-0539.

Bond, S., Léguillette, R., Richard, E.A., Couetil, L., Lavoie, J.-P., Martin, J.G. and Pirie, R.S. (2018) Equine asthma: integrative biologic relevance of a recently proposed nomenclature. *Journal of Veterinary Internal Medicine* 32, 2088–2098.

Bouchard, C., Després, J.P. and Mauriège, P. (1993) Genetic and nongenetic determinants of regional fat distribution. *Endocrine Reviews* 14(1), 72–93. doi: 10.1210/edrv-14-1-72.

Briceño, A., Méndez Sánchez, A. and Pérez Arévalo, J. (2015) Infiltrative lipomatosis in neck and colon in a Spanish pure breed horse. *Brazilian Journal of Veterinary Pathology* 8(1), 14–17.

Briceño, A., Méndez Sánchez, A., Escamilla, A. and Pérez Arévalo, J. (2017) Diagnostic tools for the study of the cresty neck in horses. *International Journal of Applied Research in Veterinary Medicine* 15(1), 41–49.

British Horse Society (2019) Advice on pasture management. Available at: https://www.bhs.org.uk/advice-and-information/horse-care/pasture-management (accessed 10 January 2023)

Bruynsteen, L., Erkens, T., Peelman, L.J. *et al.* (2013) Expression of inflammation-related genes is associated with adipose tissue location in horses. *BMC Veterinary Research* 9, 240. doi: 10.1186/1746-6148-9-240.

Bruynsteen, L., Janssens, G.P., Harris, P.A., Duchateau, L., Valle, E. *et al.* (2014) Changes in oxidative stress in response to different levels of energy restriction in obese ponies. *The British Journal of Nutrition* 112(8), 1402–1411.

Buelund, L.E., Nielsen, D.H., McEvoy, F.J. *et al.* (2011) Measurement of body composition in cats using computed tomography and dual energy x-ray absorptiometry. *Veterinary Radiology & Ultrasound* 52, 179–184.

Buff, P.R., Dodds, A.C., Morrison, C.D., Whitley, N.C., McFadin, E.L. *et al.* (2002) Leptin in horses: tissue localization and relationship between peripheral concentrations of leptin and body condition. *Journal of Animal Science* 80(11), 2942–2948.

Burke, M.A., Heiland F.W. and Nadler C.M. (2010) From 'overweight' to 'about right': evidence of a generational shift in body weight norms. *Obesity* 18(6),1226–1234.

Burkholder, W.J. (2006) Use of body condition scores in clinical assessment of the provision of optimal nutrition. *Journal of the American Veterinary Medicine Association* 217(5), 650–654.

Burns, T., Geor, R., Mudge, M., McCutcheon, L., Hinchcliff, K. *et al.* (2010) Proinflammatory cytokine and chemokine gene expression profiles in subcutaneous and visceral adipose tissue depots of insulin-resistant and insulin-sensitive light breed horses. *Journal of Veterinary Internal Medicine* 24, 932–939.

Cairns, K., Johnston, J. and Baumann, S. (2010) Caring about food: doing gender in the foodie kitchen. *Gender & Society* 24(5), 591–615. doi: 10.1177/0891243210383419.

Cairns-Haylor, T. and Fordyce, P. (2017) Mapping discussion of canine obesity between veterinary surgeons and dog owners: a provisional study. *Veterinary Record* 180(6), 149. doi: 10.1136/vr.103878.

Camhi, S.M. and Katzmarzyk, P.T. (2014) Differences in body composition between metabolically healthy obese and metabolically abnormal obese adults. *International Journal of Obesity* 38(8), 1142–1145.

Canavan, B., Salem, R.O., Schurgin, S., Koutkia, P., Lipinska, I. *et al.* (2005) Effects of physiological leptin administration on markers of inflammation, platelet activation, and platelet aggregation during caloric deprivation. *The Journal of Clinical Endocrinology and Metabolism* 90(10), 5779–5785. doi: 10.1210/jc.2005-0780.

Carow, B. and Rottenberg, M. (2014) SOCS3, a major regulator of infection and inflammation. *Frontiers in Immunology* 5, 58. doi: 10.3389/fimmu.2014.00058.

Carroll, C.L. and Huntington, P.J. (1988) Body condition scoring and weight estimation of horses. *Equine Veterinary Journal* 20(1), 41–45. doi: 10.1111/j.2042-3306.1988.tb01451.x.

Carslake, H.B., Argo, C.M., Pinchbeck, G.L., Dugdale, A.H.A. and McGowan, C.M. (2018) Insulinaemic and glycaemic responses to three forages in ponies. *Veterinary Journal* 235, 83–89.

Carslake, H.B., Pinchbeck, G.L. and McGowan, C.M. (2021) Equine metabolic syndrome in UK native ponies and cobs is highly prevalent with modifiable risk factors. *Equine Veterinary Journal* 53(5), 923–934. doi: 10.1111/evj.13378.

Carter, R.A., Treiber, K.H., Geor, R.J., Douglass, L. and Harris, P.A. (2009a) Prediction of incipient pasture-associated laminitis from hyperinsulinaemia, hyperleptinaemia and generalised and localised obesity in a cohort of ponies. *Equine Veterinary Journal* 41(2), 171–178.

Carter, R.A., Geor, R.J., Staniar, WB., Cubitt, T.A. and Harris, P. (2009b) Apparent adiposity assessed by Standardised scoring systems and morphometric measurements in horses and ponies. *The Veterinary Journal* 179(2), 204–210.

Carvalheira, J.B., Qiu, Y. and Chawla, A. (2013) Blood spotlight on leukocytes and obesity. *Blood* 122(19), 3263–3267. doi: 10.1182/blood-2013-04-459446.

Challis, J.R.G. and Brooks A.N. (1989) Maturation and activation of hypothalamic-pituitary adrenal function in fetal sheep. *Endocrine Reviews* 10(2), 182–204. doi: 10.1210/edrv-10-2-182.

Choe, S.S., Huh, J.Y., Hwang I.J., Kim, J.I. and Kim, J.B. (2016) Adipose tissue remodeling: its role in energy metabolism and metabolic disorders. *Frontiers in Endocrinology* 7 (Suppl. 2), Article 30. doi: 10.3389/fendo.2016.00030.

Christifano, D.N., Taylor, M.K., Carlson, S.E., Colombo, J. and Gustafson, K.M. (2020) Higher maternal weight is related to poorer fetal autonomic function. *Journal of Developmental Origins of Health and Disease* 12(3), 354–356. doi: 10.1017/S2040174420000653

Churchill, J. (2010) Increase the success of weight loss programs by creating an environment for change. *Compendium: Continuing Education for Veterinarians* 32(12), 1–4.

Churchill, J. and Ward, E. (2016) Communicating with pet owners about obesity: roles of the veterinary health care team. *Veterinary Clinics: Small Animal Practice* 46(5), 899–911. doi: 10.1016/j.cvsm.2016.04.010.

Clark, I.A. (2007) How TNF was recognized as a key mechanism of disease. *Cytokine & Growth Factor Reviews* 18(3–4), 335–343.

Clement, K., Viguerie, N., Poitou, C., Carette, C., Pelloux, V. *et al.* (2004a) Weight loss regulates inflammation-related genes in white adipose tissue of obese subjects. *FASEB J* 18, 1657–1669.

Clement, S., Braithwaite, S.S., Magee, M.F., Ahmann, A., Smith, E.P., Schafer, R.G., Hirsch, I.B. and Diabetes in Hospitals Writing Committee (2004) Management of diabetes and hyperglycemia in hospitals. *Diabetes Care* 27(2), 553–591.

Coleman, M.C., Whitfield-Cargile, C.M., Madrigal, R.G. and Cohen, N.D. (2019) Comparison of the microbiome, metabolome, and lipidome of obese and non-obese horses. *PLoS ONE* 14(4), e0215918. doi: 10.1371/journal.pone.0215918.

Cornell, K. and Kopcha, M.K. (2007) Client-veterinarian communication: skills for client centered dialogue and shared decision making. *Veterinary Clinics: Small Animal Practice* 37(1), 37–47.

Coverdale, J.A., Hammer, C. J. and Walter, K.W. (2015) Horse Species Symposium: Nutritional programming and the impact on mare and foal performance. *Journal of Animal Science* 93(7), 3261–3267. doi: 10.2527/jas.2015-9057.

Curtis, G.C., Barfoot, C.F., Dugdale, A.H.A., Harris, P.A. and Argo, C.M. (2011) Voluntary ingestion of wood shavings by obese horses under dietary restriction. *British Journal of Nutrition* 106, S178–S182.

Czech, M.P. (2020) Mechanisms of insulin resistance related to white, beige, and brown adipocytes. *Molecular Metabolism* 34, 27–42. doi: 10.1016/j.molmet.2019.12.014.

Danielzik, S., Langnäse, K., Mast, M., Spethmann, C. and Müller, M.J. (2002) Impact of parental BMI on the manifestation of overweight 5–7 year old children. *European Journal of Nutrition* 41(3), 132–138. doi: 10.1007/s00394-002-0367-1.

de Luca, C. and Olefsky, J.M. (2008) Inflammation and insulin resistance. *FEBS Letters* 582(1), 97–105. doi: 10.1016/j.febslet.2007.11.057.

DeVault, M.L. (1991) Family discourse and everyday practice: gender and class at the dinner table. *Syracuse Scholar (1979–1991)* 11(1), 2.

Dosi, M., Kirton, R., Hallsworth, S., Keen, J.A. and Morgan, R.A. (2020) Inducing weight loss in native ponies: is straw a viable alternative to hay? *The Veterinary Record* 187, e60–e60. doi: 10.1136/vr.105793

Dua, A., Hennes, M.I., Hoffmann, R.G., Maas, D.L., Krakower, G.R. *et al.* (1996). Leptin: a significant indicator of total body fat but not of visceral fat and insulin insensitivity in African-American women. *Diabetes* 45(11), 1635–1637.

Dugdale, A.H.A. (2011) Aspects of adiposity in ponies. PhD thesis. The University of Liverpool.

Dugdale, A.H., Curtis, G.C., Cripps, P.J., Harris, P.A. and Argo, C.M. (2011a) Effects of season and body condition on appetite, body mass and body composition in ad libitum fed pony mares. *Veterinary Journal* 190(3), 329–337. doi: 10.1016/j.tvjl.2010.11.00.

Dugdale, A.H., Curtis, G.C., Harris, P.A. and Argo, C.M. (2011b) Assessment of body fat in the pony: part I. Relationships between the anatomical distribution of adipose tissue, body composition and body condition. *Equine Veterinary Journal* 43(5), 552–561.

Duška, F., Andel, M., Kubena, A. and Macdonald, I.A. (2005) Effects of acute starvation on insulin resistance in obese patients with and without type 2 diabetes mellitus. *Clinical Nutrition* 24(6), 1056–1064.

Eades, S.C. (2010) Overview of current laminitis research. *Veterinary Clinics of North America: Equine Practice* 26(1), 51–63.

Elwyn, G., Durand, M.A., Song, J., Aarts, J., Barr, P.J. *et al.* (2017) A three-talk model for shared decision making: multistage consultation process. *British Medical Journal* 359, 1–7.

Elzinga, S., Wood, P. and Adams, A. (2016) Plasma lipidomic and inflammatory cytokine profiles of horses with equine metabolic syndrome. *Journal of Equine Veterinary Science* 40, 49–55.

Emanuelli, B., Peraldi, P., Filloux, C., Sawka-Verhelle, D., Hilton, D. *et al.* (2000) SOCS-3 is an insulin-induced negative regulator of insulin signaling. *Journal of Biological Chemistry* 275, 15985–15991. doi: 10.1074/jbc.275.21.15985.

Erskine, R.M., Tomlinson, D.J., Morse, C.I., Winwood, K., Hampson, P. *et al.* (2017) The individual and combined effects of obesity- and ageing-induced systemic inflammation on human skeletal muscle properties. *International Journal of Obesity* 41(1), 102–111. doi: 10.1038/ijo.2016.151.

Ertelt, A., Barton, A.K., Schmitz, R.R. and Gehlen, H. (2014) Metabolic syndrome: is equine disease comparable to what we know in humans? *Endocrine Connections* 3(3), R81–R93. doi: 10.1530/EC-14-0038.

Fasol, R., Schindler, M., Schumacher, B. *et al.* (1992) The influence of obesity on perioperative morbidity: retrospective study of 502 aortocoronary bypass operations. *The Thoracic and Cardiovascular Surgeon* 40, 126–129.

Faty, A., Ferré P. and Commans, S. (2012) The acute phase protein serum amyloid A induces lipolysis and inflammation in human adipocytes through distinct pathways. *PLoS ONE* 7(4), e34031. doi: 10.1371/journal.pone.0034031.

Fazakerley, D.J., Krycer, J.R., Kearney, A.L., Hocking, S.L. and James, D.E. (2019) Muscle and adipose tissue insulin resistance: malady without mechanism? *Journal of Lipid Research* 60(10), 1720–1732.

Feijóo-Bandín, S., Aragón-Herrera, A., Moraña-Fernández, S., Anido-Varela, L., Tarazón, E. *et al.* (2020) Adipokines and inflammation: focus on cardiovascular diseases. *International Journal of Molecular Sciences* 21(20), 7711. doi: 10.3390/ijms21207711.

Fitzgerald, D.M., Anderson, S.T., Sillence, M.N. and de Laat, M.A. (2019) The cresty neck score is an independent predictor of insulin dysregulation in ponies. *PLoS ONE* 14(7), e0220203. doi: 10.1371/journal.pone.0220203.

Fleisch, A.F., Agarwal, N., Roberts, M.D., Han, J.C., Theim, K.R. *et al.* (2007) Influence of serum leptin on weight and body fat growth in children at high risk for adult obesity. *The Journal of Clinical Endocrinology & Metabolism* 92(3), 948–954. doi: 10.1210/jc.2006-1390.

Fowden, A.L., Jellyman, J.K., Valenzuela, O.A. and Forhead, A.J. (2013) Nutritional programming of intrauterine development: a concept applicable to the horse? *Journal of Equine Veterinary Science* 33, 295–304.

Fowden, A.L., Giussani, D.A. and Forhead, A.J. (2020) Physiological development of the equine fetus during late gestation. *Equine Veterinary Journal* 52(2), 165–173. doi: 10.1111/evj.13206.

Frasca, D. and Blomberg, B.B. (2016) Inflammaging decreases adaptive and innate immune responses in mice and humans. *Biogerontology* 17(1), 7–19.

Frasca, D., Diaz, A., Romero, M. and Blomberg, B.B. (2017) Ageing and obesity similarly impair antibody responses. *Clinical and Experimental Immunology* 187(1), 64–70. doi: 10.1111/cei.12824.

Frühbeck, G., Catalán, V., Rodríguez, A. *et al.* (2017) Involvement of the leptin-adiponectin axis in inflammation and oxidative stress in the metabolic syndrome. *Scientific Reports* 7, 6619. doi: 10.1038/s41598-017-06997-0.

Fureix, C., Benhajali, H., Henry, S. *et al.* (2013) Plasma cortisol and faecal cortisol metabolites concentrations in stereotypic and non-stereotypic horses: do stereotypic horses cope better with poor environmental conditions? *BMC Veterinary Research* 9, 3.

Furtado, T., Perkins, E., Pinchbeck, G. *et al.* (2020) Exploring horse owners' understanding of obese body condition and weight management in UK leisure horses. *Equine Veterinary Journal* 53, 752–762. doi: 10.1111/evj.13360.

García, O.P., Long, K.Z. and Rosado, J.L. (2009) Impact of micronutrient deficiencies on obesity. *Nutrition Reviews* 67(10), 559–572.

Gardner, D.S., Tsintzas, K. and Symonds, M.E. (2005) Programming of insulin sensitivity in lean and obese sheep. *Endocrine Abstracts* 10, 35.

Gee, E.K., Fennessy, P.F., Morel, P.C.H., Grace, N.D., Firth, E.C. *et al.* (2003) Chemical body composition of 20 Thoroughbred foals at 160 days of age, and preliminary investigation of techniques used to predict body fatness. *New Zealand Veterinary Journal* 51(3), 125–131.

Gentry, L.R., Thompson, D.L., Gentry, G.T., del Vecchio, R.P., Davis, K.A. *et al.* (2004) The relationship between body condition score and ultrasonographic fat measurements in mares of high versus low body condition. *Journal of Equine Veterinary Science* 24, 198–203.

Geor, R. and Frank, N. (2009) Metabolic syndrome-From human organ disease to laminar failure in equids. *Veterinary Immunology and Immunopathology* 129(3–4), 151–154. doi: 10.1016/j.vetimm.2008.11.012.

German, A.J. and Morgan, L.E. (2008) How often do veterinarians assess the bodyweight and body condition of dogs? *The Veterinary Record* 163(17), 503–505. doi: 10.1136/vr.163.17.503.

Graham-Thiers, P.M. and Bowen, L.K. (2013) Improved ability to maintain fitness in horses during large pasture turnout. *Journal of Equine Veterinary Science* 33(8), 581–585. doi: 10.1016/j.jevs.2012.09.001.

Harker, I.J., Harris, P.A. and Barfoot, C.F. (2011) The body condition score of leisure horses competing at an unaffiliated championship in the UK. *Journal of Equine Veterinary Science* 31, 253–254.

Henneke, D.R., Potter, G.D., Kreider, J.L. and Yeates, B.F. (1983) Relationship between condition score, physical measurements and body fat percentage in mares. *Equine Veterinary Journal* 15, 371–372.

Hill, J.O. (2006) Understanding and addressing the epidemic of obesity: an energy balance perspective. *Endocrine Reviews* 27(7), 750–761. doi: 10.1210/er.2006-0032.

Holbrook, T.C., Tipton, T. and McFarlane, D. (2012) Neutrophil and cytokine dysregulation in hyperinsulinemic obese horses. *Veterinary Immunology and Immunopathology* 145(1–2), 283–289.

Hollands, T., Ellis, J.M., Allen, D.E. and Salonen, L. (2009) An assessment of 2 visual methods of fat scoring in the equine to determine the most suitable for client recognition of obesity in their horses. In: *Proceedings of 48th BEVA Congress*, p. 247.

Honce, R. and Schultz-Cherry, S. (2019) Impact of obesity on influenza A virus pathogenesis, immune response, and evolution. *Frontiers in Immunology* 10, 1071. doi: 10.3389/fimmu.2019.01071.

Horohov, D.W., Adams, A.A. and Chambers, T.M. (2010) Immunosenescence of the equine immune system. *Journal of Comparative Pathology* 142(Suppl. 1), S78–S84.

Hosogai, N., Fukuhara, A., Oshima, K., Miyata, Y., Tanaka, S. *et al.* (2007) Adipose tissue hypoxia in obesity and its impact on adipocytokine dysregulation. *Diabetes* 56(4), 901–911.

Hotamisligil, G.S., Shargill, N.S. and Spiegelman, B.M. (1993) Adipose expression of tumor necrosis factor-alpha: direct role in obesity-linked insulin resistance. *Science* 259, 87–91.

Hultén, C., Grönlund, U., Hirvonen, J., Tulamo, R.M., Suominen, M.M. *et al.* (2002) Dynamics in serum of the inflammatory markers serum amyloid A (SAA), haptoglobin, fibrinogen and alpha2-globulins during induced noninfectious arthritis in the horse. *Equine Veterinary Journal* 34(7), 699–704. doi: 10.2746/042516402776250405.

Ireland, J.L., Clegg, P.D., McGowan, C.M., McKane, S.A. and Pinchbeck, G.L. (2011) A cross-sectional study of geriatric horses in the United Kingdom. Part 2: Health care and disease. *Equine Veterinary Journal* 43(1), 37–44.

Jahan-Mihan, A., Rodriguez, J., Christie, C., Sadeghi, M. and Zerbe, T. (2015) The role of maternal dietary proteins in development of metabolic syndrome in offspring. *Nutrients* 7(11), 9185–9217.

Jamaluddin, M.S., Weakley, S.M., Yao, Q. and Chen, C. (2012) Resistin: functional roles and therapeutic considerations for cardiovascular disease. *British Journal of Pharmacology* 165(3), 622–632. doi: 10.1111/j.1476-5381.2011.01369.x.

Jansson, A., Stefansdottir, G.J. and Ragnarsson, S. (2016) Plasma insulin concentration increases linearly with body condition in Icelandic horses. *Acta Veterinaria Scandinavica* 58, 76. doi: 10.1186/s13028-016-0258-8.

Jensen, R.B., Rockhold, L.L. and Tauson, A.H. (2019) Weight estimation and hormone concentrations related to body condition in Icelandic and Warmblood horses: a field study. *Acta Veterinaria Scandinavica* 61, 63. doi: 10.1186/s13028-019-0498-5.

Joe, A.W.B., Yi, L., Even, Y., Vogl, A.W. and Rossi, F.M.V. (2009) Depot-specific differences in adipogenic progenitor abundance and proliferative response to high fat diet. *Stem Cells* 27(10), 2563–2570.

Jung, C., Gerdes, N., Fritzenwanger, M. and Figulla, H.R. (2010) Circulating levels of interleukin-1 family cytokines in overweight adolescents. *Mediators of Inflammation* 2010, 958403. doi: 10.1155/2010/958403.

Kaneko, N., Kurata, M., Yamamoto, T. *et al.* (2019) The role of interleukin-1 in general pathology. *Inflammation and Regeneration* 39, 12. doi: 10.1186/s41232-019-0101-5.

Kang, S.M., Yoon, J.W., Ahn, H.Y., Kim, S.Y., Lee, K.H. *et al.* (2011) Android fat depot is more closely associated with metabolic syndrome than abdominal visceral fat in elderly people. *PLoS ONE* 6(11), e27694. doi: 10.1371/journal.pone.0027694.

Karpe, F. and Pinnick, K.E. (2015) Biology of upper-body and lower-body adipose tissue--link to whole-body phenotypes. *Nature Reviews Endocrinology* 11(2), 90–100. doi: 10.1038/nrendo.2014.185.

Kealy, R.D., Lawler, D.F., Ballam, J.M., Mantz, S.L., Biery, D.N. *et al.* (2002). Effects of diet restriction on life span and age-related changes in dogs. *Journal of the American Veterinary Medical Association* 220(9), 1315–1320.

Kearns, C.F., McKeever, K.H., Roegner, V., Brady, S.M. and Malinowski, K. (2006) Adiponectin and leptin are related to fat mass in horses. *The Veterinary Journal* 172(3), 460–465. doi: 10.1016/j.tvjl.2005.05.002.

Kelemen, Z., Grimm, H., Vogl, C., Long, M., Cavalleri, J. *et al.* (2021) Equine activity time budgets: the effect of housing and management conditions on geriatric horses and horses with chronic orthopaedic disease. *Animals* 11(7), 1867. doi: 10.3390/ani11071867.

Kenny, R., Dinan, T., Cai, G. and Spencer, S.J. (2014) Effects of mild calorie restriction on anxiety and hypothalamic-pituitary-adrenal axis responses to stress in the male rat. *Physiological Reports* 2(3), e00265. doi: 10.1002/phy2.265.

Kershaw, E.E. and Flier, J.S. (2004) Adipose tissue as an endocrine organ. *The Journal of Clinical Endocrinology & Metabolism* 89(6), 2548e2556. doi: 10.1210/jc.2004-0395.

Kim, D., Noh, D., Oh, T. and Lee, K. (2018) Body fat assessment by computed tomography and radiography in normal Beagle dogs. *The Journal of Veterinary Medical Science* 80(9), 1380–1384. doi: 10.1292/jvms.18-0216.

Kim, J.J. and Sears, D.D. (2010) TLR4 and insulin resistance. *Gastroenterology Research and Practice 2010*, Article ID 212563, 11 pages. doi: 10.1155/2010/212563.

Larson, J.A. and Villaverde, C. (2016) Obesity – scope of the problem and perception by owners and veterinarians. *Veterinary Clinics: Small Animal Practice* 46, 761–772. doi: 10.1016/j.cvsm.2016.04.001.

Lauten, S.D., Cox, N.R., Brawner, W.R. Jr and Baker, H.J. (2001) Use of dual energy x-ray absorptiometry for non-invasive body composition measurements in clinically normal dogs. *American Journal of Veterinary Research* 62(8), 1295–1301.

Lee, M.K.S., Laurent, Y.C., Masters, S.L. and Murphy, A.J. (2016) The modern interleukin-1 superfamily: Divergent roles in obesity. *Seminars in Immunology* 28(5), 441–449.

Levenhagen, D.K., Borel, M.J., Welch, D.C., Piasecki, J.H., Piasecki, D.P. *et al.* (1999) A comparison of air displacement plethysmography with three other techniques to determine body fat in healthy adults. *Journal of Parenteral and Enteral Nutrition* 23, 293–299.

Loftus, J.P. and Wakshlag, J.J. (2014) Canine and feline obesity: a review of pathophysiology, epidemiology, and clinical management. *Veterinary Medicine (Auckland, NZ)* 6, 49–60. doi: 10.2147/VMRR.S40868.

Longland, A.C., Barfoot, C. and Harris, P.A. (2011) Effects of soaking on the water-soluble carbohydrate and crude protein content of hay. *The Veterinary Record* 168(23), 618. doi: 10.1136/vr.d157.

Longland, A.C., Barfoot, C. and Harris, P.A. (2014) Effect of period, water temperature and agitation on loss of water-soluble carbohydrates and protein from grass hay: implications for equine feeding management. *The Veterinary Record* 174(3), 68. doi: 10.1136/vr.101820.

Lopez-Castejon, G. and Brough, D. (2011) Understanding the mechanism of IL-1β secretion. *Cytokine & Growth Factor Reviews* 22(4), 189–195. doi: 10.1016/j.cytogfr.2011.10.001.

Lu, Y.C., Lin, Y.C., Yen, A.M.F. *et al.* (2019) Dual-energy X-ray absorptiometry-assessed adipose tissues in metabolically unhealthy normal weight Asians. *Scientific Reports* 9, 17698. doi: 10.1038/s41598-019-53557-9.

Lumeng C.N., Bodzin J.L. and Saltiel A.R. (2007) Obesity induces a phenotypic switch in adipose tissue macrophage polarization. *The Journal of Clinical Investigation* 117, 175–184. doi: 10.1172/JCI29881.

Lynden, J., Ogden, J. and Hollands, T. (2018) Contracting for care – the construction of the farrier role in supporting horse owners to prevent laminitis. *Equine Veterinary Journal* 50, 658–666. doi: 10.1111/evj.12950

Lynden, J., Hollands, T. and Ogden, J. (2020) A farrier making every contact count: a microlevel analysis of farrier-client interaction for partnership working in managing a horse with laminitis. *Journal of Equine Veterinary Science* 87, 102924. doi: 10.1016/j.jevs.2020.102924.

Mabuchi, T., Yatsuya, H., Tamakoshi, K., Otsuka, R., Nagasawa, N. *et al.* (2005) Association between serum leptin concentration and white blood cell count in middle-aged Japanese men and women. *Diabetes/Metabolism Research and Reviews* 21(5), 441–447. doi: 10.1002/dmrr.540.

Mann, R.P. (2018) Collective decision making by rational individuals. *Proceedings of the National Academy of Sciences* 115, E10387–E10396.

Mann, S., Nydam, D.V., Abuelo, A., Yepes, F.L., Overton, T.R. and Wakshlag, J.J. (2016) Insulin signaling, inflammation, and lipolysis in subcutaneous adipose tissue of transition dairy cows either overfed energy during the prepartum period or fed a controlled-energy diet. *Journal of Dairy Science* 99(8), 6737–6752.

Manu, H., Lee, S., Keyes, M.C., Cairns, J. and Baidoo, S.K. (2020) Behavioral and cortisol responses to feeding frequency in pregnant sows under isocaloric intake. *Journal of Animal Science* 98(8), skaa226. doi: 10.1093/jas/skaa226.

Martin-Gimenez, T., de Blas, I., Aguilera-Tejero, E., Diez de Castro, E. and Aguirre-Pascasio, C N. (2016) Endocrine, morphometric, and ultrasonographic characterization of neck adiposity in Andalusian horses. *Domestic Animal Endocrinology* 56, 57–62.

Mazaki-Tovi, M., Bolin, S.R. and Schenck, P.A. (2016) Differential secretion of adipokines from subcutaneous and visceral adipose tissue in healthy dogs: association with body condition and response to troglitazone. *Veterinary Journal* 216, 136–141.

McLaughlin, T., Deng, A., Yee, G. *et al.* (2010) Inflammation in subcutaneous adipose tissue: relationship to adipose cell size. *Diabetologia* 53, 369–377.

Meyers, M.G. Jr, Leibel, R.L., Seeley, R.J. and Schwartz, M.W. (2010) Obesity and leptin resistance: distinguishing cause from effect. *Trends in Endocrinology and Metabolism: TEM* 21(11), 643–651. doi: 10.1016/j.tem.2010.08.002.
Milner, J.J. and Beck, M.A. (2012) The impact of obesity on the immune response to infection. *The Proceedings of the Nutrition Society* 71(2), 298–306. doi: 10.1017/S0029665112000158.
Min, K.B. and Min, J.Y. (2015) Android and gynoid fat percentages and serum lipid levels in United States adults. *Clinical Endocrinology* 82, 377–387.
Moore, B.A., Bemben, D.A., Lein, D.H. *et al.* (2020) Fat mass is negatively associated with muscle strength and jump test performance. *The Journal of Frailty & Aging* 9, 214–218 doi: 10.14283/jfa.2020.11.
Moore-Colyer, M.J., Lumbis, K., Longland, A. and Harris, P. (2014) The effect of five different wetting treatments on the nutrient content and microbial concentration in hay for horses. *PLoS ONE* 9(11), e114079. doi: 10.1371/journal.pone.0114079.
Moore-Colyer, M., Longland, A., Harris, P., Zeef, L. and Crosthwaite, S. (2020) Mapping the bacterial ecology on the phyllosphere of dry and post soaked grass hay for horses. *PLoS ONE* 15(1), e0227151.
Morgan, R.A., McGowan, T.W. and McGowan, C.M. (2014) Prevalence and risk factors for hyperinsulinaemia in ponies in Queensland, *Australia. Australian Veterinary Journal* 92(4), 101–106.
Morrison, P.K., Harris, P.A., Maltin, C.A., Grove-White, D. and Argo, C.M. (2017) EQUIFAT: a novel scoring system for the semi-quantitative evaluation of regional adipose tissues in Equidae. *PLoS ONE* 12(3), e0173753. doi: 10.1371/journal.pone.0173753.
Muhammad, I.F., Borné, Y., Hedblad, B., Nilsson, P.M., Persson, M. and Engström, G. (2016) Acute-phase proteins and incidence of diabetes: a population-based cohort study. *Acta diabetologica* 53(6), 981–989. doi: 10.1007/s00592-016-0903-8.
Munday, H.S., Booles, D., Anderson, P. *et al.* (1994) The repeatability of body composition measurements in dogs and cats using dual energy X-ray absorptiometry. *The Journal of Nutrition* 124(Suppl.), S2619–S2621.
Murano, I., Barbatelli, G., Parisani, V., Latini, C., Muzzonigro, G. *et al.* (2008) Dead adipocytes, detected as crown-like structures, are prevalent in visceral fat depots of genetically obese mice. *Journal of Lipid Research* 49(7), 1562–1568.
Murray, M.J. and Eichorn, E.S. (1996) Effects of intermittent feed deprivation, intermittent feed deprivation with ranitidine administration, and stall confinement with ad libitum access to hay on gastric ulceration in horses. *American Journal of Veterinary Research* 57(11), 1599–1603.
Murray, J.A.M., Bloxham, C., Kulifay, J., Stevenson, A. and Roberts, J. (2015) Equine nutrition: a survey of perceptions and practices of horse owners undertaking a massive open online course in equine nutrition. *Journal of Equine Veterinary Science* 35(6), 510–517.
Nedoszytko, B., Sokołowska-Wojdyło, M., Ruckemann-Dziurdzińska, K. Roszkiewicz, J. and Nowicki, R.J. (2014) Chemokines and cytokines network in the pathogenesis of the inflammatory skin diseases. *Advances in Dermatology and Allergology/Postępy Dermatologii I Alergologii* 31(2), 84–91.
Nijland, M.L., Stam, F. and Seidell, J.C. (2010) Overweight in dogs, but not in cats, is related to overweight in their owners. *Public Health Nutrition* 13(1), 102–106. doi: 10.1017/S136898000999022X.
NRC (National Research Council) (2007) *Nutrient Requirements of Horses, 6th* rev. edn. National Academies Press, Washington DC.
Ogden, J. and Arulgnanaseelan, J. (2017) Medically managing obesity: offering hope or a disincentive to change? *Patient Education and Counseling* 100(1), 93–97.
Ogden, J. and Flanagan, Z. (2008) Beliefs about the causes and solutions to obesity: a comparison of GPs and lay people. *Patient Education and Counseling* 71(1), 72–78.
Ogden, J., Bandara, Cohen, H., Farmer, D., Hardie, J. *et al.* (2001) General practitioners' and patients' models of obesity: whose problem is it? *Patient Education and Counseling* 44(3), 227–233.
Okada, Y., Kobayashi, M., Sawamura, M. and Arai, T. (2017) Comparison of visceral fat accumulation and metabolome markers among cats of varying BCS and novel classification of feline obesity and metabolic syndrome. *Frontiers in Veterinary Science*, 4, 17.
Okada, Y., Ueno, H., Mizorogi, T., Ohara, K., Kawasumi, K. and Arai, T. (2019) Diagnostic criteria for obesity disease in cats. *Frontiers in Veterinary Science* 6, 284. doi: 10.3389/fvets.2019.00284.
Okosun, I.S., Seale, J.P. and Lyn, R. (2015) Commingling effect of gynoid and android fat patterns on cardiometabolic dysregulation in normal weight American adults. *Nutrition & Diabetes* 5(5), e155. doi: 10.1038/nutd.2015.5.
Okura, T., Nakata, Y., Yamabuki, K. and Tanaka, K. (2004) Regional body composition changes exhibit opposing effects on coronary heart disease risk factors. *Arteriosclerosis, Thrombosis, and Vascular Biology* 24, 923–929.
Owens, T.G., Barnes, M., Gargano, V.M., Julien, L., Mansilla, W.D. *et al.* (2019) Nutrient content changes from steaming or soaking timothy-alfalfa hay: effects on feed preferences and acute glycemic response in Standardbred racehorses. *Journal of Animal Science* 97(10), 4199–4207.
Owers, R. and Chubbock, S. (2013) Fight the fat! *Equine Veterinary Journal* 45, 5–5.
Palanivel, R., Fullerton, M.D., Galic, S., Honeyman, J., Hewitt, K.A. *et al.* (2012) Reduced Socs3 expression

in adipose tissue protects female mice against obesity-induced insulin resistance. *Diabetologia* 55, 3083–3093. doi: 10.1007/s00125-012-2665-3.
Parameswaran, N. and Patial, S. (2010) Tumor necrosis factor-α signaling in macrophages. *Critical Reviews in Eukaryotic Gene Expression* 20(2), 87–103. doi: 10.1615/critreveukargeneexpr.v20.i2.10
Park, M.H., Kim, D.H., Lee, E.K., Kim, N.D., Im, D.S., Lee, J., Yu, B.P. and Chung, H.Y. (2014) Age-related inflammation and insulin resistance: a review of their intricate interdependency. *Archives of Pharmaceutical Research* 37(12), 1507–1514. doi: 10.1007/s12272-014-0474-6.
Patterson, C. and Hilton, S. (2013) Normalisation and stigmatisation of obesity in UK newspapers: a visual content analysis. *The Open Obesity Journal* 5, 82–91.
Pawluski, J., Jego, P., Henry, S., Bruchet, A., Palme, R. *et al.* (2017) Low plasma cortisol and fecal cortisol metabolite measures as indicators of compromised welfare in domestic horses (*Equus caballus*). *PLoS ONE* 12(9), e0182257. doi: 10.1371/journal.pone.0182257.
PDSA (2020) *Animal wellbeing (PAW) report 2020*. Available at: https://www.pdsa.org.uk/media/10540/pdsa-paw-rport-2020.pdf
Pérez, L.M., Pareja-Galeano, H., Sanchis-Gomar, F., Emanuele, E., Lucia, A. *et al.* (2016) 'Adipaging': aging and obesity share biological hallmarks related to a dysfunctional adipose tissue. *The Journal of Physiology* 594(12), 3187–3207. doi: 10.1113/JP271691.
Pérez-Pérez, A., Sánchez-Jiménez, F., Vilariño-García, T. and Sánchez-Margalet, V. (2020) Role of leptin in inflammation and vice versa. *International Journal of Molecular Sciences* 21(16), 5887. doi: 10.3390/ijms21165887.
Peugnet, P., Robles, M., Wimel, L., Tarrade, A. and Chavatte-Palmer, P. (2016) Management of the pregnant mare and long-term consequences on the offspring. *Theriogenology* 86(1), 99–109. doi: 10.1016/j.theriogenology.2016.01.028.
PFMA (2019) *Pet obesity report 2019*. Available at: www.ukpetfood.org/resource/pet-obesity-report-2019.html
Pinnick, K.E., Nicholson, G., Manolopoulos, K.N., McQuaid, S.E., Valet, P. *et al.* (2014) Distinct developmental profile of lower-body adipose tissue defines resistance against obesity-associated metabolic complications. *Diabetes* 63(11), 3785–3797.
Pleasant, R.S., Suagee, J.K., Thatcher, C.D., Elvinger, F. and Geor, R.J. (2013) Adiposity, plasma insulin, leptin, lipids, and oxidative stress in mature light breed horses. *Journal of Veterinary Internal Medicine* 27(3), 576–582. doi: 10.1111/jvim.12056.
Pond, C. (1978) Morphological aspects and the ecological and mechanical consequences of fat deposition in wild vertebrates. *Annual Review of Ecology and Systematics* 9, 519–570.
Popko, K., Gorska, E., Stelmaszczyk-Emmel, A. *et al.* (2010) Proinflammatory cytokines IL-6 and TNF-α and the development of inflammation in obese subjects. *European Journal of Medical Research* 15, 120. doi: 10.1186/2047-783X-15-S2-120.
Porsani, M.Y.H., de Oliveira, V.V., de Oliveira, A.G., Teixeira, F.A., Pedrinelli, V. *et al.* (2020a) What do Brazilian owners know about canine obesity and what risks does this knowledge generate? *PLoS ONE* 15(9), e0238771. doi: 10.1371/journal.pone.0238771.
Porsani, M., Teixeira, F.A., Amaral, A.R., Pedrinelli, V., Vasques, V. *et al.* (2020b) Factors associated with failure of dog's weight loss programmes. *Veterinary Medicine and Science* 6(3), 299–305. doi: 10.1002/vms3.229.
Post, R.E., Mainous, A.G., Gregorie, S.H., Knoll, M.E., Diaz, V.A. *et al.* (2011) The influence of physician acknowledgment of patients' weight status on patient perceptions of overweight and obesity in the United States. *Archives of Internal Medicine* 171(4), 316–321.
Primeau, V., Coderre, L., Karelis, A.D., Brochu, M., Lavoie, M.E. *et al.* (2011). Characterizing the profile of obese patients who are metabolically healthy. *International Journal of Obesity* 35(7), 971–981. doi: 10.1038/ijo.2010.216.
Quaresma, M., Payan-Carreira, R. and Silva, S.R. (2013) Relationship between ultrasound measurements of body fat reserves and body condition score in female donkeys. *The Veterinary Journal* 197, 329–334.
Ragnarsson, S. and Jansson, A. (2011) Comparison of grass haylage digestibility and metabolic plasma profile in Icelandic and Standardbred horses. *Journal of Animal Physiology and Animal Nutrition* 95(3), 273–279. doi: 10.1111/j.1439-0396.2010.01049.x.
Redsell, S.A., Atkinson, P., Nathan, D., Siriwardena, A.N., Swift, J.A. *et al.* (2010) Parents' beliefs about appropriate infant size, growth and feeding behaviour: implications for the prevention of childhood obesity. *BMC Public Health* 10(1), 711.
Reilly, J., Wilson, M., Summerbell, C. and Wilson, D. (2002) Obesity: diagnosis, prevention, and treatment; evidence based answers to common questions. *Archives of Disease in Childhood* 86(6), 392–394.
Reynolds, A., Keen, J.A., Fordham, T. and Morgan, R.A. (2019) Adipose tissue dysfunction in obese horses with equine metabolic syndrome. *Equine Veterinary Journal* 51(6), 760–766.
Rizza, R.A., Mandarino, L.J. and Gerich, J.E. (1982) Cortisol-induced insulin resistance in man: impaired suppression of glucose production and stimulation of glucose utilization due to a postreceptor defect of insulin action *The Journal of Clinical Endocrinology & Metabolism* 54(1), 131–138.
Robb, J., Harper, R.B., Hintz, H.F., Reid, J.T., Lowe, J.E., Schryver, H.F. and Rhee, M.S.S. (1972) Chemical

composition and energy value of the body, fatty acid composition of adipose tissue, and liver and kidney size in the horse. *Animal Science* 14(1), 25–34.

Robin, C.A., Ireland, J., Wylie, C.E., Collins, S.N., Verheyen, K.L.P. and Newton, J.R. (2013). Prevalence and risk factors for owner-reported obesity in horses and ponies in Great Britain. *Equine Veterinary Journal* 45, 12–13.

Rogero, M.M. and Calder, P.C. (2018) Obesity, inflammation, toll-like receptor 4 and fatty acids. *Nutrients* 10(4), 432. doi: 10.3390/nu10040432.

Rønn, S.G., Billestrup, N. and Mandrup-Poulsen, T. (2007) Diabetes and suppressors of cytokine signaling proteins. *Diabetes* 56(2), 541–548. doi: 10.2337/db06-1068.

Ruan, H., Hacohen, N., Golub, T.R., Van Parijs, L. and Lodish, H.F. (2002) Tumor necrosis factor-α suppresses adipocyte-specific genes and activates expression of preadipocyte genes in 3T3-L1 adipocytes: nuclear factor-kB activation by TNF-α is obligatory. *Diabetes* 51(5), 1319–1336. doi: 10.2337.diabetes.51.5.1319.

Rutkowski, J.M., Davis, K.E. and Scherer, P.E. (2009) Mechanisms of obesity and related pathologies: the macro- and microcirculation of adipose tissue. *The FEBS Journal* 276(20), 5738–5746. doi: 10.1111/j.1742-4658.2009.07303.x.

Saddi-Rosa, P., Oliveira, C.S., Giuffrida, F.M. and Reis, A.F. (2010) Visfatin, glucose metabolism and vascular disease: a review of evidence. *Diabetology & Metabolic Syndrome* 2, 21. doi: 10.1186/1758-5996-2-21.

Salinas, C., Espinosa, G., Morales, N., Henríquez, C., Morán, G. *et al.* (2020) Assessment of peripheral blood neutrophil respiratory burst, phagocytosis and apoptosis in obese non-insulin dysregulated horses. *Research in Veterinary Science* 132, 127–132.

Salonen, L.K., Hollands, T., Piercy, R.J. and Verheyen, K.L.P. (2009) Epidemiology of equine obesity in south east England: preliminary findings. In: *Proceedings of 48th BEVA Congress*. University of Surrey, p. 247.

Samsell, L., Regier, M., Walton, C. and Cottrell, L. (2014) Importance of android/gynoid fat ratio in predicting metabolic and cardiovascular disease risk in normal weight as well as overweight and obese children. *Journal of Obesity* 2014, 846578. doi: 10.1155/2014/846578.

Sánchez, M.J., Azor, P.J., Molina, A., Parkin, T., Rivero, J.L. *et al.* (2017) Prevalence, risk factors and genetic parameters of cresty neck in Pura Raza Español horses. *Equine Veterinary Journal* 49(2), 196–200. doi: 10.1111/evj.12569.

Santarossa, A., Parr, J.M. and Verbrugghe, A. (2018) Assessment of canine and feline body composition by veterinary health care teams in Ontario, *Canada. The Canadian Veterinary Journal* 59(12), 1280–1286.

Sarvas, J.L., Khaper, N. and Lees, S.J. (2013) The IL-6 paradox: context dependent interplay of SOCS3 and AMPK. *Journal of Diabetes & Metabolism* (Suppl. 13). doi: 10.4172/2155-6156.S13-003.

Sato, M., Ohkawa, R., Yoshimoto, A., Yano, K., Ichimura, N. *et al.* (2016) Effects of serum amyloid A on the structure and antioxidant ability of high-density lipoprotein. *Bioscience Reports* 36(4), e00369. doi: 10.1042/BSR20160075.

Scheibe, K.M. and Streich, W.J. (2003) Annual rhythm of body weight in Przewalski horses (*Equus ferus przewalskii*). *Biological Rhythm Research* 34(4), 383–395.

Schröder, U.J. and Staufenbiel, R. (2006) Invited review: methods to determine body fat reserves in the dairy cow with special regard to ultrasonographic measurement of backfat thickness. *Journal of Dairy Science* 89(1), 1–14. doi: 10.3168/jds.S0022-0302(06)72064-1.

Schryver, H.F., Hintz, H.F., Lowe, J.E., Hintz, R.L., Harper, R.B. and Reid, J.T. (1974) Mineral composition of the whole body, liver and bone of young horses. *The Journal of Nutrition* 104(1), 126–132.

Sears, B. and Perry, M. (2015) The role of fatty acids in insulin resistance. *Lipids in Health and Disease* 14, 121. doi: 10.1186/s12944-015-0123-1.

Shi, H., Tzameli, I., Bjørbaek, C. and Flier, J.S. (2004) Suppressor of cytokine signaling 3 is a physiological regulator of adipocyte insulin signaling. *The Journal of Biological Chemistry* 279(33), 34733–34740. doi: 10.1074/jbc.M403886200.

Shoveller, A.K., DiGennaro, J., Lanman, C. and Spangler, D. (2014) Trained vs untrained evaluator assessment of body condition score as a predictor of percent body fat in adult cats. *Journal of Feline Medicine & Surgery* 16(12), 957–965. doi: 10.1177/1098612X14527472.

Siciliano, P.D. and Schmitt, S. (2102) Effect of restricted grazing on hindgut pH and fluid balance. *Journal of Equine Veterinary Science* 32(9), 558–561. doi: 10.1016/j.jevs.2012.01.004.

Siegers, E.W., de Ruijter-Villani, M., van Doorn, D.A., Stout, T. and Roelfsema, E. (2018) Ultrasonographic measurements of localized fat accumulation in Shetland pony mares fed a normal v. a high energy diet for 2 years. *Animal: An International Journal of Animal Bioscience* 12(8), 1602–1610.

Silva, S.R., Payan-Carreira, R., Guedes, C.M., Coelho, S. and Santos, A.S. (2016a) Correlations between cresty neck scores and post-mortem nape fat measurements in horses, obtained after photographic image analysis. *Acta veterinaria Scandinavica* 58(Suppl. 1), 60.

Silva, S.R., Payan-Carreira, R., Quaresma, M., Guedes, C. and Santos, A. (2016b) Relationships between body condition score and ultrasound skin-associated subcutaneous fat depth in equids. *Acta Veterinaria Scandinavica* 58, 62. doi: 10.1186/s13028-016-0243-2.

Simon, M.C., Bilan, S., Nowotny, B., Dickhaus, T., Burkart, V. and Schloot, N.C. (2013) Fatty acids modulate cytokine and chemokine secretion of stimulated human whole blood cultures in diabetes. *Clinical and Experimental Immunology* 172(3), 383–393. doi: 10.1111/cei.12071.

Singh, R., Laflamme, P. and Sidebottom-Nielsen, M. (2002) Owner perceptions of canine body condition score. *Journal Veterinary Internal Medicine* 16, 362.

Smith, D.G., Cuddeford, D., Mayes, R. and Hollands, T. (2007a) The dry matter intake of grazing horses. In: *Proceedings of 46th BEVA Congress*, p. 295.

Smith, D., Mayes, R., Hollands, T., Cuddeford, D., Yule, H. *et al*. (2007b) Validating the alkane pair technique to estimate dry matter intake in equids. *The Journal of Agricultural Science* 145(3), 273–281. doi: 10.1017/S0021859607006788.

Smoliga, J.M. (2014) If an animal looks obese, precise estimation of body composition is of limited clinical value. *Journal of the American Veterinary Medical Association* 245(5), 484–485.

Snijder, M.B., Visser, M., Dekker, J.M. *et al*. (2005) Low subcutaneous thigh fat is a risk factor for unfavourable glucose and lipid levels, independently of high abdominal fat. *The Health ABC Study. Diabetologia* 48, 301–308. doi: 10.1007/s00125-004-1637-7.

Sokolowska, E. and Blachnio-Zabielska, A. (2019) The role of ceramides in insulin resistance. *Frontiers in Endocrinology* 10, 577. doi: 10.3389/fendo.2019.00577.

Spangenburg, E.E. (2007) Interleukin-6 does/does not have a beneficial role in insulin sensitivity and glucose homeostasis. *Journal of Applied Physiology* 102(2), 820–823.

Speakman, J., Booles, D. and Butterwick, R. (2001) Validation of dual energy X-ray absorptiometry (DXA) by comparison with chemical analysis of dogs and cats. *International Journal of Obesity* 25, 439–447.

Staub, C., Venturi, E., Cirot, M., Léonard, L., Barrière, P. *et al*. (2019) Ultrasonographic measures of body fatness and their relationship with plasma levels and adipose tissue expression of four adipokines in Welsh pony mares. *Domestic Animal Endocrinology* 69, 75–83. doi: 10.1016/j.domaniend.2019.02.002.

Stephenson, H.M., Green, M.J. and Freeman, S.L. (2011) Prevalence of obesity in a population of horses in the UK. *The Veterinary Record* 168(5), 131. doi: 10.1136/vr.c6281.

Suagee, J.K., Burk, A.O., Quinn, R.W., Petersen, E.D., Hartsock, T.G. *et al*. (2008) Effects of diet and weight gain on body condition scoring in thoroughbred geldings. *Journal of Equine Veterinary Science* 28(3), 156–166.

Suagee, J.K., Corl, B.A., Hulver, M.W., McCutcheon, L.J. and Geor, R.J. (2011) Effects of hyperinsulinemia on glucose and lipid transporter expression in insulin-sensitive horses. *Domestic Animal Endocrinology* 40(3), 173–181. doi: 10.1016/j.domaniend.2010.11.002.

Suagee, J., Corl, B.A. and Geor, R.J. (2012) A potential role for pro-inflammatory cytokines in the development of insulin resistance in horses. *Animals* 2(2), 243–260.

Suagee, J., Corl, B., Crisman, M., Pleasant, R., Thatcher, C. and Geor, R. (2013) Relationships between body condition score and plasma inflammatory cytokines, insulin, and lipids in a mixed population of light-breed horses. *Journal of Veterinary Internal Medicine* 27, 157–163.

Sun, K., Kusminski, C.M. and Scherer, P.E. (2011) Adipose tissue remodeling and obesity. *The Journal of Clinical Investigation* 121(6), 2094–2101. doi: 10.1172/JCI45887.

Swift, J.A., Choi, E., Puhl, R.M. and Glazebrook, C. (2013) Talking about obesity with clients: preferred terms and communication styles of UK pre-registration dieticians, doctors, and nurses. *Patient Education and Counseling* 91(2), 186–191.

Tadros, E.M., Frank, N., Newkirk, K.M., Donnell, R.L. and Horohov, D.W. (2012) Effects of a ‘two-hit’ model of organ damage on the systemic inflammatory response and development of laminitis in horses. *Veterinary Immunology and Immunopathology* 150(1–2), 90–100.

Tailor, A. and Ogden, J. (2009) Avoiding the term ‘obesity’: an experimental study of the impact of doctors’ language on patients’ beliefs. *Patient Education and Counseling* 76(2), 260–264.

Trayhurn, P. and Wood, I.S. (2004) Adipokines: inflammation and the pleiotropic role of white adipose tissue. *British Journal of Nutrition* 92(3), 347–355.

Treiber, K.H., Kronfeld, D.S. and Geor, R.J. (2006) Insulin resistance in equids: possible role in laminitis. *The Journal of Nutrition* 136(7), 2094S–2098S.

Treiber, K., Carter, R., Gay, L., Williams, C. and Geor, R. (2009) Inflammatory and redox status of ponies with a history of pasture-associated laminitis. *Veterinary Immunology and Immunopathology* 129(3-4), 216–220.

Trim, W., Turner, J.E. and Thompson, D. (2018) Parallels in immunometabolic adipose tissue dysfunction with ageing and obesity. *Frontiers in Immunology* 9, 169. doi: 10.3389/fimmu.2018.00169.

Turner, R.B.S., Tyrrell, D., Hepworth, G., Dunshea, F.R. and Mansfield, C.S. (2020) Compartmental fat distribution in the abdomen of dogs relative to overall body fat composition. *BMC Veterinary Research* 16, 104. doi: 10.1186/s12917-020-02327-1.

Vargas, E., Podder, V. and Carrillo Sepulveda, M.A. (2020) Physiology, glucose transporter type 4 (GLUT4). In: *StatPearls [Internet]*. StatPearls Publishing, Treasure Island, Florida. Available at: https://www.ncbi.nlm.nih.gov/books/NBK537322/.

Vaz, J., Narayan, E.J., Dileep Kumar, R., Thenmozhi, K., Thiyagesan, K. *et al*. (2017) Prevalence and determinants of stereotypic behaviours and physiological stress among tigers and leopards in Indian zoos. *PLoS ONE* 12(4), e0174711. doi: 10.1371/journal.pone.0174711.

Via, M. (2012) The malnutrition of obesity: micronutrient deficiencies that promote diabetes. *ISRN Endocrinology* 2012, 103472.

Vick, M.M., Adams, A.A., Murphy, B.A., Sessions, D.R., Horohov, D.W. *et al.* (2007) Relationships among inflammatory cytokines, obesity, and insulin sensitivity in the horse. *Journal of Animal Science* 85(5), 1144–1155.

Vick, M.M., Murphy, B.A., Sessions, D.R., Reedy, S.E., Kennedy, E.L. *et al.* (2008) Effects of systemic inflammation on insulin sensitivity in horses and inflammatory cytokine expression in adipose tissue. *American Journal of Veterinary Research* 69(1), 130–139.

Visser, E.K. and Van Wijk-Jansen, E.E. (2012) Diversity in horse enthusiasts with respect to horse welfare: an explorative study. *Journal of Veterinary Behavior* 7(5), 295–304.

Waller, A.P., Huettnera, L., Kohlera, K. and Lacombeb, V.A. (2012) Novel link between inflammation and impaired glucose transport during equine insulin resistance. *Veterinary Immunology and Immunopathology* 149(3–4), 208–215.

Webb, A.I. and Weaver, B.M. (1979) Body composition of the horse. *Equine Veterinary Journal* 11(1), 39–47. doi: 10.1111/j.2042-3306.1979.tb01295.x.

Westervelt, R.G., Stouffer, J.R., Hintz, H.F. and Schryver, H.F. (1976) Estimating fatness in horses and ponies. *Journal of Animal Science* 43(4), 781–785.

White, G.A., Hobson-West, P., Cobb, K., Craigon, J., Hammond, R. and Millar, K.M. (2011) Canine obesity: is there a difference between veterinarian and owner perception? *The Journal of Small Animal Practice* 52(12),622–626.doi:10.1111/j.1748-5827.2011.01138.x.

Wiesenthal, S.R., Sandhu, H., McCall, R.H., Tchipashvili, V., Yoshii, H. *et al.* (1999) Free fatty acids impair hepatic insulin extraction *in vivo*. *Diabetes* 48(4), 766–774. doi: 10.2337/diabetes.48.4.766.

Williams, S., Tucker, C.A., Green, M.J. and Freeman, S.L. (2011) Investigation of the effect of pasture and stable management on large intestinal motility in the horse, measured using transcutaneous ultrasonography. *Equine Veterinary Journal* 43, 93–97. doi: 10.1111/j.2042-3306.2011.00399.x.

Williams, S., Horner, J., Orton, E., Green, M., McMullen, S. *et al.* (2014) Water intake, faecal output and intestinal motility in horses moved from pasture to a stabled management regime with controlled exercise. *Equine Veterinary Journal* 47(1), 96–100. doi: 10.1111/evj.12238.

Wilson, C.A., Bekele, G., Nicolson, M., Ravussin, E. and Pratley, R.E. (1997) Relationship of the white blood cell count to body fat: role of leptin. *British Journal of Haematology* 99(2), 447–451. doi: 10.1046/j.1365-2141.1997.3873201.x.

Witkowska-Piłaszewicz, O.D., Żmigrodzka, M., Winnicka, A., Miśkiewicz, A., Strzelec, K. *et al.* (2019) Serum amyloid A in equine health and disease. *Equine Veterinary Journal* 51(3), 293–298. doi: 10.1111/evj.13062.

Witzel, A.L., Kirk, C.A., Henry, G.A., Toll, P.W., Brejda, J.J. *et al.* (2014) Use of a novel morphometric method and body fat index system for estimation of body composition in overweight and obese dogs. *Journal of the American Veterinary Medical Association* 244(11), 1279–1284.

Wood, P.L., Steinman, M., Erol, E., Carter, C., Christmann, U. *et al.* (2018) Lipidomic analysis of immune activation in equine leptospirosis and Leptospira-vaccinated horses. *PLoS ONE* 13(2), e0193424. doi: 10.1371/journal.pone.0193424.

Wyse, C.A., McNie, K.A., Tannahil, V.J., Murray, J.K. and Love, S. (2008) Prevalence of obesity in riding horses in Scotland. *Veterinary Record* 162(18), 590. doi: .10.1136/vr.162.18.590.

Yaissle, J.E., Holloway, C. and Buffington, C.A. (2004) Evaluation of owner education as a component of obesity treatment programs for dogs. *Journal of the American Veterinary Medical Association* 224(12), 1932–1935. doi: 10.2460/javma.2004.224.1932.

Yu, C., Chen, Y., Cline, G.W., Zhang, D., Zong, H. *et al.* (2002) Mechanism by which fatty acids inhibit insulin activation of insulin receptor substrate-1 (IRS-1)-associated phosphatidylinositol 3-kinase activity in muscle. *The Journal of Biological Chemistry* 277(52), 50230–50236. doi: 10.1074/jbc.M200958200.

Zak, A.N., Siwinska, S., Elzinga, V.D., Barker, T., Stefaniak, B.J. *et al.* (2020a) Effects of advanced age and pituitary pars intermedia dysfunction on components of the acute phase reaction in horses. *Domestic Animal Endocrinology* 72,106476, doi: 10.1016/j.domaniend.2020.106476.

Zak, A., Siwinska, N., Elzinga, S., Barker, V.D., Stefaniak, T. *et al.* (2020b) Effects of equine metabolic syndrome on inflammation and acute-phase markers in horses. *Domestic Animal Endocrinology* 72, 106448, 1–8.

Zammit, C., Liddicoat, H., Moonsie, I. and Makker, H. (2010) Obesity and respiratory diseases. *International Journal of General Medicine* 3, 335–343. doi: 10.2147/IJGM.S11926.

Zdrojewicz, Z., Popowicz, E., Szyca, M., Michalik, T. and Śmieszniak, B. (2017) TOFI phenotype – its effect on the occurrence of diabetes. *Pediatric Endocrinology, Diabetes, and Metabolism* 23(2), 96–100. doi: 10.18544/PEDM-23.02.0079.

Zhang, Y., Proenca, R., Maffei, M., Barone, M., Leopold, L. *et al.* (1994) Positional cloning of the mouse obese gene and its human homologue. *Nature* 372(6505), 425–432. doi: 10.1038/372425a0.

16 Feeding the Aged Horse

Teresa Hollands

School of Veterinary Medicine, University of Surrey

Learning Objectives

LO1 Provide an overview of ageing in the horse.
LO2 Summarise the common feeding practice of owners of old horses in the UK.
How to feed the 'fit' older horse
LO3 Review common clinical conditions of the old horse that can be supported through diet.
How to feed the older horse with muscle loss
How to feed the older horse with weight loss
LO4 Describe the feeding management of forage for the older horse with dental disease.
How to feed a horse that quids or has difficulty chewing
How to feed a horse with diastemas/periodontal disease
LO5 Review supplements fed to the older horse.
When and how to recommend supplements for the older horse
LO6 Summarise feeds and feeding management for the older horse.

At the end of this chapter, you will be able to advise the way that diet and ration need to be adapted for the older horse to maximise healthy longevity.

Introduction

The older horse is often overlooked in practice, despite their numbers increasing from 2.2% (1989) to 12.5% (1999) in the USA (Brosnahan and Paradis, 2003b) and in the UK to 26% (Mellor *et al.*, 1999); 29% of the UK horse population were 15 years or older in 2011 (Ireland *et al.*, 2011). A 55% increase in patients older than 20 years of age was recorded between 1990 and 1995 at a south-eastern referral clinic, USA (McFarlane *et al.*, 2001). The number of equine patients 20 years of age or older seen at a New England (USA) referral clinic increased sixfold over a period of 10 years (Brosnahan and Paradis, 2003b).

Ageing is an inevitable physiological consequence of living organisms; nutrition can prolong healthy ageing, maintain physical health and reduce the risk of diseases that might typically be associated with ageing in the horse. The rate of ageing can vary between horses, depending on fitness levels, breed and environmental factors, of which nutrition is one. Not all tissues experience ageing at the same rate nor to the same extent and appropriate management and feeding may reduce the rate of ageing. Muscle mass can either increase or decrease in response to metabolic demands like exercise or following a period of inactivity. Older horses on reduced exercise will lose muscle (Paradis, 2002), commonly described as loss of 'topline' by your clients (Fig. 16.1). Please explain to clients that attempting to maintain the outline associated with work and muscle development by increased feed results in fat deposition that is detrimental to their horse's health and longevity (see Chapter 15).

It is important to note that 'owners seem to under-recognise some of the most prevalent diseases identified in geriatric horses' (Ireland, 2016), including differentiation of muscle and fat (obesity),

DOI: 10.1079/9781789245134.0016

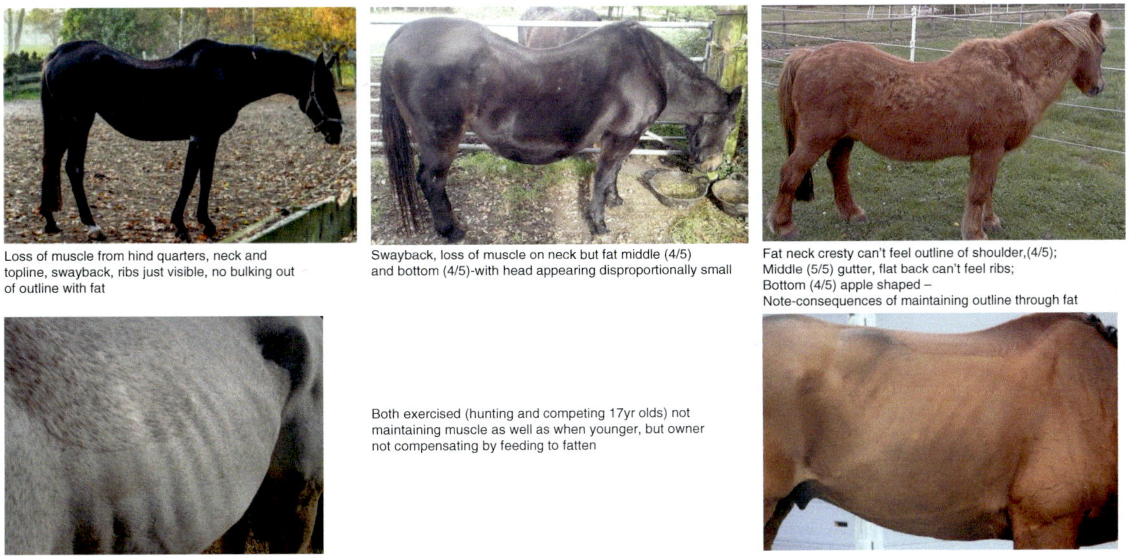

Fig. 16.1 The visual appearance of aged unexercised and exercised horses.

lameness, and respiratory and dental disease. The risk of all these diseases can be prevented, supported or minimised by appropriate diets.

Perception of ageing

Ageing is not well defined in the horse – unlike dogs and cats, where the chronological definition of age varies with breed (Michell, 1999). In horses, an increase in disease provides the indicator of physiological ageing defined as > 15 years in the UK (Ireland *et al.*, 2012a,b). A full veterinary examination of horses more than 15 years old (n = 200) found that over 95% had physiological changes typical of ageing in other species: 71% of horses had a dermatological abnormality, 22% hirsutism, 83.5% stiffness/lameness in at least one joint and 95.4% had dental abnormalities (Ireland *et al.*, 2012a,b); over 25% of the horses were carrying too much fat (> 3/5). These clinical characteristics are similar to those recorded by other researchers (Table 16.1) and most can be supported by diet.

Risk factors that reduce healthy longevity

There is a tendency for owners to keep their older horse fat to disguise the inevitable decrease in muscle mass. Total muscle mass in people decreases by nearly 50% between 20 and 90 years of age (Kalyani *et al.*, 2014) which, together with a higher fat mass, characterises older adults (Kim *et al.*, 2017). Ageing is also associated with an increase in low-grade chronic inflammation (LGCI) (Ilich *et al.*, 2014), which is further exacerbated by obesity (see Chapter 15: 'Ageing and obesity'). Consider using other species to help owners change their visual perception of an aged, out-of-work horse (Fig. 16.2). Ask them to imagine Mo Farah as he ages and loses muscle but maintains his slim outline as he does not eat excess calories and get fat. Think about dairy cows, who do not develop bulky muscle and, if they get fat, get very ill from metabolic diseases; please discourage them from keeping fat aged animals.

It is important to remind owners that ageing does not have to be associated with disease; many top Olympic horses would fall into the chronological group of aged (Table 16.2).

Only 26% of aged horses in the UK are retired (Ireland *et al.*, 2011); 74% are still being ridden. Exercise maintains muscle mass and reduces insulin resistance across age groups and species. The diet that you recommend for the old horse needs in part to reflect their exercise levels and other management practices.

Common Management Practices Related to Feeding Requirements of the Old Horse

It is always helpful to have an overview of the 'typical' management of the older horse in the UK, but because clients will have their own way of doing

Table 16.1 Clinical characteristics and signs of ageing in the older horse that can be supported through diet

Reference	Number of horses	Mean age in years (range)	BCS	Dental disease	PPID	Gastrointestinal tract (GIT)	Musculo-skeletal (MSK)	Respiratory
Brosnahan and Paradis (2003a)	165	26.5 (20–44)	28% 4–5/5	25%	8% Vet diagnosed			
Brosnahan and Paradis (2003b)	467	24 (20–45)		8%	11%	54% (39% colic)	24% (72% lame; 40% degenerative lesions of MSK) 86% laminitis	16%
Ireland *et al.* (2012a,b)	200	20 (17–24)	26% > 3.5/5	95.4%	22% hirsutism		83.5% reduced motion in at least one joint	7.5% spontaneous cough 18.5% nasal discharge 22% abnormal respiratory sounds at rest 13.6% LAD
McGowan *et al.* (2010)	974	> 15 years		10%, of which 6.6% had difficulty in eating Teeth/dental care 18%	16.8% hirsutism	Colic 7.7%, diarrhoea 8.5% Reduced appetite 5.8% Weight loss 28%	Muscle stiffness 33.4%; lameness 28% Arthritis 24%	Coughing 18.7% Nasal discharge 12.8%
Ireland *et al.* (2012a,b)	87	> 30 years	16% < 2.5/5 10% < 3/5	Quidding 33.3% 100% examined had one abnormality 75% periodontal disease, 43% missing teeth	39% hirsutism		97% reduced motion, 44.8% muscle loss Sway back 28.7%	Cough 13%

[a]% of study population

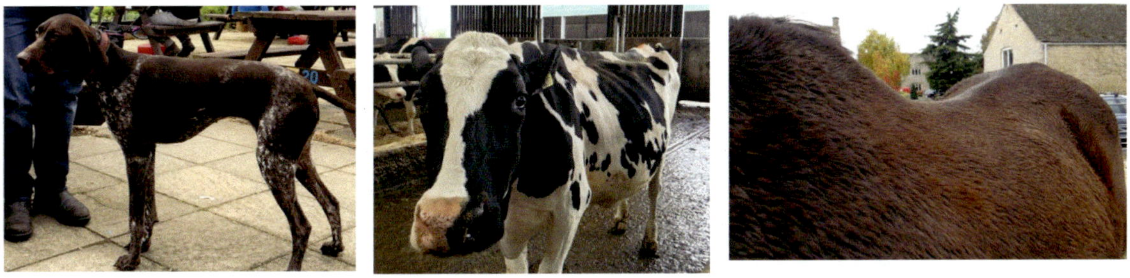

Solid muscle, lean outline, no fat

No muscle and kept slim to minimise disease so outline very slim

Bones are easily felt, but not seen, Lost muscle as not being ridden

Fig. 16.2 Cross-species comparisons of visual perception of 'good' ageing.

Table 16.2 Ageing is not a disease; many old horses successfully compete at high levels

	London 2012	Tokyo 2021
Eventing	• 23% horses were 15 years or older • 40% Germany Gold medal team 15 years or older • Highest placed individual horses (Imperial Cavalier) 15 years • Lenamore (NZL) 20 years old won team bronze	• Tayberry (HING King) 20 years old
Dressage	• Donnperignon, 17-year-old Finnish Warmblood, Danish Team • Parzival, 19-year-old KWPN, Netherlands • Chablis, 19-year-old Danish Warmblood, Italy	• 19-year-old Ramoneur (ruled out due to laminitis)
Paradressage	• Noki – 16 years (Sophie Wells) won team gold and two individual silvers	

things, a full dietary history would be appropriate as part of your old horse clinic (see Chapter 2).

Workload

In the UK, 74% of horses over 15 years of age are still exercised (Ireland *et al.*, 2011) (Fig. 16.3), of which 25% are competed.

Feeding management

Many owners make changes to the diet of their older horses, feeding less than recommended quantities of complementary feed with a greater reliance on feeding chaff and sugar beet (Ireland *et al.*, 2011). resulting in micronutrient deficiencies (Fig. 16.4 and Table 16.3). The change in feeding likely reflects the lighter workload, the horse being out at grass for longer than it was when it was younger and so obtaining more of its nutrition from grass, or it might simply be economics.

Access to grazing

Grazing times of old horses varies across the year, reflecting those of other leisure horses; at least 90% of UK old horses are turned out at some time of the year (Ireland *et al.*, 2011) (Fig. 16.5 and Table 16.3) with 73% out during the day and in at night over a 12-month period.

Do encourage daily turnout, even in the winter. Pastured horses stay fitter than horses kept stabled – horses kept on pastures of 29,166 m^2 during the winter to minimise dietary differences and trained, compared with stabled and trained horses, needed less time for fittening and conditioning (Rivera *et al.*, 2002). Pastured horses turned out onto hilly 100 acres stayed as fit as stabled horses exercised 1–2 h of light-to-moderate work, 5 days/week (walking, trotting and cantering under saddle) with paddock turnout onto 1 acre at night (Graham-Thiers and Bowen, 2013). A reduction in exercise is a risk factor for laminitis (Wylie *et al.*, 2013); whereas increasing exercise and decreasing calories reduces insulin resistance (IR) (Freestone *et al.*, 1992); however, if the horse is fat, exercise alone does not always reduce IR (Carter *et al.*, 2010). Any form of exercise, whether ridden or otherwise, will help maintain muscle mass whatever the age of the horse. The key is to match the diet to the exercise level.

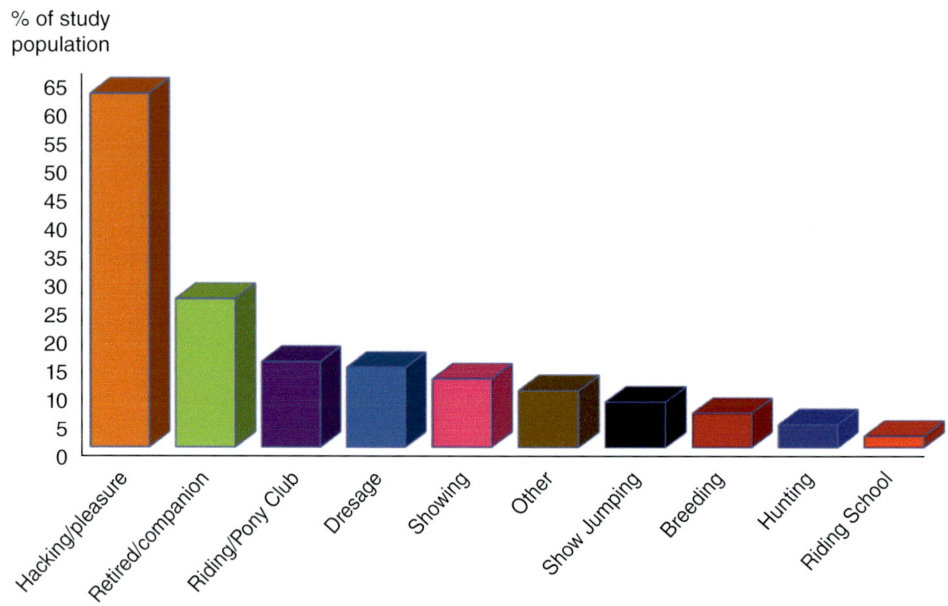

Fig. 16.3 The workload of old horses in the UK (exercised 1–4 days/week for 20–60 min/day). Source: Ireland *et al.* (2011).

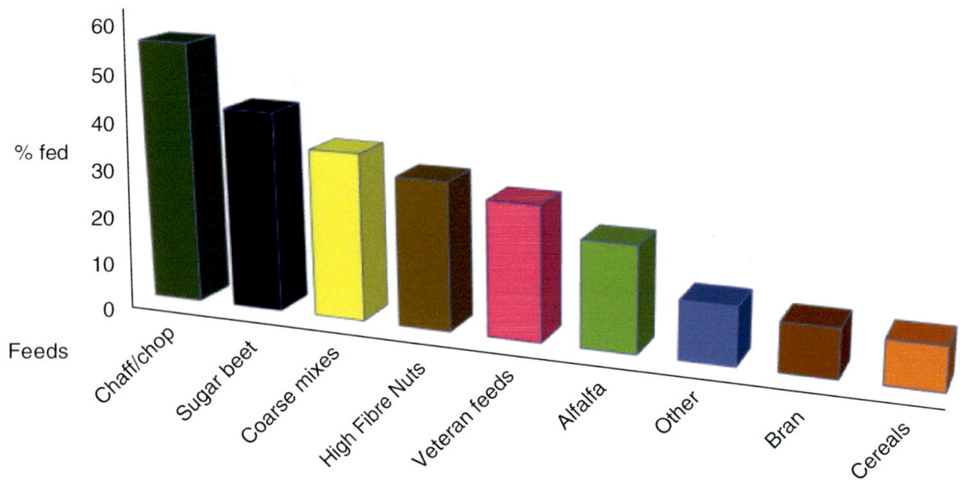

Fig. 16.4 The percentage of UK old horses (median age 22.7 years) eating common feeds. Source: Ireland *et al.* (2011).

Feeding for the Older Horse

Assuming the horse is not showing signs of physiological ageing, the feed you would advise would depend upon the workload, the fat score, how the horse is being managed and what forage the horse is eating

'Fit' Old Horse

There is often no need to recommend any specialised feed for these older horses, but they might benefit from a higher protein intake to maintain muscle mass. Do remind owners that feeding protein alone will not improve muscle mass; an increase in muscle mass will only occur alongside exercise. The same thing happens in people: physical inactivity (common in elderly people) combined with inadequate protein intake has been shown to aggravate muscle loss (Houston *et al.*, 2008).

Table 16.3 A summary of feeds and feeding management of aged horses (% of surveyed sample): a comparison across the literature

Reference	Workload	Access to grazing	Grazing hours summer	Grazing hours winter	Forage fed (%)	Hay replacers (%)	Chaff as complementary feed (%)	Feed fed	Supplements
Ireland *et al.* (2011)	65% kept/ ridden for pleasure 25% retired	90.4%	45% out 24 h/ day	<20% out grazing 24/7	Haylage 52 Dry hay 38 Dampened hay 22 Soaked hay 11.5 Steamed hay 1.7	15	55	Fig. 16.4	
Brosnahan and Paradis (2003a)		66% mostly outside 21% mostly in stalls			Alfalfa hay 89	7		37% leisure feeds 51% geriatric feeds	54% 66% vits/mins 47% joint
McGowan *et al.* (2010)		24 h grazing 68%	95% some of the time		Lucerne hay 75 Grass hay 39			Stud mixes 62 Coarse mix 26	71% Vitamins 29 Hoof 7 Joint 6 Minerals 58 Oil/fat 29%
Bushell and Murray (2016)		66% pasture			93% in winter Grass hay 78% Alfalfa hay 29% Dry 73% Dampened 15% Soaked 9% Steamed 3%		Sugar beet pulp 46%	7C% in winter 62% manufactured feeds 23% home mixed	86% Vits/mins 78% Slat/electrolytes 46% Joint 43% Hoof 23% Oil/fat 35%
Muller and Linberg (2020)					42% adlib; 57% in meals Mean 1.5 kg DM/100 kg BW 19% just forage		34% sugar beet pulp	81% fed hard feed 57% commercial concentrates Mean intake 0.11 kg/100 kg BW 7% of ration	

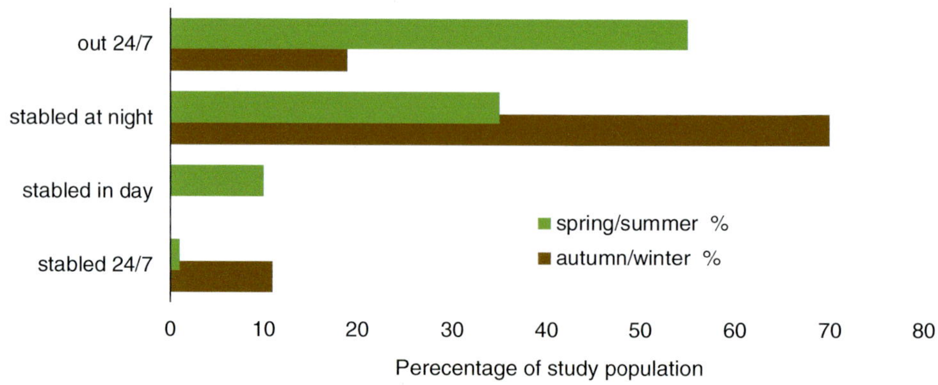

Fig. 16.5 Annual pattern of grazing and stabling management of a UK population of aged horses. Grazing median 22 h during spring/summer and 8 h autumn/winter; 16% never stabled. (Modified from Ireland *et al.*, 2011.)

Light work

Maximise grazing

Encourage owners to keep the horse out grazing for as many hours as possible, using a muzzle if there is excess grass and the horse is at risk of getting fat. The time of year and availability of grass will clearly affect the feed and forage that you would advise (see Chapter 11: Fig. 11.1).

Forage replacers

The type of forage that you would recommend is dependent on several factors, including dental health, body fat score (see Chapter 3: 'Body fat scoring') and forage hygiene (see Chapter 9: 'Soaking or steaming for dust suppression').

Conserved forages should be advised when the horse is stabled or when grass is not growing; 52% of older horses in the UK are fed haylage and 22% are fed hay replacers. It is important that clients understand the implication of forages in terms of the amount of fibre (dry matter) (see Chapter 9: Tables 9.9 and 9.10) to ensure that fibre intake is maintained to support gut health – including minimising the risk of colic (see Chapter 12: 'Colic').

Top tips for clients who have horses that are not showing signs of ageing

- Continue to feed for the work of the horse.
  - Regular exercise maintains muscle mass.
- Accept weight (fat) gain in the summer if just in light work.
  - This fat gain needs to be lost in the winter.
- Balance energy intake with adequate protein and vitamins and minerals.
  - If feeding less than manufacturer's recommended quantities, change feed.
  - Often a balancer suffices in summer.
  - Chaff and sugar beet are useful calorie sources but low in quality protein.
- Soak hay ensuring fat loss to 3, 3, 3 in winter.
  - Might be FS 2.5 in places at end of winter.
- Accept winter muscle loss if in light work.
  - The horse's outline will look weaker due to decreased exercise.
  - Discourage maintaining an outline through just feeding: you do not want an increased BFS increasing the risk of many age-related diseases, such as PPID, osteoarthritis.
- Regular dental care.
- Regular worm counts.

Balancing vitamins and minerals

All old horses in work that put fat on easily will in most instances be obtaining excess calories from grazing or other forages, but they will be deficient in vitamins and minerals and quality protein.

If the horse has access to nutritious grazing, then advise a good-quality general vitamin and mineral supplement that is normally fed at 12 g/100 kg BW mixed with a small quantity of dampened low-calorie chaff. If the horse is on conserved forages/winter grazing/soaked hay, then recommend a good-quality balancer (100 g/100 kg BW) with alfalfa chaff (100–500 g/100 kg BW), divided into two meals (Table 16.4). Individuals with higher protein intake lose less lean mass with ageing (Houston *et al.*, 2008).

Table 16.4 How to check a diet of a 'fit aged' horse

Horse signalment	20-year-old, 15 hh cob type gelding	Tendency to put weight on easily – weight tape indicates 525 kg
Horse history	Generally light exercise	Owner was worried that horse had lost too much weight in the winter, particularly on its neck and hindquarters
Differentials		
Results of any tests	BFS 4, 4, 4	Fat carrying too much weight

Current diet	Grazing 6 h/day;soaked hay;
	large haynet at night;
	½ scoop horse and pony nuts
		• Grass intake varied
		  ◦ Sparse and not managed so feed value low
		• Soaked hay leaches minerals
		  ◦ Quantity of feed not sufficient to provide daily requirements of any micronutrients

Advice	Overfed but undernourished –not fit enough for the work as is fat
	Provide a suggestion for fittening
	• Walk out briskly daily for 30 min with heart rate to 80 bpm
	  ◦ At the pace of walking if you saw a bus in the distance and thought you were going to miss it
	Use muzzle in field and increase turnout – improves fitness
		• Continue with soaking hay.
		  ◦ Advise weighing out 6 kg before soaking for 12 h.
		• 0.5 kg alfalfa chaff to improve protein quality
		• High spec balancer fed at 100 g/100 kg BW (525 g/day) split into two feeds

Horses that do show signs of ageing will need dietary support targeted to their differentials.

Common Clinical Conditions of the Old Horse That Can Be Supported Through Diet

Muscle loss in the aged horse

It has been reported that 28% of aged horses suffer from weight loss (McGowan *et al.*, 2010) whereas 44% exhibit muscle loss (28% noted as sway back) (Ireland *et al.*, 2012a,b) (see Table 16.1).

In older people, lean body mass was associated with better strength, mobility and performance in daily activities compared with people with a high body mass index with a high percentage of body fat (Kim *et al.*, 2017). Ageing in all animals causes changes in body composition, with a decrease in muscle mass and an increase in adiposity, specifically fat infiltration in muscles (see Chapter 15, Fig. 15.1: 'Intra and intermuscular fat in a pony').

Ageing has been associated with a decline in muscle fibre number, which is thought to be the principal cause of age-related loss of muscle mass in humans. Similar age-associated changes in skeletal muscle have been measured in the horse (Li *et al.*, 2016).

When different-aged horses (1.8 years old versus 17–25 years old) from the same breed and same fat score were compared, skeletal muscle ageing was accompanied by a shift in fibre type composition towards a higher percentage of type I and IIA muscle fibres, and a decrease in mitochondrial density. Additionally, the muscle oxidative capacity, measured by cytochrome c oxidase (COX), was 47% lower in aged gluteus ($P < 0.001$) and 30% lower in aged triceps muscle ($P = 0.003$). The researchers postulated that 'despite some age-associated changes, there was no overt mitochondrial dysfunction in skeletal muscle from aged American Quarter Horses. If a transition age exists in the horse, defining it might provide insights about a beneficial time point to apply interventions aiming to delay the onset of overt muscle oxidative dysfunction and decline in physical performance' (Li *et al.*, 2016) – such as diet.

The cross-sectional area of the longissimus muscle is smaller in aged (≥ 16 years old) compared with adult horses (1–21 years old) (Reed *et al.*, 2015). Age appears to be accompanied by an increase in muscle glycolytic capacity and a decrease in muscle oxidative capacity in horses (Kim *et al.*, 2005). A reduction in muscle mass will compromise the ability of the older horse to exercise. It is important that you establish if the muscle loss is due to lack of exercise before you look at dietary support.

There is no difference in body composition (measured by ultrasound of rump fat and muscle biopsies

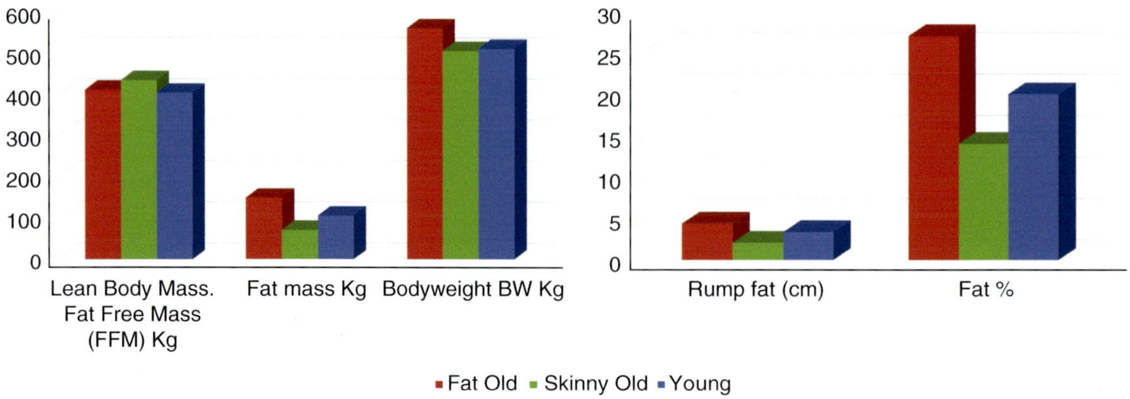

Fig. 16.6 The difference in body composition between aged and young unexercised mares. Older horses divided into two phenotypes: skinny and fat.

of the gluteals) between young unfit mares (4–8 years) and old unfit mares (> 20 years) (Lehnhard *et al.*, 2004). When the old horses were classified by their fat score (Fig. 16.6) the skinny old mares had less fat and greater lean bodyweight compared with the young mares, with a similar bodyweight. However, the fat old mares were heavier, due to their increased body fat mass. It seems that if an older horse puts on weight, that weight is due to an increase in fat, not muscle tissue.

Support client's understanding that if old horses gain weight, they gain fat mass at a faster rate than muscle and will have a greater body fat percentage compared with a younger horse of comparable weight.

Top Tips

Ageing in the horse results in:

- decline in concentrations of insulin growth-like factor (Malinowski *et al.*, 2006);
- alterations in metabolic control, immune function (Petersson *et al.*, 2010);
- changes in endocrine function, both at rest and following exercise (McKeever and Malinowski, 1999); and
- excess adipose tissue exacerbating the changes (Carter *et al.*, 2010) (see Chapter 15).

It is important that your clients understand that being fat, old and unexercised will have a negative effect on health and exacerbate the changes, regardless of dietary support.

Protein requirements

Exercise is vital for maintaining muscle mass; equally important is the protein quality of the horse's diet. The typical diet of the older horse – forages, chaff and sugar beet -– is low in essential amino acids; clearly this type of diet will not support muscle mass even with exercise.

Historically, protein requirements for aged horses were determined to be higher than for young horses (Ralston *et al.*, 1989). The improvement in husbandry means that it is generally accepted that 'the reduction in apparent digestion of protein, phosphorus and fibre reported previously in aged horses may have been due in part to chronic parasitic damage to the large colons and/or abnormal dentition rather than caused by aging per se in the equine animal' (Ralston *et al.*, 1989) and, as such, there is no need for you to be advising extra protein for the older horse.

Amino acids

Protein quality is a different issue. Adding amino acids (lysine 20 g/day; threonine 15 g/day) to the diet of young (mean 9 years) and old horses (mean 22 years) to a standard coarse mix and hay diet was compared with controls whose feeding and management was the same minus the supplementary amino acids. All horses in the study were similar bodyweight and fat score. The supplemented horses, regardless of age, had lower fat scores and better subjective muscle scores compared with the unsupplemented (Graham-Thiers and Kronfield, 2005).

It does appear that, if the diet meets NRC 2007 requirements for amino acids, there is no advantage in adding amino acids (Latham *et al.*, 2019), but these horses were not compared with a younger age group and appeared to be having less exercise than those in Graham-Thiers and Kronfield (2005).

When checking the evidence base, it is important to note both the analysis of the diet and the intake, to compare rations on a bodyweight basis.

How to check protein intake

Follow the steps in Table 16.5 and then use PCHorse or similar to compare with requirements (see Chapter 10). Table 16.6 gives diet advice for an aged horse with muscle loss.

Weight loss

If the horse has lost weight as well as muscle (fat score < 3, 3, 3), then you need to advise increasing calories as well as protein. All manufacturers produce feeds for the older horse that has lost weight and they are normally formulated to be fed at more than 400 g/100 kg BW.

Assuming that the horse is being exercised but struggling with maintaining muscle and body fat, then consider some specialised feeds for the older horse. These should contain better-quality protein with higher lysine, but lower starch compared with a leisure feed (Table 16.7).

Before you advise increasing the concentrate part of the diet, it is important that you check the forage intake as many old horses lose weight simply because they are no longer able to chew forages.

Forage for the Old Horse with Dental Disease

Dental disease and abnormalities dominate in the aetiology of weight loss in the older horse. Over 95% of aged horse in the UK suffered at least one dental abnormality (see Table 16.1) (Ireland *et al.*, 2012a,b); similar incidence has been recorded in Australia (McGowan *et al.*, 2010). Windsucking or quidding results in unequal wearing of the incisors, meaning that the horse has difficulty prehending grass and other forage.

Owners often economise on dental consults with the older horse and do not recognise dental disorders in their horses (Ireland, 2016). There is an increasing risk for simple colonic obstruction and distension colic with an increasing duration since the horse last received dental care. 'Dental care has not been previously associated with colic ... Ingestion of longer length fibre maybe important' (Hillyer *et al.*, 2002).

If dental care is neglected, chewing will be compromised, exacerbating the uneven wearing of teeth, which might offer an explanation as to why Ireland *et al.* (2012a,b) reported that the most prevalent dental pathologies in horses more than 15 years old are mandibular lingual enamel points (64%) and maxillary buccal enamel points (51%).

The older horse's teeth are more worn and as enamel decreases then the horse becomes less able to chew fibre (Dixon and Dacre, 2005). A reduction in fibre intake is also associated with an increased risk of colic (Tinker *et al.*, 1997).

Forage is the main calorie source for the older horse, so anything that compromises intake will result in weight loss. Clearly it is not appropriate to simply replace fibre with starch as the calorie supply – the effect on gastrointestinal health is well documented in the literature and commonly appreciated by your clients.

One of the first signs of inadequate fibre processing is quidding and if this continues after dental treatment, then a fibre substitute is usually fed; a higher proportion of horses with loss of teeth, known dental disease or displaying quidding or difficulty eating were fed a hay replacer (Ireland *et al.*, 2011). But this does not always mean your clients feed forage replacers correctly; consequently they often resort to old horse complementary feeds, which is not appropriate.

Advising a forage replacer for a horse that quids or has difficulty chewing

- Introduce slowly.
- Explain that this is replacing hay or grass usually fed at 2–2.5% BW/kg DM.
- Although fed in buckets, it is not a complementary feed.
- It is higher in calories compared with hay, so complementary feed (hard feed) normally not fed.
  - But may need vitamin/mineral supplement.
- Horses tend to rush forage replacers, so consider ways of slowing intake:
  - multiple containers around the stable;
  - feeding small quantities more frequently;
  - use feed balls;
  - put large boulders in container to reduce bite size.

Table 16.5 Working out the protein contribution of various feedstuffs available for horses in the UK from their analytical declarations[a,b]

Step 1 Check the label for the protein declaration-make a note	Step 2 Check the feeding rate	Step 3 Check the amino acid content from data sheet or call the manufacturer	Step 4 Work out the intake of protein and lysine using the declaration and feed rate to provide grammes/day
Product	Feed rate per 100 kg BW	Lysine content[c] (g/kg feed)	Intake[d] g lysine/day
Alfalfa Chaff 16% protein 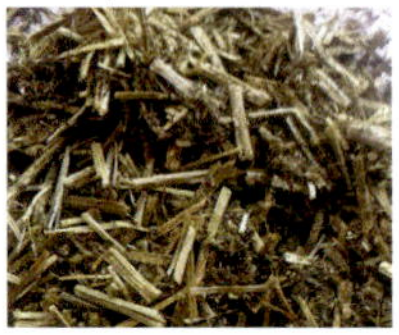	100–500g	8.2	4.15–20.5
Muscle Builder 48% protein 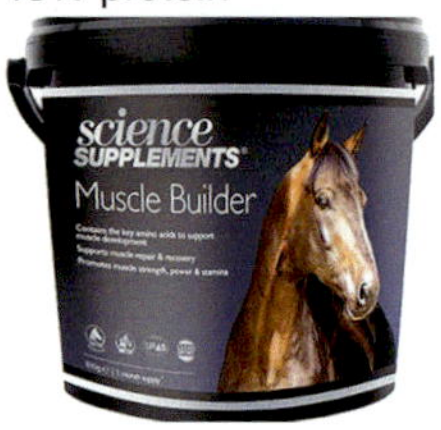 	Daily dose 55 g for 500kg horse	181 g	10
Pony Nuts 10% protein 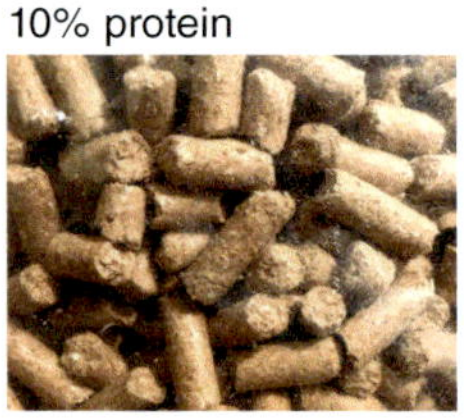	500 g	4	10
Typical general vitamin and mineral– supplement- 0% protein	10 g	15	0.75
Competition Cubes- 12% protein 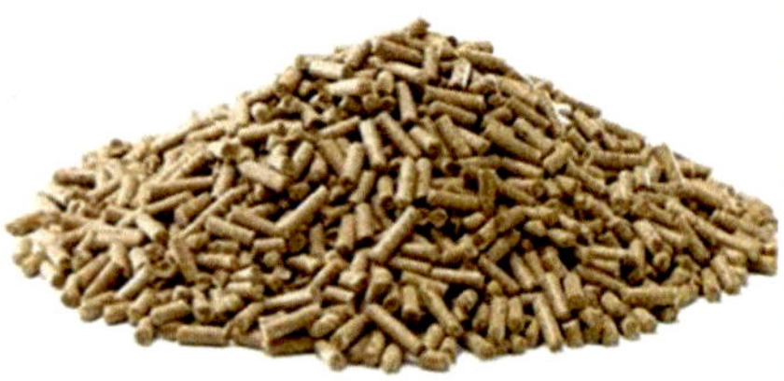	500 g	5.4	13.5

[a]Check label for protein declaration
[b]Or call feed company for data sheet
[c]Check the amino acid content
[d]Work out intake of protein and lysine in g/day, not %

Table 16.6 How to check a diet for an aged horse with muscle loss

Horse signalment	25-year-old, 12.2 hh pony	Lacking muscle, specifically on gluteals and neck
Horse history	Generally light exercise but only in school holidays	Owner was worried that horse is thin, particularly on its neck and hindquarters
Differentials		
Results of any tests	BFS 3, 3, 3	ideal fat score
Current diet	• Grazing 6 h/day; haylage (easier to chew) • Small haynet at night • Scoop of chaff • Double handful of soaked sugar beet • Glucosamine supplement • Vitamin and mineral supplement • ½ scoop conditioning mix	
Advice	• Fed enough calories, as carrying ideal fat ◦ Main protein supply is forage, which is low quality. ◦ Need to improve protein intake without increasing calories. • Provided a suggestion for fittening: ◦ Walk out briskly daily for 30 min with heart rate to 80 bpm (the pace of walking if you saw a bus in the distance and thought you were going to miss it) • Use muzzle in field if plenty of grass ◦ Increase turnout – improves fitness	Change diet to: • 0.25 kg alfalfa chaff to improve protein quality • High-spec Balancer fed at 100 g/100 kg BW (250 g/day) split into two feeds (replacing vit/min supplement) • Check weighed out haylage ◦ Explain DM vs as-fed (see Chapter 9) ◦ Should be eating 3.75 kg DM haylage (7.5 kg fresh weight if small-bale haylage).

Table 16.7 A comparison of lysine content of different complementary horse feeds and the effect of recommended intake on daily intake of lysine for 500 kg horse (websites information correct, summer 2020)

Product	Protein % (as fed)	Lysine g/kg (as fed)	Starch %	Digestible energy (estimated as fed) MJ/kg	Feeding rate /100 kg BW/ day	Lysine intake/ day (g)
Dodson & Horrell Sixteen Plus	13	5	17 (sugar 5.5)	11	400 g–1 kg	10–25
Pure Veteran mix	13	5.8	3	10	400–600 g	11.6–17.4
Dodson & Horrell Senior Support	22	14	10	10.5	100–200 g	7–14
Baileys no. 15 Senior Mix	12.5	6	27	11.5	500 g	15
Saracen Veteran Mix	14	6	16.5	12.6	500–830 g	15–25
Spillers Senior Complete Care Mix	13	–	18	11	580–600 g	
Spillers Supple and Senior Balancer	25	–	9 (sugar 5)	10.5	100 g	

- Need large containers, such as half water butts
- Feed by weight.
  - Tell clients not to be overwhelmed by volume.
- Weigh out equal quantities of:
  - unmolassed sugar beet shreds;
  - Just Grass/Alfalfa Chaff; and
  - High-Fibre Nuts (Fig. 16.7).
- The horse needs to be eating a minimum of 2% BW as dry matter in kg (Fig. 16.7):
  - unmolassed sugar beet shreds (kwik beet) – soak overnight: 660 g/100 kg BW;
  - Just Grass/Alfalfa Chaff: 660 g/100 kg BW;
  - High Fibre Nuts – add ½ h before feeding: 660 g/100 kg BW.
- Mix together and divide into smaller amounts
  - Provide biggest quantity when stabled.

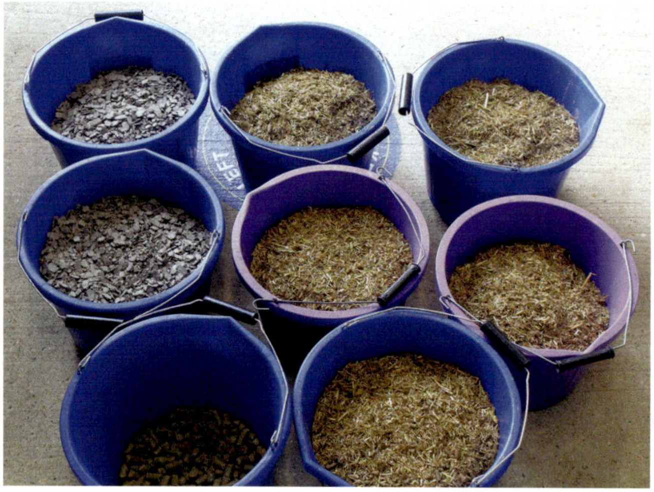

Product	Quantity	How to feed
Unmolassed sugar beet shreds or kwik beet	2.6kg 2 buckets once soaked	Weigh out 2.6kg, then soak – add to hay replacer 1/2hr before feeding
Alfalfa or grass chaff	2.6kg 5 buckets	Mix with nuts and sugar beet Add large boulders to slow intake
High-fibre nuts	2.6kg ¼ bucket	Add to sugar beet 10 mins before feeding

Fig. 16.7 Example hay replacer for 400 kg horse fed at 2% BW (8 kg in total)

Alternatively, many horse owners choose to feed a product that is sold as a hay replacer. Ireland *et al.* (2012a,b) established that 15% of owners fed hay replacers such as Hi Fi or Readigrass (Table 16.8). The feeding advice varies according to the manufacturer and it is always helpful to work with their nutritionists to work out the best ration. Do not forget that these horses normally do well on well-maintained grass but struggle more during the winter or if grass gets too long.

How to feed a horse with diastemas or periodontal disease

At a UK referral hospital, 75% of horses undergoing dental investigation between November 2006 and December 2009 had a minimum of one diastema (Ramzan and Palmer, 2011). Over a 12-month period (2008–2009), 49.9% of horses (n = 471) in Scotland undergoing routine dental examination were recorded as having cheek teeth diastemas, of which 91.4% had food trapped in them (Walker *et al.*, 2012); the authors noted that horses over 15 years old had a greater incidence of the disease. Nuttall and Ravenhill (2019) only recorded 13.9% periodontal disease, 8.7% and 8.2% peripheral caries in first-opinion practice in south-west England (n = 932) but also noted that increasing age was a significant risk for both periodontal disease and diastemas.

Collins and Dixon (2005) indicated that after cleaning diastemas, chaffs that are < 5 mm can be recommended for feeding but cautioned that short-chop changes the chewing action of the horse from predominantly vertical to horizontal.

You will need to be more vigilant in checking cheek teeth overgrowth when you do your regular health checks. There will always be groups of horses when none of the above products are suitable because the chaff still gets impacted. These horses should be fed ground fibre (Fig. 16.8).

If the horse continues to lose fat and muscle (weight) having rectified the forage intake, then you will need to discuss the specialised feeds (Table 16.9) formulated for weight gain in the older horse. These products are higher in calories, predominantly from fibre and oil; they usually have higher-quality protein and may well contain antioxidants and some form of joint support. The intake rate is also higher than balancers, to ensure adequate calorie intake. If the weight/fat gain is rapid on the recommended intake and the owner feeds less than recommended intake, the protein and vitamin/mineral requirements will be inadequate.

You should encourage your clients to base their choice on the macro nutrients (protein, calories and fibre), because the levels of antioxidants and joint support are usually below those needed for efficacy. Should the horse need additional micronutrients, then from a cost perspective encourage your client to consider supplements.

Table 16.8 Products available in the UK that are marketed as hay replacers suitable for old horses

Product	Feed guide	Composition	Digestible energy (DE) MJ/kg Analytical constituents (%)
*Spillers Speedy Mash Super-fast soaking sugar beet blend for all horses and ponies	500 kg horse: 11.5 kg as hay replacer	Nutritionally improved straw Oat feed Unmolassed sugar beet Rape and sunflower oils Wheat feed	DE 8 Oil 3.5 Protein 10.0 Fibre 24.0
*Spillers Happy Hoof	As above	Nutritionally improved straw Straw Alfalfa Molasses Rice bran Oat feed	DE 8.8 Oil 3.5 Protein 9 Fibre 25 Starch and Sugar 5.5
*Spillers Senior Super Mash	As above	Soya hulls (GM) Oat feed Unmolassed sugar beet Wheat feed Nutritionally improved straw Rice bran	DE 11 Oil 4.5 Protein 12.0 Fibre 20.0 Starch 8.0 Sugar 2.5
Dengie Hi Fi Senior	2.5% BW	Grass, alfalfa, molasses, rape seed oil	Protein 10 Oil 2 Fibre 30 Sugar & Starch 11.6
Dengie Hi Fi Lite	Replacing weight for weight for hay 0.8–1.1 kg/100 kg	Cereal straw, alfalfa, molasses mould inhibitor	DE 7.5 Protein 10 Oil 1.5 Fibre 35 Starch & sugar 8.5
Dengie Pure Grass	2–2.5% BW	100% grass	DE 10 Protein 18 Oil 3 Fibre 20 Sugar and starch 14
[a]Allen & Page Fast Fibre	Soak before feeding 750 g–1 kg/100 kg BW	Nutritionally improved straw, oat feed, unmolassed beet pulp, linseed expeller (6.1%), grass meal	Protein 7.5 Oil 3.0 Fibre 26 , Sugar & starch 7.5
Baileys Light Chaff	N/A	Oat straw, alfalfa, soya oil	DE 8 Protein 10 Oil 6 Fibre 30 Starch & Starch 5

*Contain vitamin and mineral premix
[a]Provides information on additives but no vitamin/mineral premix in composition
Details correct on company websites June 2020

The Role of Supplements in the Diet of the Older Horse

Old horses in the UK are fed a variety of supplements (Fig. 16.9). The percentage of owners feeding joint supplements closely reflects the percentage of horses that were identified as having stiff joints or lack of joint flexibility (41.8%) by Ireland *et al.* (2011).

Supplements to minimise the risk of osteoarthritis

It is always useful for clients to have an understanding of the physiology behind osteoarthritis (OA) to help them distinguish between supplements that potentially could be efficacious and legal (see Chapter 6: 'Advising a joint nutraceutical'). Skeletal

Primary aim is to maintain fibre intake at 2% BW		
1.	Recommend feeding each ingredient at 0.66% BW	Sugar Beet Pellets (SBP) Grass Nuts Alfalfa pellets
2.	Soak SBP	For 12 hrs
3.	Add other pellets	30mins before feeding
4.	Make a mash of all ingredients and add Performance Vitamins and Minerals (10g/100kgBW)	Add bricks to prevent drinking Divide into 'small haynets' and feed throughout the day

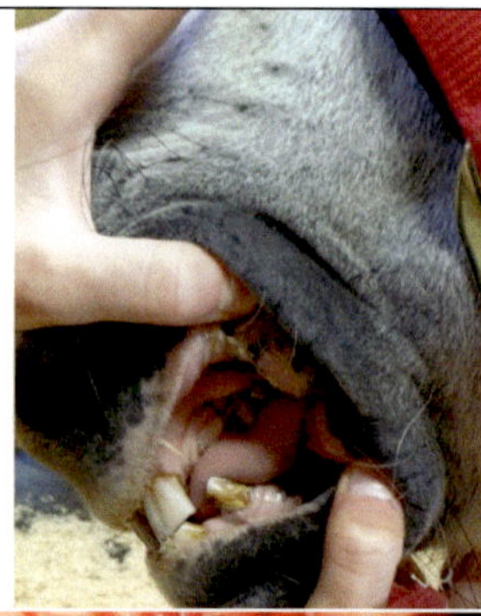

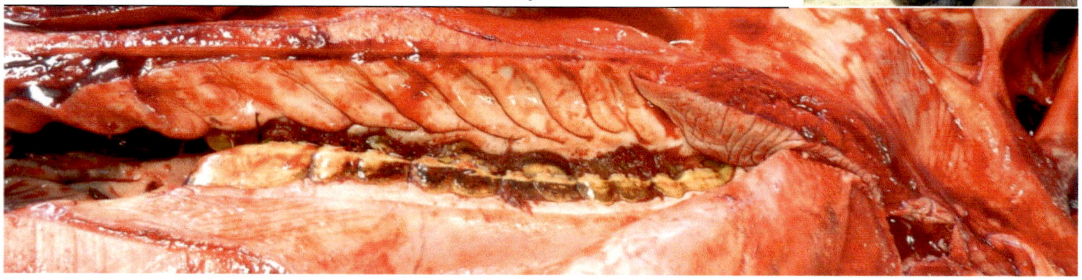

Fig. 16.8 Forage replacer for horses with (1) periodontal disease or (2) diastemas, examples of dental diseases where a mash of forage replacers would minimise further progression of disease.

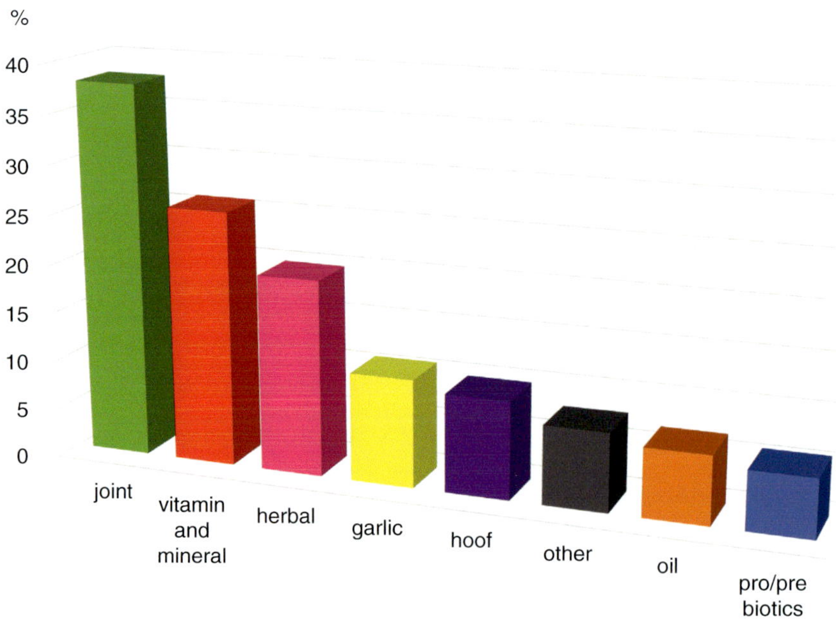

Fig. 16.9 The percentage of owners feeding supplements (by type) to old horses in the UK. (Based on Ireland *et al*., 2011.)

Table 16.9 Products formulated for old horses that are losing weight (information correct from company websites, June 2020)

Product	Protein %	Fibre %	Oil %	Starch and sugar %	Calories MJ DE/kg	Ingredients	Feeding rate /100 kg BW
Allen and Page Old Faithful Special Blend	10	5	3	47.5	11.5	Barley, Molasses, Maize, Alfalfa, Field Beans, Calcium Carbonate, Linseed Expeller, Oat Straw, Salt, Di-calcium Phosphate, Organic Soya Oil, Mint, Yeast, Fructo-oligosaccharides, Mannan-oligosaccharides, Garlic, Fenugreek Cloves	100–300 g
Allen and Page Veteran Vitality	12	16	4	14.7	11	Unmolassed Beet Pulp, Wheat Feed, Nutritionally Improved Straw, Linseed (9%), Grass Meal, Field Beans, Calcium Carbonate, Salt, Mint, Di-calcium Phosphate, Yeast, Organic Soya Oil, Nettle, Dandelion, Garlic, Fenugreek, Cloves, Fructo-oligosaccharides, Mannan-oligosaccharides	100–300 g
Spillers Conditioning Mix	14	10	5	30	12.2	Flaked barley, Wheatfeed, Sunflower extract, Flaked maize, Oatfeed, Molasses, Flaked peas, Rice bran, Calcium carbonate Rapeseed oil, Salt, Vitamin & mineral premix, Di calcium phosphate, Glucosamine (0.18%), Lysine, Live yeast	600–800 g
Saracen Veteran Mix	14	15.5	7	16.5	12.6	lucerne Pellets, Barley Flakes, Soya Flakes, Soya Hulls, Oatfeed Molasses, Pea Flakes, Maize Flakes Vitamins, Soya Oil, Dried Sugar Beet Pulp, Herbs, Dicalcium Phosphate Minerals, Yeast, Mixture of flavouring compounds	500 g
Dodson & Horrell 16+	13	12	4.5	22.5	10.9	Oatfeed, Wheatfeed, Barley, Grass, Soya, Sunflower seed meal, dehulled, Cane molasses, Maize, Calcium carbonate, Soya bean meal, dehulled, Peas, Linseed, Rapeseed oil, Linseed expeller, Carrot, dried, Sodium chloride, Unmolassed sugar beet, Magnesium oxide, Dicalcium phosphate, Monocalcium phosphate, Mint, Basil, Glucosamine (0.2%), Garlic granules, Potassium chloride, Methyl sulphonyl methane (0.1%), Dandelion leaves, Mixture of: Blackcurrant, Kale, Spinach, Beetroot, Rosemary, Rosehip, Pomegranate (0.03%), Nettle leaves	400 g–1 kg
Baileys no 15 Senior Mix	12.5	14	4.5	32.5	11.5	Micronised Barley, Micronised Wheat, Oatfeed (by-product of the oat milling industry), Alfalfa Meall, Distillers' Grains, Nutritionally Improved Straw, Molasses, Micronised Maize, Extracted Sunflower Meal, Micronised Peas, Soya Bean Meal, Calcium Carbonate, Soya Oil, Dicalcium Phosphate, Vitamins and Minerals, Sodium Chloride, Calcined Magnesite, Garlic supplement 0.3%, ScFOS (Digest Plus prebiotic) 2.5g/kg,Yea-Sacc ® yeast culture	N/A

ageing in the horse has been extensively researched, in part because it reflects a similar trajectory to us. Obesity, excess joint trauma or joint malalignment increases the risk of the ageing horse developing OA. Human medicine considers that ageing does not necessarily cause OA but that individuals with specific OA risk factors undergo an accelerated rate of certain changes that would eventually be associated with ageing (Lotz and Loeser, 2012).

Collagen provides tensile strength to the joint but in OA the collagen molecules are degraded and there is a change in the cartilage matrix because of an increase in the proteolytic activity of the cartilage and synovial fluid. The biomechanical properties of cartilage are also reduced because of an increase in the amount of advanced glycation end-products (AGEs), increasing cross-linking of collagen molecules; the horse will show clinical signs of increased stiffness and susceptibility to fatigue.

In healthy joints, the articular chondrocyte produces the cartilage extra-cellular matrix (ECM). The ECM provides compressive stiffness, elastic properties and lubrication at its surface and the large proteoglycan aggrecan ensures the resilience of cartilage to withstand compressive loads. As the load is removed from the joint, water that was squeezed out during loading is attracted back in by the highly negatively charged hydrophilic proteoglycans. Platt *et al.* (1998) reported that it was the cellularity of equine cartilage and changes in sulphation pattern of chondroitin sulphate chains rather than an alteration in the proteoglycan content of the matrix that decreased with a horse's ageing.

Cartilage calcification common in ageing joints seems to trigger the chondrocyte to produce inflammatory mediators and start the onset and progression of OA (Lotz and Loeser, 2012). It appears that OA chondrocytes produce increased levels of nitric oxide (NO) linked to chondrocyte apoptosis (programmed cell death); horses with OA have a greater number of apoptotic chondrocytes compared with those without, which was associated with areas that stained as high for nitrotyrosine – an indirect measure of NO (Kim *et al.*, 2003). Glucosamine but not chondroitin sulphate added to cultured chondrocytes at concentrations found in equine plasma after supplementation reduced levels of NO (Neil *et al.*, 2005). Similarly, glucosamine HCl but not chondroitin sulphate reduced the degradative changes as well as the reduction of NO release that had been induced by added interleukin when added to bovine cartilage explants (Bascoul-Colombo *et al.*, 2016).

Which supplement?

Glucosamine is the supplement most commonly fed to both performance (Agar *et al.*, 2016) and old horses. There are three main sources of glucosamine commercially available: glucosamine hydrochloride, glucosamine sulphate and *N*-acetyl-D-glucosamine. There is a mixed message from the literature as to efficacy, with positive effects being described *in vitro* and some clinically published evidence (Table 16.10).

It is difficult to compare the research because different doses and formulations are used, trial designs vary, and measures of efficacy are not consistent. Across the species, there is some evidence to support advising glucosamine HCl over sulphate, although not all researchers agree. Fenton *et al.* (2000), using cultures from equine articular cartilage, concluded that 'glucosamine sulfate also has the potential to prevent or reduce articular cartilage degradation similar to glucosamine HCl *in vitro*. The amine group at the carbon-2 position appears important for the effectiveness of the glucosamine derivative. The therapeutic value of *N*-acetyl-glucosamine remains questionable.'

A Cochrane review concluded that the most favourable results are associated with the prescription of glucosamine sulphate (GS) in humans (Towheed *et al.*, 2005).

Following encouraging work by Laverty *et al.* (2005) that showed that a dose of 20 mg of glucosamine HCL (GHCL) in the horse reached the synovial fluid, the group compared GS and GHCL uptake in horses. Meulyzer *et al.*, 2008 compared 20mg/kg BW of a human grade glucosamine sulphate (GS) or glucosamine hydrochloride (GHCl) administrated either intravenously or via nasogastric intubation (NG). After NG admin, GS resulted in significantly higher levels in the synovial fluid (but supplement used was not practically translatable and cost would be prohibitive) compared to baseline but GHCl did not, (Table 16.20).

Factors to consider when advising joint supplements

- Both glucosamine and chondroitin are bioavailable after oral supplementation (Du *et al.*, 2004).
- Avoid supplements that are labelled incorrectly (see Chapter 7). Glucosamine is considered a feed ingredient, so functional but not medicinal claims can be made.

Table 16.10 A comparison of trials published in the scientific literature investigating the efficacy of joint supplements fed to horses

Horses (*n*)	Design	Glucosamine	Chondroitin	Other	Result	Reference
(20) Veteran	Randomised, blinded, placebo-controlled study (*n* = 15) or placebo group (*n* = 5) 12 weeks Pre-treatment gait characteristics recorded at trot using digital video footage (50 Hz). Range of joint motion, stride length, and swing and stance duration assessed using 2-dimensional motion analysis. Gait was reassessed every 4 weeks using the pre-treatment protocol. Double blind procedure was implemented throughout.	Loading dose • 1–1.5 g hydrochloride & 1–1.5 g acetyl D Maintenance • 0.5 g hydrochloride & 0.5 g acetyl D • Mean 0.15 g/100 kg BW/day of each	Loading dose • 4–6 g sulphate Maintenance 2 g • Mean 0.6 g/100 kg BW/day		Differences occurred in the treated horses by week 8. Range of joint motion increased significantly in the elbow ($P<0.05$), stifle and hind fetlock ($P<0.01$). Stride length increased significantly ($P<0.05$) with treatment. Swing duration was significantly increased at week 12 ($P<0.05$), whilst stance duration remained constant.	Forsyth *et al.* (2006)
(24) 29 ± 4 y	3 months oral supplementation. Kinematic outcome criteria (primary: stride length; secondary: carpal flexion, fore fetlock extension and tarsal range of motion) were objectively quantified on a treadmill at a walk and trot before and after treatment	• 9.96 g /500 kg BW sulphate • 1.93 g/100 kg BW/day	• 2 g/500 kg BW sulphate • 0.4 g/100 kg BW	• 2.5 g/500 kg BW MSM • 0.5 g/100 kg BW	No indications of effect of the supplement on gait characteristics	Higler *et al.* (2014)
(24) Mature horses	Fed for 21 days triple-blind crossover design – random allocation clinical orthopaedic evaluation for straight line and lungeing circle (walk and trot) and during ridden exercise (walk, trot and canter); handler field evaluation, during groundwork and while ridden, grading-specific criteria; grading of range of motion (ROM) and muscle tone based on standardised physiotherapy criteria	• glucosamine 1.9 g/100 kg BW	• sulphate 1.62 g/100 kg BW	vitamin C • 0.8 g/100 kg BW MSM • 2.56 g/100 kg BW DHA • 0.66 g/100 kg BW, EPA • 0.34 g/100 kg BW	Significantly lower lameness grade in a straight line and circle. Improved ridden/groundwork scores and improved 'ease-of-movement' in the field	Murray *et al.* (2013)

Continued

Table 16.10 Continued.

Horses (*n*)	Design	Glucosamine	Chondroitin	Other	Result	Reference
(26) Horses with primary fetlock lameness	56-day controlled, randomised and double-blinded, multi-centre clinical trial. Partial crossover with a washout period and consisted of 19 horses treated with LPPC and 20 with a placebo. Efficacy was evaluated by clinical assessment of lameness, passive flexion, pain, swelling and heat in the affected joint.			25 mg/kg BW/day green lipped mussel (GLM) Supplement = 100% GLM • BW 300 kg one scoop ◦ 7.5 g/day. • > 300–< 500 kg 1.5 scoops ◦ 11.25 g = 28 mg/kg BW daily • over 500 kg 2 scoops ◦ 15 g = 30 mg/kg BW daily.	Significant improvement in lameness and flexion scores and greater reduction in pain for the horses given the GLM compared with horses treated with the placebo	Cayzer *et al.* (2012)

Table 16.11 A comparison of plasma[a] and synovial fluid concentrations of two types of glucosamine after nasogastric administration[b] to eight horses

Plasma or synovial fluid	Glucosamine hydrochloride	Glucosamine sulphate[c]
Plasma 12 h after treatment	305.0 ± 136.4 ng/ml	433.3 ± 245.1 ng/ml
Synovial fluid concentrations 1 h after	92.7 ± 34.9 ng /ml	153.6 ± 32.9 ng/ml
Synovial fluid 12 h after treatment	12.3 ± 6.2 ng /ml	36.4 ± 25.0 ng/ml

[a]Peak plasma 2 h after dose
[b]Nasogastric dose 20 mg/kg BW
[c]DONA 5 days supply =£94

- Be aware of the work that showed that of 23 commercially available oral supplements for joints, only 14 contained quantities stated on the label (Oke *et al.*, 2006).
- Owners provide anecdotal evidence as to the success of herbal supplements for joint pain in dogs and horses.
- Green-lipped mussel as a source of omega-3 appears to be an effective anti-inflammatory in humans (Brien *et al.*, 2008) and dogs (Hielm-Björkman *et al.*, 2009) as well as horses.
- Check doses – 20 mg/kg BW has been shown to be absorbed and appear in the synovial fluid.
- Think about collecting evidence – *in vivo* effects of supplementation following joint pathology would be useful.
- Check the weight (g) of actual active ingredient.

And of course, in line with all other species, advise the owner to keep the horse moving regardless of which joint supplement they choose.

Exercise will also reduce the risk of the old horse getting fat. Recent experimental evidence has shown an increased inflammatory potential of adipose tissue in aged animals causing insulin resistance (Alicka *et al.*, 2020).

Feeds and Feeding Management of the Old Horse

As with any other group of horses, there are a number of options that you might advise and your choice will depend upon the clinical history of the horse as well as the willingness of the client to work with you.

Spend time to show the owner the options (Table 16.12) and work through a label including the feeding guides to find a solution that is manageable for them as well as suitable for their aged horse. Sometimes the decision must be based on economic reality, but correct nutrition and feeding management will reduce costs later down the line.

Summary

In all species, the only scientific validated intervention for healthy longevity is the maintenance of lean body mass and reduction of fat mass. This is easily achievable for the older horse if you can support your client in recognising the difference between muscle and fat mass, ensure a balanced diet in terms of micronutrients as well as protein and calories, ensure fibre first and foremost and keep the horse moving. To share a human analogy, 'you don't stop dancing because you are old; you get old because you have stopped dancing' (adapted from G.B. Shaw).

Table 16.12 A summary of feeding options for the older horse

Options	In work, not showing signs of ageing	Light or no work, overweight (fat score > 3.5, 3.5, 3.5)	Underweight but no differentials of disease (fat score > 2.5 in summer on neck, middle or bottom)	Unable to chew fibre
Overview	No obvious signs of ageing	Will be at greater risk of developing PPID, OA and other age-related diseases. Encourage increased exercise if possible. Encourage natural seasonal fat loss in winter	Re-assure that muscle loss through winter (if not been ridden, will result in weak outline) should not be compensated for by getting fat. Fat loss through winter is fine and should be supported	Check if dental disease or simply compromised chewing
Forage	Grazing in summer, hay or haylage in winter	Use muzzle in field, limit time in stable, use bare paddocks or turnout schools. Soak hay overnight and maintain 2% BW DMI. If still not losing fat, then replace with lower-calorie forage, not reduced DMI. Increase exercise, remove rugs	Assuming no dental issues, advise hay (soaked for 30 min only) or haylage as long as owner feeds at correct weight to meet DMI by taking water content into account	Advise hay replacers to provide 1.8% DMI BW Quidding but no underlying dental disease 600 g/100 kg BW of each Sugar beet shreds or equivalent Alfalfa or grass chaff Grass nut and vit/min supplement or high-fibre cube and products described in Table 16.8
Hard feed	Feed formulated for the workload – most light work formulations will be fibre and oil based	Balancer 100 g/100 kg BW	Specialised feed for weight gain in old horses – intake usually 600–800 g/100 kg BW/day (see Table 16.8)	Unless still losing weight, unlikely to need hard feed because of the higher nutritive value of the hay replacer
Supplements	Might need a vit/min supplement if feed less than recommended intake of feed	None required	If owner reports slightly stiff, then recommend joint supplement	Vit/min supplement needed unless using high fibre nuts as above or hard feed at recommended intake (unlikely)
Management	Encourage regular turnout Check feeding recommended quantities – if on less, then recommend change feed or add vit/min supplement Fat score fortnightly	No rugging in winter unless being ridden and clipped and then lightweight rugs in field only Feed forage on the ground using grids to slow intake Ridden work should increase heart rate to 80 bpm (speed that walk if about to miss the bus) – minimum 30 min/day	Rug in winter Maximise good-quality grazing Feed forage at floor level Hard feed to be split into minimum two meals to keep starch intake to < 1 g starch/kg BW/meal. Add 50 g/100 kg BW alfalfa chaff to feed Soaked sugar beet in winter helps maintains water intake Regular faecal worm test Exercise daily to maintain lean body mass	Reassure owner that v large volume because replacing hay Introduce slowly Quantities will depend upon grazing Mix components together before feeding Sugar beet needs soaking Divide into multiple 'meals' hay buckets with largest at night

Bibliography

Agar, C., Gemmill, R., Hollands, T. and Freeman, S.L. (2016) The use of nutritional supplements in dressage and eventing horses. *Veterinary Record Open* 3, e000154. doi: 10.1136/vetreco-2015-000154.

Alicka, M., Kornicka-Garbowska, K., Kucharczyk, K. *et al.* (2020) Age-dependent impairment of adipose-derived stem cells isolated from horses. *Stem Cell Research & Therapy* 11, 4. doi: 10.1186/s13287-019-1512-6.

Aulisio, J., Liburt, N., Malinowski, K. and McKeever, K. (2010) Training-induced alterations in rump fat thickness and plasma leptin concentration in young mature and old Standardbred mares. *Comparative Exercise Physiology* 7(3), 127–132. doi: 10.1017/S1755254011000018.

Bascoul-Colombo, C., Garaiova, I., Plummer, S.F., Harwood, J.L., Caterson, B. *et al.* (2016) Glucosamine hydrochloride but not chondroitin sulfate prevents cartilage degradation and inflammation induced by interleukin-1α in bovine cartilage explants. *Cartilage* 7(1), 70–81.

Brien, S., Prescott, P., Coghlan, B., Bashir, N. and Lewith, G. (2008) Systematic review of the nutritional supplement *Perna canaliculus* (green-lipped mussel) in the treatment of osteoarthritis. *QJM: An International Journal of Medicine* 101(3), 167–179. doi: 10.1093/qjmed/hcm108.

Brosnahan, M.M. and Paradis, M. (2003a) Assessment of clinical characteristics, management practices, and activities of geriatric horses. *Journal of the American Veterinary Medical Association* 223(1), 99–103.

Brosnahan, M.M. and Paradis, M. (2003b) Demographic and clinical characteristics of geriatric horses: 467 cases (1989–1999). *Journal of the American Veterinary Medical Association* 223(1), 93–98.

Bushell, R. and Murray, J. (2016) A survey of senior equine management: owner practices and confidence. *Livestock Science* 186, 69–77.

Carter, R.A., McCutcheon, J.L., Valle, E., Meilahn, E.N. and Geor, R.J. (2010) Effects of exercise training on adiposity, insulin sensitivity, and plasma hormone and lipid concentrations in overweight or obese, insulin-resistant horses. *American Journal of Veterinary Research* 71(3), 314–321.

Cayzer, J., Hedderley, D. and Gray, S. (2012) A randomised, double-blinded, placebo-controlled study on the efficacy of a unique extract of green-lipped mussel (*Perna canaliculus*) in horses with chronic fetlock lameness attributed to osteoarthritis. *Equine Veterinary Journal* 44(4), 393–398.

Collins, N.M. and Dixon P.M. (2005) Diagnosis and management of equine diastemata. *Clinical Techniques in Equine Practice* 4(2), 148–154.

Dixon, P.M. and Dacre, I. (2005) A review of equine dental disorders. *The Veterinary Journal* 169(2), 165–187.

Du, J., White, N. and Eddington, N.D. (2004) The bioavailability and pharmacokinetics of glucosamine hydrochloride and chondroitin sulfate after oral and intravenous single dose administration in the horse. *Biopharmaceutics & Drug Disposition* 25, 109–116. doi: 10.1002/bdd.392.

Fenton, J.I., Chlebek-Brown, K.A., Peters, T.L., Caron, J.P. and Orth, M.W. (2000) The effects of glucosamine derivatives on equine articular cartilage degradation in explant culture. *Osteoarthritis and Cartilage* 8, 444–451.

Forsyth, R.K., Brigden, C.V. and Northrop, A.J. (2006) Double blind investigation of the effects of oral supplementation of combined glucosamine hydrochloride (GHCL) and chondroitin sulphate (CS) on stride characteristics of veteran horses. *Equine Veterinary Journal* 38, 622–625.

Freestone, J.F., Beadle, R., Shoemaker, K. *et al.* (1992) Improved insulin sensitivity in hyperinsulinaemic ponies through physical conditioning and controlled feed intake. *Equine Veterinary Journal* 24, 187–190.

Graham-Thiers, P.M. and Bowen, L.K. (2013) Improved ability to maintain fitness in horses during large pasture turnout. *Journal of Equine Veterinary Science* 33(8), 581–585.

Graham-Thiers, P.M. and Kronfeld, D.S. (2005) Amino acid supplementation improves muscle mass in aged and young horses. *Journal of Animal Science* 83(12), 2783–2788. doi: 10.2527/2005.83122783x.

Hielm-Björkman, A., Tulamo, R.M., Salonen, H. and Raekallio, R. (2009) Evaluating complementary therapies for Canine osteoarthritis part I: green-lipped mussel (*Perna canaliculus*). *Evidence-Based Complementary and Alternative Medicine* 6(3), 365–373. doi: 10.1093/ecam/nem136.

Higler, M.H., Brommer, H., L'Ami, J.J., de Grauw, J., van Weeran, P. *et al.* (2014) The effects of three-month oral supplementation with a nutraceutical and exercise on the locomotor pattern of aged horses. *Equine Veterinary Journal* 46(5), 611–617.

Hillyer, M.H., Taylor, F.G., Proudman, C.J., Edwards, G.B., Smith, J.E. *et al.* (2002) Case control study to identify risk factors for simple obstructive and distension colic in horses. *Equine Veterinary Journal* 34(5), 455–463.

Houston, D.K., Nicklas, B.J., Ding, J., Harris, T.B., Tylavsky, F.A. *et al.* (2008) Dietary protein intake is associated with lean mass change in older, community dwelling adults: the Health, Aging, and Body Composition (Health ABC) Study. *American Journal of Clinical Nutrition* 87, 150–155.

Ilich, J.Z., Kelly, O.J., Inglis, J.E., Panton, L.B., Duque, G. *et al.* (2014) Interrelationship among muscle, fat, and bone: connecting the dots on cellular, hormonal, and whole-body levels. *Ageing Research Reviews* 15, 51–60.

Ireland, J. (2016) Demographics, management, preventive health care and disease in aged horses. *Veterinary Clinics: Equine Practice* 32, 195–214.

Ireland, J.L., Clegg, P.D., McGowan, C.M., McKane, S. and Pinchbeck, G.L. (2011) A cross-sectional study of geriatric horses in the United Kingdom Part 1: demographics and management practices. *Equine Veterinary Journal* 43, 30–36.

Ireland, J.L., Clegg, P.D., Mcgowan, C.M., Mckane, S.A., Chandler, K.J. *et al.* (2012a) Disease prevalence in geriatric horses in the United Kingdom: Veterinary clinical assessment of 200 cases. *Equine Veterinary Journal* 44, 101–106.

Ireland, J.L., McGowan, C.M., Clegg, P.D., Chandler K.J. and Pinchbeck, G.L. (2012b) A survey of health care and disease in geriatric horses aged 30 years or older. *The Veterinary Journal* 192(1), 57–64.

Kalyani, R.R., Corriere, M. and Ferrucci, L. (2014) Age-related and disease-related muscle loss: the effect of diabetes, obesity, and other diseases. *Lancet* 2, 819–829.

Kim, D.Y., Taylor, H.W., Moore, R.M., Paulsen, D.B. and Cho, D.Y. (2003) Articular chondrocyte apoptosis in equine osteoarthritis. *The Veterinary Journal* 166, 52–57.

Kim, J.S., Hinchcliff, K.W., Yamaguchi, M., Beard, L.A., Markert, C.D. *et al.* (2005) Age-related changes in metabolic properties of equine skeletal muscle associated with muscle plasticity. *The Veterinary Journal* 169, 397–403.

Kim, S., Leng, X.I. and Kritchevsky, S.B. (2017) Body composition and physical function in older adults with various comorbidities. *Innovation in Aging* 1(1), 1–9.

Latham, C.M., Wagner, A.L. and Urschel, K.L. (2019) Effects of dietary amino acid supplementation on measures of whole-body and muscle protein metabolism in aged horses. *Journal of Animal Physiology and Animal Nutrition* 103(1), 283–294.

Laverty, S., Sandy, J.D., Celeste, C., Vachon, P., Marier, J.F. and Plaas, A.H. (2005) Synovial fluid levels and serum pharmacokinetics in a large animal model following treatment with oral glucosamine at clinically relevant doses. *Arthritis and rheumatism* 52(1), 181–191. https://doi.org/10.1002/art.20762

Lehnhard, R.A., McKeever, K.H., Kearns, C.F. and Beekley, M.D. (2004) Myosin heavy chain profiles and body composition are different in old versus young Standardbred mares. *The Veterinary Journal* 167, 59–66.

Li, C., White, S.H., Warren, L.K. and Wohlgemuth, S.E. (2016) Effects of aging on mitochondrial function in skeletal muscle of American Quarter Horses. *Journal of Applied Physiology (1985) 2016*, 121(1), 299–311. doi: 10.1152/japplphysiol.01077.2015.

Lotz, M. and Loeser, R.F. (2012) Effects of aging on articular cartilage homeostasis. *Bone* 51(2), 241–248.

Malinowski, M., Shock, E.J., Rochelle, P., Kearns, C.F., Guirnalda, P.D. *et al.* (2006) Plasma P-endorphin, cortisol and immune responses to acute exercise are altered by age and exercise training in horses. *Equine Veterinary Journal* (Suppl. 36), 267–273.

McFarlane, D., Sellon, D.C. and Gibbs, S.A. (2001) Age-related quantitative alterations in lymphocyte subsets and immunoglobulin isotypes in healthy horses. *American Journal of Veterinary Research* 62, 1413–1417.

McGowan, T.W., Pinchbeck, G.L., Phillips, C., Perkins, N., Hodgson, D.R. *et al.* (2010) A survey of aged horses in Queensland, Australia. Part 2: clinical signs and owner perceptions of health and welfare. *Australian Veterinary Journal* 88, 465–471.

McKeever, K.H. and Malinowski, K. (1999) Endocrine response to exercise in young and old horses. *Equine Veterinary Journal* 31(S30), 561–566.

Mellor, DJ., Love, S., Gettinby, G. and Reid, S.W.J. (1999) Demographic characteristics of the equine population of northern Britain. *Veterinary Record* 145(11), 299–304.

Meulyzer, M., Vachon, P., Beaudry, F., Vinardell, T., Richard, H., Beauchamp, G. and Laverty, S. (2008) Comparison of pharmacokinetics of glucosamine and synovial fluid levels following administration of glucosamine sulphate or glucosamine hydrochloride. *Osteoarthritis and Cartilage* 16, 973–979.

Michell, A.R. (1999) Longevity of British breeds of dog and its relationships with sex, size, cardiovascular variables and disease. *Veterinary Record* 145, 625–629.

Muller, C.E. and Lindberg, J.E. (2020) Demographics, body condition scores and feeding of aged horses (>20 years of age) – a Swedish survey. *Livestock* 233, 103949.

Murray, R., Adams, V., Walker, V., Tranquille, C., Copeman, S. *et al.* (2013) To determine the effect of an oral joint supplement on orthopaedic, physiotherapy and handler evaluation scores in horses. *Clinical Research Abstracts of the British Equine Veterinary Association Congress* 45(S44), 3.

Neil, K.M., Orth, M.W., Coussens, P.M., Chan, P.S. and Caron, J.P. (2005) Effects of glucosamine and chondroitin sulfate on mediators of osteoarthritis in cultured equine chondrocytes stimulated by use of recombinant equine interleukin-1beta. *American Journal of Veterinary Research* 66(11), 1861–1869.

Nuttall, H.E. and Ravenhill, P.J. (2019) Prevalence and analysis of equine periodontal disease, diastemata and peripheral caries in a first-opinion horse population in the UK. *The Veterinary Journal* 246, 98–102.

Oke, S., Aghazadeh-Habashi, A., Wees, J.S. and Jamali, F. (2006) Evaluation of glucosamine levels

in commercial equine oral supplements for joints. *Equine Veterinary Journal* 38(1), 93–95
Paradis, M.R. (2002) Demographics of health and disease in the geriatric horse. *Veterinary Clinics: Equine Practice* 18(3), 391–401.
Petersson, K.H., Burr, D.B., Gomez-Chiarri, M. and Petersson-Wolfe, C.S. (2010) The influence of vitamin E on immune function and response to vaccination in older horses. *Journal of Animal Science* 88(9), 2950–2958. doi: 10.2527/jas.2008-1724.
Platt, D., Bird, J.L.E. and Bayliss, M.T. (1998) Ageing of equine articular cartilage: structure and composition of aggrecan and decorin. *Equine Veterinary Journal* 30(1), 43–52.
Ralston, S.L., Squires, E.L. and Nockels, C.F. (1989) Digestion in the aged horse. *Journal of Equine Veterinary Science* 9(4), 203–205.
Ramzan, P.H.L. and Palmer, L. (2011) The incidence and distribution of peripheral caries in the cheek teeth of horses and its association with diastemata and gingival recession. *The Veterinary Journal* 190(1), 90–93.
Reed, S.A., LaVigne, E.K., Jones, A.K., Patterson, D.F. and Schauer, A.L. (2015) Horse Species Symposium: the aging horse: effects of inflammation on muscle satellite cells. *Journal of Animal Science* 93, 862–870.
Rivera, E., Benjamin, S., Nielsen, B., Shelle, J. and Zanella, A.J. (2002) Behavioral and physiological responses of horses to initial training: the comparison between pastured versus stalled horses. *Applied Animal Behaviour Science* 78, 235–252.
Tinker, M.K., White, N.A., Lessard, P., Thatcher, C.D., Pelzer, K.D. *et al.* (1997) A prospective study of equine colic risk factors. *Equine Veterinary Journal* 29, 454–458.
Towheed, T.E., Maxwell, L. Anastassiades, T.P., Shea, B., Houpt, J. *et al.* (2005) Glucosamine therapy for treating osteoarthritis. *Cochrane Database of Systematic Reviews* 2, CD002946.
Walker, H., Chinn, E., Holmes, S., Barwise-Munro, L., Robertson, V., Mould, R., Bradley, S., Shaw, D.J. and Dixon, P.M. (2012) Prevalence and some clinical characteristics of equine cheek teeth diastemata in 471 horses examined in a UK first-opinion equine practice (2008 to 2009). *Veterinary Record* 171(2), 44.
Wylie, C.E., Collins, S.N., Verheyen, K.L. and Newton, J.R. (2013) Risk factors for equine laminitis: a case-control study conducted in veterinary-registered horses and ponies in Great Britain between 2009 and 2011. *The Veterinary Journal* 198(1), 57–69.

17 Feeding the Donkey

Nikki Bell and Faith A. Burden

The Donkey Sanctuary, Sidmouth, Devon

Learning Objectives

LO1 Outline the metabolic and physiological differences between donkeys and other equids.
LO2 Describe adaptations to feedstuffs and diets.
LO3 Provide examples of common diets and the advantages and disadvantages in the UK and in low- and middle-income countries (LMICs).
LO4 Describe how diets can be adapted to minimise the risk of common nutritional diseases.

At the end of this chapter, you will be able to provide an evidence-based summary of the adaptations to feeding and management for donkeys in the UK and in low- and middle-income countries (LMICs).

Introduction

The domestic donkey (*Equus asinus*) is a descendant of the African wild ass (*Equus africanus*), a species that evolved to survive in some of the most inhospitable parts of the world. There are currently about 50 million donkeys and 8 million donkey hybrids globally (FAOSTAT, 2020) with the vast majority of these living and working in low- and middle-income countries (LMICs). A knowledge of the nutrition of donkeys in LMICs will be essential if you work with non-government organisations (NGOs).

Domesticated in approximately 3000 BC (Rossel *et al.*, 2008), the donkey has proved vital to many communities throughout the world particularly for transport and draught power (Ali *et al.*, 2014a). Donkeys are also increasingly being farmed on an intensive scale for production purposes for their meat and milk (Souroullas *et al.*, 2018) and for products made from their skin, particularly within China (Zhu and Weng, 2018). Donkeys have more recently found a role as pets and companion animals with a growing interest in their use for therapeutic purposes for vulnerable children and adults. Despite donkeys having a rich and important role in human development and history and featuring in many religious texts and historical stories, they have often unfairly been described as 'beasts of burden' and seen as the poor relation compared to their close relation, the horse (Burden and Thiemann, 2015).

Although there is a shared heritage between the donkey and horse, they are remarkably different in their physical traits, behaviour and nutritional requirements. To avoid compromising their health and welfare, you should avoid treating them as if they are a small horse, as otherwise their innate needs are unlikely to be met (Burden and Bell, 2019).

Origins of the donkey

The African wild ass (*E. africanus*), from which domestic donkeys are descended from, evolved to live in semiarid, often mountainous environments with steep terrain, sparse vegetation, dispersed water sources and often widely fluctuating temperatures. They learnt to thrive in an environment where food resources were very limited and of poor quality, maximising food quality over quantity

DOI: 10.1079/9781789245134.0017

using a selective feeding strategy. The donkey's natural environment contrasts significantly with the grassy plains of the ancestral home of their cousin, the horse, and explains some of the nutritional differences between the two species. Although certain characteristics have changed since the donkey was first domesticated, they have retained much of their ancestor's behaviour, for example social and feeding behaviour.

Feeding behaviour

In their natural environment, donkeys are trickle feeders, typically spending around 14–18 h/day foraging on lignin-rich, low-energy fibrous plants whilst travelling distances of up to 20–30 km/day (Klingel, 1977; Moehlman, 1998; Smith and Pearson, 2005). To increase their potential source of food in their natural environment, donkeys have evolved to be browsers as well as grazers (Aganga and Tsopito, 1998), with woody shrubs and trees being potential food sources when grasses and other low vegetation are in short supply. Donkeys kept in domestic environments rarely have the opportunity to exhibit the same kinds of natural feeding behaviours without significant input to enrich their environment and provide appropriate exercise.

Feeding in a domestic setting

Donkeys generally tolerate the presence of other equids well and can successfully be kept either in pairs or in larger groups (Fig. 17.1). When kept as part of larger groups, care should be taken to provide ample feeder space (the Donkey Sanctuary recommends a minimum of 0.75 m width feeding space per equid) to prevent dominant animals bullying those lower in the hierarchy, which could lead to submissive animals having a reduced feed intake. Donkeys will often be bullied at feed times if kept with horses, ponies or mules, which can lead to injury or donkeys may not be able to access sufficient food to satisfy their requirements. Provision of straw can be used to the donkey's advantage in such situations, as many other equids will be less inclined to bully for access to low-quality fibre sources.

Whatever environment a donkey is kept in, close observation should always be made of their feeding behaviour. 'Sham eating' is a unique trait often seen in sick donkeys whereby they will appear to mouth and swallow food, or they might nudge and nuzzle through it, but they invariably intake very little. Such behaviour is often a sign of a serious illness, which should prompt full investigation by a veterinarian, who must be particularly mindful of hyperlipaemia (Evans and Crane, 2018).

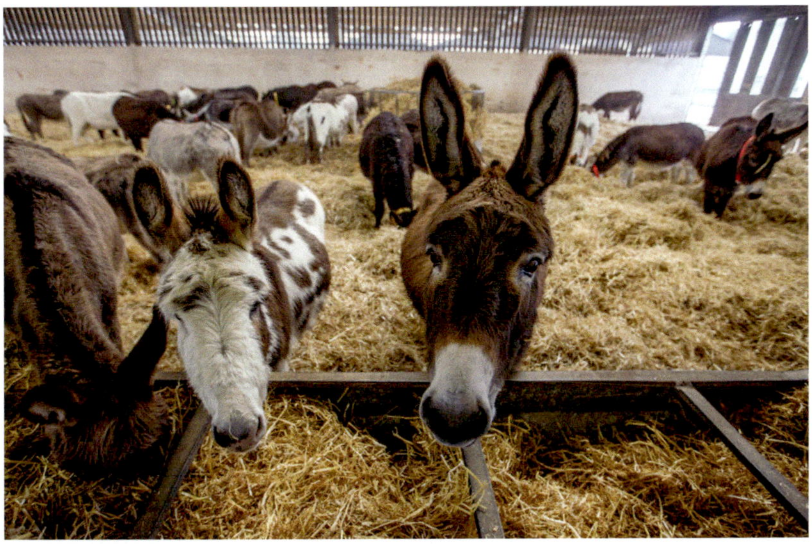

Fig. 17.1 Group-feeding of straw to donkeys. Donkeys are better able to digest straw compared with other equids. Check that there is enough space for donkeys: minimum of 0.75 m trough space per donkey. Watch for sham feeding.

Dietary adaptations

When compared with horses, donkeys are highly efficient at digesting poor nutritional quality fibre; in particular, they possess a superior digestive efficiency when digesting highly fibrous roughages such as straw (Pearson *et al.*, 2001; Wood, 2010). When fed on the same diet as ponies, donkeys have been shown to chew their food less and have a faster rate of intake relative to body size (Smith, 1999) (see Chapter 4).

Whilst the large intestine (caecum and colon) is generally considered the main site of fibre digestion in equids, pre-caecal fibre digestion in donkeys might actually contribute over 50% of the total tract digestion (Liu *et al.*, 2020a). High-fibre diets (70% rice straw) have the lowest mean retention time at the ileo-caecal junction in donkeys as measured by the retention time of nylon bags through the pre-caecal phase (Liu *et al.*, 2020a). Fibre content of feeds is the main factor affecting the pre-caecal digestibility contribution in relation to the total digestive tract, though lack of fibrolytic enzyme activity in pre-caecal digestion is commonly believed to be the cause. Although pre-caecal retention times have also been studied in horses fed timothy hay along with varying amounts of whole cereal grains (Macheboeuf *et al.*, 1995; Rosenfeld and Austbo, 2009; Brokner *et al.*, 2012) and ponies fed grass hay and grass nuts (Moore-Colyer *et al.*, 2002), differences in diet compositions between studies makes direct comparisons between horses/ponies and donkeys fed chopped rice straw and alfalfa along with varying levels of soyabean meal, corn meal and cottonseed meal (Liu *et al.*, 2020a) difficult.

Digesta passes through the donkey's whole gastrointestinal tract (GIT) at a slower rate to that in horses and ponies when fed similar diets (Pearson and Merritt, 1991; Cuddeford *et al.*, 1995; Pearson *et al.*, 2001). The longer mean retention time in donkeys is likely to be more favourable for anaerobic fungi growth (Cuddeford *et al.*, 1995).

Until recently, knowledge of the horse gut microbiota has tended to be extrapolated across to donkeys. However, with diet and gut transit times being key influencing factors of the hind-gut microbiome, the validity of direct translation has been questionable. Although Liu *et al.* (2014) provided some initial evidence relating to the donkey gut microbiota, their focus was solely on the bacterial communities rather than any of the other microbes. A core faecal microbiota exists across all equid types, but there are core differences in both faecal microbial concentrations and community compositions, with donkeys generally being most distinct from the other equid types (Edwards *et al.*, 2020a,b).

Donkeys have a sixfold higher anaerobic fungal concentration compared with horses (Edwards *et al.*, (2020b). Anaerobic fungi are one of the primary degraders of fibre in mammalian herbivores and they are particularly good at degrading plant cell walls. The high concentrations of anaerobic fungi found by Edwards *et al.* would therefore be consistent with the reported higher fibre digestibility of donkeys compared with horses and may explain why they can digest highly lignified forages such as straw. Clearly these dietary adaptations enable donkeys to survive working in areas where food is of poor quality and/or limited and allows them to thrive on rations that horses could not. This should be borne in mind when providing nutritional advice, particularly for domesticated donkeys living in temperate climates and leading a sedentary lifestyle.

Nutritional Requirements

Before formulating rations for donkeys, it is important to understand their unique nutritional requirements and to be aware of how they differ from those of horses and ponies. Extrapolating across recommendations from horses will result in an overestimate of the donkey's nutrient requirements for maintenance and work. Failure to take into account the donkey's differing nutritional requirements is likely to lead to disease or behavioural issues.

Energy requirements

Digestible energy requirements for maintenance in the donkey are significantly overestimated. Studies conducted in tropical and temperate climates have found the maintenance energy requirements of donkeys are 50–75% less than those of a horse of the same size, depending upon the season (Carretero-Roque *et al.*, 2005; Wood, 2010). Mature donkeys kept at maintenance require between 0.080 and 0.095 MJ of digestible energy (DE) per kilogram of live weight per day (Table. 17.1).

Table. 17.1 Digestible energy requirements and dry matter intake of donkeys of different body weights fed on a low energy density diet such as straw (5.5–6.5 MJ/kg DM). (Adapted from Carretero-Roque *et al.*, 2005; Wood, 2010.)

Donkey liveweight (kg)	Daily requirement for digestible energy[a] (MJ/day)	Daily dry matter intake (kg/day)
150	12–14	2.3
175	14–17	2.6
200	16–19	3
225	18–22	3.4
250	20–24	3.8

[a]Lower value = when daytime temperatures are higher than 18°C.

Overfeeding energy

Domesticated donkeys are typically overweight and, like fat horses, have higher basal insulin levels. Insulin resistance is an adaptive response when energy is limited, and donkeys might be more insulin resistant than horses, in part due to having lower nutrient requirements and higher metabolic efficiency (McLean *et al.*, 2009).

Research in this area is limited. Donkeys have similar insulin sensitivity to adult horses of similar body condition score, unlike adult ponies who have lower levels of insulin sensitivity when compared with both groups (McLean *et al.*, 2009). Obese donkeys have higher basal insulin levels when compared with moderate or thin donkeys (Pritchard *et al.*, 2019), a finding similar to previous work in horses (Curtis *et al.*, 2010). Excess weight gain and obesity is of welfare concern, because high circulating insulin interferes with cellular mechanisms in glucose-insulin dynamics.

> **Top tip**
>
> Encourage clients to body condition/fat score (see Chapter 3: 'Body fat scoring') as a measure for energy balance to determine if a donkey is at risk for high insulin concentrations and potentially insulin resistance.

Dry matter appetite

Donkeys have a lower dry matter intake (DMI) relative to their metabolic body size (Tisserand *et al.*, 1991; Pearson and Merritt, 1991; Pearson *et al.*, 2001) compared with ponies. Typical daily DMIs in UK donkeys fed straw (ad lib) and hay are 1.3–1.7% of live weight (Wood 2010). Intakes can vary between 0.9% and 2.5% (Smith and Pearson, 2005; Liu *et al.*, 2020b), depending on the type of forage given, which is likely a reflection of the NDF content (see Chapter 4). Donkeys fed chopped lucerne have the highest intake levels (Smith, 1999). Donkeys fed unchopped forage have appetite limits of approximately 1.5% of their live weight in dry forage per day (Smith and Pearson, 2005).

Protein requirements

Protein metabolism and utilisation in the donkey appear to be complex, and experience would indicate that donkeys are better able to survive on low-quality protein-containing diets than horses, as evidenced by the donkey's ability to breed, grow and work on forages containing low-quality protein.

The estimated digestible crude protein (DCP) requirements for adult UK donkeys are 26 ± 1.3 g DCP per 100 kg bodyweight (BW) per day (approximately 40 g CP/100 kg BW) (Wood, 2010). Diets based around ad lib straw/stover and if necessary supplemental hay/haylage will supply the desired amount of DCP. If a donkey's energy requirements are satisfied, so are their protein requirements. Estimations of the DCP requirements of pregnant, lactating and growing donkeys have yet to be established.

Vitamin and mineral requirements

Little research has been carried out to establish the vitamin and mineral requirements of donkeys (Smith and Burden, 2013) but the levels advised by the National Research Council (NRC) for horses appear to provide optimal levels for donkeys and can be safely extrapolated (NRC, 2007).

Whilst pasture-fed donkeys or those fed fresh forages are unlikely to suffer from vitamin deficiencies, those with more restricted access or who are housed for long periods eating conserved dried forages may be more vulnerable, especially if young or geriatric. Allowing donkeys some time to graze may be beneficial for their vitamin intake, otherwise provision of an appropriate vitamin supplement would be advisable.

Whilst the exact mineral requirements of donkeys have not been established, as with vitamins the NRC guidelines for horses are considered optimal; it is likely donkeys have slightly lower requirements (Smith and Burden, 2013).

If you are working in LMICs, donkeys fed large quantities of wheat bran, crop by-products such as rice bran and cotton seed and/or the feeding of some tropical grasses such as *Panicum maximum*, *Setaria anceps*, *Digitaria* spp., *Pennisetum clandestinum* and *Cenchrus ciliaris* (Stewart, 2018) will have a deficiency of calcium and phosphorus.

Although evidence is limited (Faillace *et al.*, 2017), prolonged deficiencies of calcium and phosphorus will weaken bones and are likely to cause developmental orthopaedic disease resulting in permanent bone deformity and weakness in young donkeys. Diets containing excessively high levels of phosphorus or oxalates can interfere with the absorption of calcium, which can lead to secondary nutritional hyperparathyroidism (also known as Miller's disease, big head disease, or bran disease) in equids (McDowell, 2003; Luthersson *et al.*, 2005).

Mineral provision can take many forms, from lick blocks to supplements and pelleted ration balancers. Daily intake can be difficult to monitor with licks, but they are often the only feasible way for donkeys (particularly those in LMICs) to obtain minerals. To avoid problems, the mineral lick provided should be one specifically designed for equids and should have a full statement of ingredients. Free-choice access to salt is also advisable, particularly for donkeys working in hot environments, as demands for sodium chloride are likely to be higher (McDowell, 2003). Salt levels of 0.25–1.0% of the total diet are considered adequate even for donkeys working under hot conditions (McDowell, 2003). Maximum tolerable salt should not exceed 3% of the total diet; free access to clean water should always be available.

Water requirements

Water requirements for donkeys are similar to those of horses at about 5–9% of bodyweight daily (Martin-Rosset, 2018); however, their intake varies considerably depending on workload, ambient temperature, water content of feed and during pregnancy and lactation. Fresh, clean water should be provided at all times and care should be taken to ensure that water sources are regularly cleaned and functioning correctly. Self-filling water troughs are ideal to ensure a constant supply of water but the water intake of individual animals will be more difficult to monitor. Working donkeys should be taken to water points as frequently as possible during the day, at least once every 4 h.

In tropical countries, donkeys may be forced to drink highly saline ground water, which can become more concentrated if left to stand in troughs for long periods of time (McDowell, 2003). Ideally, total soluble salt content of drinking water should not exceed 3000 ppm; levels above this are likely to cause digestive upsets and may initially be refused by animals. Levels of total soluble salt in drinking water above 7000 ppm are not fit for donkeys, especially animals that are heavily worked or heat stressed.

In the donkey's natural, semiarid environment, water is often in short supply and widely dispersed, which has led to them being well adapted to tolerate thirst and rapid rehydration (Maloiy, 1973). Donkeys can tolerate body water losses of up to 30% of their normal bodyweight and are able to rehydrate rapidly by drinking 20–30 litres of water within a few minutes without apparent ill effect (Maloiy, 1973). Donkeys are more thirst tolerant than ponies and will maintain appetite and even choose food over water after water withdrawal even when dehydrated (Houpt, 1993; Mueller *et al.*, 1997). This trait can lead to a late diagnosis of dehydration and concurrent issues such as impaction colic (Burden and Bell, 2019).

Donkeys wary of drinking from unfamiliar water sources and fussy about the temperature may suffer impaction colic. If you are dealing with domesticated donkeys, advise owners that provision of warmed water in winter can be beneficial, particularly for vulnerable or geriatric donkeys (Evans and Crane, 2018). During periods of particularly cold weather, water sources should be checked several times a day to ensure they are kept free from ice. Donkeys living in routinely cold climates will appreciate the provision of heated troughs or buckets.

How to Monitor the Donkey

Bodyweight

Monitoring a donkey's weight (ideally monthly) is extremely useful for assessing their general condition and health status. Weight can be measured using electronic scales, a weight estimation calculator/chart or by use of a weight tape. For the latter two options, it is important that donkey-specific estimators[i] and tapes[ii] are used (Fig. 17.2); those designed for horses and ponies tend not to be accurate, due to species-specific differences.

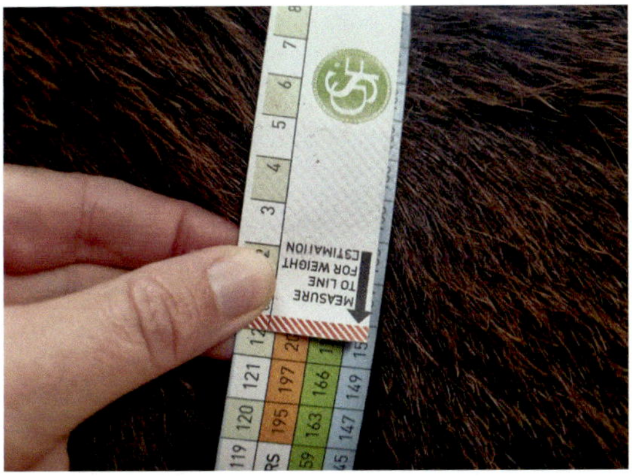

Fig. 17.2 Illustration of weight tape. Don't put your fingers behind the tape.

Body condition/fat scoring

Whilst the Henneke system of body scoring is generally used for horses (Henneke *et al.*, 1983), a species-specific body scoring tool should be used for donkeys (Fig. 17.3) as they lay down fat stores in more localised areas and have a different body shape than horses and ponies (Valle *et al.*, 2017; Burden, 2012).

It is essential for carers to get hands-on and feel the amount of fat and muscle covering a donkey's bones, especially when donkeys have thick coats. Donkeys tend to have quite an angular frame and often have a pendulous abdomen. The pendulous abdomen may be due to increased retention of fibre (Pearson *et al.*, 2001) within the gut and the related increased volume of the large intestine, or it can be due to abdominal fat, or in sedentary animals a slackness of the abdominal muscles.

Donkeys frequently develop fat pads when allowed to become overweight. Fat pads are common on the neck, buttocks and the dorsal and lateral thorax (Fig. 17.4). Donkeys often carry significant

FACTSHEET: Animal Health Professionals and Owners

DONKEY BODY CONDITION SCORE CHART

THE DONKEY SANCTUARY

Accurate Body condition scoring is a hands-on process for feeling the amount of muscle and fat that are covering the donkey's bones. Using this chart as a guide, feel the coverage over the bones in five specific areas listed below. Fat deposits may be unevenly distributed especially over the neck and hindquarters. Some resistant fat deposits may be retained in the event of weight loss or may calcify (harden). Careful assessment of all areas should be made and combined, to give an overall score. When deciding on the correct course of action following condition scoring, you might have to take into consideration the age of the donkey and any veterinary conditions they have. Aged donkeys can be hard to condition score due to lack of muscle bulk and tone giving thin appearance dorsally with dropped belly ventrally, while overall condition may be reasonable. If in doubt, get advice from your vet.

Condition score	Neck and shoulders	Withers	Ribs and belly	Back and loins	Hindquarters
1. Poor (very thin) 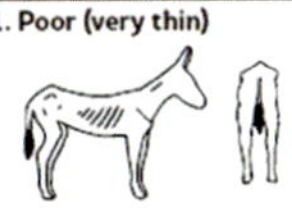	Neck thin, all bones easily felt. Neck meets shoulder abruptly, shoulder bones felt easily, angular.	Dorsal spine and withers prominent and easily felt.	Ribs can be seen from a distance and felt with ease. Belly tucked up.	Backbone prominent, can feel dorsal and transverse processes easily.	Hip bones visible and felt easily (dock and pin bones). Little muscle cover. May be cavity under tail.
2. Moderate (underweight) 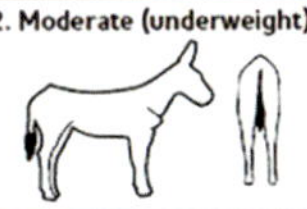	Some muscle development overlying bones. Slight step where neck meets shoulders.	Some cover over dorsal withers, spinous processes felt but not prominent.	Ribs not visible but can be felt with ease.	Dorsal and transverse processes felt with light pressure. Poor muscle development either side of midline.	Poor muscle cover on hindquarters, hip bones felt with ease.
3. Ideal 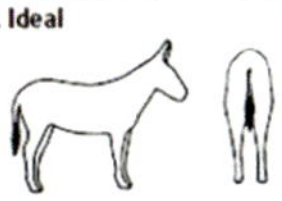	Good muscle development, bones felt under light cover of muscle/fat. Neck flows smoothly into shoulder, which is rounded.	Good cover of muscle/ fat over dorsal spinous processes, withers flow smoothly into back.	Ribs just covered by light layer of fat/muscle, ribs can be felt with light pressure. Belly firm with good muscle tone and flattish outline.	Can feel individual spinous or transverse processes with pressure. Muscle development either side of midline is good.	Good muscle cover over hindquarters, hip bones rounded in appearance, can be felt with light pressure.
4. Overweight (fat) 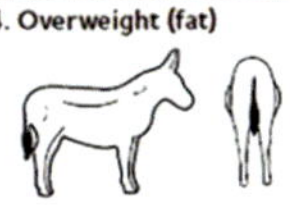	Neck thick, crest hard, shoulder covered in even fat layer.	Withers broad, bones felt with pressure.	Ribs dorsally only felt with firm pressure, ventral ribs may be felt more easily. Belly over developed.	Can only feel dorsal and transverse processes with firm pressure. May have slight crease along midline.	Hindquarters rounded, bones felt only with pressure. Fat deposits evenly placed.
5. Obese (very fat) 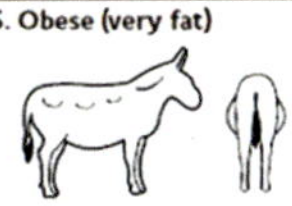	Neck thick, crest bulging with fat and may fall to one side. Shoulder rounded and bulging with fat.	Withers broad, bones felt with firm pressure.	Large, often uneven fat deposits covering dorsal and possibly ventral aspect of ribs. Ribs not palpable dorsally. Belly pendulous in depth and width.	Back broad, difficult to feel individual spinous or transverse processes. More prominent crease along mid line fat pads on either side.Crease along midline bulging fat either side.	Cannot feel hip bones, fat may overhang either side of tail head, fat often uneven and bulging.

Research and Operational Support | © The Donkey Sanctuary | Published: 2013 | Revised: October 2018 | Phone: 01395 578222

Fig. 17.3 Body fat score chart for donkeys.

abdominal fat (often up to 8 cm but increasing up to 14 cm in the obese donkey). Once in situ these fat pads rarely disappear even with dieting and may remain in a donkey that has ideal fat scores elsewhere on the body.

Whilst body condition scoring is generally assumed to be the most practical way of monitoring fat reserves in equines, the ability of untrained operators to accurately assess BCS has been raised as a cause for concern (Mottet *et al.*, 2009). Real-time ultrasonography (RTU) has shown potential as another non-invasive tool for assessing body fat and has been trialled successfully in horses (Gee *et al.*, 2003; Superchi *et al.*, 2014; Silva *et al.*, 2016), donkeys (Quaresma *et al.*, 2013; Silva *et al.*, 2016) and mules (Velasquez-Mosquera and Corrales-Alvarez, 2019).

When devising diets for donkeys, their body condition *must* be taken into account to determine whether the individual needs to gain, maintain or lose weight. The aim should be for donkeys to be maintained at around condition/fat score 2.5–3 out of 5 (Evans and Crane, 2018).

Practical Feeding for the Healthy Donkey

Formulating a donkey's ration and deciding on which foods to offer requires knowledge of the donkey's requirements and the nutrient value of the foods available. Consideration should also be given to the donkey's natural feeding behaviour to ensure digestive health and to reduce behavioural stress. Diets that are high in fibre but low in energy and non-structural carbohydrates (NSC) tend to be the most ideal (Smith and Burden, 2013).

Checking dental health is key for successful feeding and regular dental examinations (a minimum of once yearly) should be carried out to ascertain the individual's ability to chew and digest fibre sources (Fig. 17.5).

Straw as forage

For donkeys with good dental function, straw (barley or wheat – checked to have few seed heads or retained loose grain) or other fibrous forage such as stover (the leaves and stalks of field crops such as corn, maize or sorghum) should make up at least 70–75% of the diet. Provision of straw on an *ad libitum* basis should help prevent boredom and unwanted behaviours such as chewing of fences and other wooden structures. When transitioning donkeys to this type of diet the straw/stover will need to be introduced very gradually to avoid the risk of gastrointestinal impaction (Cox *et al.*, 2009).

In specific circumstances, such as the older donkey or those with fat loss, small amounts (about 25–30% of the diet) of mature, coarse grass hay, haylage and/or grazing can be given in addition to straw to top up energy levels. The amount given will need adjusting depending on the donkey's body condition, the time of year and the prevailing weather conditions. Safe logs and branches should also be provided to satisfy the donkey's natural browsing behaviours.

As the donkey's digestive system is adapted to a more or less continuous intake of fibrous food,

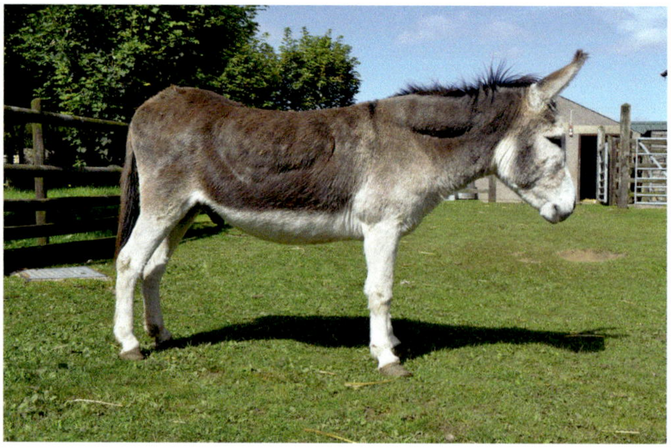

Fig. 17.4 Defined fat deposits on an obese donkey.

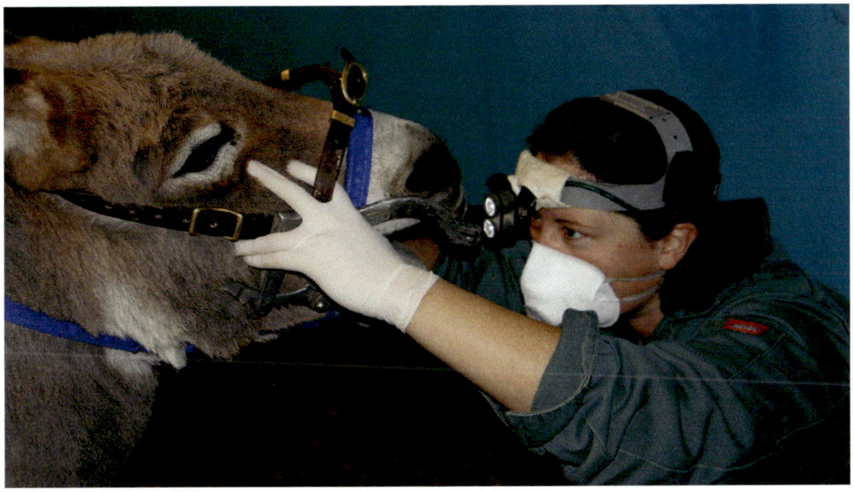

Fig. 17.5 Dental examination being carried out by a fully qualified BAEDT equine dental technician (EDT).

trickle-feeding the ration throughout a 24 h period is ideal to ensure sufficient chewing time throughout the day and night. Chewing promotes production of saliva, which acts as a lubricant and acts to neutralise the continuous production of acid in the stomach, in turn helping reduce the risk of gastric ulcer development (Burden and Bell, 2019).

> **Top tip**
>
> Straw is not a risk factor for gastric ulceration syndrome in donkeys, with only 7% incidence within a sanctuary population (Burden and Stradling, 2013).

Supplementary feeding and compound feeds

Certain individuals, such as pregnant and lactating jennies, young growing donkeys, working donkeys, stallions kept for breeding purposes and underweight individuals (Fig. 17.6), might need their diet supplementing to meet their higher energy requirements (Pearson, 1991; Martin-Rosset, 2018). Although many donkeys can live on a diet of straw along with supplemental grass and hay or haylage, vitamins and minerals may be necessary.

A thorough clinical assessment should be carried out on underweight individuals to check for any underlying causes before too many dietary changes are made.

Dietary assessments

Dietary assessments should include the following.

- Observation of feeding behaviour – ensure the donkey is prehending, masticating and swallowing effectively and not sham eating.
- Feeding and management practices.
- A thorough dental examination.
- A blood sample to assess the overall health of the donkey, with particular attention to liver and kidney function, pituitary pars intermedia dysfunction (PPID) and equine metabolic syndrome (EMS).
- An assessment of the potential parasitic burden (Burden, 2012).

The amount of fibre or oil-based compound fibre (e.g. alfalfa, unmolassed beet pulp or rice bran) can be fed in small meals mixed with appropriate roughage such as an unmolassed short chopped fibre if required (Burden, 2012; Evans and Crane, 2018) to meet but not exceed the donkey's energy requirements.

Forage feeds can be given at a rate of 0.5 kg/100 kg BW for large-breed donkeys or 0.25 kg/100 kg BW for miniatures and small breeds. However, the maximum amount recommended per feed is 1 kg and this may mean dividing into at least two to three small feeds a day.

The use of cereal grain-based compound feed is discouraged in donkeys as this would increase the

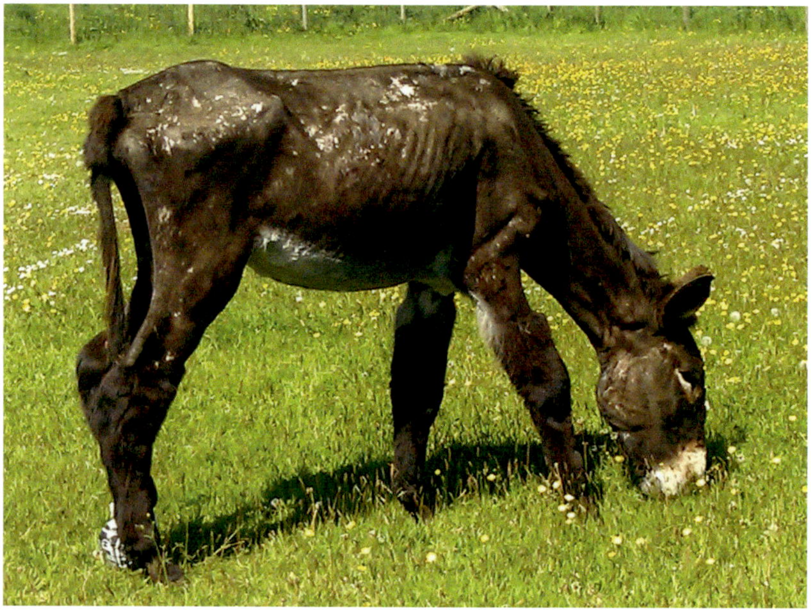

Fig. 17.6 Underweight donkeys may require extra feeds in order to help gain condition.

risk of gastric ulcers (Burden *et al.*, 2009), laminitis and colic (Cox *et al.*, 2009). Where cereal grains or molasses are included to increase the palatability or energy density of feeds, it is advised that combined starch and sugar levels do not exceed 15% and ideally should be < 10% on a dry matter basis.

> **Top tip**
>
> When dealing with donkeys with different nutritional needs there may be times when companions need separating for short periods in order to allow one to receive additional food. In such circumstances it is important to keep bonded companions at least within sight (some donkeys will not even tolerate being separated by a fence), otherwise one or both animals may refuse to eat in spite of their hunger.

Feeding Working Donkeys in Lower- and Middle-income Countries (LMICs)

Educating owners on suitable, locally available feedstuffs and the importance of frequent body condition/fat scoring is essential to the nutritional management of the working donkey. Nutrition is an important component of preventive healthcare and must be addressed alongside matters such as parasite control, harnessing and infectious diseases.

- Assessment should include an assessment of workload and the availability of feedstuffs during working hours.
- The energy requirements for working donkeys are likely to be higher than for maintenance but will vary according to the type of work done, the length of the working period, access to food and the quality of it.
  - Working donkeys unable to access adequate feedstuffs are prone to a poor body condition score.
  - Donkeys in poor body condition have been found to suffer from work-related harness sores more frequently than those in good condition (Burden *et al.*, 2009).

Energy requirements

An average donkey with a pack, or pulling a cart travelling 20 km, will require 100% more energy than a sedentary animal, and one travelling 30 km will require 160% more energy (Pearson, 2005).

> **Top tip**
>
> Where distances are difficult to estimate, the length of time that the donkey is worked for can be used as a guideline: 4 h work will require 50% more energy and 6 h work will require 100% more energy (Pearson, 2005).

Forages

Working donkeys may be unable to eat enough forage due to either lack of digestive tract capacity or lack of time to physically eat to obtain all their requirements.

Grazing is often limited in tropical areas for much of the year so locally available crop by-products or standing hay crops are frequently fed along with supplementary rations of cereal grains such as barley, oats, maize and sorghum.

Cereals

Working donkeys may require higher-energy feedstuffs but cereal grains should not be fed in excess. Physical processing such as crushing, cracking or rolling helps improve small-intestine digestion (Smith and Burden, 2013), particularly for donkeys with poor dentition.

Other ingredients

Molasses and oils

Molasses or oils increase the energy level of the diet but must be added gradually to a base feed of cereal or vegetable matter to avoid feed refusal. Addition of up to 150 ml of oil, split in to two feeds, for a 180 kg donkey or 250 ml for a large donkey or mule is sufficient to make a significant contribution to the energy content of the diet.

Legumes

Protein-rich legumes such as alfalfa (lucerne), berseem and faba (broad) beans can be fed alongside roughages to enhance the energy and protein content of the diet; all are highly palatable to donkeys and mules.

- Donkeys or mules working 4–6 h/day can be fed lucerne at inclusion rates of up to 25% of the dry matter intake.
  - Higher inclusion rates are likely to oversupply energy and protein and are therefore wasteful (Smith and Burden, 2013).
- Broad/faba beans should only be considered for donkeys working very hard and it is important that they are fed slowly and in small amounts.
  - They typically contain 25–33% protein/kg DM, 7–11% crude fibre/kg DM and 40–48% starch/kg DM (Feedipedia[iii]).

Water

Under certain conditions, working donkeys may require five times more water than a sedentary individual (up to 35 litres per day) (Aganga *et al.*, 2000).

- Ensuring adequate water intake is particularly important for working donkeys to enable them to work and digest their food effectively. Water will be lost through sweating.
- The donkey's ability to continue to work and maintain appetite despite water deprivation makes them more suitable for working in hot environments than horses (Smith and Burden, 2013).

Feeding Donkey Hybrids

Mules are the hybrid resulting from a mating between a horse or pony mare and a donkey jack. Less frequently encountered are hinnies, the result of a mating between a donkey jenny and a horse or pony stallion. Mules are physically strong and make excellent working animals (Fig. 17.7). They are able to survive working in harsh conditions, tolerating adverse weather in which donkeys would not thrive (Ali *et al.*, 2014b, 2015) on limited food resources, often out-surviving horses and oxen on long journeys.

There has been little research to determine the actual nutritional needs of mules but experience has shown they will thrive on rations similar to those described for the donkey. Do not advise feeding the same as a horse, as this has been associated with significant behavioural changes. Whilst the occurrence of conditions such as obesity and laminitis is generally lower in mules than in horses, ponies and donkeys, obese laminitic mules do occur so care is needed over their diet (Burnham, 2002; Taylor and Matthews, 2002).

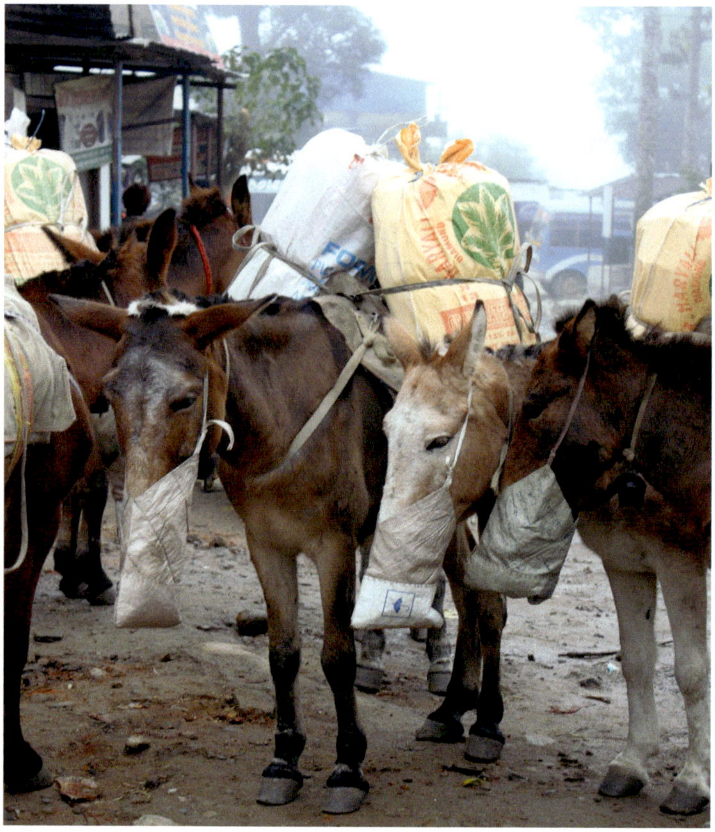

Fig. 17.7 Mules are ideally suited to working in challenging environments.

Feeding Donkeys in Production

Donkeys are increasingly being farmed on an intensive scale for production purposes, due to an increase in the popularity of products such as donkey meat, milk (Souroullas *et al.*, 2018; Altomonte *et al.*, 2019; Aspri *et al.*, 2019) and products made from their skins, particularly within China (Mayers, 2017; Kohle, 2018; Zhu and Weng, 2018).

The nutritional needs of donkeys kept for such purposes are similar to those of all other donkeys; you need to take into account the animal's body condition, their health and dental status and their breeding status, with consideration given to their environment and the climate.

Ideally donkeys with similar nutritional needs should be housed together to ensure the most appropriate diet can be given. The provision of adequate feeding space is important; a suitable source of fibre should be freely available for a minimum of 14–18 h/day. If supplementary feeds are required, individuals should be removed from their group but kept within sight of their companions. Where available, access to turnout should be encouraged, as it can be beneficial to the physical and mental wellbeing of the animals.

Feeding in Pregnancy and Lactation

Nutrient requirements for pregnancy and lactation in the donkey have yet to be established (Martin-Rosset, 2018) so guidelines tend to make use of practical experience along with recommendations extrapolated from horse and pony data (Burden, 2012; Evans and Crane, 2018).

Pregnancy

Similar to all breeding animals, the majority of pregnant donkeys will not need their diet altering until the final trimester, at which point the energy density and quality of forages should be increased in order to meet the female donkey's increasing nutrient requirements to support foetal development (Martin-Rosset, 2018). The provision of fibre sources should change from straw to hay, haylage or grazing, depending on fat score, and advise a balancer to meet vitamin, mineral and protein requirements.

If the jenny is losing fat or if grazing is very poor, then supplementation with chopped alfalfa or high-fibre compound feeds may also be indicated to satisfy energy requirements. Pregnant and lactating donkeys will be at high risk for developing hyperlipaemia, so their dry matter appetite should be monitored closely and care should be taken to ensure that their energy requirements are met (Durham and Thiemann, 2015).

Feeding the foal

The growth rate of foals should be steady and measured fortnightly (weight and body fat/condition score); growth curves are not yet available for donkey foals (Martin-Rosset, 2018). If the rate of growth is too rapid, any supplementary nutritional intake should be restricted, but with appropriate vitamin and mineral supplementation. If the foal's growth is stunted, appropriate supplementary feeding may be required. Fat scoring will aid in this decision. Foals should be allowed to pick at their dam's feed in preparation for weaning, which can be carried out from 6 months of age.

Dietary Adaptations for Common Nutritional Problems

Obesity

Obesity is a significant welfare problem for donkeys and is commonly caused by overfeeding and lack of exercise (Wood, 2010). Obesity predisposes to a number of diseases and has been shown to be influential to metabolic and hormonal imbalances (Mendoza *et al.*, 2015), hyperlipaemia (Burden *et al.*, 2011) and laminitis (Morrow *et al.*, 2011).

In all of these conditions, an excess storage of energy as metabolically active adipose tissue can lead to inappropriate mobilisation of lipid, insulin resistance, and enzyme dysregulation (see Chapter 15).

Dieting obese donkeys is extremely difficult and potentially dangerous and will often require ongoing support from yourself. The donkey's diet is often just one of several factors involved; a lack of exercise, companion issues and mental stimulation will often need addressing too. Before embarking on a management plan for an obese donkey you should carry out a dental check, to ensure that the donkey can be given the most appropriate diet, and an assessment of the donkey's ability to exercise. In some cases, it may also be appropriate for you to take a blood sample to check for underlying disease, in particular assessing triglyceride levels before dietary change to help prevent hyperlipaemia.

Dietary management for obese donkeys should be based on high-fibre, low-energy, low-NSC forages (Evans and Crane, 2018). Maintaining dry matter/fibre intake is essential even in overweight donkeys, as starvation is likely to result in hyperlipaemia. For donkeys with good dental function, diets comprising predominantly long-stem straw or stover tend to be most ideal. A proprietary vitamin, mineral and protein supplement, TopSpec Donkey Forage Balancer[iv], should be provided if there are concerns about nutritional deficiency.

Pasture management will be an important part of a weight reduction programme. Evidence suggests that fructan levels in grass are unlikely to trigger ration induced laminitis due to disrupted fermentation in the hind gut. It is more likely that high NSC such as simple sugars from the grass when enzymically digested in the small intestine may lead to increased insulin resistance and the development of endocrine-related laminitis (Katz and Bailey, 2016). It is therefore extremely important to maintain a healthy grass sward (see Chapter 4).

Reducing the time at grazing has a limited effect on the total dietary intake of donkeys and instead is more likely to lead to them spending every minute at pasture eating, rather than exercising and carrying out social behaviours (Wood, 2010). A more ideal way to reduce grass intake is to reduce the amount of grass that is made available, by means of strip grazing or by creating track systems; however, suitable forage such as straw or stover should be freely available at all times.

Donkeys should be encouraged to exercise as much as possible and they should be regularly condition scored and have their weight checked on a monthly basis. Progress of dieting donkeys may be slow, and perseverance is essential. It often takes weeks or months for the first weight to be lost. However, once this process begins, weight loss should be gradual. The aim should be to lose 2–3% of bodyweight monthly.

Laminitis

Laminitis is a common cause of lameness in non-working donkeys but often goes undetected until the condition is advanced, due to the donkey's stoic nature and subtlety of changes in behaviour in response to pain (Evans and Crane, 2018). Do make sure that clients understand that donkeys with dropped pedal bones might not show pain, but nonetheless may have laminitis (Collins *et al.*, 2009).

In the acute stages, it is essential to remove any contributory dietary issues. Fibre from pasture is replaced by a high-fibre, low-NSC diet (Evans and Crane, 2018). Fibre intake should be maintained to reduce the risk of hyperlipaemia. Whilst straw may be fed to laminitic donkeys, those with decreased mobility should have frequent checks made of their gut motility and faecal output (Burden and Bell, 2019). A short-chopped forage with an NSC level of < 10% may need to be considered in the short term to reduce the risk of impaction.

Hay and haylage can be considered for laminitics that have hind gut disruption (as opposed to metabolic aetiology) to provide substrate for the cellulytic bacteria. Forage analysis (see Chapter 9), ideally by means of wet chemistry, can be a useful tool for assessing the suitability of available forage. Sloppy feeds of unmolassed beet pulp can be useful to encourage water intake and assist with the administration of drugs. Long-term management of the chronic laminitic is the same as described above for obese animals.

Hyperlipaemia

Donkeys are particularly prone to developing hyperlipaemia, especially with increasing age (Reid and Mohammed, 1996). Incidence rates vary from 3% (Reid and Mohammed, 1996) to 7% in older donkeys (Burden *et al.*, 2011.) The condition is triggered in response to a negative energy balance resulting in mobilisation of body fat stores to fuel essential organs. The disorder can accompany almost any other disease of the donkey; colic, respiratory disease and laminitis are particularly common concurrent diseases (Evans and Crane, 2018).

Many 'stressors' can contribute to the development of hyperlipaemia and prevention through reduction of stress and maintenance of appetite is important (Burden *et al.*, 2011). A dull, inappetent donkey is a clinical emergency requiring prompt intervention; serum triglycerides can help confirm the diagnosis (Fig. 17.8).

More severe cases are likely to need treating in a hospital environment where companion(s) should accompany the sick donkey in order to limit any additional stress from separation and to encourage appetite. If a donkey's appetite is significantly

> **Top tip**
>
> Maintaining appetite is crucial in sick donkeys and tempters such as safe fruit and vegetables, dried mint, unmolassed beet pulp, peppermint cordial or yeast extracts can be added to a base fibre feed to try to stimulate appetite (Evans and Crane, 2018). Donkeys should also be given the opportunity to browse and graze; taking them to a hedgerow will often spark some interest.

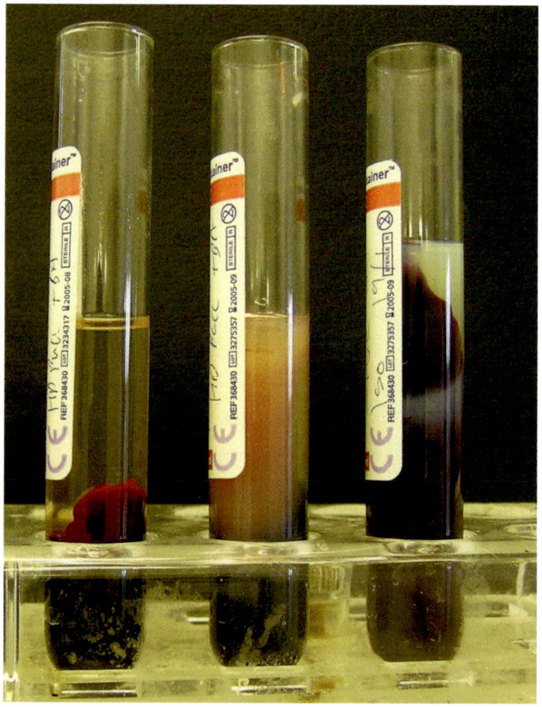

Fig. 17.8 Clotted blood samples. Normal clear serum (left); moderately cloudy serum (middle) with elevated triglycerides; and milky white serum (right) with triglycerides severely elevated. Note that clear serum does not rule out mild hyperlipaemia.

reduced or absent, consideration may be given to nasogastric tubing, IV fluids, or total parenteral nutrition to maintain a positive energy balance until voluntary feeding is re-established (Thiemann, 2013; Durham and Thiemann, 2015).

Dental disease

Dental abnormalities (Fig. 17.9) have a prevalence of 73–93% in donkeys globally (Evans and Lilly, 2019), particularly geriatrics (du Toit *et al.*, 2008, 2009; Rodrigues *et al.*, 2013). Dental problems can result in pain and discomfort or an inability to chew and masticate food properly, significantly affecting the animal's behaviour, health and diet. Clinical signs include quidding (food dropped from the mouth in a partially chewed state), weight loss, impacted digesta in the digestive tract, halitosis, choke, associated depression and lethargy; or varying levels of inappetence, predisposing donkeys to hyperlipaemia (Burden *et al.*, 2011).

Dental disease is often at an advanced stage by the time donkeys start to show symptoms. It is especially important for them to receive regular dental examinations so that interventions or preventive care can be started promptly if needed. Examination of faeces can also provide clues regarding the impact of dental pathologies on digestion, with excessive faecal fibre length (FFL) typically indicating that dental abnormalities are present. The optimum faecal fibre length for donkeys is just short of 2 mm (Evans and Lilly, 2019).

Johnson *et al.* (2017) found slight differences in the association between FFL and dental abnormalities in horses and donkeys, but an average FFL > 3.6mm is generally thought indicative of dental disease, with FFL > 4.5mm indicative of severe dental disease (Evans and Lilly, 2019).

Donkeys with only mild or correctable dental abnormalities may require few changes being made to their diet, as long as you or an equine dentist is seeing them regularly. As long as donkeys are not quidding and choke is not a problem, they may still be able to be maintained on suitable long-fibre forages along with small, frequent meals of high-fibre chaffs/compound feeds and unmolassed soaked beet pulp (Evans and Lilly, 2019).

Advanced dental disease

Donkeys with more advanced dental disease or more severe dental abnormalities who are struggling to chew long fibres effectively or those showing a reduction in food intake are likely to benefit from changes to their diet (Evans and Lilly, 2019). Long-fibre forages are likely to need replacing with alternative fibre sources than can be chewed and digested more easily (Fig. 17.10). Low in energy and NSCs, short-chopped products should be provided throughout the day and be fed to DMI requirements. Although feeding of such products *ad libitum* may lead to gorging in the short term, intake should self-regulate after a few weeks. Care should be taken to monitor weight throughout this period, with restrictions put in place if unwanted weight is gained (Evans and Crane, 2018).

Gastric ulcers

Whilst the prevalence of gastric ulceration in horses is known to be quite high, there is limited information in donkeys. Non-working donkeys leading a

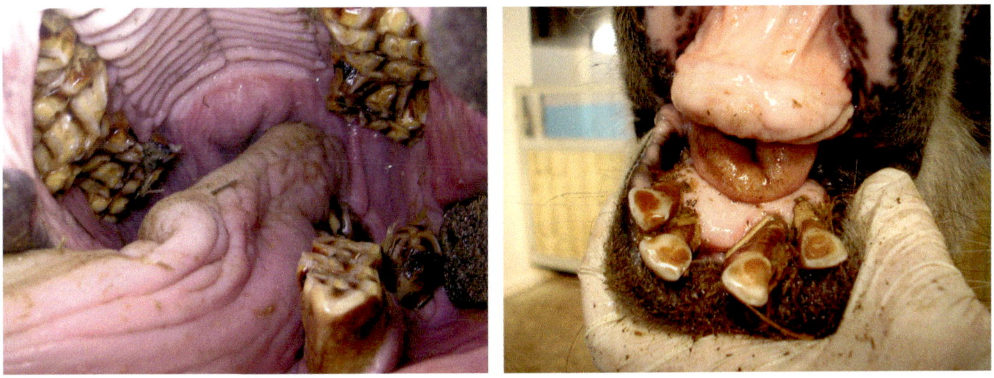

Fig. 17.9 Dental disease in the donkey.

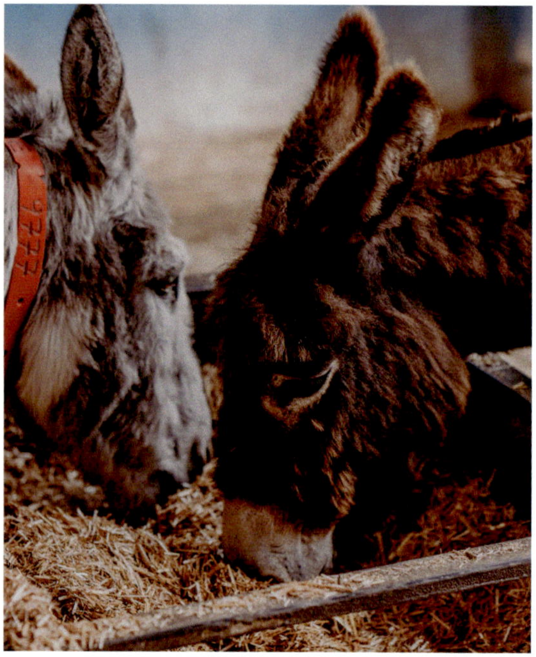

Fig. 17.10 Short-chop material is easier for donkeys to chew.

sedentary lifestyle with access to *ad libitum* forage would have traditionally been considered low risk for gastric ulcer development. Post-mortem data (The Donkey Sanctuary) highlighted that donkeys being fed cereal-based supplementary rations were at risk (Burden *et al.*, 2009); replacing cereal-based with fibre-based alternatives reduced the incidence of gastric ulcers at post mortem from 41% in 2005 to 7% in 2011 (Burden and Stradling, 2013).

Summary

The donkey is well adapted to survive on food that would be inadequate for most other equines. The donkey's ability to digest highly fibrous forages, its thirst tolerance and ability to maintain appetite even when dehydrated enables survival in some of the world's most inhospitable places. These natural characteristics have led to the donkey and its hybrid, the mule, being invaluable working animals for communities in LMICs across the world. Whilst still commonly found working across the globe, the donkey also faces new challenges as a production and companion animal where environmental conditions and feed provision are very different to those found in the species' natural environment and thus obesity becomes a welfare issue. The donkey should be fed a diet high in fibre and low in energy and non-structural carbohydrates, which is best supplied using straws and moderate-quality hay and grazing. Such a diet should be complemented with an enriched natural environment allowing opportunities to browse and exercise and carry out other natural behaviours. Dietary management of the donkey is essential to avoid health issues and ensure wellbeing and should be seen as the foundation of a healthy animal experiencing a high welfare state.

Notes

[i] https://www.thedonkeysanctuary.org.uk/sites/uk/files/2018-10/donkey-weight-estimator-chart.pdf
[ii] http://www.donkeyweightape.com
[iii] https://www.feedipedia/org/node/4926
[iv] https://www.topspec.com/topspec-donkey-forage-balancer

Bibliography

Aganga, A.A., Letso, M. and Aganga, A.O. (2000) Feeding Donkeys. *Livestock Research for Rural Development* 12(2). Available at: http://www.fao.org/livestock/agap/frg/lrrd/lrrd12/2/agan122.htm (accessed 23 June 2020).

Aganga, A.A. and Tsopito, C.M. (1998) A note on the feeding behaviour of domestic donkeys: a Botswana case study. *Applied Animal Behaviour Science* 60, 235–239.

Ali, M., Baber, M., Hussain, T., Awan, F. and Nadeem, A. (2014a) The contribution of donkeys to human health. *Equine Veterinary Journal* 46, 766–767.

Ali, B.A.A., Matoock, M.Y., Fouad, M.A., Heleski, C.R. (2014b) Are mules or donkeys better adapted for Egyptian brick kiln work? (Until we can change the kilns). *Journal of Veterinary Behavior* 10, 158–165.

Ali, A., Matoock, M.Y., Fouad, M.A. and Heleski, C.R. (2015) A welfare assessment scoring system for working equids—A method for identifying at risk populations and for monitoring progress of welfare enhancement strategies (trialed in Egypt). *Applied Animal Behaviour Science* 176, 52–62.

Altomonte, I., Salari, F., Rosario, L. and Martini, M. (2019) Donkey and human milk: insights into their compositional similarities. *International Dairy Journal* 89, 111–118.

Aspri, M., Souroullas, K., Ioannou, C. and Papademas, P. (2019) Physico-chemical composition and antimicrobial protein content of early lactation donkey milk. *International Journal of Food Studies* 8, 68–75.

Brokner, C., Austbo, D., Naesset, J.A., Knudsen, K.E. and Tauson, A.H. (2012) Equine pre-caecal and total tract digestibility of individual carbohydrate fractions and their effect on caecal pH response. *Archives of Animal Nutrition* 66, 490–506.

Burden, F. (2012) Practical feeding and condition scoring for donkeys and mules. *Equine Veterinary Education* 24, 589–596.

Burden, F. and Bell, N. (2019) Donkey nutrition and malnutrition. *The Veterinary Clinics of North America. Equine Practice* 35(3), 469–479.

Burden, F.A. and Stradling, N. (2013) Dietary management to improve the gastrointestinal health of the donkey. In: *6th European Equine Health and Nutrition Congress* (1–2 March 2013). Ghent, Belgium.

Burden, F. and Thiemann, A. (2015) Donkeys are different. *Journal of Equine Veterinary Science* 35(5), 376–382.

Burden, F.A., Gallagher, J., Thiemann, A.K. and Trawford, A.F. (2009) Necropsy survey of gastric ulcers in a population of aged donkeys: prevalence, lesion description and risk factors. *Animal* 3, 287–293.

Burden F.A., Du Toit, N., Hazell-Smith, E. and Trawford, A. (2011) Hyperlipemia in a population of aged donkeys: description, prevalence, and potential risk factors. *Journal of Veterinary Internal Medicine* 25, 1420–1425.

Burnham, S.L. (2002) Anatomical differences of the donkey and mule. *American Association of Equine Practitioners* 48, 102–109.

Carretero-Roque, L., Colunga, B. and Smith, D.G. (2005) Digestible energy requirements of Mexican donkeys fed oat straw and maize stover. *Tropical Animal Health and Production* 37, 123–142.

Collins S.N., Murray, M.C., Burden, F.A. and Trawford, A.F. (2009) *Radiographic anatomy of the donkey foot: objective characterisation of the normal and laminitic donkey foot. BEVA Congress Proceedings*, p. 109.

Cox, R., Burden, F., Gosden, L., Proudman, C., Trawford, A. *et al.* (2009) Case control study to investigate risk factors for impaction colic in donkeys in the UK. *Preventive Veterinary Medicine* 92(3), 179–187.

Cuddeford, D., Pearson, R.A., Archibald, R.F. and Muirhead, R.H. (1995) Digestibility and gastro-intestinal transit times of diets containing different proportions of alfalfa and oat straw given to Thoroughbreds, Shetland ponies, Highland ponies and donkeys. *Animal Science* 61, 407–417.

Curtis, G.C., Barfoot, C.F., Dugdale, A.H.A., Harris, P.A., Grove-White, D. *et al.* (2010) Comparison of two practical weight loss protocols for the management of overweight and obese horses and ponies. In: Ellis, A.D., Longland, A.C., Coenen, M. and Miraglia, N. (eds) *The Impact of Nutrition on the Health and Welfare of Horses.* Proceedings 5th European Workshop Equine Nutrition Cirencester, UK 19–22 September 2010. European Association Animal Production (EAAP) Vol. 128. Wageningen Academic Publishers, Wageningen, The Netherlands, p. 237.

du Toit, N., Gallagher, J., Burden, F.A. and Dixon, P.M. (2008) Post mortem survey of dental disorders in 349 donkeys from an aged population (2005–2006). Part 1: prevalence of specific dental disorders. *Equine Veterinary Journal* 40, 204–208.

du Toit, N., Burden, F.A. and Dixon, P.M. (2009) Clinical dental examinations of 357 donkeys in the UK. Part 1: prevalence of dental disorders. *Equine Veterinary Journal* 41, 390–394.

Durham, A.E. and Thiemann, A.K. (2015) Nutritional management of hyperlipaemia. *Equine Veterinary Education* 27(9), 482–488.

Edwards, J.E., Shetty, S.A., van den Berg, P., Burden, F., van Doorn, D.A. *et al.* (2020a) Multi-kingdom characterization of the core equine fecal microbiota based on multiple equine (sub) species. *Animal Microbiome* 2(1), 1–16.

Edwards, J.E., Schennink, A., Burden, F., Long, S., van Doorn, D.A. *et al.* (2020b) Domesticated equine species and their derived hybrids differ in their fecal microbiota. *Animal Microbiome* 2(1), 1–13.

Evans, L. and Crane, M. (2018) *The Clinical Companion of the Donkey*. Matador Publishing, London.

Evans, L. and Lilly, G. (2019) *Clinical Companion of Donkey Dentistry*. Troubador Publishing, Leicester, UK.

Faillace, V., Tambella, A. M., Fratini, M., Paggi, E., Dini, F. *et al.* (2017) Use of autologous platelet-rich plasma for a delayed consolidation of a tibial fracture in a young donkey. *The Journal of Veterinary Medical Science* 79(3), 618–622. doi: 10.1292/jvms.16-0400.

FAOSTAT (2020) Live animals (data). Available at: http://www.fao.org/faostat/en/#data/QA (accessed 23 June 2020).

Gee, E.K., Fennessy, P.F., Morel, P.C.G., Grace, N.D., Firth, E.C. *et al.* (2003) Chemical body composition of 20 Thoroughbred foals at 160 days of age, and preliminary investigation of techniques used to predict body fatness. *New Zealand Veterinary Journal* 51(3), 125–131.

Henneke, D.R., Potter, G.D., Kreider, J.L. and Yeates, B.F. (1983) Relationship between condition score, physical measurements and body fat percentage in mares. *Equine Veterinary Journal* 15(4), 371–372.

Houpt, T.R. (1993) Water and electrolytes. In: Dukes, H.H., Swenson, M.J. and Reece, W.O. (eds) *Physiology of Domestic Animals*. Cornell University Press, New York, p. 9.

Johnson, C., Williams, J. and Phillips, C. (2017) Effect of routine dentistry on fecal fibre length in donkeys. *Journal of Equine Veterinary Science* 57, 41–45.

Katz, L.M. and Bailey, S.R. (2016) The pathogenesis of equine acute laminitis. *Equine Veterinary Journal* 44, 752–761.

Klingel, H. (1977) Observations on social organization and behaviour of African and Asiatic wild asses (*Equus africanus* and *E. hemionus*). *Zeitschrift für Tierpsychologie* 44, 323–331.

Köhle, N. (2018) Feasting on donkey skin. In: Smith, C.A., Kohle, N. and Jaivin, L. (eds) *Conspicuous Consumption*, 1st edn. ANU Press, Canberra, Australia. ISBN (ebook)9781760462031.

Liu, X., Fan, H., Ding, X., Hong, Z., Nei, Y. *et al.* (2014) Analysis of the gut microbiota by high-throughput sequencing of the v5-v6 regions of the 16s rRNA gene in donkey. *Current Microbiology* 68, 657–662.

Liu, L.L., Zhou, X.L. and Yang, H.J. (2020a) Effect of dietary forage: concentrate ration on pre-caecal and total digestive tract digestibility of diverse feedstuffs in donkeys as measured by the mobile nylon bag technique. *Animals* 10(6), 1070.

Liu, L.L., Zhou, X.L., Yang, H.J. and Chen, R. (2020b) Effect of dietary forage/concentrate ration on nutrient digestion and energy and protein metabolism in adult donkeys. *Animals* 10(6), 1025.

Luthersson, N., Chunekamrai, S., Estepa, J.C. *et al.* (2005) Secondary nutritional hyperparathyroidism in ponies in Northern Thailand. *Pferdeheilkunde* 21, 97–98.

Macheboeuf, D., Marangi, M., Poncet, C. and Martin-Rosset, W. (1995) Study of nitrogen digestion from different hays by the mobile nylon bag technique in horses. *Acoustics, Speech, and Signal Processing Newsletter, IEEE* 44(Suppl. 1), 219.

Maloiy, G.M.O. (1973) The effect of dehydration and heat stress on intake and digestion of food in the Somali donkey. *Environment, Physiology and Biochemistry* 3, 36–39.

Martin-Rosset, W. (2018) Donkey nutrition and feeding: nutrient requirements and recommended allowances—a review and prospect. *Journal of Equine Veterinary Science* 65, 75–85.

Mayers, A. (2017) *Under the Skin*. The Donkey Sanctuary, Sidmouth, UK.

McDowell, L.R. (2003) *Minerals in Animal and Human Nutrition*, 2nd edn. Elsevier, Amsterdam, The Netherlands.

McLean, A., Nielsen, B., Yokoyama, M., O´Connor-Robison, C., Hengemuehle, S. *et al.* (2009) Insulin resistance in standard donkeys (*Equus asinus*) of three body conditions – thin, moderate, and obese. *Journal of Equine Veterinary Science* 29(5), 406–407.

Mendoza, F.J., Estepa, J.C., Gonzalez-De Cara, C.A., Aguilera-Aguilera, R., Toribio, R.E. *et al.* (2015) Energy-related parameters and their association with age, gender, and morphometric measurements in healthy donkeys. *The Veterinary Journal* 204, 201–207.

Moehlman, P.D. (1998) Behavioral patterns and communication in feral asses (*Equus africanus*). *Applied Animal Behaviour Science* 60, 125–169.

Moore-Colyer, M.J., Hyslop, J.J., Longland, A.C. and Cuddeford, D. (2002) The mobile nylon technique as a method for determining the degradation of four botanically diverse fibrous feedstuffs in the small intestine and total digestive tract of ponies. *British Journal of Nutrition* 88, 729–740.

Morrow, L.D., Smith, K.C., Piercy, R.J., du Toit, N., Burden, F.A. *et al.* (2011) Retrospective analysis of post-mortem findings in 1,444 aged donkeys. *Journal of Comparative Pathology* 144, 145–156.

Mottet, R., Onan, G. and Hiney, K. (2009) Revisiting the Henneke body condition scoring system: 25 years later. *Journal of Veterinary Science* 29, 417–418.

Mueller, P.J., Brockmann, K.A., Houpt, K.A. *et al.* (1997) Water intake by donkeys: is it affected by accessibility? In: *Proceedings of the Fifteenth Equine Nutrition and Physiology Symposium*, Fort Worth, Texas, USA, pp. 193–194.

NRC (National Research Council) (2007) Donkeys and other equids. In: *Nutrient Requirements of Horses*. 6th revised edn. National Academy of Sciences, Washington DC, pp. 268–279.

Pearson, R.A. (ed.) (1991) *Donkeys, Mules and Horses in Tropical Agricultural Development*. University of Edinburgh Press, UK, pp. 86–95.

Pearson, R.A. (2005) Nutrition and feeding of donkeys. In: Mathews, N.S. and Taylor, T.S. (eds) *Veterinary Care of Donkeys*. International Veterinary Information Service, Ithaca, NY, pp. 1–5. Available at: http://www.ivis.org.

Pearson, R.A. and Merritt, J.B. (1991) Intake, digestion and gastrointestinal transit time in resting donkeys and ponies and exercised donkeys given ad libitum hay and straw diets. *Equine Veterinary Journal* 23, 339–342.

Pearson, R.A., Archibald, R.F. and Muirhead, R.H. (2001) The effect of forage quality and level of feeding on digestibility and gastrointestinal transit time of oat straw and alfalfa given to ponies and donkeys. *British Journal of Nutrition* 85, 599–606.

Pritchard, A., Nielsen, B., McLean, A., Robison, C., Yokoyama, M. *et al.* (2019) Insulin resistance as a result of body condition categorised as thin, moderate and obese in domesticated US donkeys (*Equus asinus*). *Journal of Equine Veterinary Science* 77, 31–35.

Quaresma, M.N.P., Payan-Carreira, R. and Silva, S. (2013) Relationship between ultrasound measurements of body fat reserves and body condition score in female donkeys. *The Veterinary Journal* 197(2), 329–334.

Reid, S.W. and Mohammed, H.O. (1996) Survival analysis approach to risk factors associated with hyperlipaemia in donkeys. *Journal of the American Veterinary Medical Association* 209(8), 1449–1452.

Rodrigues, J.B., Dixon, P.M., Bastos, E., San Roman, F. and Viegas, C.A. (2013) A clinical survey on the prevalence and types of cheek teeth disorders present in 400 Zamorano-Leonés and 400 Mirandês donkeys (*Equus asinus*). *Veterinary Record* 173, 581.

Rosenfeld, I. and Austbo, D. (2009) Digestion of cereals in the equine gastrointestinal tract measured by the mobile bag technique on caecally cannulated horses. *Animal Feed Science and Technology* 150, 249–258.

Rossel, S., Marshall, F., Peters, J., Pilgram, T., Adams, M.D. *et al.* (2008) Domestication of the donkey: timing, processes, and indicators. *Proceedings of the National Academy of Sciences* 105, 3715–3720.

Silva, S.R., Payan-Carreira, R., Quaresma, M., Guedes, C.M and Santos, A.S. (2016) Relationships between body condition score and ultrasound skin-associated subcutaneous fat depth in equids. *Acta Veterinaria Scandinavica* 58(Suppl. 1), 62.

Smith, D.G. (1999) The impact of grazing time allowance on the dry matter intake and foraging behaviour of cattle and donkeys managed under traditional African grazing systems. PhD Thesis, University of Edinburgh.

Smith, D.G. and Burden, F.A. (2013) Practical donkey and mule nutrition. In: Geor, R., Coenen, M. and Harris, P. (eds) *Equine Applied and Clinical Nutrition*. Saunders, Philadelphia, Pennsylvania, pp. 304–316.

Smith, D.G. and Pearson, R.A. (2005) A review of the factors affecting the survival of donkeys in semi-arid regions of sub-Saharan Africa. (Special issue: Nutrition and health of donkeys in the tropics). *Tropical Animal Health and Production* 37(Suppl. 1), 1–19.

Souroullas, K., Aspri, M. and Papademas, P. (2018) Donkey milk as a supplement in infant formula: benefits and technological challenges. *Food Research International* 109, 416–425.

Stewart, J.H. (2018) *Big Head or Bran Disease (Nutritional Secondary Hyperparathyroidism)*. Available from: http://www.mitavite.com/kb/big_head_or_bran_disease_nutritional_secondary_hyperparathyroidism (accessed 14 February 2020).

Superchi, P., Vecchi, I., Beretti, V and Sabbioni, A. (2014) Relationship among BCS and fat thickness in horses of different breed, gender and age. *Annual Research & Review in Biology* 4, 354–365.

Taylor, T.S. and Matthews, N.S. (2002) Donkey and Mule Scenarios: When to stop, think, read or call. *The American Association of Equine Practitioners* 48, 115–116.

Thiemann, A. (2013) Clinical approach to the dull donkey. *In Practice* 35(8), 470–476.

Tisserand, J.L., Faurie, F. and Toure, M. (1991) A comparative study of donkey and pony digestive physiology. In: Fielding, D. and Pearson, R.A. (eds) *Donkeys, Mules and Horses in Tropical Agricultural Development*. Alexander Ritchie & Son, Edinburgh, UK, pp. 67–72.

Valle, E., Raspa, F., Giribaldi, M., Barbero, R., Bergagna, S. *et al.* (2017) Functional approach to the body condition assessment of lactating donkeys as a tool for welfare evaluation. *Peer J* 5, 3001.

Velasquez-Mosquera, J. and Corrales-Alvarez, J. (2019) Anatomical distribution of subcutaneous fat and its relationship with body condition score in pack mules from the Central Andean Area of Colombia. *Revista Veterinaria y Zootecnia* 13(2), 1–13.

Wood, S.J. (2010) Some factors affecting the digestible energy requirements and dry matter intake of mature donkeys. PhD Thesis. University of Edinburgh, Edinburgh, UK.

Zhu, M. and Weng, Q. (2018) China: Will the donkey become the next pangolin? *Equine Veterinary Journal* 50(2), 276.

Index

Note: Page numbers in **bold** type refer to **figures**, page numbers in *italic* type refer to *tables*